Mastering the Presbyopic Surgery Lenses and Phakic IOLs

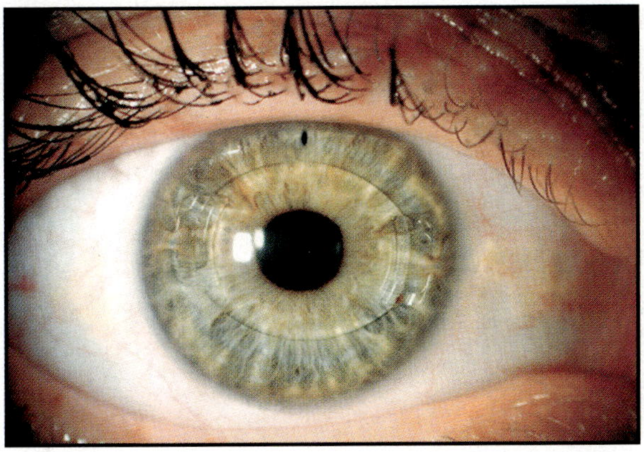

System requirement:

- **Windows XP or above**
- **Power DVD player (Software)**
- **Windows media player 10.0 version or above (Software)**

Accompanying DVD Rom is playable only in Computer and not in DVD player.

Kindly wait for few seconds for DVD to autorun. If it does not autorun then please do the following:

- Click on my computer
- Click the **DVD drive labelled JAYPEE** and after opening the drive, kindly double click the file **Jaypee**

DVD Contents

Mastering the Presbyopic Surgery Lenses and Phakic IOLs

Editors

Ashok Garg
MS, PhD, FIAO (Bel)
FRSM, ADM, FAIMS, FICA
International and National Gold Medalist
World Record Holder in
Guinness and Limca Books
Chairman and Medical Director
Garg Eye Institute and Research Centre
235-Model Town, Dabra Chowk
Hisar-125 005 (India)

JT Lin PhD
Technical Director
New Vision, Inc.
4532, Old Carriage Trail
Oviedo, FL 32765 (USA)

Carlo F Lovisolo MD, PhD
Medical Director
QuattroElle Eye Center
Via Cusani, 709, 20121
Milano (Italy)

Emanuel Rosen MD
Medical Director
Rosen Eye Associates
Harbour City
Salford Quays
M50 3BH (UK)

Frank Jozef Goes MD
Medical Director
Goes Eye Centre
W Klooslaan 6 B2050
Antwerp (Belgium)

Boris Malyugin MD
Chief of Department of Cataract
and Implant Surgery
Dy Director General
S Fyodorov Eye Microsurgery
Complex State Institution
127486 Moscow
Beskundnikovsky blvd 59A
Russia

Foreword
Georges Baikoff

JAYPEE BROTHERS
MEDICAL PUBLISHERS (P) LTD
New Delhi

Published by

Jitendar P Vij
Jaypee Brothers Medical Publishers (P) Ltd
B-3 EMCA House, 23/23B Ansari Road, Daryaganj
New Delhi 110 002, India
Phones: +91-11-23272143, +91-11-23272703, +91-11-23282021, +91-11-23245672, Rel: 32558559
Fax: +91-11-23276490, +91-11-23245683
e-mail: jaypee@jaypeebrothers.com
Visit our website: www.jaypeebrothers.com

Branches

- 2/B, Akruti Society, Jodhpur Gam Road Satellite
  Ahmedabad 380 015
  Phones: +91-079-26926233, Rel: +91-079-32988717, Fax: +91-079-26927094
  e-mail: ahmedabad@jaypeebrother.com
- 202 Batavia Chambers, 8 Kumara Krupa Road, Kumara Park East
  Bengaluru 560 001
  Phones: +91-80-22285971, +91-80-22382956, Rel: +91-80-32714073
  Fax: +91-80-22281761. e-mail: bangalore@jaypeebrothers.com
- 282 IIIrd Floor, Khaleel Shirazi Estate, Fountain Plaza, Pantheon Road
  Chennai 600 008
  Phones: +91-44-28193265, +91-44-28194897, Rel: +91-44-32972089
  Fax: +91-44-28193231. e-mail: chennai@jaypeebrothers.com
- 4-2-1067/1-3, 1st Floor, Balaji Building, Ramkote Cross Road
  Hyderabad 500 095, Phones: +91-40-66610020, +91-40-24758498,
  Rel:+91-40-32940929. Fax:+91-40-24758499, e-mail: hyderabad@jaypeebrother.com
- No. 41/3098, B & B1, Kuruvi Building, St. Vincent Road
  Kochi 682 018, Kerala, Phones: 0484-4036109, +91-0484-2395739, +91-0484-2395740
  e-mail: kochi@jaypeebrothers.com
- 1-A Indian Mirror Street, Wellington Square
  Kolkata 700 013, Phones: +91-33-22451926, +91-33-22276404, +91-33-22276415,
  Rel: +91-33-32901926. Fax: +91-33-22456075, e-mail: kolkata@jaypeebrothers.com
- 106 Amit Industrial Estate, 61 Dr SS Rao Road, Near MGM Hospital, Parel
  Mumbai 400 012
  Phones: +91-22-24124863, +91-22-24104532, Rel: +91-22-32926896
  Fax: +91-22-24160828, e-mail: mumbai@jaypeebrothers.com
- "KAMALPUSHPA" 38, Reshimbag
  Opp. Mohota Science College, Umred Road
  Nagpur 440 009 (MS)
  Phones: Rel: 3245220, Fax: 0712-2704275
  e-mail: nagpur@jaypeebrothers.com

Mastering the Presbyopic Surgery Lenses and Phakic IOLs

First Edition: **2008**

ISBN 81-8448-076-8

Typeset at JPBMP typesetting unit
Printed at Paras Offset Pvt. Ltd., New Delhi-28

To

- *My Respected Param Pujya Guru Sant Gurmeet Ram Rahim Singh Ji for his blessings & motivation*
- *My Respected Parents, teachers, my wife Dr Aruna Garg, son Abhishek and daughter Anshul for their constant support and patience during all these days of hard work*
- *My dear friend Dr Amar Agarwal, a leading International ophthalmologist from India for his continued support & guidance.*

— Ashok Garg

The memory of my step-daughter Nicola Ross who enjoyed benefits from refractive surgery were cut short by a tragic fatal illness.

— Emanuel Rosen

My wife, Jeanette and my sons Alex and Tao, who have been giving me constant support and love.

— JT Lin

My wife, Rita, for the support in my Professional Career and to my four grandchildren — Stephanie, William, Louise and Vincent — with the hope that at least one of them will become an ophthalmologist — as their father and their Daddy did.

— Frank Jozef Goes

My kids Alessandro and Luca Ghigo, the last comers, two potentially brilliant researchers in the field of nanotechnology.

— Carlo F Lovisolo

To my father Edvard Malyugin for everything and to my wife Natalia for her continuous support and love.

— Boris Malyugin

Contributors

Anand Aggarwal MS
Sr Registrar
Dr RP Centre for Ophthalmic
Science (AIIMS)
New Delhi, India

Antonio A Marinho MD, PhD
Professor of Ophthalmology
University of Porto
R Crasto, 708
4150-243, Porto
Portugal

Antonio Calossi MD
Via 2 Giugno 52
50053, Certaldo (FI)
Italy

Ashok Garg MS, PhD, FRSM
Chairman and Medical Director
Garg Eye Institute and Research
Centre, 235-Model Town
Dabra Chowk
Hisar-125 005 (India)

Birgit Lackner MD
Medical University Vienna
Deptt of Ophthalmology
Waehringer Guertel 18-20
A, 1090 Vienna, Austria

Boris Malyugin MD, PhD
Chief of Department of Cataract and
Implant Surgery
Dy Director General
S Fyodorov Eye Microsurgery
Complex State Institution,
127486 Moscow
Beskudnikovsky blvd 59A
Russia

Carlo F Lovisolo MD
Medical Director
QuattroElle Eye Center
Via Cusani, 7-9, 20121
Milano, Italy

Claes Feinbaum MD
Professor Emeritus Optometry
OkoMedica, Ul. Marywilska 34
03-228 Warsaw
Poland

Christa Gore MD
Rosen Eye Associates
Harbour City
Salford Quays
M50 3 BH
UK

Cyres K Mehta MD, FAGE, FSVH
The Mehta's International Eye
Institute, Sea Side
147, Shahid Bhagat Singh Road
Colaba, Mumbai-400 005
India

David Brown MD
Eye Centre of Florida
Ft Myers, Florida
USA

David Dulaney MD
Barnet Dulaney Perkins Eye Center
Phoenix, Arizona
USA

David Schneider MD
Midwest Eye Centre
Cincinnati, Ohio
USA

Dimitrii Dementiev MD
Chief & Medical Director
Blue Eye Centro di
Michro Chirurgia Oculare Eye Clinic
Arese 20020 (MI)
Via Campo Gallo 21/10
Italy

Donald R Sanders MD
Dept of Ophthalmology
University of Illinois at
Chicago College of Medicine
Chicago, Illinois
USA

Elbland Klinik Radebeul MD
Consultant Ophthalmologist
Germany

Emanual Rosen MD
Rosen Eye Associates
Harbour City, Salford Quays
M50 3 BH
UK

Elizabeth Kowaleski MD
Rosen Eye Associates
Harbour City
Salford Quays
M50 3 BH
UK

Frank Jozef Goes MD
Director Goes Eye Centre
W Klooslaan 6 B2050
Antwerp, Belgium

GU Auffarth MD, PhD
Vice Chairman
Chief Surgeon
Dept of Ophthalmolgoy
University of Heidelberg
INF 400
69120, Heidelberg
Germany

Gerald Schmendinger MD
Department of Ophthalmology
Medical University of Vienna
AKH-Vienna
Waehringer Guertel 18-20
1090 Vienna, Austria

Georges Baikoff MD
Clinique Monticelli
88, Rue du Commandant Rolland
13008, Marsielle, France

Harinder S Sethi MD
Research Officer
Dr RP Centre for Ophthalmic
Sciences (AIIMS)
Ansari Nagar, New Delhi-110 029
India

I Howard Fine MD, FACS
Oregon Eye Surgery Centre
1550, Oak Street
5, Eugene, OR - 97401, USA

Ioannis G Pallikaris MD
Professor and Head,
University of Crete - School of
Health Sciences
Institute of Vision and Optics (IVO)
Vardinoyiannion Eye Institute of
Crete (VEIC), GR 71 003 Voutes
Heraklion, Crete
Greece

Jairo E Hoyos MD, PhD
Instituto Oftalmologico Hoyos
Rambla de Sabadell 62 1°
8201 Sabadell
Barcelona, Spain

Jairo Hoyos-Chacon MD
Instituto Oftalmologico Hoyos
Rambla de Sabadell 62 1°
08201 Sabadell
Barcelona, Spain

Javier A Montero MD
Vitreo-Retional Unit
Instituto Oftalmologico de Alicante
Alicante, Spain

Johan A de Lange MD
Ocumed Building
Vaal Drive
Vanderbijlpark
Gauteng, South Africa

John Vukich MD
Department of Ophthalmology
University of Wisconsin School of Medicine and Davis Duehr Dean Medical Center, Madison
Wisconsin, USA

Jose M Ruiz-Moreno MD
Department of Ophthalmology
Miguel Hernandez University School of Medicine, 03550, Alicante
Spain

JT Lin PhD
Technical Director
New Visiion, Inc.
4532 Old Carriage Trail
Oviedo, FL 32765, USA

Juan C Rocco MD
Medical Director
Centro de Miopia y Astigmastismo
Jujuy 167 (Sur)
San Juan
Argentina J5402EMC

Kayo Nishi MD
Nishi Eye Hospital
Osaka, Japan

Keiki R Mehta MS
Medical Director
The Mehta's International Eye Institute, Sea Side, 147
Shahid Bhagat Singh Road, Colaba
Mumbai (India)-400 005

K Takhchidi MD
Director General
S Fyodorov Eye Microsurgery
Complex State Institution
127486 Moscow
Beskudnikovsky blvd 59A
Russia

Lalik Alok MD
Research Associate
Dr RP Centre for Ophthalmic Science (AIIMS), New Delhi, India

Manoj Gupta MD
Registrar
Dr RP Centre for Ophthalmic Science (AIIMS), Ansari Nagar
New Delhi-110 029

Maria I Kalyvianaki MD
University of Crete
Dept of Ophthalmology
VEIC, PO Box 2208
Heraklion 71003
Crete, Greece

Mark Wevill MD
Rosen Eye Associates
Harbour City
Salford Quays
M50 3 BH, UK

Mark Packer MD
Oregan Eye Surgery Centre
1550, Oak Street
5, Eugene, OR- 97401, USA

Melania Cigales-Jirout MD
Instituto Oftalmologico Hoyos
Sabadell (Barcelona)
Spain

M Shaju Asokan DO,MS,DNB
Vasan Eye Care Hospital
Thillai Nagar Main Road
Trichy-620 018
India

O Kravchuk MD
S Fyodorov Eye Microsurgery
Complex State Institution
127486 Moscow
Beskudnikovsky blvd 59A
Russia

Okihiro Nishi MD
Director
Nishi Eye Hospital
Osaka
Japan

Oliver Findl MD
Department of Ophthalmology
Medical University of Vienna
Waehringer Guertel 18-20
1090 Vienna
Austria

Oliver Stachs MD
Universitat Rostock
Medizinische Fakultat
Augenklinik
Doberraner Str. 140
18055, Rostock
Germany

Paul Rolf Preussner MD
Professor of Ophthalmology
University Eye Hospital
Langenbecksts-1
D-55101, Mainz
Germany

Ramiro Salgado MD
Consultant Ophthalmologist
University of Porto
Portugal

Richard S Hoffman
Oregon Eye Surgery Centre
1550, Oak Street, # 5 Eugene
OR- 97401
USA

Rishi Mohan MD,DNB
Director
M M Eyetech
29, Link Road, Lajpat Nagar-III
New Delhi-110024, India

Robert Martin MD
Consultant Ophthalmologist
Carolina Eye Associate
Southern Pines, NC
USA

Sanjay Chaudhary MS
Chaudhary Eye Centre and
Laser Vision
4802, Bharat Ram Road
Ansari Road, 24, Darya Ganj
New Delhi-110 002

Shiao Chang MD
Nishi Eye Hospital
Osaka
Japan

Stephen Slade MD
The Laser Center
Houston, Texas, USA

Steven Schallhorn MD
Dept of Ophthalmology
Navy Medical Center San Diego
San Diego, California
USA

Swati Phuljhele MD
Sr Registrar
Dr RP Centre for Ophthalmic
Sciences (AIIMS), Ansari Nagar
New Delhi (India)-110 029

Tanuj Dada MD
Additional Professor,
Dr RP Centre for Ophthalmic
Sciences, AIIMS, Ansari Nagar
New Delhi-110 029, India

T Morozova MD
S Fyodorov Eye Microsurgery
Complex State Institution
127486 Moscow
Beskudnikovsky blvd 59A
Russia

Ulrich M Klemen MD
NA
Auhofstrasse 213
1130, Vienna, Austria

V Cherednik MD
S Fyodorov Eye Microsurgery
Complex State Institution
127486 Moscow
Beskudnikovsky blvd 59A
Russia

Wolf Buehl MD
Department of Ophthalmology
Medical University of Vienna
Waehringer Guertel 18-20
1090 Vienna, Austria

Yoshiaki Nawa MD
Associate Professor
Dept of Ophthalmology
Nara Medical University
Kashihara
Nara 6348522
Japan

Yutaro Nishi MD
Nishi Eye Hospital
Osaka
Japan

Foreword

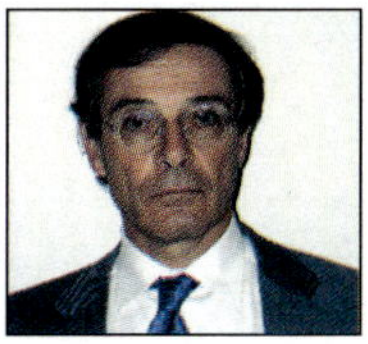

Refractive surgery is now part of everyday ocular surgery. To date, it is the second most important surgical activity in ophthalmology just behind cataract surgery; thus, making it essential to frequently update progress made in this field.

Today, refractive surgery is divided into different fields: First of all corneal surgery (PRK, LASIK, LASEK, EPILASIK, etc.) which is based on reshaping the corneal diopter. The quality of optical treatment software is being improved constantly adapting itself to patient optical aberrations and/or topography and femtolaser has replaced microkeratome sections.

The second aspect of refractive surgery is the use of intraocular lenses either as an addition or in replacement of the crystalline lens. The field of intraocular lenses is more confined but as our knowledge regarding the limits of corneal surgery improves, indications for this type of surgery is steadily increasing.

Dr Ashok Garg's merit lies in having brought together the most prominent authors in the field of such hot topics as phakic implants and clear lens exchange. He has succeeded in obtaining an international panel to review the progress made on this very delicate subject. Twenty years ago, along with Svyatoslav Fyoderov, Paul Fechner and Jan Worst I was lucky to be one of the pioneers of the new generation of modern phakic implants. Their importance is recognised today.

However, considering that this kind of surgery requires a great deal of skill and is constantly changing, surgeons wishing to improve their knowledge in this field will reap a huge benefit from reading this remarkable work.

I am most grateful to Ashok Garg for his constant friendship and would like to take this opportunity to congratulate him for his dedication and contribution to this excellent book.

Georges Baikoff
MD
Centre D'Ophtalmologie Clinique Monticelli
88, rue du Commandant Rolland-13008 Marseille
France
Tel. 04 91 16 22 28
Fax. 04 91 16 22 25
E-mail: g.baik.opht@wanadoo.fr

Preface

Since the introduction of bifocal spectacles by Benjamin Franklin in 1784 for the treatment of presbyopia technology it has come a long way with various treatment options. Today presbyopic population expects high quality functional vision pretty much like any other age group. Today presbyopic lens implantation focuses on restoring functional vision and enhancing quality of life. Either an accommodative IOL or a multifocal IOL can provide distance and near correctioin following the removal of an early cataract or clear lens. Lenticular Refractive Surgery achieve optimal refractive outcomes specially with new designs and techniques of phakic IOLs. Phakic IOLs provide an excellent quality of vision without altering the curvature and anatomy of the cornea in the center. They also provide predictable, precise and stable refractive results.

The present International book has been formated with an aim to provide complete uptodate information regarding presbyopia lenses and phakic IOLs. Forty-nine chapters of this book have been written by Internationally known Refractive Surgeons who are masters in Lenticular Refractive Surgery field. Detailed information regarding history, various types of presbyopia lenses and phakic IOLs, surgical techniques, complication management, recent advances and insight into future possibilities have been provided into this book in a comprehensive manner. Futuristic technique for restoring near vision function by refilling the capsular bag with a deformable gel (injectable polymer) is specially included in this book.

An Interactive DVD is being given with this book showing various lenticular refractive surgery techniques by International masters of this field.

We deeply appreciate the efforts of Sh Jitendar P Vij (CEO), Mr Tarun Duneja, General Manager (Publishing) and staff of M/s Jaypee Brothers Medical Publishers (P) Ltd., New Delhi who took active interest in this project and published it expeditiously.

With ongoing research works and modifications in presbyopic lenses and phakic IOLs, lenticular refractive and presbyopia surgery shall be available in the armamentarium of every refractive surgeon to correct entire range of refractive errors to provide safe and stable refractive vision in near future. We are hopeful, this book shall be desktop reference for refractive surgeons worldwide.

Editors

Contents

SECTION 1 : LENS HISTORY, PRELIMINARY CONSIDERATIONS AND IOL POWER CALCULATIONS

SECTION 2 : PRESBYOPIA (ACCOMMODATING AND ASPHERIC) LENSES : TYPES AND SURGICAL TECHNIQUES

Section 1

Lens History, Preliminary Considerations and IOL Power Calculations

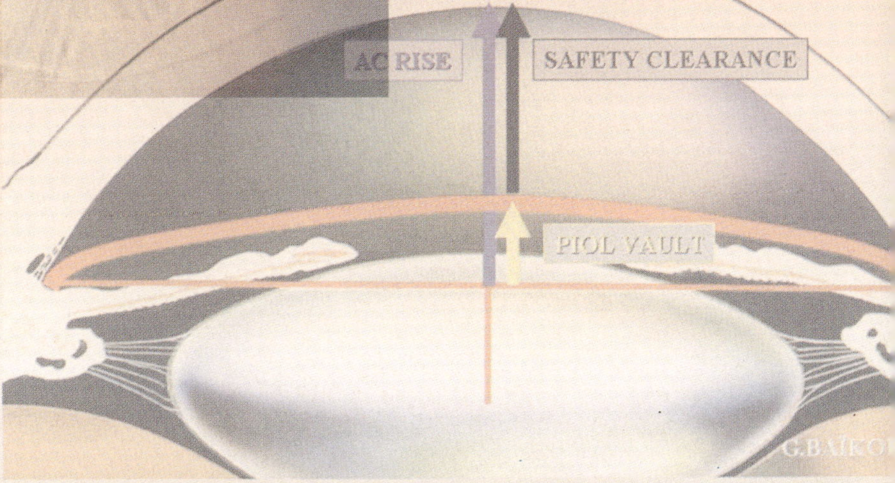

CHAPTER

1

António Marinho, Ramiro Salgado (Portugal)

History of Phakic IOLs

EARLY DEVELOPMENTS

The first phakic Iols were designed in the sixties in Spain (Barraquer), Italy (Strampelli) and England (Choyce). The idea of introducing a lens in a phakic eye to correct high myopia was a consequence of 2 factors. First, there was a wave of enthusiasm after the implantations of pseudophakic IOLs by Harold Ridley in 1949, proving that the eye could tolerate an intraocular lens and second, the work of Jose I.Barraquer showing the correction of high ametropias with corneal remodelling, laying the foundations of modern refractive surgery.

However this early experience with phakic IOLs was short lived. These early designs were rigid angle-supported phakic IOLs, associated with many complications such as: uveitis, glaucoma, hyphaema, extreme pupil distortion and endothelial decompensation.

The concept was totally abandoned during almost 20 years, and the refractive surgery of high ametropias stayed with corneal surgery (different modalities of keratomileusis) with low predictability and requiring complicated machinery and technical skills.

ORIGIN OF MODERN PHAKIC IOLs

In 1986/87 three different investigators looked again to the issue of phakic IOLs and designed 3 different models of IOLs, that are forefathers of our present phakic IOLs.

Georges Baikoff (France) presented the ZB lens,[1,2] that was an angle-supported phakic IOL, following the Kelman design of a pseudophakic IOL. Although this IOL still caused endothelial problems due to proximity of corneal endothelium[3,4] the next model ZB5M overcome this problem and must be considered the origin of actual models of angle supported phakic IOL.

At the same time, in the Netherlands, Jan Worst develops the first iris-supported phakic IOL. This model was biconcave (the present models are planoconcave) and was derived from the "Lobster Claw" pseudophakic IOL developed in Pakistan in 1978 by Jan Worst and Singh. The first implantation of the biconcave phakic IOL was done by Paul Fechner in Germany in 1986.[5]

The present Artisan, Toric Artisan and Artiflex, the most implanted type of phakic IOLs today, come from this model.

Meanwhile,in Russia, Fyodorov presented a silicone posterior chamber phakic IOL.[6]Although this implant was associated with complications, such as: uveitis, cataract and corneal endothelial cell loss,[7] it paved the way for future developments, like the Adatomed IOL (still associated with high rate of cataracts) and to the modern posterior chamber phakic IOLs (ICL and PRL).

REFERENCES

1. Baikoff G, Arne JL, Bokobza Y, et al. Angle-fixated anterior chamber phakic intraocular lens for myopia of -7 to -19 diopters. J Refract Surg,1998; 14 (3): 282-93
2. Baikoff G, Joly P. Correction chirurgicale de la forte myopie par les implants phakes de chambre antérieure. Concepts et resultants. Bull Soc Belge Ophtalmol,1989;233:109-25
3. Mimouni F, Colin J, Koffi V, Bonnet P. Damage to the corneal endothelium from anterior chamber intraocular lenses in phakic myopic eyes. Refract Corneal Surg,1991; 7 (4): 277-81
4. Saragoussi JL, Cotinat J, Renard G, et al. Damage to the corneal endothelium by minus power anterior chamber intraocular lenses. Refract Corneal Surg,1991; 7 (4): 282-85
5. Fechner PU, Strobel J, Wichmann W. Correction of myopia by implantation of a concave Worst iris-claw lens into phakic eyes. Refract Corneal Surg,1991; 7 (4): 286-89
6. Fyodorov SN, Zuev VK, Aznabayev BM. Intraocular correction of high myopia with negative posterior chamber lens. Ophthalmosurgery, 1991; 3: 57-8
7. Fyodorov SN, Zuev VK, Tumanyan NR, Suheil AJ. Clinical and functional follow-up of minus IOL implantation in high grade myopia. Ophthalmosurgery, 1993; 2: 12-7

CHAPTER

2

António Marinho, Ramiro Salgado (Portugal)

Patient Preoperative Evaluation and Selection

INTRODUCTION

The goal of refractive surgery is to alter the refractive condition of the eye in order to eliminate or reduce refraction errors.[1] This purpose normally serves other than medical indications, such as professional requirements or cosmetic desire, eliminating the need for glasses or contact lenses. Nevertheless, exceptionally, medical conditions such as high anisometropias in young patients with the risk of developing amblyopia, may constitute one indication for refractive surgery.[2,3] The modification of the refractive status may be achieved by means of several different techniques, after a careful assessment of the patient candidate and a thorough explanation of the procedure itself and risks or complications involved. This particular point is of paramount importance in creating, for the patient, an environment of realistic expectations over the final outcome.

Regarding the refraction error, for it is the reason for which the patient seeks the refractive surgeon, the approaches vary according to the type of error (spherical and/or cylindrical), its amount (i.e. the value in diopters), and anatomical criteria such us pachimetry, keratometry and topography.[4-6] Begining with myopic defects, the implantation of phakic IOL's is indicated for the correction of myopia above the LASIK range, that is, -10 D, but lower defects can be corrected in cases where the required criteria are not met for the corneal procedure. Being the fact that, for most phakic IOL's, the upper limit is around –22 D, it is, however, possible to correct even higher ametropias through a combined procedure (phakic IOL implantation+Lasik), designated as Bioptics[7] or Adjustable Refractive Surgery,[8] which broadens considerably our spectrum of action up to –30 to –35 D.

Other indications of this combined technique are the treatment of residual refractive defects and the refinement of the quality of vision outcome (like the use of wider optical zones).[9,10] Of course, clear lens extraction remains a mainstay of the treatment of very high myopia,[11,12] still haunted by the fear of retinal detachment and the loss of accommodation;[13,14] this counterback is being addressed to, more recently, by the implantation of IOL's capable of some degree of accommodation, a procedure designated by Refractive Lens Exchange.[15]

Regarding hyperopia, a defect above +5 D is an indication for phakic implants, as it is a more effective, predictable and safer procedure than LASIK or other techniques in this range of ametropia.[16,17]

As to cylindrical defects, there are anterior chamber phakic IOL's designed to correct astigmatism up to 7 D,[18-20] a procedure with a somewhat lesser degree of predictability dependent on a large incision and suturing. This counterback is prone to be overcome with the advent of foldable AC phakic IOL's. Again, a combined procedure such as Bioptics, if possible, may be an eligible surgical option, associated with an higher predictable outcome.

Beyond the type and amount of the refractive error, the selection of the candidates for a phakic implantation procedure obligates to a selective assessment englobing a comprehensive anatomical evalution, which will be the scope of a further section in this chapter.

GENERAL FEATURES

Patient Profile

The motive that directs a patient towards a phakic implant procedure is very often a cosmetic one, that is, an intolerance to wearing spectacles. This may be in fact more than a cosmetic worry since, for high ametropias, the optical aberrations and image size alterations associated with glasses usually leads to a lower than optimal vision. Also, very often, however, the contact lens alternative is not suitable because an intolerance to contact lenses wear is present.

Another subset of candidates is the group of professional reason, where either the use of spectacles or contact lenses is not indicated, such as pilots, workers of industry exposed to dust.

Of paramount importance is the education of patient, which assures the final satisfaction of the patient. Elucidation of the procedure, explaining the alternatives when it is the case, mentioning the possibility of complications and its approach, and evidence-based prognosis of the final outcome are, in sum, the steps that provide the patient with realistic expectations about the all process involving this surgical procedure.

Systemic Conditions

There are some requisites a patient should fulfill in order to become a candidate for phakic implantation. Age is one of them. Normally, the minimum age is 18, as the eyeball is not yet fully developed before this age. Again, in extreme cases of amblyopic risk, the surgery can be performed earlier. As to the upper limit, patients older than 45 years old in general do not fully benefit from the procedure, as the limited accommodation thereafter demands the use for near vision additional correction (i.e. spectacles).

Systemic conditions may constitute a contraindication for phakic implantation. Thus, listed as contraindications, are the following conditions: pregnancy, diabetes mellitus, autoimmune diseases, neopalsy/ immunosuppression and any severe systemic pathology.

Ocular Conditions

At first hand, any of the following conditions are absolute contraindications for phakic implantations: lens opacity or developing cataract, glaucoma or ocular hypertension, personal history of uveitis, retinal detachment or maculopathy and chronic infection of ocular adnexa. Some corneal disorders like scars, keratoconus or degenerative conditions are only relative contraindications and may, in selected cases, constitute elective indications. Also, patients with postoperative high ametropia following previous corneal surgery such as penetrating keratoplasty or residual ametropia post-keratorefractive surgery such as LASIK or PRK, may be eligible candidates for a phakic implantation; this technique, i.e. following any kind of primary procedure, is an extended approach of the phakic IOL implantation and is designated by Phakic IOL's as a Secondary Procedure (PISP).

One-eyed patients or with severe amblyopic fellow eye are always a contraindication for phakic implants. A carefull approach is advised when dealing with eyes with best corrected vision worse than 20/40.

General Ophthalmic Examination

Every candidate for phakic IOL implantation should undergo a general ophthalmic examination. This englobes a thorough refraction study, comprising not only the measurement of uncorrected and best-corrected visual acuity by an optotype chart (i.e. Snellen chart), but also the assessment of the quality of vision, envolving parameters such as mesopic vision, glare and contrast sensitivity.

For refractive and topographical purposes, every patient should remove contact lenses before the preoperative examination. This period should be a minimum of four weeks for rigid gas-permeable lenses, and two weeks for soft lenses; eventually, a longer period is required depending on the corneal status (i.e. corneal warpage).

Manifest refraction should be obtained for all patients, and cycloplegic refraction for hyperopia and dubious cases (accommodative spasms, young patients), measured on the spectacle plane. This particular aspect, together with a proper standard vertex distance of 12 mm, is essential to the accuracy of the procedure,[21] as small variations may give rise to large variations in the final refraction due to the the high refractive error in these patients. Stability of refraction for a period of at least 12 months, is mandatory.

Keratometric values can be obtained with manual or automated keratometry, videokeratography or, with anterior segment analysis systems such as Orbscan or Pentacam.

Automated keratometers only measure the paracentral cornea (4.0 mm) and along two perpendicular axis, presenting a non negligeable error. These latter topographic devices extend the concept of corneal morphology, beyond the conventional assessment based on specular technology (Placido's disks), providing invaluable information on corneal refractive status and pathology.

A moto-sensorial study should be performed, in order to assess binocular balance (for example, the existence of tropias), most particularly in high anisometropia cases.

A mandatory slit-lamp examination of the anterior segment, with biomicroscopy performed with both undilated pupil and in mydriasis, with special attention given to the cornea and crystalline lens.

Gonioscopy with Goldmann's three-mirror lens is in order so as to verify the criteria for implantation of angle-supported and posterior phakic IOL's: an angle ≥30º corresponding to grade 0 to 1 under the Scheie grading, or 3 to 4 according to the Shaffer classification.

Intraocular pressure should be measured by applanation tonometry. An IOP greater than 21 mm Hg contraindicates the implantation of any phakic lens.

Fundus examination is mandatory and divides into the peripherinal retina and vitreous examination and the macula observation.

The fundus examination should be performed under dilation and indirect ophthalmoscopy, or a three-mirror Goldman contact lens, in order to evaluate the posterior pole and peripheral retina thus identifying any lesion requiring prophylactic laser retinal treatment preoperatively. High myopic eyes have predisposing lesions to retinal detachment,[22] such as lattice degeneration, in as much as 6.5 to 13%.[23] Retinal dehiscence and atropic holes are also very frequent in this population. Overall, the risk of retinal detachment in patients with high pyopia (>-6.0 D) is as high as 3.2%.[24] The preventive role of laser coagulation is emphasized in several series, showing a decrease of retinal detachment incidence in argon laser treated eyes post-phakic IOL implantation.[25]

The examination of the macula is equally important, since highly myopic eyes are prone to the appearance of staphyloma, more easily identified in contrast sensitivity testing, and CNV. The incidence of the latter in myopia above -6.0 D varies from 4 to 11%,[26-28] according to different studies. An important issue is that, according to some authors (Pollack et al,[29] Blair et al[30]), surgery may induce wet AMD progression or CNV formation. Notwithstanding the fact that, nowadays, OCT proved reliable in studying the macula[31] (specially in the detection of macular edema), performing a fluorescein, and, exceptionally, an indocyanine (hidden CNV in macular hemorrhages) angiography, are still clearly indicated when CNV is suspected.

SPECIFIC OPHTHALMIC EXAMINATION

Pupillometry

In order to avoid secondary visual phenomena occurring in lower illumination conditions, such as glare, halos and ghosting, the scotopic pupil size must never exceed the optical zone of the phakic lens. Being the fact that the diameter of any phakic IOL is, at most, 6.0 mm wide, candidates with a pupil size larger than 6.0 mm in scotopic conditions should be excluded. Notwithstanding the fact that, although posterior chamber lenses are generally smaller, their effective optical zone is increased, because of their location behind the iris diaphragm.

The pupil size assessment has been performed in several ways, depending the patient postoperative satisfaction on the reliability of the measurement. It should be present that pupil size diminishes with age and normally is slightly smaller in males.

A most important aspect regarding different luminosity conditions, is the evaluation of quality of vision. Actually, more than 60% of a person's normal activity is performed under mesopic conditions.

One of the easiest measurement procedures, is the use of pocket cards (Rosenbaum, Holladay) with different pupil sizes that should match the patient´s pupil size under different illumination conditions (not possible a scotopic evaluation) by dimming the room; this little controlled variable, and the subjectivity inherent to the observer renders this procedure a low reproducibility.

Another method is the infrared based technology used in devices such as the Colvard Pupillometer (Oasis Medical)[32] (Fig. 2.1), which provides a semi-quantitative assessment of the scotopic pupil size; the examiner matches the pupil diameter image with a grading scale; the same technology is used in Pupil Scan II 12 A, in which the reading is digital.

There are devices in which the measurement is fully automatic, i.e. quantitative, eliminating the examiner bias. Computerized systems, such as the Procyon PS2000SA,[33] accomplishes the goal of precise quantification of pupil size, under mesopic high (4.0 lux), mesopic low (0.4 lux) and scotopic (0.04 lux) and in binocularity. One recent study (Kurz et al)[34] has shown statistically significant differences between monocular and binocular pupil size. The binocular pupil size appears, in that series, to be larger than in monocular conditions, and further work is in order to may bring some enlightening on this selection criteria.

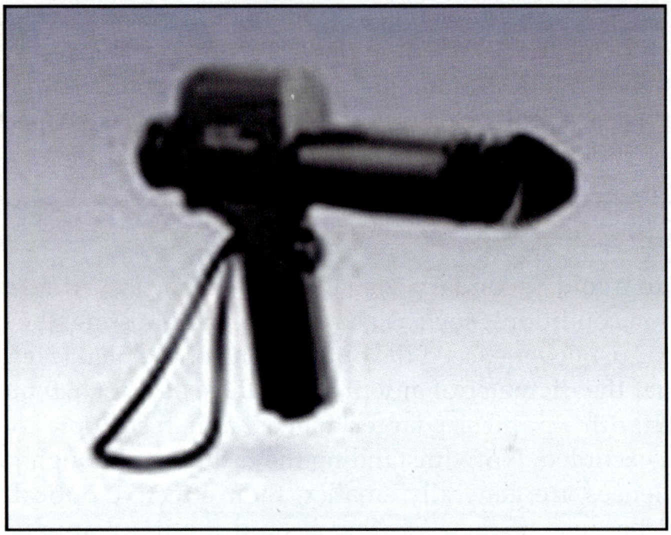

Fig. 2.1: Colvard pupillometer

Most of anterior segment analysis system devices, like videokeratographers or even Orbscan, which also uses specular reflection, when used in evaluating pupil size, underestimate the effect of high luminance of the apparatus itself, thus requiring a correction factor, generally accepted as +2.6 mm[35] in order to correlate to mesopic conditions as measured on more precise devices (i.e. computerized pupillometers).

Anatomical Evaluation

Endothelial Study

In order to implant a phakic IOL, it is mandatory to assess the condition of corneal endothelium; this involves both counting and morphology. For safety purposes it is consensual that a count inferior to 2200 cells/ mm^3 is a contraindication for phakic lens implantation (Fig. 2.2).[36] Less strict but still relevant to endothelium condition, is the existence of anomalies in cell shape or size, such as pleomorphism or polymegatism.

Endothelial cells at birth are generally 4400 to 6000 per mm^3, with a loss of 40% in the first year. Thereafter, the loss is of about 25% until adulthood, diminishing about 0.57% per year until the age of 80.[37]

Contact lens users of long date normally have lower values for their age when compared to normal subjects. This stress is not to be overlooked and an evidence of the magnitude of this phenomena when compared to the potential damage of a phakic implant, is the apparent postoperative gain in cell count in these patients' eyes following a phakic implant procedure in most refractive centers.

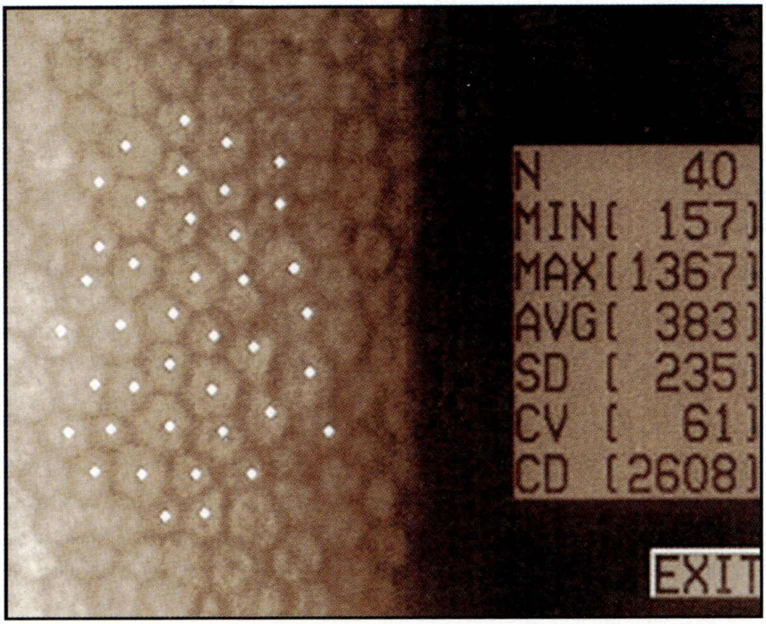

Fig. 2.2: Normal endothelial cell count and morphology

Corneal Pachymetry and Topography

In phakic IOL surgery, pachymetry provides general information on corneal health. Topographic devices such as Orbscan II or Pentacam, provide extended information on corneal thickness along with anterior and posterior elevation with thorough mapping, enabling the detection of pathologies like keratoconus or pellucid marginal degeneration, very often selecting refractive candidates for phakic implantation as an alternative to corneal surgery.

Anterior Chamber Internal Dimensions

Angle-to-angle/sulcus-to-sulcus distance: The adequate size of an angle-supported anterior chamber phakic IOL or posterior phakic IOL depends on the accuracy of the angle-to-angle and sulcus-to-sulcus distances measurement. [38,39] Too large angle-supported implants may lead to iris ischemia, angle recession, raise intraocular pressure, low-grade recurrent inflammation, anterior synechiae and sectorial atrophy. These complications, in turn, can lead to pupil distorsion. Too short lenses, on the other hand, tend to rotate or decentrate and may be associated with excessive movement in the anterior chamber causing endothelial damage through intermittent contact.[40]

For this matter it has been shown that there is no adequate correspondance between the linear external white-to-white measurement and actual internal anterior segment dimensions.[41] The former "rule of thumb", applied to angel-supported and posterior implants, was: IOL size = external measurement of the horizontal white-to-white distance (W-to-W) + 0.5 or 1.0 mm in myopia, or -0.5 mm (in hyperopia). Iris-supported implants and posterior PRL lenses are "one size fits all", and do not require this parameter. The mean value, for Caucasian populations, of the horizontal W-to-W distance, is 11.7 ± 0.4 mm, as measured with a surgical calliper or ruler, intraoperatively. Taking this method as the gold standard one, several other tests have different reproducibility tolerances. Hence, the Holladay and Godwin Corneal Gauge (Asico, USA), in which the observer matches, at a distance, the more suitable half-moons (varying between 9.0 and 14.0 mm in diameter) with patient's horizontal corneal diameter, has a reproducibility tolerance of ± 0.5 mm. Other less subjective methods, are digital photography based videokeratographers. For instance, the EyeSys 2000, CSO EyeTop, and Tomey-2, have reproducibility tolerances of nearly 0.2 mm; as to the W-to-W module of Orbscan has a lower value of 0.4 mm.

However still in use, the W-to-W distance is liable of non-adequate evaluation of the internal anterior segment dimensions, resulting in a loss of safety regarding the implantation of phakic IOL's. Thus, measurement of the angle-to-angle and sulcus-to-sulcus should be a demand for phakic lenses implantation.

Ultrasonography, while effective in providing anterior chamber depth measures and a detailed imaging of linear and angular structures,[42] was not able, until not long ago, to obtain a full image of the anterior segment.

Devices like Ultrasound BioMicroscope (UBM, Humphrey Zeiss/ Paradigm),[43] using 50 to 100 MHz frequencies, "form" one full anterior segment composite image by pasting three separate images together. This procedure lacks accuracy in angle-to-angle or sulcus-to-sulcus measurement. Latter in the year 2002, another ultrasound-based device, the Artemis 2 (Ultralink, LLC) (Fig. 2.3),[44] became available. This arc-scannig device is capable of taking a full anterior segment scan in one plane, visualizing corneal structures (such as epithelium or LASIK flaps) with 1 μm precision.[45]

This device further allowed to verify a long time ago forseen evidence: a comparision between W-to-W and angle-to-angle or sulcus–to-sulcus (Reinstein et al) has shown that weak or no statistical correlation whatsoever existed between W-to-W and the other two parameters. Furthermore, the predictability of a statistically regression formula for myopes, produced an unacceptable tolerance error of 0.9 mm.

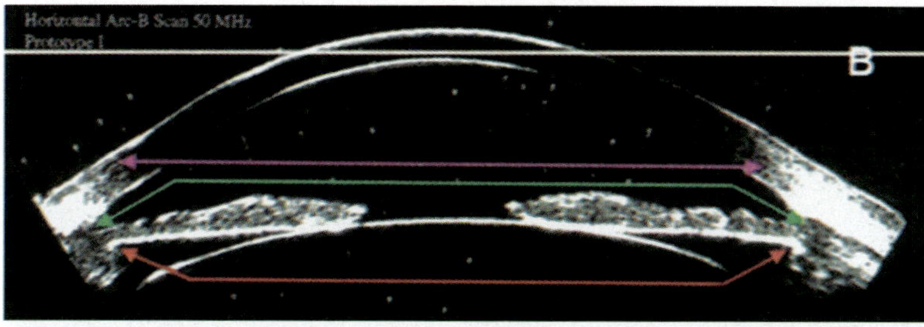

Fig. 2.3: Very high frequency ultrasonography with Artemis 2 (UltraLink LLC) providing full anterior segment image (lines show anterior segment diameters)

Orbscan II register 40 independent images by a calibrated video-camera, analyzing about 9,000 points in anterior cornea, posterior cornea, anterior iris and anterior lens.[46] It is through interpolation routines that an estimation of the angle and angle-to-angle distance are obtained.

Devices based in Scheimpflug photography, such as the EAS-1000 Computerized Anterior Segment Evalution System (Nidek, Japan), allow a the visualization of the angle.[47] A more recent and performant device, Pentacam, enables the visualization, in 50 images and 25,000 points, of the anterior segment, and consequently, the angle-to-angle measurement (Fig. 2.4).

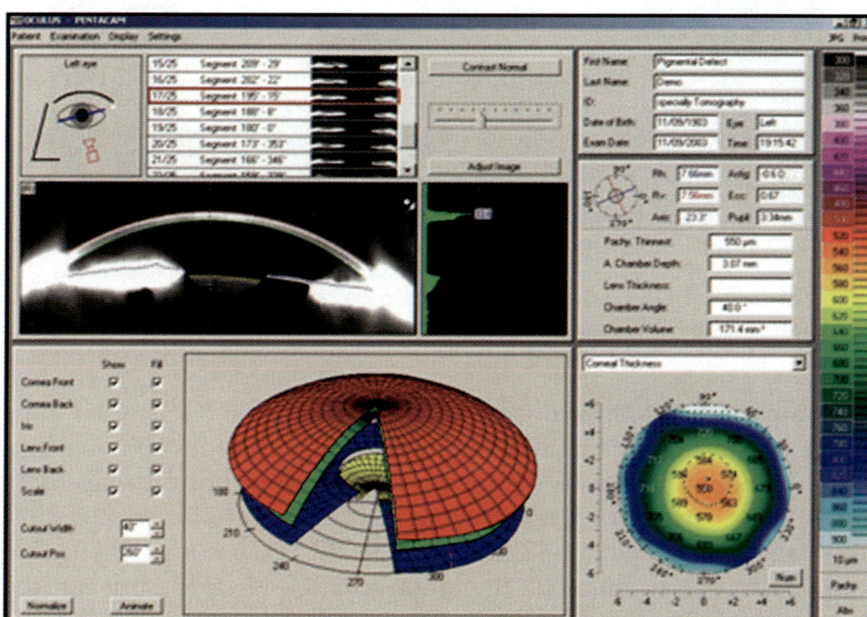

Fig. 2.4: Anterior segment pentacam image. Topographic and pachymetric maps also displayed

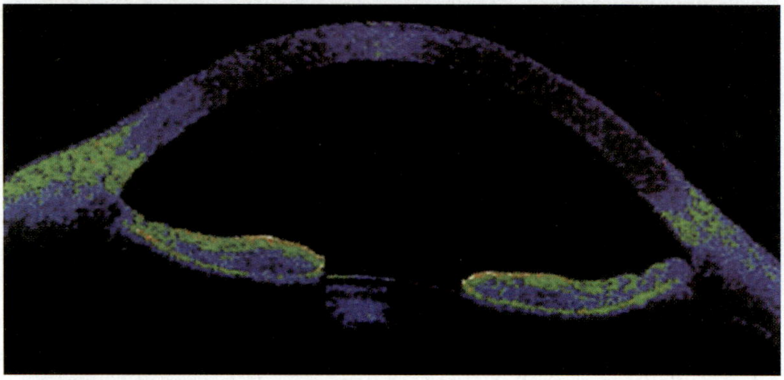

Fig. 2.5: Cross-sectional anterior segment image with optical coherence topography (OCT)

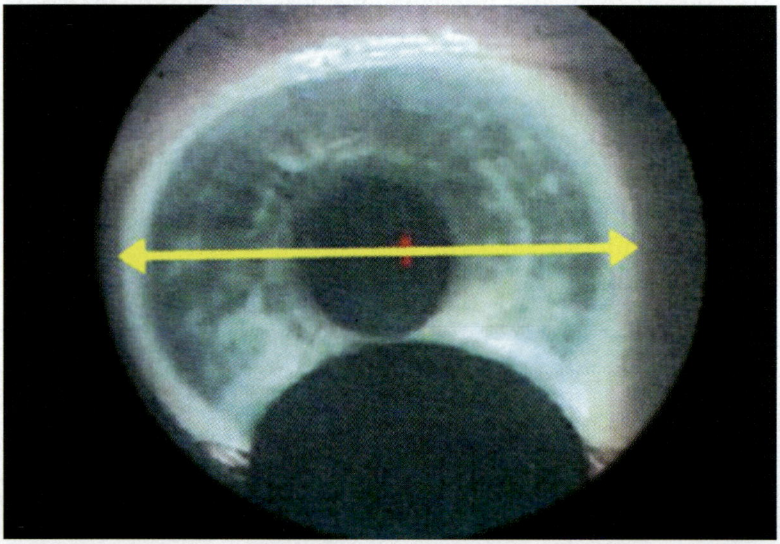

Fig. 2.6: The LED sizer (IOLTech, France). The contrast difference analysis after illumination of the eye shows three peaks; one central peak corresponds to the pupil contour and two peripheral correspond to the lateral trabeculum. Hence, the distance between the central and lateral peak measures the radius; consequently the diameter of angle-to-angle is easily calculated

More recently, Optical Coherence Tomography (OCT, Carl Zeiss Meditec, Germany) (Fig. 2.5) can perform precise morphometrical measurements in a cross-sectional way, based in optical reflectivity differences between the microstructures of the anterior segment.[48,49] Another optical device, the Led Sizer (IOLTECH, La Rochelle) (Fig. 2.6) is equally able to measure the angle-to-angle distance but not the sulcus-to-sulcus diameter. The method applies an oblique (18°) diode visible light illuminating the eye, enhancing the contrast difference between sclera and trabecular region.

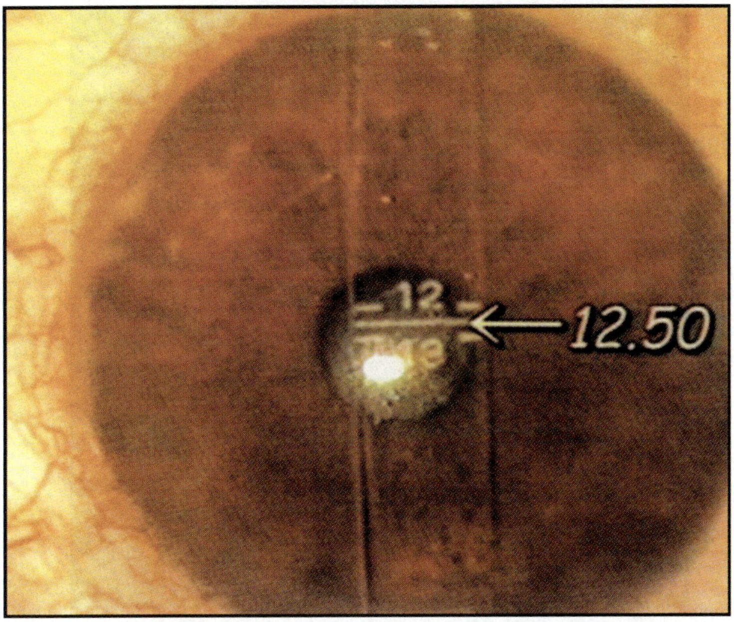

Fig. 2.7: Intraoperative ruler. Careful perpendicularity between microscope axis and iris plane is necessary in order to avoid paralaxis error

Finally, a direct way of measuring the angle-to-angle distance is the use of an intraoperative ruler (Fig. 2.7), by reading the measure correspondant to the center of the temporal pupillary border. Because of paralaxis error, the microscope axis must be aligned at 90° of the iris plane.

Anterior chamber depth: This parameter is crucial to the implantation of any phakic IOL. Its importance relies not only on evaluating the capacity of the anterior segment to safely shelter a phakic IOL, but, very particularly, it is essential to the calculation of the IOL potency (Van der Heijde's formula).

It is a well-known fact that anterior chamber depth decreases with age.[50] This decrease centrally varies between 0.2 and 1.0 mm over a 50-year period, due to slow constant increase in crystalline lens and progressive anterior displacement.

In general, AC depth should have a minimum value of 2.8 mm, as mesured from the corneal endothelium to the anterior surface of the crystalline lens.

Ultrasonography has long been used in anterior chamber depth measurement, besides the more common use in pachimetry and axial length evaluation.[51] A-scan provides a better assessment due to the higher frequencies involved (20 MHz) than B-scan (10 MHz), being that

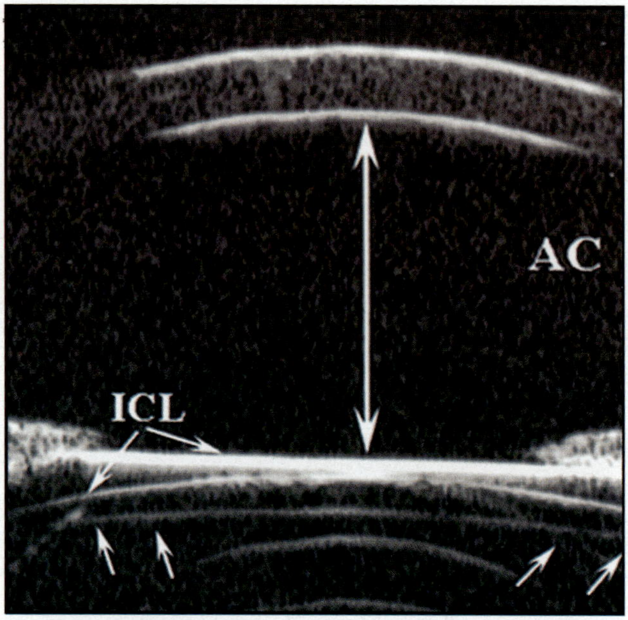

Fig. 2.8: UBM (Humphrey Zeiss/Paradigm). AC depth measurement in an eye with ICL implant

the immersion technique ensures no foreshortening of the axial measurement by pressure on the cornea, an advantage over contact biometry.

Improved accuracy is provided by very high frequency ultrasound (50 to 100M Hz) devices like UBM (Humphrey Zeiss/Paradigm) (Fig. 2.8).[52] Likewise, Artemis 2 (Ultralink LLC) enables a fine measurement of AC depth.

Optical devices like Orbscan II utilizes hybrid technology (specular reflection + slit-scanning) in order to calculate anterior chamber depth,[53] whose measurement correlates well with Scheimpflug photography-based devices, such as EAS-1000 (Nidek, Japan); we have examined this correlation in a study, which results were presented in the ESCRS 2003 Congress. More recently, a rotating Scheimpflug camera, Pentacam (Oculus), has broadened the range of utility of such operating instruments.

Another recent optical device is the IOLMaster (Humphrey Zeiss), which uses partial coherence interferometry; it measures AC depth based in the distance between corneal and crystalline lens optical sections.

OCT (Carl Zeiss Meditec) is another way of obtaining the AC depth, however dependent on the transparency level of the structures, a feature that is common to any optical device.

SUMMARY

In order to achieve the goal of refractive surgery, i.e. the correction of refractive error, a sequence of various steps is mandatory.

It is determinant to the patient's postoperative satisfaction, to keep in mind that an adequate candidate is a well-motivated and educated one. The education of the patient, regarding the many preoperative, operative and postoperative aspects, should aim at the creation of realistic expectations towards the the final outcome.

General ophthalmic and systemic pathology must be excluded. Age, as a factor of exclusion, may be broadened in its limits of range (normaly between 18 and 45 years old) in selected cases.

A careful refraction assessment should be performed, keeping in the mind that this step is fundamental to the accuracy and efficacy of the surgical procedure.

Specific ocular examination, involving pupillometry, endothelial study and the evaluation of anterior chamber dimensions, is the corner step of this selection path in terms of safety. Criteria such as scotopic pupil size ≤ 6.0 mm, endothelial cell count ≥ 2200 cells/mm^3, AC depth ≥ 2.80 mm, must be met. Furthermore, the angle-to-angle or sulcus-to-sulcus distance (the use of W-to-W is no longer acceptable) must be assessed in order to adequate the size of phakic angle-supported or posterior chamber IOL's, respectively. This dependence on these internal diameters, which do not exist in iris-supported phakic IOL's and PRL ("one size fits all") is prone to the development of new imaging devices, together with the stimulus of challenging upcoming techniques and insights in refractive surgery.

Most relevant to the accuracy of the phakic implantation procedure, anatomical evaluation provides, through AC depth measurement, a parameter fundamental to the IOL power calculation.

It is appropriate to state, as a final comment, that most of the success of phakic IOL refractive surgery, as measured both in terms of surgeon's projected outcome and, most determinantly, patient satisfaction, is dependent on the accurate selection of the candidate.A careful and thorough examination is the mainstay of this selection.

REFERENCES

1. Barraquer JL. Bases de la Queratoplastia Refractiva. Arch Soc Amer Oftal Optom 1965; 5; 179-224.
2. Lesueur LC, Arne JL. Phakic posterior chamber lens implantation in children with high myopia. J Cataract Refract Surg 1999; 25:1571-5.
3. BenEzra D, Cohen E, Karshai I. Phakic posterior chaber intraocular lens for the correction of anisometropia and treatment of amblyopia. Am J Ophthalmol 2000; 130:292-6.

4. Pallikaris IG, Siganos DS. Excimer laser *in situ* keratomileusis and photorefractive keratectomy for correction of high myopia. J Cataract Refract Surg 1994; 10:498-510.
5. Perez-Santonja JJ, Bellot J, Claramonte P, et al. Laser in situ keratomileusis to correct high myopia. J Cataract Refract Surg 1997;23 :372-85.
6. Güell JL, Muller A. Laser in situ keratomileusis (LASIK) for myopia from -7 to -18 diopters. J Cataract Refract Surg 1996; 12:222-8.
7. Zaldivar R, Davidorf JM, Oscherow S, et al. Combined posterior chamber phakic intraocular lens and laser in situ keratomileusis: Bioptics for extreme myopia. J Refract Surg 1999; 15:299-308.
8. Güell JL, Vasquez M, Gris O. Adjustable refractive surgery: 6-mm Artisan lens plus laser insitu keratomileusis for the correction of high myopia. Ophthalmology 2001: 108:945-52.
9. Mutyala S, McDonald M, Scheinblum K. Contrast sensitivity evaluation after laser in situ keratomileusis. Ophthalmology 2000; 107:1864-7.
10. Malecaze F, Hulin H, Bierer P, et al. A randomised paired eye comparison of two techniques for treating moderatly high myopia; LASIK and Artisan phakic lens. Ophthalmology 2002; 109:1622-30.
11. Gris O, Güell JL Manero F, et al. Clear lens extraction to correct high myopia. J Cataract Refract Surg 1996; 22:686-9.
12. Colin J, Robinet A. Clear lensectomy and implantation of low-power posterior chamber intraocular lens for the correction of high myopia. Ophthalmology 1994; 101:107-12.
13. Barraquer C, Cavelier C, Mejia LF. Incidence of retinal detachment following clear-lens extraction in myopic patients; retrospective analysis. Bases de la Queratoplastia Refractiva. Arch Ophthalmol 1994; 112:336-9.
14. Colin J, Robinet A, Cochener B. Retinal detachment after clear lens extraction for high myopia. Seven-year follow-up. Ophthalmology 1999; 106:2281-5.
15. Fine H, Hoffman RS, Packer M, Refractive lens exchange. In Garg A, Alió, Dementiev D, Marinho A, (Eds): Mastering the Techniques of Lens Based Refractive Surgery. New Delhi, Jaypee Brothers, 2005; 180-5.
16. Alió JL, Mulet ME, Shalaby AM. Artisan phakic iris claw intraocular lens for high primary and secondary hyperopia. J Refrat Surg 2002; 18:697-707.
17. Singh D. Phakic intraocular lens implantation for hyperopia. In Shear NA, (Eds): Surgery for Hyperopia and Presbyopia. Baltimore, MD, Williams and Wilkins, 1997; 183-91.
18. Dick HB, Alió JL, Bianchetti M, et al. Toric Phakic intraocular Lens: European Multicenter Study. Ophthalmology 2003; 110:150-62.
19. Budo C, Hessloehl JC, Izak M, et al. Multicenter study of Artisan phakic intraocular lens. J Cataract Refract Surg 2000; 26:1163-71.
20. Marinho A, Salgado R. Toric phakic IOL's. In Garg A, Alió, Dementiev D, Marinho A (Eds): Mastering the Techniques of Lens Based Refractive Surgery. New Delhi, Jaypee Brothers, 2005; 124-7.
21. van der Heijde GL, Fechner PU, Worst JGF. Optische konsequenzen der implantation einer negativen intraokularlinse bei myopen patienten. Klin Mbl Augenheilk 1988; 99-102.
22. Burton TC. The influence of refractive errors and lattice degeneration on the incidence of retinal detachment. Trans Am Ophthalmology Soc 1990; 87:143-55.
23. Arné JL. Correction chirurgicale de la myopie forte. In Saragoussi JJ, Arné JL, Colin, J, Montard M (Eds): Chirugie réfractive. Paris, Masson ed, 2001 : 457-62.

24. Schepens CL, Marden D. Data on the natural history of retinal detachment : Further characterization of certain unilateral non-traumatic cases. Am J Ophthalmol 1966; 61:213-26.
25. Ruiz-Moreno JM, Alió JL, Pérez-Santonja JJ, de la Hoz F. Retinal detachment in phakic eyes with anterior chamber intraocular lenses to correct severe myopia. Am J Ophthalmol 1999; 127:270-75.
26. Grossniklaus HE, Green WR. Pathologic findings in pathologic myopia. Retina 1992;12 :127-33.
27. Curtin BJ. The posterior staphyloma of pathologic myopia. Trans Am Ophthalmol Soc 1977; 75:67-86.
28. Curtin BJ, Karlin DB. Axial length measurements and fundus changes of the myopic eye. Am J Ophthalmol 1971; 71:42-53.
29. Pollack A, Marcovich A, Bukelman A, Oliver M. Age-related macular degeneration after extracapsular cataract extration with intraocular implantation. Ophthalmology 1996; 103:1546-54.
30. Blair CJ, Ferguson JJR. Exacerbation of senile degeneration following cataract extraction. Am J Ophthalmol 1979; 87:77-83.
31. Puliafito C, Hee MR, Schuman JS, et al. Optical Coherence Tomography of Ocular Diseases. Thorofare NJ Slack Inc, 1996.
32. Colvard M. Preoperative measurement of scotopic pupil dilation using an office pupillometer. J Cataract Refract Surg 1998; 24:1594-7.
33. Muller A, Schnaidt A, Buchwald HJ, Kampmeier J. Comparison of different methods for pupillometry for mesopic and scotopic conditions. Klin Monatsbl Augenheilkd 2004; 221:843-8.
34. Kurz S, Krummenauer F, Pfeiffer N, Dick HB. Monocular versus binocular pupillometry. J Cataract Refract Surg 2004; 30:2551-6.
35. Perlman LM, Ambrósio RJ, Harrison DA, Wilson SE. Correlation of pupil sizes measured with a mesopic infrared pupillometer and a photopic topographer. J Refrat Surg 2004; 19:555-9.
36. Werblin TP. Long-term endothelial cell loss following phacoemulsification: Model for evaluating endothelial damage after intraocular surgery. Refract Corneal Surg 1993; 9:29-35.
37. Tuft SJ, Coster DJ. The corneal endothelium. Eye 1990; 4:389-424.
38. Leroux les Jardins, Hélicon JP, Ozdemir N, et al. Medium-term tolerance of anterior chamber implants in surgical treatment of severe myopia. J Fr Ophthalmol 1995; 18:45-9.
39. Baikoff G, Arne JL, Bokobza Y, Colin J, George J, Lagoutte F, Lesure P, Montard M, Saragoussi J, Scheyron P. Angle-fixated anterior chamber phakic intraocular lens for myopia of -7 to -19 diopters. J Refract Surg 1998; 282-93.
40. Marinho A, Salgado R. Complications of phakic IOLs. In Garg A, Alió, Dementiev D, Marinho A, (Eds): Mastering the Techniques of Lens Based Refractive Surgery. New Delhi, Jaypee Brothers, 2005; 139-45.
41. Werner L, Izak AM, Pandey SK, Apple DJ, Trivedi RH, Schmidbauer JM Correlation between different measurements within the eye relative to phakic intraocular lens implantation. J Cataract Refract Surg. 2004;30(9):1982-8.
42. Radhakrishnan S, Goldsmith J, Huang D, Westphal V, Dueker DK, Rollins AM, Izatt JA, Smith SD. Comparison of optical coherence tomography and ultrasound biomicroscopy for detection of narrow anterior chamber angles. Arch Ophthalmol 2005;123(8):1053-9.
43. Barraquer JL. Bases de la Queratoplastia Refractiva. Arch Soc Amer Oftal Optom 1965; 5; 179-224.

44. Cusumano A, Coleman DJ, Silverman RH, et al. Three dimensional ultrasound imaging. Clinical applications. Ophthalmology 1998; 105:300-6.
45. Reinstein DZ, Silverman RH, Raevsky T, et al. A new arc-scanning very high –frequency ultrasound system for 3D pachymetric mapping of corneal epithelium, lamellar flap and residual stromal layer in situ keratomileusis. J Refract Surg 2000; 16:414-30.
46. OrbscanBarraquer JL. Bases de la Queratoplastia Refractiva. Arch Soc Amer Oftal Optom 1965; 5; 179-224.
47. Boker T, Shequem J, Rauwolf M, et al. Anterior chamber angle biometry: a comparison of Scheimpflug photography and ultrasound biomicroscopy. Ophthalmic Res 1995; 27 Suppl 1:104-9.
48. Goldsmith JA, Li Y, Chalita MR, Westphal V, Patil CA, Rollins AM, Izatt JA, Huang D. Anterior chamber width measurement by high-speed optical coherence tomography. Ophthalmology. 2005 Feb;112(2):238-44.
49. Baikoff G, Luton E, Ferraz C, et al. Static and dynamic analysis of the anterior segment with optical coherence tomography. J Cataract Refract Surg 2004; 30:1843-50.
50. Fontana ST, Brubaker RF. Volume and depth of the anterior chamber in the normal aging human eye. Arch Ophthalmol 1980; 98:1803.
51. Nemeth J, Fekete O, Pesztenlehrer N. Optical and ultrasound measurement of axial length and anterior chamber depth for intraocular lens power calculation. J Cataract Refract Surg. 2003;29(1):85-8.
52. Souza Filho EC, Marigo Fde A, Oliveira C, Cronemberger S, Calixto N. Intraobserver reproducibility in anterior segment morphometry of normal eyes using ultrasound biomicroscopy (UBM) Arq Bras Oftalmol 2005; 68(2):177-83. Epub 2005 May 18.
53. Auffarth GU, Tetz MR, Biazid Y, Volcker HE. Measuring anterior chamber depth with the Orbscan Topography System. J Cataract Refract Surg 1997; 23:1351-5.

CHAPTER

3

M Shaju Asokan (India)

Informed Consent for Phakic Implant Surgery: ICL™

INTRODUCTION

This information and the *Patient Information Booklet* are being provided to you so that you can make an informed decision about having eye surgery to reduce or eliminate your nearsightedness. Only you and your ophthalmologist can determine if you should have phakic implant surgery based upon your own visual needs and medical considerations. Take as much time as you wish to make your decision before signing this consent form. You have the right and are encouraged to ask your doctor questions about this procedure before agreeing to have it.

The ICL™ (Implantable Contact Lens) is a lens that is permanently implanted in the eye behind the iris and in front of the natural lens. It is called a phakic intraocular lens (IOL) because the eye still has its natural lens. The ICL™ has been approved by the Food and Drug Administration (FDA) for the treatment of patients with moderate to severe nearsightedness (myopia). Myopia, the clinical term for nearsightedness, is a condition that causes light rays to focus in front of the retina, causing distant objects to look blurry or distorted. It can be caused by an eyeball that is too long for its optical power or by curvature of the cornea or lens that is too high for the actual length of the eyeball. The amount of myopia is measured in "diopters," a technical term used to describe the power of a lens. The ICL™ is approved for treatment of myopia between the ranges of –3 to –20 diopters, with up to 5 diopters of astigmatism.

Phakic implant surgery is an elective procedure: there is no emergency condition or other reason that requires or demands that you have it performed. You could continue wearing contact lenses or glasses and have adequate visual acuity. This procedure, like all surgery, presents some risks, many of which are listed below. You should also understand that there may be other risks not known to your doctor, which may become known later. Despite the best of care, complications and side effects may occur. Should this happen in your case, your vision could be affected, and might even be worse than before surgery.

ALTERNATIVES TO PHAKIC IMPLANT SURGERY

You are under no obligation to have phakic implant surgery. If you decide not to have phakic implant surgery, there are other methods of correcting your nearsightedness:

Non-surgical Alternatives

Contact lenses or glasses are non-surgical, extremely accurate, permit easy changes in prescription, and also allow the eye to retain its focusing power for near vision.

1. *Spectacles (glasses):* Although there are essentially no risks to wearing glasses, the quality of vision with strong nearsighted glasses is not normal because of the smaller appearance of images ("minification") and the slight decrease in peripheral vision caused by the thickness of the lenses.
2. *Contact lens:* While contact lenses provide higher quality and more normal vision, they have a slight risk of complications, especially if they are worn overnight. The risks of contact lenses include infection, allergies, irritation, and discomfort.

Surgical Alternatives including Laser

There are several other procedures for the correction of moderate to high myopia. Unlike phakic implant surgery, PRK and LASIK do not require an incision into the inside of the eye.

1. *Photorefractive Keratectomy (PRK)* uses an excimer laser to reshape the cornea to refocus light rays on the cornea. PRK may be used to correct low to higher amounts of myopia (generally –1 D to –12 D).
2. *LASIK* is a two-phase operation. First, a thin layer of cornea is either surgically cut with the microkeratome or a flap is created using a laser. Then the exposed surface of the cornea is reshaped with an excimer laser, and the flap is returned to its original position. LASIK has been found to be quite successful and relatively safe for the correction of moderate and high myopia up to –12 D. Above 12 diopters, LASIK is known to have a high incidence of complications involving the quality of vision, especially at night, and has proven to be less accurate than it is with the treatment of lower levels of nearsightedness. For these reasons, many surgeons have stopped performing LASIK for extremely nearsighted eyes.
3. *Refractive Lens Exchange (RLE)* is an intraocular procedure in which the natural lens is removed and replaced with a synthetic lens of a more accurate power. Patients age 40 or over may request a multifocal lens that corrects for both near and distance vision. Because of the increased risk of retinal detachment, refractive lens exchange is done very selective.
4. *Other refractive surgery procedures* include keratomileusis, corneal inlays, and radial keratotomy (RK). These procedures are rarely performed, and RK is generally effective only for patients with low to moderate degrees of myopia.

GENERAL DESCRIPTION OF TREATMENT WITH PHAKIC IMPLANT SURGERY

If you wear contact lenses, you will be required to leave them out of the eyes for a period of time prior to having your preoperative eye examination and before your surgery. This is done because the contact lens rests on the cornea, distorting its shape, and this distortion will have an effect on the accuracy of the doctor's measurements of the power of surgical correction needed. Discontinuing contact lens use allows the corneas to return to their natural shape. Soft contact lens wearers should leave lenses out of the eyes for at least one week. Rigid (including gas permeable and standard hard lenses) contact lens wearers should leave lenses out of the eyes for at least three weeks. Rigid contact lens wearers usually experience fluctuating vision once their lenses have been discontinued due to changes in the shape of the cornea. Although the cornea usually returns to its natural state within three weeks, this process may take longer, and you will need to remain contact lens free until stabilization is complete.

The surgeon will make two small holes in the colored portion of your eye (the iris) to help ensure that intraocular fluid does not build up behind the phakic lens; this procedure is called an iridotomy. It will take place either at the time of surgery by using an instrument (a surgical iridotomy) or within two weeks before the placement of the phakic implant by using a laser (YAG-laser iridotomy).

Before phakic implant surgery begins, your pupils will be dilated and you will be given an anesthetic to minimize your pain during surgery. You may undergo light sedation administered by an anesthesiologist or nurse anesthetist while your eye is made numb by your surgeon with either drops or an injection (local anesthesia); you may elect to have the surgery with local anesthesia only, without sedation; or, if your surgeon determines that it is in your best interest, you may undergo general anesthesia, in which case you will not be awake during the operation. All methods of anesthesia have risks, and although not common, may include the risk of serious bodily injury or death. Your ophthalmologist or other qualified health care professional will explain the method of anesthesia that has been selected for you as well as the associated risks. You have the right and are encouraged to ask your doctor or health care professional any questions you have related to the anesthesia.

After your pupil has been dilated, and your eye has been anesthetized, the surgeon will make a small incision in your cornea to allow insertion of the lens. The ICL™ phakic IOL is inserted in the posterior chamber of the eye, behind the iris and in front of the natural lens. The incision required to perform this operation is usually self-sealing but it may require closure with very fine stitches (sutures) which will gradually dissolve over time or may require removal later in the office. A temporary shield may be placed over the eye to protect it during the immediate postoperative period.

You will return to your ophthalmologist the next day for an examination. The shield will be removed and your eye will be examined with a microscope to make sure the lens is positioned correctly and that there are no complications. You will return for additional post-operative exams as instructed by your ophthalmologist. Although you may see some improvement in your vision as early as the first post-operative day, the visual effects of phakic implant surgery may take several weeks to stabilize. Patients are generally able to return to their normal activities within 2 or 3 days following phakic implant surgery.

Only one eye will be treated at a time. If you decide to have the second eye treated with phakic implant surgery, you will need to wait until your ophthalmologist has determined that the first eye has healed sufficiently. You will be required to wait a minimum of one week and possibly as much as three months following surgery on your first eye before receiving an implant in the second eye.

BENEFITS OF PHAKIC IMPLANT SURGERY

If you have moderate to high myopia, phakic implant surgery may improve your natural distance vision without the use of glasses or contacts.

LIMITATIONS OF PHAKIC IMPLANT SURGERY

1. This procedure does not treat presbyopia, a condition common in patients age 40 or older in which the eye loses its ability to change power to allow focusing of both near and distant objects. Even with a successful surgery and an accurate intraocular lens calculation targeted to correct the eye's distance vision, close vision will usually remain blurred for presbyopic patients. Patients age 40 or older are likely to require bifocals or reading glasses to improve their near vision.
2. The ICL™ phakic lens also corrects astigmatism.
3. The results of this surgery cannot be guaranteed, and glasses may still be required for sharpest vision for distance, for night driving or other activities performed in low light, for reading or, for all of these activities.
4. With increasing age, patients are likely to develop cataracts. If the cataracts are significant enough to cause visual problems, the phakic

implant may need to be removed so that the eye can undergo cataract removal with or without implantation of an artificial intraocular lens.

PATIENT RESPONSIBILITY FOR COSTS

Health insurance generally does not pay for elective phakic implant surgery for the purpose of correcting natural vision. Therefore, the patient is responsible for the cost of the surgery, including the surgeon's fee, anesthesiologist's fee, (if any), and the surgical center's or hospital's fee. In the event of a complication, it may be possible that other surgery, eye drops, or even hospitalization may be required. Some or even all of these costs may be covered by health insurance. The patient is responsible for the costs of any uncovered surgery-related injuries.

PATIENT CONSENT

I give my ophthalmologist permission to perform either a YAG-laser iridotomy or a surgical iridotomy and phakic implant surgery, and acknowledge that I understand the following: the foreseeable risks of phakic implant surgery are not fully known. I have received no guarantee as to the success of my particular case and I understand that I may still need glasses, contact lenses, or a laser procedure such as LASIK for further improvement of my vision. I understand that during the surgical procedure, the doctor may decide not to implant the lens even though I have given permission to do so. Furthermore, I understand that the following risks are associated with the procedure:

Complications of Iridotomy

Potential complications of either a YAG-laser iridotomy or a surgical iridotomy are very rare but include damage to the natural lens; inflammation inside the eye; temporary increases in the pressure in the front part of the eye; cataract formation; bleeding (usually a small amount but can be a large amount); scar formation between the iris and phakic IOL (synechia) that prevents the pupil from moving correctly; corneal damage; and vision disturbances such as double vision (diplopia), glare, or halos.

Vision-threatening Complications

1. In most cases, the surgery will be accomplished with numbing drops, but in some cases the eye surgeon may elect to use an injection around the eye for anesthesia. Very rare complications from injections include damage to the eye muscles, perforation of

the eye, and damage to the retina or optic nerve leading to loss of vision.

2. I understand that mild or severe infection is possible. Mild infection can usually be treated with antibiotics and usually does not lead to permanent visual loss. Severe infection, even if treated with antibiotics, could lead to permanent scarring and loss of vision that may require corrective laser surgery or, if very severe, corneal transplantation, blindness, or even loss of the eye.
3. I understand that I could experience damage to the iris (the colored portion of the eye) or develop a rise in the pressure in the front of my eye (secondary glaucoma). I may require another iridotomy or eye drops to control the pressure if this occurs.
4. I understand that I could develop a retinal detachment, a separation of the retina from the inside wall of the eye, which usually results from a tear in the retina and could lead to vision loss. Patients with moderate to high levels of nearsightedness have a higher risk of retinal detachment when compared to the general population. This risk level may be increased with implantation of the phakic IOL.
5. I understand that I may develop a cataract, or a clouding of the eye's natural lens, which impairs normal vision, and may require removal of the lens, the phakic implant, and insertion of an artificial lens. Patients with high levels of nearsightedness are at higher risk for cataract development, and that risk may be increased with implantation of the phakic IOL.
6. I understand that I may develop corneal swelling (edema) and/or ongoing loss of cells lining the inner surface of my cornea (endothelial cells). These cells play a role in keeping the cornea healthy and clear. Corneal edema and loss of endothelial cells may result in a hazy and opaque appearance of the cornea, which could reduce vision. It is not yet known how much endothelial cell loss will occur and what effect the cell loss and phakic implant will have on the long-term health of the cornea. If too many cells are lost over time, I may need a corneal transplant.
7. I understand that I may develop glaucoma, which is an increase in the pressure of the eye caused by slowed fluid drainage. Glaucoma can lead to vision loss, and may require treatment with long-term medications or surgery. Patients with high levels of nearsightedness are at an increased risk for the development of glaucoma, and that risk may be increased by implantation of the lens. The effect of the ICL™ Phakic IOL on the future risk of glaucoma is not known.

8. I understand that other complications could threaten my vision, including, but not limited to, iritis or inflammation of the iris (immediate and persistent), uveitis, bleeding, swelling in the retina (macular edema), and other visual complications. Though rare, certain complications may result in total loss of vision or even loss of the eye. Complications may develop days, weeks, months, or even years later.

Non-vision-threatening Complications

1. I understand that I may be given sedation in conjunction with the procedure and that my eye may be patched afterward. I have been advised not to drive immediately after receiving sedation and for a period of eight hours thereafter. I understand that my life and health and the life of others will be at risk if I drive during this period. This is because I may be impaired by the sedative. I also understand that driving while impaired may violate traffic laws.
2. I understand that there may be increased sensitivity to light or night glare. I also understand that at night there may be a "starbursting" or halo effect around lights. The risk of this side effect may be related to the size of my pupil, and larger pupils may put me at increased risk.
3. I understand that an overcorrection or undercorrection could occur, causing me to become farsighted, remain nearsighted, or increase my astigmatism and that this could be either permanent or treatable with either glasses, contact lenses, or additional surgery.
4. I understand that the phakic lens may need to be repositioned, removed surgically, or exchanged for another lens implant. The lens may change position (decentration), or I may require a different size or power of lens than that of the implanted lens. In rare instances, lens power measurements may significantly vary, resulting in the need for corrective lenses or surgical replacement of the phakic lens. Potential complications of additional surgery include all of the complications possible from the original surgery.
5. I understand that there may be a difference in vision between my two eyes after the phakic implant surgery has been performed on one eye but not the other. This imbalance is called anisometropia. I understand this would cause eyestrain and make judging distance or depth perception more difficult. Because of the marked difference in the prescriptions, vision correction using glasses most likely would not be comfortable or provide good vision. In order to have balanced vision in both eyes, I may need to wear a contact

lens in the eye without the phakic implant or consider a phakic implant or another type of surgery for that eye.

6. I understand that, after phakic implant surgery, the eye may be more fragile to trauma from impact. Evidence has shown that, as with any scar, a corneal incision will not be as strong as the cornea originally was at that site. I understand that the treated eye, therefore, is somewhat more vulnerable to all varieties of injuries, at least for the first year following phakic implant surgery. I understand it would be advisable for me to wear protective eyewear when engaging in sports or other activities in which the possibility of a ball, projectile, elbow, fist, or other traumatizing object contacting the eye may be high.
7. I understand that there is a natural tendency of the eyelids to droop with age and that eye surgery may hasten this process.
8. I understand that there may be pain or a foreign body sensation, particularly during the first 48 hours after surgery.
9. I understand that the long-term effects of phakic implant surgery are unknown and that unforeseen complications or side effects could possibly occur.
10. I understand that the correction that I can expect to gain from phakic implant surgery may not be perfect. I understand that it is not realistic to expect that this procedure will result in perfect vision, at all times, under all circumstances, for the rest of my life. I understand I may need glasses to refine my vision for some purposes requiring fine detailed vision after some point in my life, and that this might occur soon after surgery or years later.
11. I understand that if I currently need reading glasses, I will still likely need reading glasses after this treatment. It is possible that dependence on reading glasses may increase or that reading glasses may be required at an earlier age if I have this surgery.
12. I understand that, as with all types of surgery, there is a possibility of complications due to anesthesia, drug reactions, or other factors that may involve other parts of my body. I understand that, since it is impossible to state every complication that may occur as a result of any surgery, the list of complications in this form is not complete.

PATIENT'S STATEMENT OF ACCEPTANCE AND UNDERSTANDING

The details of phakic implant surgery have been presented to me in detail in this document and in the *Patient Information Booklet* and have been explained to me by my ophthalmologist. Although it is impossible for the doctor to inform me of every possible complication that may occur, my ophthalmologist has answered all my questions to my satisfaction. In signing this informed consent for YAG-laser iridotomy or surgical iridotomy, and phakic implant surgery, I am stating that I have read this informed consent and *Patient Information Booklet* (or they have been read to me), fully understand the possible risks, complications, and benefits that can result from the surgery and the alternatives available to me, and hereby give my consent to have phakic implant surgery performed on my:

Left Eye Right Eye

My personal reason(s) for choosing to have phakic implant surgery are as follows:

____

____

____

I give permission for my ophthalmologist to record on video or photographic equipment my procedure, for purposes of education, research, or training of other health care professionals. I also give my permission for my ophthalmologist to use data about my procedure and subsequent treatment to further understand phakic implant surgery. I understand that my name will remain confidential, unless I give subsequent written permission for it to be disclosed outside my ophthalmologist's office or the center where my phakic implant surgery will be performed.

____________________________ ____________________________

Patient Name Date Witness Name Date

I have been offered a copy of this consent form (please initial) _____

CHAPTER

4

Georges Baikoff (France)

AC-OCT Preoperative Evaluation of the Anterior Chamber for Phakic IOLs

INTRODUCTION

Today, the increasingly popular development of phakic implants as well as the FDA agreement obtained for the VERISYSE implant, means that a very precise preoperative evaluation of the dimensions of the anterior chamber is essential.

Axial measurements are evaluated with ultrasonography (A-scan, B-scan),[1,2] with optical procedures (Slit Lamp,[3] IOLMaster[4]). The relationship between different eye structures can be studied in reduced areas with ultrasonography (A-scan, B-scan) ultrasound biomicroscopy (UBM),[5] and posterior segment optical coherence tomographer.[6]

The Scheimpflug technique[7] gives a complete image of the anterior chamber, but the complex and inaccurate mathematical reconstructions make it difficult to evaluate the anterior segment precisely. The disparities in the obliquity of the cross sectional and projection plane of photographic images can sometimes lead to measurements being obtained through extrapolation.

It is only recently that complete axial cross sections of the anterior segment are possible with ultra high frequency ultrasound equipment (Artemis)[8] and with the anterior chamber optical coherence tomographer (AC-OCT).[9]

Not only is the OCT simple to use but it is possible to obtain a very precise analysis of anterior segment modifications during accommodation and ageing of the eye. Development of this new imaging technique has enabled us not only to show that in certain cases there is a possibility of contact between a phakic implant and the anatomical structures of the eye but also to evaluate the internal dimensions of the anterior chamber with precision.

OPTICAL COHERENCE TOMOGRAPHY TECHNOLOGY FOR THE ANTERIOR CHAMBER

Today, the AC-OCT with its 820 nm wavelength, is a well-known posterior segment imaging device,[6] and by 1994 Izatt et al[9] had already suggested using it for anterior segment imaging. It was only in 2001, with the introduction of a high speed AC-OCT using a 1310 nm wavelength that good quality, easy to interpret images, were obtained.[10,11]

Analysis of the eye is a non-contact procedure during which the patient fixes an optical target. The target's focus can be adjusted with positive or negative lenses to compensate the patient's spherical ametropia and obtain images of the eye unaccommodated. The target can be defocused by using negative lenses to induce natural accommodation of the studied eye.

There is no undue pressure on the anterior segment because there is no contact, the images are obtained in just a few seconds and only modifications to the studied eye are taken into account under physiological conditions. This examination is, therefore, very different from the ultrasound explorations which require stimulation of the fellow eye or the Scheimpflug technique where pilocarpine drops are used to obtain an artificial accommodation.

The image acquisition system provides a video image of the examined zone and stores the last seven images taken at a rate of 8 frames per second. At the end of the examination, the images are reviewed by the examiner and only the best shots are retained.

The chosen image is then interpreted with specific software which re-adjusts the dimensions of the images by eliminating the distortions induced by corneal optical transmission differences. After reconstruction of the image, all the required anterior chamber measurements can be done : anterior chamber diameter, anterior chamber depth, corneal pachymetry, crystalline lens radius of curvature, crystalline lens thickness, irido-corneal angle opening. The prototype's resolution is approximately 14 µm. The infrared light beam is stopped by the pigments, therefore a satisfactory view of the different structures situated behind the epithelium pigment layer of the iris or of the anterior uvea is not possible.

INTEREST OF THE AC-OCT AND THE STUDY OF ACCOMMODATION WHEN IMPLANTING PHAKIC IOLs

Measurement of the Anterior Chamber's Internal Diameter

One of the key points in improving anterior chamber angle-supported implant tolerance lies in correctly adapting its size with the anterior chamber's internal diameter. Until today, we had to rely on approximate measuring methods, such as white-to-white, sometimes improved by using a graduated plastic sizer when inserting the implant. However, these measuring means are relatively inaccurate and do not give a precise evaluation of the anterior chamber diameter.

Figure 4.1 clearly demonstrates the interest of this type of anterior segment preoperative imaging (AC-OCT, Scheimpflug, ultra-high frequency ultrasound) to evaluate the internal diameter dimensions before surgery.

We were surprised[12] when we compared the anterior chamber's diameter on the 0°, 45°, 90° and 135° axes. The vertical diameter appeared larger than the horizontal diameter in 74% of the cases. The mean difference between the vertical and horizontal axis is more

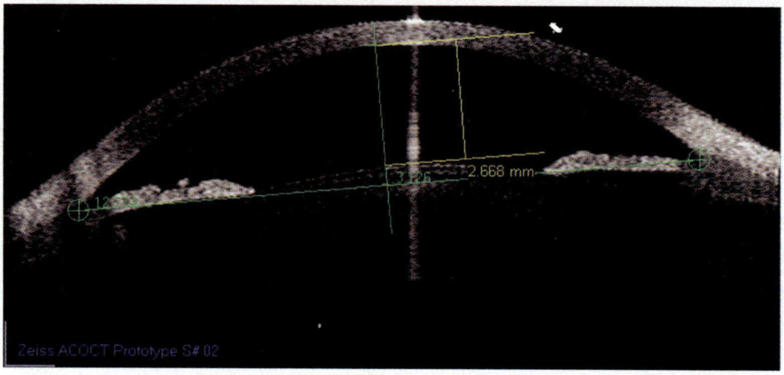

Fig. 4.1: Aspect/dimension of the anterior segment photographed with the AC-OCT

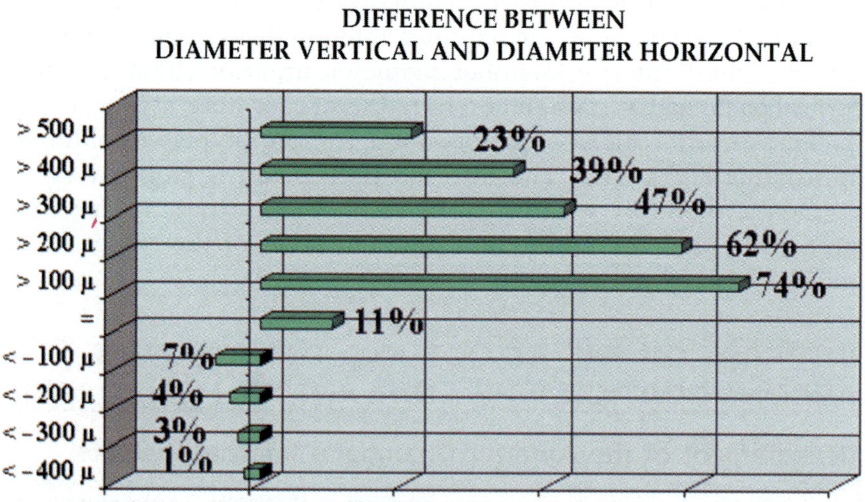

Fig. 4.2: In 74% of normal non-operated eyes, the vertical diameter is greater than the horizontal diameter

significant for eyes with small diameters than eyes with large diameters. The average difference is approximately 300 μm (Fig. 4.2), which is more than the examination measuring or reproducibility error which is not more than 50 μm. In the future, this phenomenon must be taken into account in order to chose the implant. The largest diameter must be taken into account when choosing a angle-supported implant. Indeed, if one chooses an implant with an overall diameter equal to the eye's horizontal diameter, which is generally the smaller of the two diameters, there is a risk that the implant rotates or is unstable. On the contrary, to avoid implant rotation and ensure its stability, it is essential that the implant is fitted both in size and orientation to the largest diameter, i.e. generally the vertical one. This is to avoid an implant that is too big being placed on the smaller diameter which would inevitably lead to oversizing and pupil ovalisation.

Endothelium Safety Distance

Retrospective studies have shown that a 1.5 mm distance must be respected between the edge of the IOLs optic and the corneal endothelium. This minimum safety distance avoids the risk of endothelial cell loss secondary to contact between the implant and the endothelium in particular when the patient rubs his eyes. Anterior segment imaging software should therefore include this safety distance.

Studying accommodation and crystalline lens ageing[13,14] has shown that the crystalline lens increases in volume with age and during accommodation. Developing software that simulates anterior segment distortions with the variations of the crystalline lens volume should allow us to define a safety free zone in the anterior chamber where the optic of the implant should be situated in order to reduce the risk of complications, because of contact with the endothelium or with the crystalline lens (Fig. 4.3).

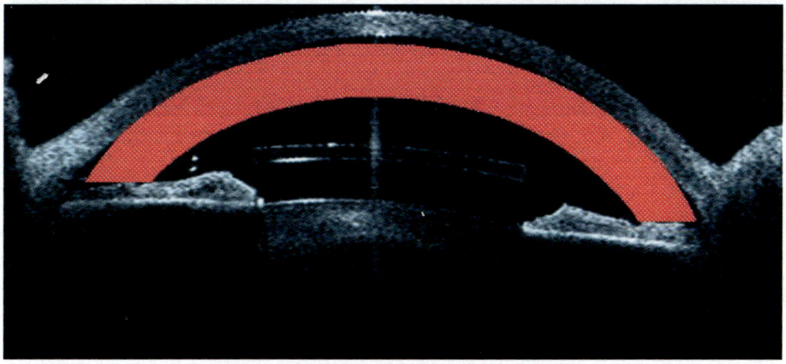

Fig. 4.3: Endothelial safety distance

Possibility of Contact Crystalline Lens/Implant

Having studied numerous series of phakic implants,[15] we were able to show evidence of contact of different models of implants with the crystalline lens. Having dilated a hyperopic patient with an ARTISAN implant, we discovered a contact between the lower edge of the implant and the crystalline lens. Likewise, during accommodation, the posterior face of a hyperopic patient's PRL phakic implant came into contact with the crystalline lens. In a patient implanted 10 years ago with an angle-supported IOL, we noticed that the crystalline lens came into contact with the implant's posterior face because the crystalline lens had increased in volume with age (Fig. 4.4).

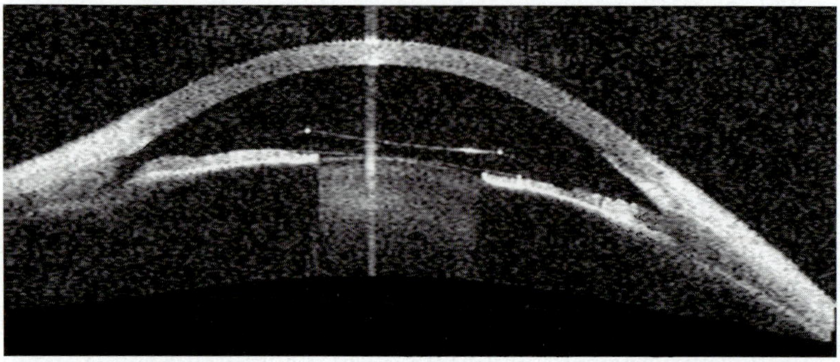

Fig. 4.4: Contact between a ZB5M implant and the crystalline lens 10 years after implantation

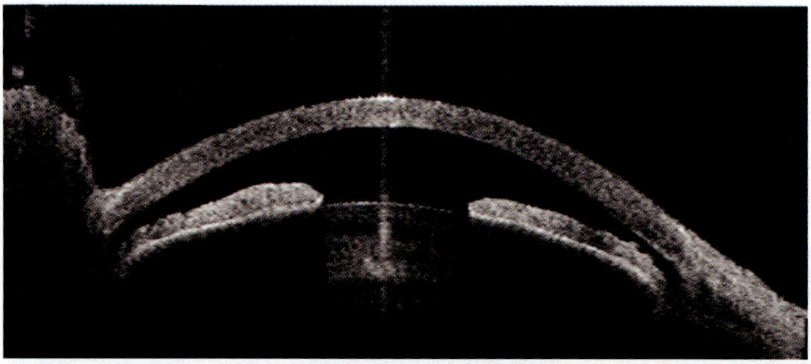

Fig. 4.5: Forward thrust of crystalline lens with aging

These different elements should encourage manufacturers to include in their software the profiles of the different implants available so as to be able to simulate their position in the anterior segment either accommodated or unaccommodated. Simulating anterior segment ageing would give us an indication of how long an implant will be tolerated (Fig. 4.5).

In a previous work,[13] we demonstrated that because the crystalline lens thickens with age, there is a forward movement of its anterior pole which reduces the depth of the anterior chamber by 18 µm to 20 µm per year. As the irido-corneal angle recesses remain fixed, the crystalline lens distorts and pushes the iris forward modifying its relationship with an angle-supported implant and or iris fixated implant. We also found[16] that with Artisan phakic implants, there was an unusually high percentage (6%) of pigment dispersions in hyperopes. This has been confirmed by Saxena and Landesz.[17]

In this study, we measured the distance between the crystalline lens' anterior pole and the line represented by the horizontal internal diameter of the anterior chamber (Fig. 4.6). In subjects having

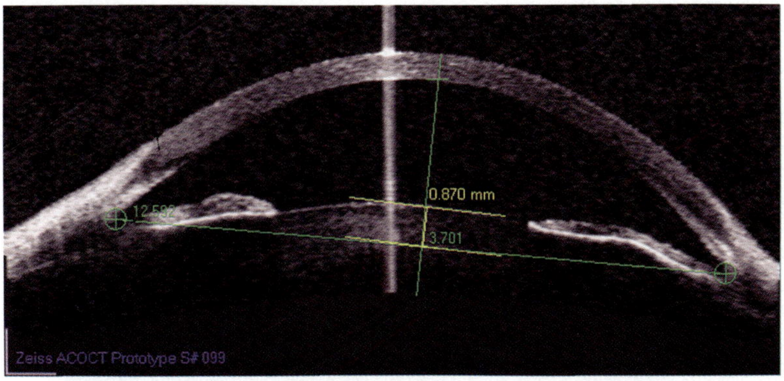

Fig. 4.6: Crystalline lens rise. Distance between anterior pole of the crystalline lens and the line connecting two angle recesses at 3 o'clock and 9 o'clock

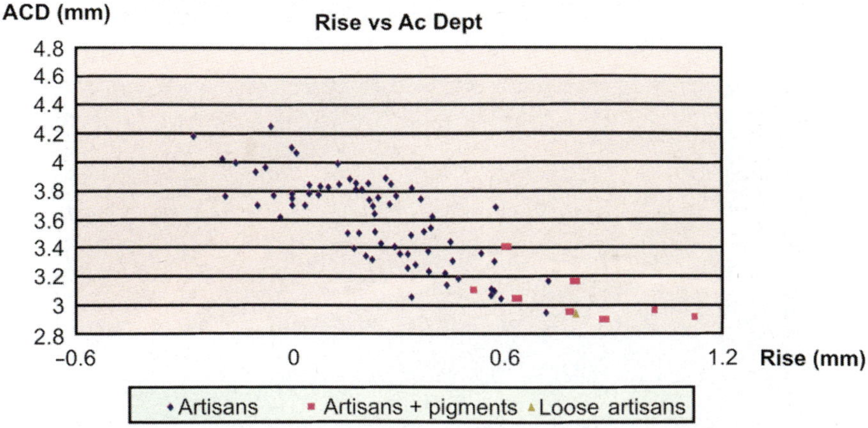

Fig. 4.7: Crystalline lens rise vs AC depth. Eyes having developed pigment dispersion are displayed in red

developed pigment dispersion, this rise was much higher than average. If the crystalline lens rise is above 600 µm, there is a 75% risk of developing pigment dispersion (Fig. 4.7), and this complication can lead to removal of the implant and even extraction of the crystalline lens. If the crystalline lens rise is known on the day of surgery, as well as the statistical forward movement of the crystalline lens, it is possible to estimate the Artisan implant tolerance period knowing that the critical level is around 600 µm according to the following formula:

$$T = \frac{S - F}{\Delta} \Rightarrow T = \frac{600 - F}{20}$$

where T = number of safe years, S = danger level in microns, F = rise measured in microns on the day of examination, Ä = yearly

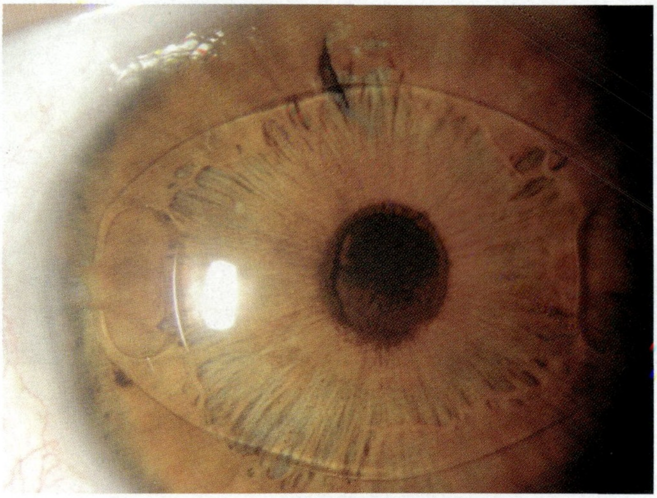

Fig. 4.8: Clinical aspect of pigment dispersion behind an Artisan implant

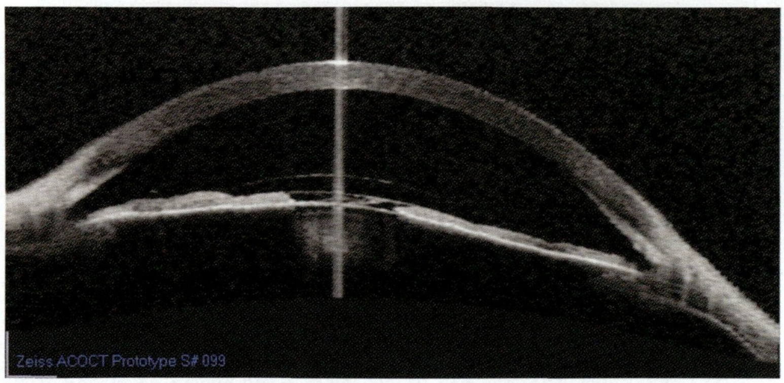

Fig. 4.9: AC-OCT anterior segment cut of an Artisan implant in a case of pigment dispersion. Note: The presence of iris pigments between the crystalline lens and the implant and flattening of iris

reduction of anterior chamber or yearly progression of crystalline lens' anterior pole in microns (Figs 4.8 and 4.9).

This notion of the crystalline lens rise should also be applied to angle-supported anterior chamber implants. The implant's vault measures the implant's posterior face rise with regards to the baseline joining the tip of the implant's footplates. It is, therefore, easy to understand that if the crystalline lens has a rise equal to or superior to the implant's vault, there will be contact between the posterior face of the implant and the crystalline lens. It is necessary today to take into account the implant's vault and the crystalline lens rise when considering surgery to know whether an angle-supported anterior chamber implant is indicated or not and for how many years it will be tolerated. We consider this notion to be just as essential as anterior

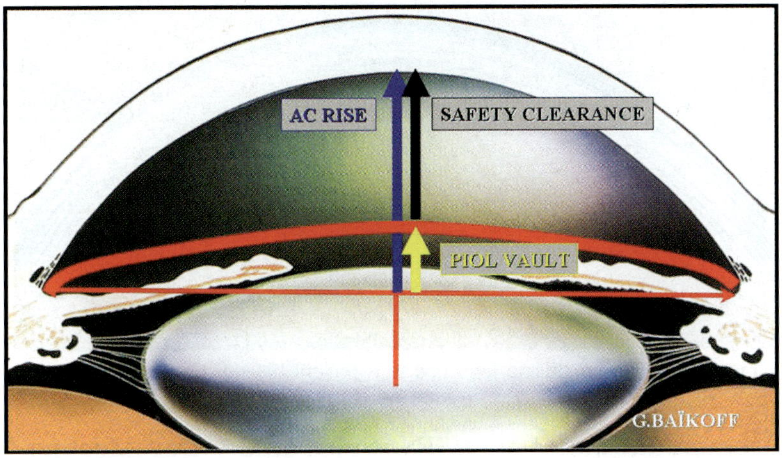

Fig. 4.10: Different anterior chamber safety distances measured from the angle recess to recess baseline

chamber depth. To ensure safe anterior chamber implantation, endothelial safety distances as well as crystalline lens safety distances must be respected. With aging, endothelial safety distances remain constant whereas the distance between implant and crystalline lens gradually decreases over the years (Fig. 4.10).

Can Anterior Segment Imaging Indicate that One Particular Implant is Preferable over Another?

Studying accommodation in an albino patient[18] showed that all the structures of the anterior uvea were malleable and mobile. The only stable elements of the anterior segment are the cornea and the uvea insertion at the corneo-scleral junction, that is to say the irido-corneal angle; the iris, the sulcus, the ciliary body and the crystalline lens show significant modifications during accommodation.

In our opinion, these elements define the irido-corneal angle as the most stable structure and the least affected by accommodation. This could be another fact in favour of angle-supported implants, as long as the problem of pupil ovalisations has been definitely solved as they are the result of inaccurate preoperative measurements.

Studying the ciliary body and the sulcus in an albino patient showed evidence of important diameter variations of these two structures during accommodation.[18] In its present state, the Visante™ OCT technology does not allow us to routinely study the posterior chamber in a normal subject.

Liliana Werner et al studied the internal diameter of the anterior chamber on 20 phakic and pseudophakic cadaver eyes with the Artemis (L Werner et al. Poster ASCRS San Diego 2004, Poster SFO Paris 2004,

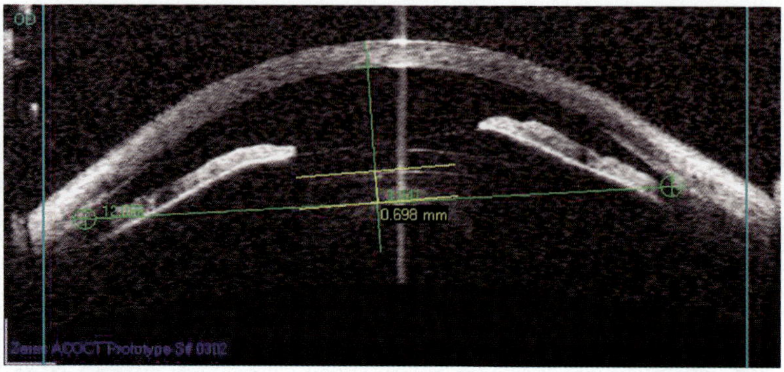

Fig. 4.11: High crystalline lens rise in a patient having developed cataract after an ICL

oral communication AAO/ISRS Subspecialty Day Meeting New Orleans 2004) and found, as we did, that in most cases, the anterior chamber's internal vertical diameter and the sulcus' vertical diameter were statistically larger than their horizontal diameters. More recently, in a patient with an ICL and having developed bilateral cataract, we were able to establish that the patient had a very high crystalline lens rise (Fig. 4.11). This complication is probably due to the forward thrust of the crystalline lens, Gonvers[19] demonstrated that in ICL patients, the risk of cataract dramatically increased with age.

SUMMARY

In the light of these studies, it appears that the AC-OCT or other similar techniques (Scheimpflug, ultra-high frequency ultrasound) available in everyday practice are going to become essential when scheduling a phakic implant in a patient where Lasik is contraindicated. Static and dynamic study of the anterior segment as well as new software are going to become necessary to simulate the anatomical relationship of the implant and the anterior chamber during accommodation and ageing. The safety distances required in the anterior segment will be specified and we will probably be able to predict a safety period during which the implant will be well tolerated and after which it will probably be necessary to remove it.

NB: Most of this article (text and illustrations) appears in the recently published book "Refractive Surgery—Second Edition, Edited by Dimitri AZAR and Damien Gatinel, courtesy of Elsevier Inc. Philadelphia USA

REFERENCES

1. Kurtz D, Manny R, Hussein M; COMET study group. Variability of the ocular component measurements in children using A-scan ultrasonography. Optom Vis Sci. 2004; 81,1: 35-43

2. Hamidzada WA, Osuobeni EP. Agreement between A-mode and B-mode ultrasonography in the measurement of ocular distances. Vet Radiol Ultrasound. 1999; 40, 5: 502-7
3. Krogsaa B, Fledelius H, Larsen J, et al. Photometric oculometry. II. Measurement of axial ocular distances with slit-lamp microscopy. Clinical evaluation and comparison with ultrasonography. Acta Ophthalmol (Copenh).1984; 62, 2:290-9
4. Sheng H, Bottjer CA, Bullimore MA. Ocular component measurement using the Zeiss IOL Master. Optom Vis Sci. 2004; 81, 1: 27-34
5. Mishima HK, Shoge K Takamatsu M, et al. Ultrasound biomicroscopic study of ciliary body thickness after topical application of pharmacologic agents. Am J Ophthalmol. 1996; 121, 3: 319-21
6. Puliafito C, Hee MR, Schuman JS, et al. Optical Coherence Tomography of Ocular Diseases, Thorofare NJ Slack Inc, 1996.
7. Boker T, Shequem J, Rauwolf M, et al. Anterior chamber angle biometry: a comparison of Scheimpflug photography and ultrasound biomicroscopy. Ophthalmic Res. 1995; 27 Suppl 1: 104-9
8. Kim DY, Reinstein DZ, Silverman RH, et al. Very high frequency analysis of a new phakic posterior chamber intraocular lens in situ .Am J Ophthalmol.1998; 125, 5:725-9
9. Izatt JA, Hee MR, Swanson EA, et al., Micrometer-scale resolution imaging of the anterior eye *in vivo* with optical coherence tomography. Arch Ophthalmology, 1994; 112,1, 584-9
10. Radhakrishnan S, Rollins AM, Roth JE, et al. Real-time optical coherence tomography of anterior segment at 1310 nm, Arch Ophthalmology, 2001;119, 8: 1179-85,
11. Huang D, Swanson EA, Lin CP, et al., Optical Coherence Tomography. Science, 1991, 254: 1178-81
12. Baikoff G, Bourgeon G, Jitsuo Jodai H, et al. Evaluation of the measurement of the Anterior Chamber's internal diameter and depth: IOL Master vs AC OCT. J Cataract Refract Surg (submitted)
13. Baikoff G, Lutun E, Ferraz C, et al. Static and dynamic analysis of the anterior segment with opticla coherence tomography. J. Cataract Refract Surg 2004; 30:1843-1850
14. Koretz J, Strenk S, Strenk L, Semmlow J. Scheimpflug and high-resolution magnetic resonance imaging of the anterior segment: A comparative study. J. Opt. Soc. Am 2004; 21:346-54
15. Baikoff G, Lutun E, Ferraz C. Contact between 3 phakic intraocular lens models and the crystalline lens: An anterior chamber optical coherence tomography study. J. Cataract Refract Surg.2004; 30:2007-12
16. Baikoff G, Bourgeon G, Jitsuo Jodai H, et al. Pigment Dispersion and Artisan Implants. The crystalline lens rise as a safety criterion. J. Cataract Refract Surg (submitted)
17. Saxena R, Landesz M, Noordzij B, Luyten G. Three-year Follow-up of the Artisan Phakic Intraocular lens for Hypermetropia.: Ophthalmology 2003; 110: 1391-5
18. Baikoff G, Lutun E, J. Wie, Ferraz C. Anterior chamber optical coherence tomography study of human natural accommodation in a 19-year-old albino. J. Cataract Refract Surg 2004; 30:696-701
19. Gonvers M, Bornet C, Othenin Girard P; Implantable contact lens for moderate to high myopia : Relation of vaulting to cataract formation; J Cataract Refract Surg.2003; 29(5): 918-24

CHAPTER

5

JT Lin (USA), Ashok Garg (India)

Comparing Methods of IOL Power Calculations

INTRODUCTION

Both classical and modern formulas have been used for the power calculation of regular IOL or accommodative IOL in aphakic, pseudophakic and phakic eyes. The modern formulas include that of Holladay, SRK/T, SRK I and II, Hoffer Q, Olson, Haigis and the more recent formulas by Odenthal et al (the historical method), Aramberri et al (the double-K method), Rosa et al (the R-factor method) and Jin et al (the Adjusted-K method). Most of these efforts were to improve the prediction of IOL-power by a better prediction of the postoperative anterior chamber depth (ACDpost) or the effective lens position (ELP) defined by ACDpre, corneal height and curvature, lens thickness and axial length. All the existing IOL-power calculations (except Lin's new formulas) are based on the classical vergence formulas (CVF) of Fyodorov (1975), and van der Heijde (1976) or their revision, the Hoffer Q formula (1981).

The CVFs assume a thin lens (for both corneal and IOL) and are all based on a 2-optics system (the cornea and the IOL) which, strictly speaking, can only apply to aphakic eyes. For pseudophakic or phakic eyes, the 3-optics systems are much more complex and the over-simplified 2-optics CVF suffers the following possible drawbacks. It excludes the effects of IOL thickness and shape (configuration) and the role of natural lens or primary IOL. Major error may result from the use of the keratometric power (Kpre or Kpost) rather than the true postoperative corneal power which requires accurate measurement of both the anterior (r1) and posterior radius (r2). In addition, the CVF assumes paraxial ray and spherical surface for the cornea and IOL. Therefore, it also excludes the effects due to corneal surface asphericity change after refractive surgery.

One of the major pitfalls of the existing IOL power calculations is the ignoring of individual true corneal power and using a mean-zero error for the postoperative refraction. Except the Haigis formula and the Lin Z^2-formula, all other optimization formulas are based on one-constant like the surgeon factor, the A-constant, the ACDpost or the ELP. The mean-zero error might be the result of the balanced errors of short and long eyes. Therefore, the validity range of axial length for various existing formulas under a linear empirical-fit could not justify their accuracy when they are applied to individual eyes. A true personalized IOL power prediction, in our opinion, should at least individualize the following parameters: the postoperative ELP, axial length, corneal anterior and posterior surface, and the IOL types (or configurations).

In this Chapter, we would up-date the IOL formulas and address the critical issues covering 4 subjects:
1. IOL power,
2. Corneal power after refractive surgery,
3. Piggyback IOL power, and
4. Accommodating IOL.

Greater details of subject (3) and (4) may be found in separate Chapters of Lin in this book.

IOL POWER FORMULAS

Theoretical Formulas

All the theoretical formulas (except Lin's formulas) for IOL power are based on a two lens systems, i.e. the cornea and the pseudophakic lens focusing images on the retina, where thin lens is also assumed. Table 5.1 summarizes these formulas.

Basic Theoretical Formulas

These include Colenbrander's, Fyodorov's and Van-der-Heijde's formula which yield approximately the same IOL powers.

Binkhorst's formula yield 0.50 D stronger lens power.

Modified Theoretical Formulas

These include Hoffer's formula, Shamman's fudged formula and Binkhorst's adjusted formula. The fudged formula is a modification of Colenbrander's formula.

The Modern Formulas

These include formulas of Haigis and Lin, where 3-constant optimization is proposed for all ranges of eye length and IOL types. In Lin's new formulas, both effective ACD and corneal power are personalized for more accurate prediction.

Regression Formulas

These formulas are derived empirically from retrospective computer analysis of data of patients who have undergone surgery before. The factors on which IOL power calculation depends are:

Axial Length Measurement

This is the most important step in calculation of lens power. The IOL Master is a recent method using PCI which gives high accuracy in measurement of axial length. An error of 1 mm affects the postoperative

Table 5.1: For emmetropic IOL power calculations	
1. Basic theoretical formulas for emmetropia:	
Colenbrander's formula	$P = \frac{1336}{L - C - 0.05} - \frac{1336}{\frac{1336}{K} - C - 0.05}$
Fyodorov's formula	$P = \frac{1336 - LK}{(L - C)\left(1 - \frac{CK}{1336}\right)}$
Van der Heijde's formula	$P = \frac{1336}{L - C} - \frac{1}{\frac{1}{K} - \frac{C}{1336}}$
Binkhorst's formula	$P = \frac{1336\ (4R - L)}{(L - C)\ (4R - C)}$
Lin's S-formula (I)	$Z'P = \frac{1336}{(L-S)} - \frac{1336}{\frac{1336}{Dc} - S}$
2. Modified formulas for ametropia:	
Hoffer's formula	$P = \frac{1336}{L - C - 0.05} - \frac{1336}{\frac{1336}{K + E} - C - 0.05}$
Shamman's fudged formula	$P = \frac{1336}{L - 0.1(L - 23) - C - 0.05} - \frac{1}{\frac{1.0125}{K} - \frac{C + 0.05}{1336}}$
Binkhorst's adjusted formula	$P = \frac{1336\ (4R - L)}{(L - C)\ (4R - C)}$
Lin's S-formula (II) (see Table 5.3)	$Z'P = \frac{1336}{(L-S)} - \frac{1336 - qE - Pn}{\frac{1336}{Dc} - S}$
	$q = (1 + kP)/Z^2$
	$Z = 1 - S\ (Dc/1336),\ Z' = 1 - p'(Pn/1336)$

refraction by (1.2 to 2.5) D approximately. It is measured in millimeters (mm).

Corneal Power

It is measured either in diopters or in mm (radius of curvature).

Keratometer measures the radius of curvature of the central part of anterior corneal surface (r1) and given by K=337.5/r1. All the conventional formulas for corneal power (Kc) is given by (see Table 5.2)

$$Kc = 1.114\ K - C,$$

with C given by a mean value of 5.1, 5.5 or 6.5 diopter to count for the mean posterior surface power. The Lin's formula using the

Table 5.2: Corneal power (Dc) calculation after refractive surgery

Method	Formula
(1) Clinical-history Method	Dc = Kpre – RC, RC = refractive correction of LASIK
(2) Contact Lens Method	DC = B + P + Rw – Rno B = base curve; P = power of CL Rw = refractive error; Rno = bare refraction
(3) Shammas Method	Dc = 1.114 Kpost – 6.8
(4) Maloney Topography Method	Dc = 1.114 Ktopo – 5.5
(5) Koch Method	Dc = 1.114 Ktopo – 6.1
(6) Shammas Refraction Method	Dc = (1.114 Kpost – 6.8) – 0.23 (RC)
(7) Hoffer Mean-value Method	Dc = 337.5 (1/r1 + 1/r2)/2
(8) Lin Gaussian-optics (I)	Dc = 1.117 Kpost – 41/r2
(II)	Dc = (377/r1)[1 – 0.109 (r1/r2)]

where,
r1 = cornea front surface radius (postop)
r2 = cornea back surface radius (postop)
Kpost = postoperative keratometry
Kpre = preoperative keratometry

personalized p–C = 41/r1 to count for the role of individual posterior corneal surface (r2) which may deviate significantly from the commonly used mean value of 6.5 mm. As pointed out by Lin, each 1.0 diopter of corneal power would result in an error of about (1.3 to 1.6) diopter of IOL power calculation.

Postoperative Anterior Chamber Depth (ACD)

It is least important factor in calculation of lens power. An error of 1 mm affects the postoperative refraction or IOL power by approximate (0.6 to 2.5) diopter depending on the ocular conditions based on Lin's M-formula.

THE ESTIMATED IOL POSITION (ELP)

The main part of highly accurate IOL power calculation is able to correctly predict the estimated IOL position (d=ELP) for any given patient and IOL. Various formulas have been presented as follows:

SRK/T,
  d = A constant
Hoffer Q,
  d = pACD
Holladay I,
  d = Surgeon factor
Holladay II,
  d = ACD
Haigis,
  d = aO + (a1 × ACD) + (a2 × AL)

Table 5.3: Lin's formula for IOL-power in aphakia and phakia

(A) 2-optics aphakia/IOL	
Effective ACD:	S = d + gT
Thin-IOL:	d = ELP (for T = 0)
Thick-IOL:	g =1/(1 + Z"P1/P2)
	Z" = 1 – T(P2/1336)
(B) 3-optics phakia/IOL	S' = (d + gT) + Gp'
	p' = p + 2.4 mm
	G = 1/(1+Z'P/Pn)
	Z' = 1 – p'(Pn/1336)
(C) Piggyback-IOL	S' = (d + gT) + g'p'
(D) IOL-power (the most generalized format for 3-optics system)	
	Z'P = 1336 [1/X – 1/Y]-Pn - q'E
	X = L – S – 0.05 mm
	Y = 1336/Dc – S
	q' = (1 + kP)/Z^2
	Z = 1 – S' (Dc/1336)

where,

d = separation of cornea and IOL (or ELP, ACD).
p = separation of piggyback and primary IOL, or IOL and natural lens
T = thickness of piggyback-IOL
P = IOL power (thin lens), or P1/P2 for front/back power (thick-lens)
Pn = power of natural lens (or primary-IOL)
Dc = corneal power
E = refractive error to be corrected (on corneal plane)
(g, G) = geometry factor for (thick IOL, subsystem).

Lin,

S = d + gT + Gp (see also Table 5.3).

In actual practice, the two eyes with same axial length and keratometric reading may have different lens power. This may be due to:

- Effective (or optical) lens position (S) which may be different from the ELP (or d).
- Individual geometry of lens types.
- Presence of the natural lens or the primary IOL.

Hoffer Q formula is best for short eyes. Holladay for long eyes and SRK/T is best for very long eyes. Overall SRK/T is probably most accurate in majority of cases. It, however, ignores the role of IOL thickness and types and only good for 2-optics aphakic-IOL like others. The Lin's formula is good for all axial length and IOL types.

ACCURACY OF IOL POWER CALCULATION

In spite of recent advances in technology, there is no single method to accurately determine the net central power of these post refractive surgery eyes. The current method available is limited by lack of clinical experience on large scale and by the theoretic nature of all the calculation methods.

The factors, which significantly affect the accuracy of IOL Power calculations, are:

1. The error in preoperative biometry with regard to the difference between post and preoperative axial length measurement.
2. The position of the implantation of intraocular lens.
3. The style of intraocular lens.
4. The preoperative corneal astigmatism.
5. Surgically induced corneal astigmatism.
6. The postoperative astigmatism.
7. The true corneal power (post Lasik).
8. The formulas used to find IOL power.
9. Assumption of thin lens or 2-optics system.

Greater details of above will be presented in a Chapter of "Error analysis of IOL power calculations" by Lin.

THE NEW GENERATION FORMULAS

Formulas to be detailed in the following include: SRK (I, II), SRK/T, Hoffer Q, Holladay (I, II), Olson and the more recently formulas of Haigis d-formula and Lin's S-formula.

SRK Formula

SRK I Formula

It is basic regression formula. It is given by:

$P = A - 0.9K - 2.5\ L$

where,

P = IOL power for emmetropia

K = Keratometric power reading

A = A constant

L = Axial length in mm.

SRK II Formula

In this formula, the A constant is adjusted to different axial length ranges. It is given by:

$P = A1 - 0.9\ K - 2.5\ L$

A1 = adjusted constant

$A1 = A + 3$, if Axial length (L) < 20 mm

$A1 = A + 2$, if L 20 - 21 mm

$A1 = A + 1$, if L 21 – 22 mm

$A1 = A$, if $L = 22 - 24.5$ mm

$A1 = A - 0.5$, if $L > 24.5$ mm

SRK/T Formula

Regression formula for ACD (or ELP) is used to calculated IOL power based on Fyodorov formula. This formula is more accurate than SRK I and II.

ACD post = ACD – 3.336 + corneal height (H),

where, ACD is related to the manufacturer's A-constant by

ACD = 0.62467 A – 68.747.

Hoffer Q Formula

The Hoffer Q formula was published in 1993 [Hoffer, 1993] and gives the IOL power

P = f (A, K, Rx, pACD) which is a function of

A: axial length

K: average corneal refractive power (K-reading)

Rx: refraction

pACD: personalized ACD (ACD - constant)

Likewise, the Hoffer Q refractive error Rx

Rx = f (A, K, P, pACD), which depends on A, K, P and pACD.

For the calculations, the corneal radii, R1C and R2C in (mm) are converted into K in (D) according to:

K = 0.5 (K1 + K2) with K1 = 337.5/R1C and K2 = 337.5/R2C.

The personalized ACD (pACD) is set equal to the manufacturer's ACD - constant, if the calculation was selected to be based on the ACD-constant. In case the A – constant was chosen, pACD is derived from the A - constant (Hoffer, 1998) according to (Holladay et al, 1988)

pACD = ACD - constant = 0.58357 A constant - 63.896

Holladay's Formulas

The components of the three part Holladay system are:

Holladay (I) Formula

1. Data screening criteria to identify improbable axial length and keratometric measurement.
2. The modified theoretical formula, which predicts the effective position of the IOL based on the axial length and the average corneal curvature.
3. Personalized Surgeon Factor (PSF) that adjusts for any consistent bias on surgeon from any source. It is advance method, which requires patient refractions.

The initial formula uses the "Basic Surgeon Factor". It can be calculated from the A-constant provided by lens manufacturer.

Holladay (II) Formula

The IOL power is calculated based on the Colenbrander or Hoffer formula for ametropic case and it is independent to the axial length (L).

P = Ppre – Pdesire,

where, the preoperative and desired refractive power is given by (for j=1, 2, respectively):

Pj = 1336 / [1336/Kj – ELP],

where, Kj is the corneal power calculated from the measured K-reading, Kj=1.114 K-C, C being a mean power of the corneal posterior surface.

Olson Formula

Olson proposed his 2003 regression formula for the predicted postoperative ACD as follows:

ACDpost = ACDmean + 0.12H + 0.33ACDpre
+0.3T^1 + 0.1L – 5.18

where, H is the corneal height, T′ is the natural lens thickness. Above formula, however, can only apply to phakic eyes. For aphakic or pseudophakic eyes, the coefficients will change.

Haigis Formula

It uses three constants to set both the position and shape of a power prediction curve. The IOL calculation according to Haigis is based on the elementary IOL formula for thin lenses.

d = a0 + [a1 × ACD] + (a2 × AL)

where,

d = the effective (or optical) lens position
ACD = measured anterior chamber depth of the eye
AL = axial length of the eye.
a0 constant = same as lens constants for the different formulas given before
a1 Constant = tied to anterior chamber depth
a2 Constant = measured axial length

Thus, the value for d is determined by a function rather than a single number.

The a0, a1 and a2 constants area derived by multi-variable regression analysis. The Haigis formula IOL constants will appear different than normal as they interact with the ACD and the AL.

The conventional optimization based on one constant (A-constant, surgeon's factor, ACD) which could only "parallel shift" the calculated curve to fit the measured data for a predicted mean zero error. Therefore, the validation range of the axial length is limited, where improvement for long eye results more errors for short eye, and vice versa. For example, SRK/T is accurate for long eye ($L > 26$ mm), but not for very short eye ($L < 22$ mm) which requires the Hoffer formula. Haigis 3-constant optimization allows the curve-fit by both parallel shift and rotation of the curve such that it covers wider range of axial length. However, the above Haigis formula also assumed thin-IOL and excludes the role of IOL configurations for different IOL types.

Lin's S Formula

Based on a generalized effective ACD ("S") derived from Gaussian optics in thick lens for 2-optics and 3-optics system valid for all range of axial length and IOL types. It also includes the effects due to natural lens and primary IOL which are totally neglected in all the other formulas presented in above A to E.

An effective (or optical) ACD is introduced as S given by, for the case of thick IOL in aphakic eye,

$$S = ELP + gT, \quad (1.a)$$
$$g = 1/[1+Z''(P1/P2)] \quad (1.b)$$
$$Z'' = 1-T(P2/1336) \quad (1.c)$$

where, T is the IOL thickness, and the geometry factor (g) is determined by the ratio of the IOL front and back surface power P1/P2. Note that g could be positive (for $P1/P2 > 0$) or negative ($P1/P2 < 0$). Therefore, S could be myopic or hyperopic shifted. Figure 5.1 shows the definition of S in a 2-optics system, where both optics can be either thin or thick lenses. Other formulas for S are summarized in Table 5.3 for both phakic and piggyback IOL. Greater details of the geometry factors g and G will be presented in a separate Chapter of Lin in this book.

IOL POWER IN APHAKIC EYE

This is a simple 2-optics system consisting of the cornea and IOL (with natural lens removed). The IOL power calculation based on S and the true corneal power (Dc) is also developed by Lin as follows:

$$P = 1336/X - 1336 / Y - qE, \quad (2.a)$$
$$X = L - S + 0.05 \quad (2.b)$$
$$Y = 1336/Dc - S \quad (2.c)$$

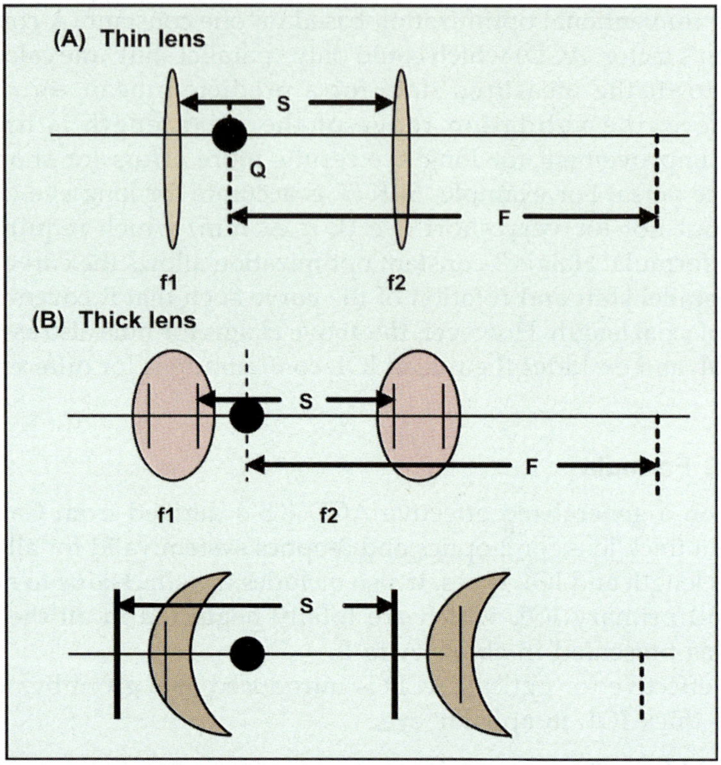

Fig. 5.1: Definition of effective (optical) separation (S) between 2 thin lenses (A) and 2 thick lenses (B). Also shown is the second principal plane position (Q) and the system effective focal length (F)

where, $q=(1+kP)/Z^2$ is a nonlinear term, with k about 0.003 and $Z=1-S(Dc/1336)$. E is the remaining refractive error after IOL implant. The above Lin's new formula contributes two improvements: the S function, defined by Eq.(1) and in Table 5.3 to include the IOL configuration and the true corneal power calculated by:

$$Dc = 1.117K - 41/r2, \qquad (3)$$

in which the true corneal power after refractive surgery is personalized by its measured front and back surface radius (r1 and r2). The K-reading is further defined as K=337.5/r1. Because that both S and Dc are personalized, accurate IOL power may be calculated for individual cases without the use of "fudge factors" to fit for mean zero error. Figure 5.2 shows the change of corneal power for various r2 values.

The individual effective ACD (the "S") may be calculated from Eq.(1) for a given function of f(P, L, Dc, E) by solving a quadratic equation of S, similar to the d-function of Haigis. The 3-constant

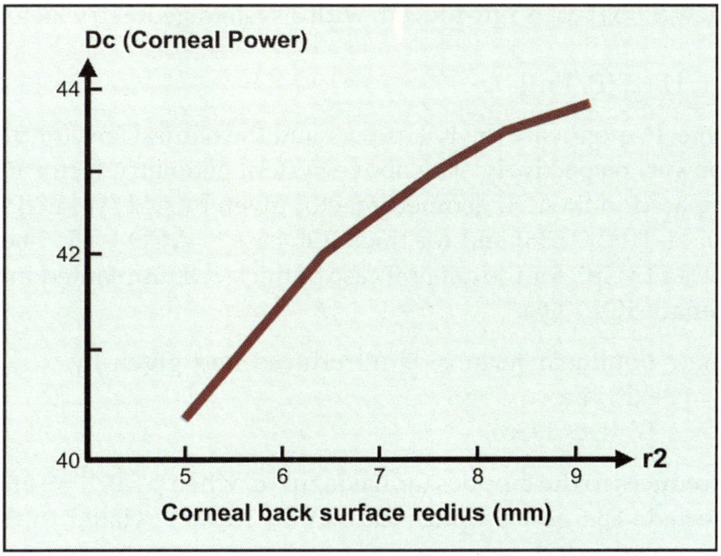

Fig. 5.2: Corneal power change at various back surface

optimization like Haigis, but using S rather than d, allows us to obtain the minimal mean error not only for all range of axial length (L), but also for all IOL types via the g-factor in Eq.(1).

IOL POWER IN PHAKIC AND PIGGYBACK IOL

For phakic IOL or piggyback IOL, the IOL power calculations involve with a 3-optics system which has been recently formulated by Lin by generalizing the Eq.(2) of 2-optics (aphakic-IOL) as follow:

$$Z'P = 1336/X - 1336/Y - q'E - Pn \quad (4)$$

which has the following revisions to count for the effects from the presence of the natural lens or the primary IOL (having a power Pn) and the separation between the cornea and IOL (ACD or ELP); and IOL and natural lens or primary IOL (p).

a. A reduction factor Z′ = 1-p′ (Pn/1336), with p′=p+2.4 mm, is introduced and has a value of Z′=0.95, for p′=6.0 mm for a typical phakic IOL implanted in front of a natural lens power of 21 D and separated by p=1.0 mm or p′=1.0+2.4=3.4 mm. In comparison, Z′ is about 0.99 for the case of piggyback IOL (with p′=p=1.0 mm). Therefore, a reduction of about 5% and 1% is expected in the IOL power term (Z′P).

b. A new S′=S+Gp′ is introduced, with a system geometry factor given by:

$$G=1/[1+Z'(P/Pn)] \quad (5)$$

where, P and Pn are the IOL power and the natural lens (or primary-IOL) power, respectively. The above system geometry factor (G) may be compared to the IOL geometry factor given by g=1/[1+Z″(P1/P2)], with Z″=1-T(P2/1336) and for thick IOL case S=ACD + gT. Therefore, S′=ACD+gT+Gp′, for the general case of thick-IOL implanted in phakic (or primary-IOL) eye.

c. A new nonlinear term q′ is introduced and given by

$$q' = (1+kP)/Za^2, \quad (6.a)$$

$$Za = 1-S' (Dc/1336), \quad (6.b)$$

which reduces to the 2-optics (aphakia) q′=q, when p′=0, S′=S and Z′=Z as expected. The new 3-optics Za may be further related to the Z in 2-optics aphakic IOL by:

$$Za = Z - Gp' (Dc/1336), \quad (7)$$

where, the second term is due to the shifted distance of the second principal plane of the IOL-natural lens or piggyback-IOL and primary IOL subsystem.

d. Conversion function (CF), one may define Zeff derived from $Zeff^2 = Z'Za$ to obtain

$$Zeff = 1 - Seff (Dc/1336), \quad (8.a)$$

$$Seff = S + 0.5p' (Pn/Dc), \quad (8.b)$$

where, Seff is defined as the shifted S by an amount proportional to p′ and the power ratio (Pn/Dc) of the natural lens or primary-IOL(Pn) and the cornea (Dc). For typical values of p′=3.0 mm, Pn=20 D, Dc=43 D, one obtains Seff = S + 0.7 mm. This 0.7 mm shift may result in IOL power difference about $(0.7/S)^2$ or about 3% to 5%, for S=3 to 4 mm.

Above Eq.(8) allows us to calculate a conversion function (CF), defined by:

CF = –(dE/dP) which may be derived from the deviative of Eq.(4) and using Eq. (8) as follows:

$$CF = 1-2k'E)Zeff^2, \quad (9)$$

Therefore, the CF in 3-optics is lower due to the natural lens (or primary IOL) about 5% to 10% less than 2-optics formula. In other words, the conventional 2-optics formulas overestimate the IOL power when it is implanted in phakia or pseudophakia.

PIGGYBACK IOL POWER

Given the CF, the piggyback IOL power to correct a residual ametropia power (E), on the corneal plane (not spectacle plane), may be calculated by:

$$P = E/CF, \qquad (10)$$

where, CF is given by Eq.(9) in general. Comparison of various formulas is shown in Table 5.4. Several critical issues on the previous formulas may be addressed as follows:

a. All the formulas, except Lin's, are based on the spectacle power (E) converted to IOL power (P). The Es of Lin is defined as E on the corneal plane.
b. Formulas of Sanders-Kraff and Feiz-Mannis are comparable. However, both are based on a mean value of CF=0.7 which may be valid only for average clinical data. Individual CF value could be 10% to 20% deviate from this mean value and would require Lin's formula.
c. Gills formula is only good for hyperopia and it is also based on average case.
d. Shammas formula might be good for low IOL power, say 5.0 D or less. It includes the dependence of ACD (or the a-constant).

Table 5.4: Piggyback IOL power (P) formulas for residual ametropia error

Formula	P
(1) Sanders and Kraff (1980) based on empirical data of over 2500 IOL lens	P = E/0.67=1.49 E
(2) Feiz and Mannis (2001)	P = E/0.7 = 1.43E
(3) Holladay II (1993) based on Hoffer (1981), Colenbrander (1973)	P = (IOL)1– (IOL)2 (IOL)j = 1336/[1336/Kj-ELP] Kj (j=1,2), for pre- and postop corneal power
for plus IOL,	P(+) =1.5E,
for minus IOL,	P(–) = 1.0E;
E is the postop refractive error at spectacle plane.	
(4) Shammas (2001) where, a = 0.03 for plus IOL, a = 0.04 for minus IOL. A = A-constant = (ACD+63.896)/0.5836	P = (E/a)/(138.3-A)-0.5
(5) Gills (1996) only for hyperopic correction	P(+) =1.4E+1.0
(6) Lin (2005) The Z^2-formula * for both plus and minus IOL.	P = Ec/(CF) = (1.25 to 1.7) Ec CF = (1–2kE)(Ec/Z^2) Z =1–S(Dc/1336) Typical value: CF = (0.6 to -0.8)

where,
Dc is the corneal power and k is a nonlinear term.
S is the effective (optical) lens position, S=ELP+gT+ Gp'
E(Ec) is the refractive error on the spectacle (corneal) plane and may be related by another conversion factor Ec=E/Zs^2, with Zs=1–0.012E.
* For simplified 2-optics system, see Eq.(9) in the text and Table 5.3 for 3-optics system

However, it does not include the effects due to corneal power or individual IOL types. It also assumes thin IOL and a 2-optics system or aphakic IOL.

e. Holladay II is based on Colenbrauder including the effect of ELP and corneal Power. It needs numerical method versus the analytic formula of Lin which also revises ELP by S.
Both Holladay II and Lin's formula for P are independent to the axial length (L) and only depend on the ACD (or ELP) or S.

f. Lin's new formula based on Gaussian optics might be the only one which includes most of the effects due to individual ocular parameter and IOL types, where the effective ACD (S, or Seff) has been rigorously defined for various systems of aphakic, aphakic or pseudophakic and for both thin and thick IOL. The roles of natural lens or primary IOL are also included in the new formula.

ACCOMMODATING IOL (AIOL)

The accommodating rate function (M) defined as the accommodation amplitude increase per 1.0 mm forward movement of a plus AIOL may be expressed by the Lin's M-formula

$$M = (Z/1336)P[2Dc+ZZ'P], \quad (11)$$

Above formula is a general form for both phakia and aphakia and also for dual-optics AIOL. As shown in Figures 5.3 to 5.8, for the thick IOL single-optics case, the M value is higher for convex-concave IOL configuration (having front and back surface power of P1 and P2) which has higher P1 for a given P1+P2, when P2 < 0 (concave). Depending on ocular conditions, M ranges from 0.5 to 2.5 (D/mm) for AIOL-power of 10 to 20 diopters. Greater details of single-optics and dual-optics AIOL may be found in other Chapters of Lin in this book.

CONCLUSION

The existing IOL power (except Lin's) based on 2-optics system could only apply to aphakia. For phakia or piggyback IOL, a 3-optics system based on Gaussian optics is required. The Lin's new formulas provide more accurate calculations for both phakia and aphakia presented by:

- The S-formula (to include IOL thickness and types)
- The Seff-formula (to include the role of natural lens and primary-IOL)
- The personalized r2-formula (including corneal posterior surface power post-LASIK)
- The M-formula (for accommodating IOL efficiency)

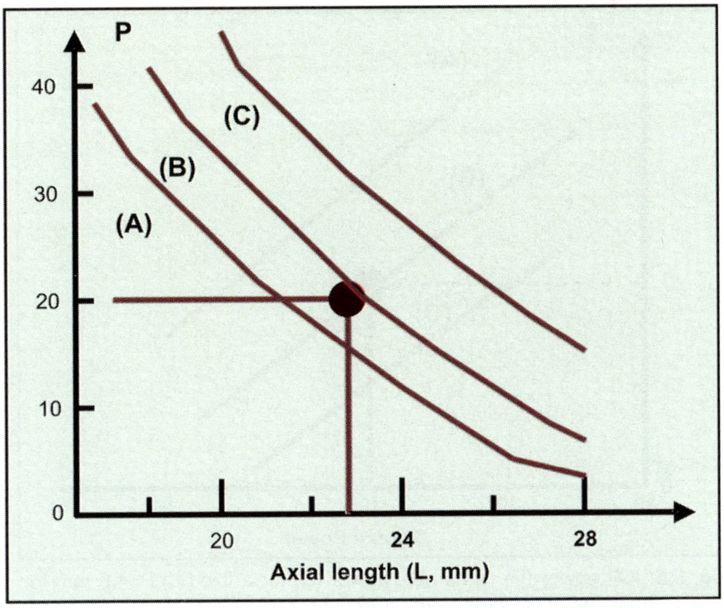

Fig. 5.3: IOL power (P) vs axial length (L) for a fixed corneal power Dc=43 diopter at various IOL position ELP=3.5, 4.5 and 5.5 mm shown by curve (A), (B) and (C), respectively

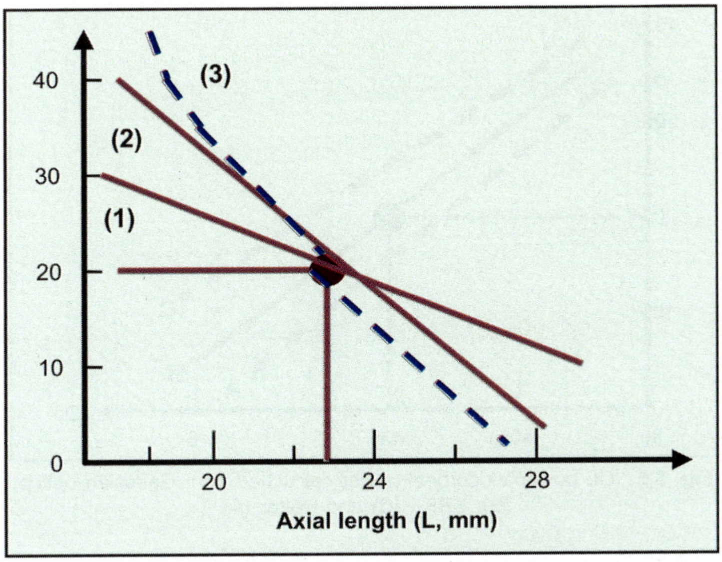

Fig. 5.4: Schematics of P vs L for SRK formula (curve 1), Gaussian optics (curve 2) and Colenbrander (curve 3)

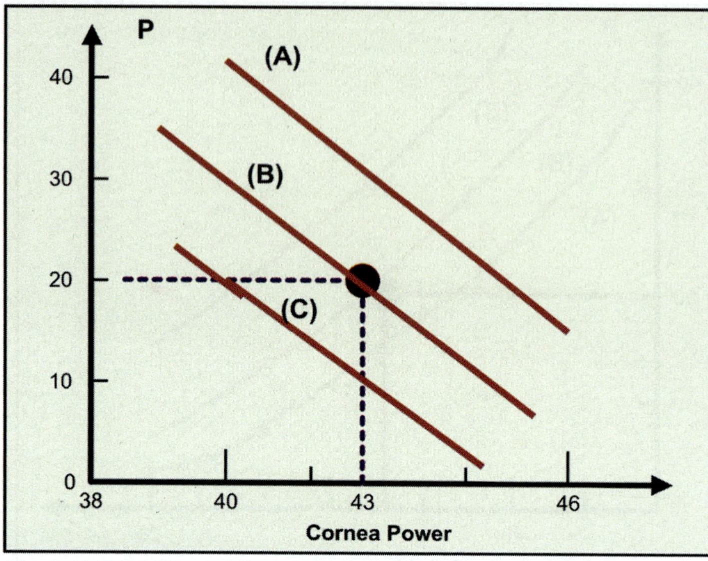

Fig. 5.5: IOL power (P) vs corneal power (D) for a fixed ELP=4.5 mm for long, normal and short eyes, with L=26, 23.5 and 21 mm shown by curves A, B, C, respectively

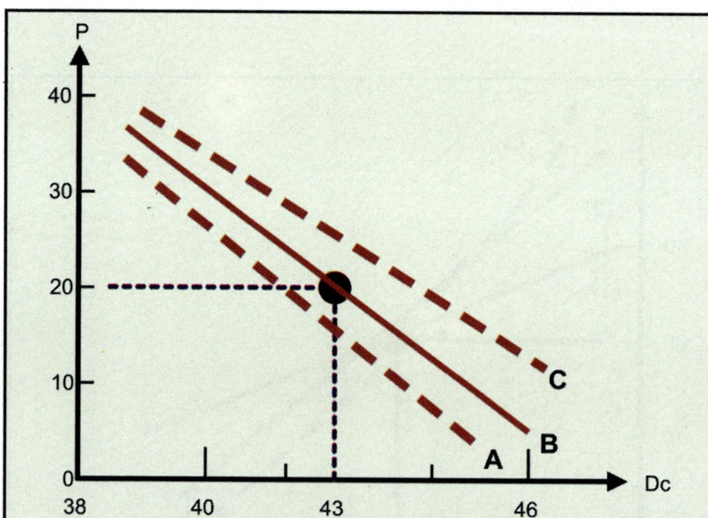

Fig. 5.6: IOL power vs corneal power calculated from Gaussian optics (B), SRK-I (C) and Hoffer (A)

- The Z^2-formula (for conversion of IOL power in 3-optics system of phakia or piggyback IOL).
  Greater details of above formulas may be found in other Chapters of Lin in this book.

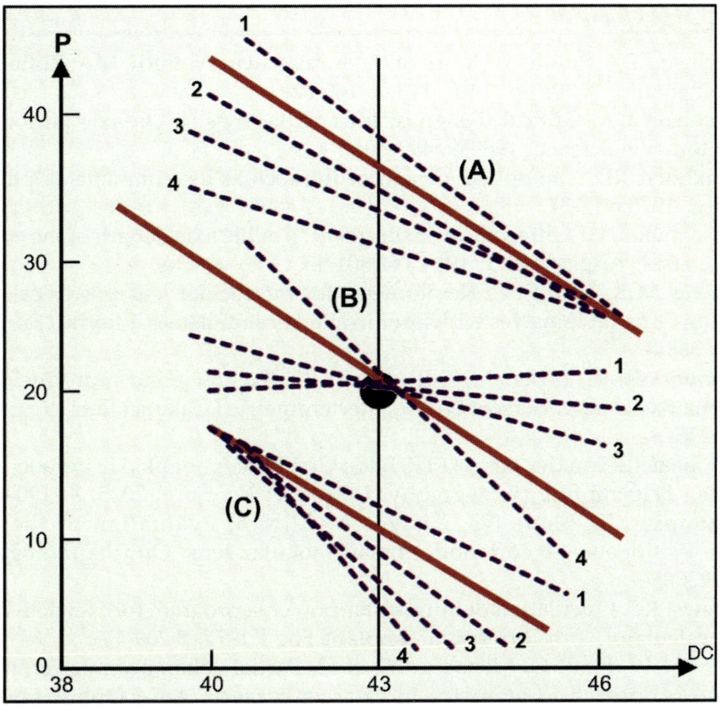

Fig. 5.7: Schematic comparison of various K-based formulas (dashed lines 1 to 4) and Gaussian-optics formulas (solid lines) at various corneal power for long (A) and short (C) eyes

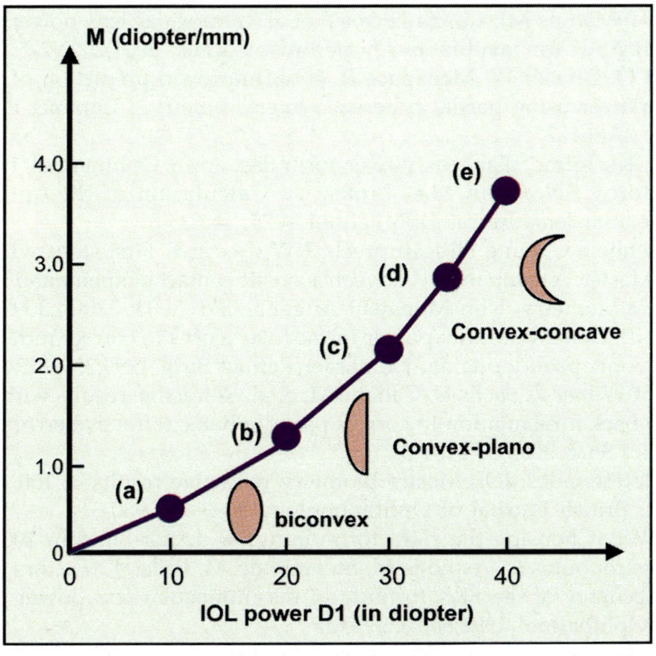

Fig. 5.8: Accommodation rate (M) vs. IOL-power in single-optics IOL at various configurations

BIBLIOGRAPHY

1. Atchison DA, Smith G. Optics of the human eye. Woburn, MA: Butterworth-Heinemann; 2000; pp. 14-6, 143-7, 160-62.
2. Atchison DA. Optical design of intraocular lens. I. On-axis performance. Optom Vis Science. 1989;66:492-506.
3. Binkhorst RD. The optical design of intraocular lens implants. Ophthalmic Surg. 1975;6:17-31.
4. Buschmann, W: Ultrasonic measurement\s of the axial length of the eye, Klin. Monatsbl. Augenheilkd. 1964;144:801-15.
5. Cheng ACK, Lam DSC. Keratometry for intraocular lens power calculation using Orbscan II in eyes with laser in situ keratomileusis. J Refract Surg. 2005; 21: 365-8.
6. Connors R, III, Boseman P, III, Olson RJ. Accuracy and reproducibility of biometry using partial coherence interferometry. J Cataract Refract Surg 2002; 28:235–8.
7. Coppens JE, van der Berg, JTTP, Bado CJ. Biometry of phakic intraocular lens using Scheimpflug photography. J Cataract Ref Surg. 2005; 31:1904-14.
8. Cumming JS, Slade SG, Chayet A. Clinical evaluation of the model AT-45 silicone. Accommodating intraocular lens. Ophthalmology 2001; 108:2005-9.
9. Drews, RC. Calculation of intraocular power, a program for Hewlett-Packard 97 calculator, Am Intraocular Implant Soc J 1977; 3:209-12.
10. Drexler W, Findl O, Menapace R, et al. Partial coherence interferometry: a novel approach to biometry in cataract surgery. Am J Ophthalmol 1998; 126:524–34.
11. Eleftheriadis H.: IOL Master biometry: Refractive results of 100 consecutive cases. Br J Ophthalmol. 2003;87(8):960-3.
12. Feiz V, Mannis MJ, Garcia-Ferrer F et al. Intraocular lens power calculation after LASIK for myopia and hyperopia. Cornea, 2001;20:792-7.
13. Findl O, Drexler W, Menapace R, et al. Improved prediction of intraocular lens power using partial coherence interferometry. J Cataract Refract Surg 2001; 27:861–7.
14. Fritz, KJ. Intraocular lens power formulas. Am J Ophthalmol 1981: 91:414.
15. Fyodorov SN, Galin MA, Linksz A. Calculation of the optical power intraocular lens. Invest Ophthalmol 1975; 14:625-8.
16. Gantenbein C, Lang HM, Ruprecht KW, Georg T. First steps with the Zeiss IOL Master: A comparison between acoustic contact biometry and non-contact optical biometry, Klin Monatsbl Augenheilkd. 2003; 220(5):309-14.
17. Gills JP, Denzl R. Minus-power intraocular lenses to correct refractive errors in myopic pseudophakia. J Cataract Refract Surg 1999;25:1205-8.
18. Habot-Wilner Z, Sachs D, Cahane M, et al. Refractive results with secondary piggyback implantation to correct pseudophakic refractive errors. J Cataract Refract Surg 2005;31:2101-3.
19. H. Eleftheriades. IOL Master Biometry refractive results of 100 consecutive cases. British Journal of Ophthalmology 2003; 87: 960-3.
20. Hill WE. Choosing the right formula. www.doctor-hill.com 2003.
21. Kalogeropoulos C, Aspiotis M, Stefaniotou M, Psilas K. Factors influencing the accuracy of the SRK formula in the intraocular less power calculation. Doc Ophthalmol 1994;85(3):223-42.
22. Kim JN, Lee DN, Joo CK. Measuring corneal power for intraocular lens power calculations after refractive surgery. J Cataract Refract Surg. 2002; 28 (II):1932-8.

23. Ho A, Manns F, Pham T et al. Predicting the performance of accommodating intraocular lens using ray tracing. J Cataract Refract Surg. 2006;32:129-36.
24. Hoffer KJ. Accuracy Ultrasound intraocular lens calculation. Arch Ophthalmol 1981;99:1819-23.
25. Holladay JT. Optics and intraocular lens power calculation for phakic intraocular lenses. In: Horden DR. Lindstrom RL. Davis EA, ed. Phakic intraocular lens: principles and practice. Thorofare NJ:SLACK; 2004.pp. 59-61.
26. Holladay JT. Refractive power calculation for intraocular lenses in the phakic eye. Am J Ophthalmol 1993;116:63-6.
27. Kraff, MC, Sanders, DR, Lieberman, HL. Determination of intraocular lens power: a comparison with and without ultrasound. Ophthalmic Surg 1978;9:81-4.
28. Kielhorn I, Rajan MS, Tesha PM, Subryan VR, Bell JA. Clinical assessment of the Zeiss IOL Master 1: J Cataract Refract Surg 2003 Mar; 29(3):518-22.
29. Liang YS, Chen TT, Chi TC, Chan YC: Analysis of intraocular lens power calculation. J Am Intraocular Implant Soc 1985; 11(3):268-71.
30. Lin, JT. Unified refractive-state analysis for customized vision correction. J. Refract Surg 2004; 20: 398-400.
31. Lin, JT. New formulas comparing accommodation in human lens and intraocular lens. J. Refract Surg 2005; 21:200-1.
32. Lin, JT. A generalized refractive state theory and effective eye model. Chin J Optom & Ophthal 2005;7:1-6.
33. Lin JT. Correcting the cornea-power measurement for intraocular lens power calculation after myopic laser in situ keratomileusis. Am J Ophthalmol. 2004; 137:786-787.
34. Lin JT. Unified formulas for phakic-aphakic IOL and spectacle-cornea power conversion. J Refract Surg 2006;22:(in press).
35. Lin, JT. The role of corneal power and anterior chamber depth on the accommodation in aphakic IOL.J. Refract Surg. 2005;21:765-6.
36. Lin, JT. Error analysis of intraocular lens power in eye after LASIK. J Refract Surg 2006; 22:127-8.
37. Lin, JT. Analytic formulas for error factors in intraocular lens power calculation. J Cataract Refract Surg 2006;32: (in press).
38. Mcleod SD, Portney V, Ting A. A dual optic accommodating fordable intraocular lens. Br J. Ophthalmol 2003;87:1083-5.
39. Missotten T, Verkamme T, Blanckaert J, et al. Optical forumula to predict outcomes after implantation of accommodating intraocular lens. J Cataract Refract Surg 2004;30:2084-7.
40. Nawa Y, Ueda T, Nakatsuka M et al. Accommodation obtained per 1.0 mm forward movement of a posterior chamber intraocular lens. J Cataract Refract Surg 2003;29:2069-72.
41. Odenthal MTP, Eggink CA, Melles G. et al. Clinical and theoretical results of intraocular lens power calculation for cataract surgery after photorefractive keratectomy for myopia. Arch Ophthalmol 2002; 120:431-8.
42. Olsen T. Corydon L. Gimbel H. Intraocular lens power calculation with an improved anterior chamber depth prediction algorithm. J. Cataract Refrqact Surg 1995;21:313-9.
43. Olsen T. Theoretical approach to intraocular lens calculation using Gaussian optics. J Cataract Refract Surg 1987; 13:141–5.
44. Olsen T. Sources of error in intraocular lens power calculation. J Cataract Refract Surg 1992; 18:125–9.

45. Olsen T, Thim K, Corydon L. Accuracy of the newer generation intraocular lens power calculation formulas in long and short eyes. J. Cataract Refract Surg 1991; 17(2):187-93.
46. Ouda B, Tawafik B, Derbala A, Youseif AB. Error correction of intraocular lens (IOL) power calculation. Biomed Instrum Technol 1999;33(5):438-45.
47. Pedrotti LS, Pedrotti FL. (1998) Optics and Vision. Liper Saddle River, NJ, Prentice Hall; pp. 74-87, 122-41.
48. Pedrotti LS, Pedrotti FL. Optics and Vision. Liper Saddle River, NJ, Prentice Hall; 1998: pp. 74-87, 92-5.
49. Pierscionek BK. Presbyopia-effect of refractive index. Chin Exp Optom. 1990;73:23-30.
48. Preussner PR, Wahl J, Weitzel D. Topography-based intraocular lens power selection. J. Cataract Refract Surg 2005; 31:525-33.
50. Rana A, Miller D, Magnante P. Understanding the accommodating IOL. J. Cataract Refract Surg 2003; 29:2284-7.
51. Rajan MS, Keilhorn I, Bell JA. Partial coherence laser interferometry vs conventional ultrasound biometry in intraocular lens power calculations. *Eye* 2002; 16:552–6.
52. Rosa N, Capasso L, Lanza M, et al. Reliability of a new correcting factor in calculating intraocular lens power after refractive corneal surgery. J Cataract Refract Surg 2005; 31:1020-4.
53. Rose LT, Moshegov CN. Comparison of the Zeiss IOL Master and applanation A-scan ultrasound: Biometry for intraocular lens calculation. Clin Experiment Ophthalmol 2003;31(2):121-4.
54. Raj PS, Ilango B, Watson A. Measurement of axial length in the calculation of intraocular lens power. Eye 1998:12(Pt2):227-9.
55. Shammas HJ. A comparison of immersion and contact techniques for axial length measurement. J Am Intra-Ocular Implant Soc 1984; 10:444–7.
56. Sanders DR, Kraff MC: Improvement of intraocular lens power calculation using empirical data, Am. Intraocular Implant Soc J 1980; 6:263-7.
57. Sanders DR, Retzlaff J, Kraff MC. Comparison of empirically derived and theoretical aphakic refraction formulas. Arch Opththal. 1983;10:965-7.
58. Sanders DR, Retzlaff J, Kraff MC. Comparison of the SRKII formulas and the other second generation formulas. J Cataract Refract Surg 1988;14:136-41.
59. Shammas HJ. Intraocular lens power calculations. Thorofare NJ: SLACK; 2004. pp. 59-61; 64-5.
60. Stachs O, Schneider H, Steve J, Guthoff R. Potentially accommodating intraocular lenses-an in vitro and in vivo study using three-dimensional high-frequency ultrasound. J Refract Surg 2005;21:37-45.
61. Suto C, Hori S, Fukuyama E, Akura J: Adjusting intraocular lens power for sulcus fixation. J. Cataract Refract Surg 2003;29(10):1913-7.
62. Telando A. Pseudo-accommodative cornea: a new concept for correction of presbyopia. J Refract Surg 2004;20(Suppl.):S714-17.
63. Twa MD, Lemback RG, Bullimore MA, Roberts C, "A prospective randomized clinical trial of laser in situ keratomileusis with two different lasers", Am J Ophthalmol 2005;140:173-83.
64. van der Heijde GL. The optical correction of unilateral aphakia. Trans Amer Academy Ophthalmol Otolarynogol 1976;81:80-8.
65. Verhulst E, Vrijghem JC. Accuracy of intraocular lens power calculations using the Zeiss IOL Master. A prospective study, Bull Soc Belge Ophthalmol 2001 (281):61-5.

66. Verhulst E, Vrijghem JC. Accuracy of intraocular lens power calculations using the Zeiss IOL Master. A prospective Study.
67. Vongthorgsri A, Phusitphoykai N, Tungsiriput T. Laser in situ keratomileusis for high myopia using a small ablation-zone and large aspheric transition zone. J. Refract Surg 2004;20(Suppl): S669-73.
68. Wainstock, M.A. Ultrasonography: Its role in the success of intraocular implant surgery, Int. Ophthalmol Clin 1979;19:43-50.
69. Wallman J. How is emmetropization controlled? Results of research on experimental myopia. In: Tokoro T. ed. Myopia updates: Proc. 6-th Inter. Conf. on Myopia, Tokyo: Spring-Verlag; 1998. p. 13-30.
70. Wang XJ, Jin CP, Wang QM. Aberration with IOLs based on different optical design. Chinese J Optom & Ophthal (in Chinese). 2003;5:209-11.
71. Wildsoet CF. Structural correlates of myopia. In: Resenfield M, Gilmartin B. eds. Myopia and Nearwork. Woburn, MA: Butterworth-Heinemann; 1998. p. 31-56.

CHAPTER

6

JT Lin (USA)

Optics Gaussian Formulas for Phakic and Piggyback IOLs

INTRODUCTION

Both classical and modern formulas have been used for the power calculation of regular IOL or accommodative IOL in aphakic, pseudophakic and phakic eyes. The modern formulas include that of Holladay, SRK/T, SRKI & II, Hoffer Q, Olson, Haigis and the more recent formulas by Odenthal et al (the historical method), Aramberri et al (the double-K method), Rosa et al (the R-factor method) and Jin et al (the Adjusted-K method). Most of these efforts were to improve the prediction of IOL-power by a better prediction of the postoperative anterior chamber depth (ACDpost) or the estimated lens position (ELP) defined by ACDpre, corneal height and curvature, lens thickness and axial length. All the existing IOL-power calculations (except the Lin's Gaussian optics formulas) are based on the classical vergence formulas (CVF) of Fyodorov (1975), and van der Heijde (1976) or their revision, the Hoffer Q formula (1981).

The CVFs assume a thin-lens (for both corneal and IOL) and are all based on a 2-optics system (the cornea and the IOL) which, strictly speaking, can only apply to aphakic eyes. For pseudophakic or phakic eyes, the 3-optics systems are much more complex and have been recently studied by Lin (2006).

The previous calculations are also based on one primary parameter of expected lens position (ELP), although some secondary variables such as axial length, anterior chamber depth (ACD), lens thickness, corneal curvature and age have been used to improve the calculations.

One of the major pitfalls of the most existing IOL power calculations[1,2] is the ignoring of individual true corneal power and using a mean-zero prediction error for the postoperative refraction. Except the Haigis formula and the Lin Z^2-formula, all other optimization formulas are based on one-constant like the surgeon factor, the A-constant, the ACDpost or the ELP. The mean-zero error might be the result of the balanced errors of short and long eyes. Therefore, the validity range of axial length for various existing formulas under a linear empirical-fit could not justify their accuracy when they are applied to individual eye. A true personalized IOL power prediction, in my opinion, should at least individualize the following parameters: the postoperative ELP, axial length, corneal anterior and posterior surface, and the IOL types (or configuration).

The existing formulas of Holladay [2] show the 1-for-1 for minus spectacle converted to IOL-power and the 1.5-for-1 for plus spectacle. The new formulas of this Chapter will demonstrate that Holladay's formulas are valid only for certain spectacle powers and can not apply to all IOL power ranges.

In this Chapter, the following areas would be covered:

- Gaussian optics for IOL-power in aphakic eye (a simple 2-optics system)
- Extension of above to piggyback IOL (a 3-optics thin lens system)
- Extension to phakic eyes (a 3-optics thick lens system)
- Conversion function (CF) which translates the required IOL-power to the refractive error in both aphakia and phakia
- Comparison of 2-optics and 3-optics
- Comments on the conventional Holladay formulas.

TWO OPTICS FORMULAS (APHAKIC EYE)

The IOL power may be calculated from the classical Vergence formulas[1] developed by Fyodorov (1975), Colenbrander (1973), van der Heijde (1976) or Binkhorst (1975) given by a general format of

$$P = 1336/(L-C) - 1336/(y-C), \quad (1.a)$$
$$y = 1336/(Kc+De), \quad (1.b)$$

where Kc is the corneal power measured by keratometer defined by K=337.5/R, with R being the front surface radius of the cornea. De is the remaining refractive error, and C=ELP. The above formula for ametropic case was also used by Hoffer (1981) and more recently by Haigis (2003), where the original formula of Colenbrander or van der Heijde (for the emmetropic case with De=0) was revised as y in (1.b) for the ametropia. Unlike the new formula of Lin (to be shown below) which is rigorously derived from Gaussian optics, the above classical formula was "phenomenally" formatted by replacing Kc by y to count for the effect of remaining refractive error (De). This procedure is accurate under the assumption that the refractive error (E) may be added to the corneal power with a 100% conversion.

By Gaussian optics theory, the residual refractive error (De) after an IOL is implanted in an aphakic eye may be described by Lin's image equation [3] (Fig. 6.1).

$$De = 1336[1/(L-L2) - 1/F]. \quad (2.a)$$

As shown by Figure 1, Eq. (2.a) may be re-expressed as

$$De = 1336/(X+P2') - 1336/F, \quad (2.b)$$

where L is the axial length, L2 is the position of the second principal plane. P2'=SF/fc, F is the effective focal length (EFL) of the cornea-IOL system related to the EFL of the cornea (fc) and IOL (f1) by

$$1/F = 1/fc + Z/f1, \quad (3)$$
$$Z=1-S/fc,$$

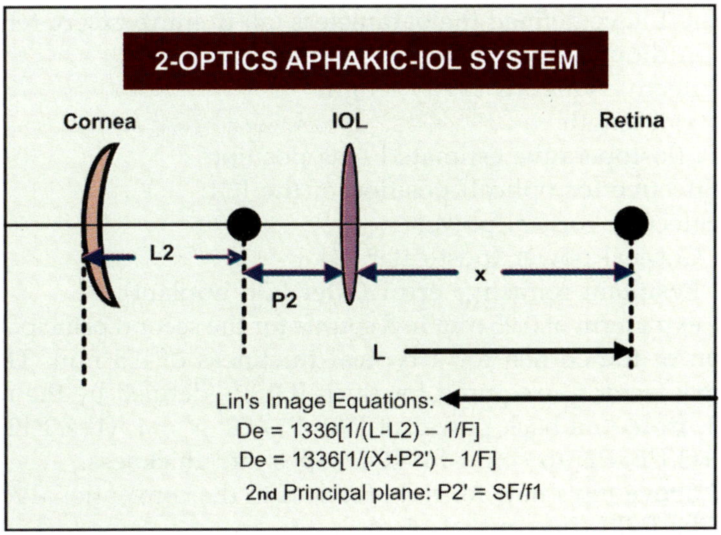

Fig. 6.1: Schematics of 2-optics (cornea and thin-IOL) aphakic system

where fc and f1 are the EFL of the cornea and IOL: S being the effective (or optical) anterior chamber depth of the IOL which equals to the postoperative estimated lens position (ELP) when a thin IOL lens is assumed. For thick IOL, it needs a revision to S=ELP + g′T, shifted by a geometry factor (g′) and IOL thickness (T). Using the relation of L2=S(1-F/fc) (for thin lens) and substituting Eq.(3) to (2.b) to decouple the F dependence of P2', one obtains the Lin's formula (2006)

$$qDe = 1336/X - Dc/Z - P, \quad (4)$$
$$q = 1/Z^2,$$

where the effective vitreous length defined by X=L-S+0.05 mm. Dc and P are the power of the cornea and IOL, respectively. It should be noted that Eq.(4) may be also derived from the second order expansion of Eq.(1.b). Note that Eq.(1) and (4) are also identical for emmetropic state (De=0), except C becomes S in Lin's formula.

THE IOL POWER IN APHAKIA

The IOL power (P) required to correct refractive error of an aphakic eye (2-optic system) after cataract surgery is given by re-arranging Eq.(4) to solve for P

$$P = 1336(1/X - 1/Y) - qDe, \quad (5.a)$$
$$X = L - S + 0.05, \quad (5.b)$$
$$Y = 1336/Dc - S, \quad (5.c)$$
$$S = ELP + g'T + 0.05 \quad (5.d)$$

where I have defined the parameters (all in mm), except refractive power in diopter in an effective eye model (EEM)[4-6]

X: Effective vitreous cavity length

L: Axial length

ELP: Postoperative estimated lens position

S: Effective (or optical) position of the IOL

Y: Effective corneal power

Dc: Corneal power (post-cataract)

De: Resultant refractive error (after IOL implant).

The extra term of 0.05 mm in S counts for the second principal plane position of the cornea for a typical thickness of 0.5 mm. The IOL geometry factor g′ (required for thick IOL) is defined by the ratio of the IOL front and back power of P12=P1/P2, g′ = 1/(1+Z′P12), with Z′= 1-T(1336/P2) to count for IOL types and thickness.

The above Lin's new formula reduces to the conventional formula under the following special cases.

a. Reduced to Colenbrander formula when De=0 (emmetropic state) and when S=ELP=constant, ignoring the IOL configuration factor (g′T=0).
b. Reduced to Hoffer formula when S=ELP.
c. Reduced to Haigis formula when g′T=0.

CONVERSION FUNCTION

The conversion function (CF) defined by the derivative (or change) ratio of the system refractive error and the IOL-power, CF=dDe/dP, may be easily derived from Eq.(5.a), the Lin's Z^2-formula

$$CF = (1 + C')Z^2, \quad (6)$$

where C′ is a nonlinear term given by C=k(dP), with k=S/1336.

Similarly, derivative of Eq.(A.4.a) w.r.t. the corneal power gives us another conversion for corneal power function CFc=dDe/dDc given by CFc=1.0 which indicates that the change of corneal power is 100% converted to the system refractive error (De).

In contrast to CFc, the CF for IOL-power is governed by the Z-function. If one ignores the small C term, the following examples for IOL conversion function (CF) are calculated for corneal power of Dc=43 diopter (or fc=31 mm).

a. Anterior implant IOL (with S=2.5 to 3.5 mm)
   CF=84.5% to 78.7%
b. Posterior implant IOL (with S=3.8 to 5.0 mm)
   CF=76.9% to 70.4%.

Above examples show that CF is a strongly decreasing function of S, or ELP. However, it is much less sensitive to the corneal power.

Clinical Application

The CF allows us to find the required IOL power to correct a refractive error (E) without knowing the axial length by the relationship of P=(E-E′)/CF, E′ being the remaining error. For example, for IOL implanted at a position S=ELP=3.5 and 5.0 mm and E=20, E′=1.0 (diopter), one may use CF=78.7% and 70.4% to calculate IOL-power of P=(20 – 1.0)/CF=24.14 and 27.0 diopter, respectively, for S=3.5 (anterior IOL) and S=5.0 (posterior IOL). Above results may be also calculated by Holladay II formula which is based on the Heijde formula. However, it requires numerical method versus the simple analytic Z^2 formula of Lin. The CF may be also used to find the power of a piggyback IOL, which however, is a 3-optics system and a revision is required. (See later section of this Chapter).

THREE-OPTICS FORMULAS (IN PHAKIC EYE)

For IOLs implanted in phakic eye, two methods may be used to reduce the 3-optics to 2-optics by combining: (a) the natural lens and the IOL as one subsystem, or (b) the IOL and cornea as a subsystem. These two methods are expected to result in the same reduced 2-optics formula within certain approximations. The parameters used for method (a) are shown in Figure 6.2.

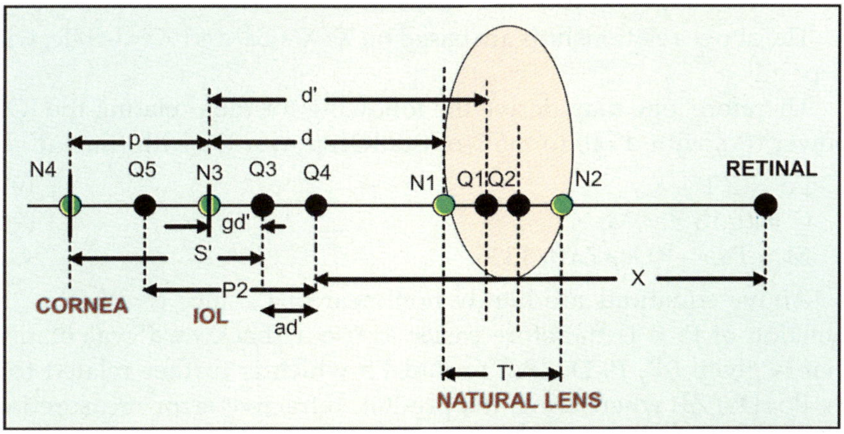

Fig. 6.2: Schematics of 3-optics system for method (a) defined in the text. Positions of the natural lens, IOL and corneal vertex surface are given by N1, N2, N3 and N4. The first and second principal plane (PP) positions are given by (Q1, Q2) for the natural lens, (Q3, Q4) for the subsystem of IOL-natural lens. Q5 is the position of the system second PP. The effective anterior chamber depth given by S=p+gd'+0.05

Similar to the method in 2-optics system, the IOL-power needed to correct refractive error of a phakic eye (3-optics system) may be derived as (see Appendix)

$$Z'P = 1336(1/X' - 1/Y') - P2, \qquad (6)$$

where the cornea (power Dc) and the natural lens (power P2) separate with the IOL (power P) by a distance of p and d′, respectively, with d′=d+2.4 mm. In comparing to Eq.(5) for 2-optics aphakic system, the new parameters of Eq.(6) for phakia are X′=X-gd′, with S=p+gd′ and Y′=1336/Dc-S. Where I had introduced the geometry factor g (for the subsystem of IOL and natural lens) given by g=1/[1+Z′P/P2] since f2/f1=P/P2 in Eq.(3.A).

COMPARISON OF 2-OPTICS AND 3-OPTICS

Above 3-optics formula reduces to that of 2-optics under the limiting case of when (i) f2=infinity (absence of natural lens P2=0), or (ii) d′=0, such that g=Z′=1.

To compare the 3-optics and 2-optics formulas, I further define the following parameters. The IOL-power (Po) when d′=0 may be calculated from

$$Po = Px - Dc/Z - P2, \quad (7)$$

where Px=1336/X related to Px′=1336/X′ by

$$Px = Px'/(1+A'), \quad (8.a)$$
$$A' = (Px'/1336)(gd'), \quad (8.b)$$
$$Z=Za/(1-A), \quad (8.c)$$
$$A=(Dc/Z)(gd'/1336). \quad (8.d)$$

The above relationships are based on X=X′+gd′ and Za=1-S/fc, with S=p+gd′.

Therefore, one may derive the following formula relating the IOL-power (Po, with d′=0) to the 3-optics IOL-power (P, with finite d′) by

$$Po = Z'P - C, \quad (9.a)$$
$$C = (gd'/Za^2)M, \quad (9.b)$$
$$M = Px'^2 - (Dc/Za)^2/1336. \quad (9.c)$$

Above equations are highly nonlinear of P, since g,=P2/P is the function of P. It is therefore easier to use a "backward" calculation, that is given (d′, P, Dc, P2) to find Po which is further related to Z by $Po=De/Z^2$, where De is the pre-IOL refractive error measured on the corneal plane (Fig. 6.3).

Substituting Eq. (8) with Eq.(9), I obtain an analytic formula

$$P = (Po + C')/(1-b)^2 \quad (10.a)$$
$$C' = [(2P'/Z)/(1-A)+P2]b \quad (10.b)$$
$$b = d'/f2 = 1 - Z'. \quad (10.c)$$

The derivative of P w.r.t. corneal power (P′) also gives us the conversion function CF = dP′/dP = dDe/dP since the refractive error change (De) equals the change of corneal power, or dDe=dP′,

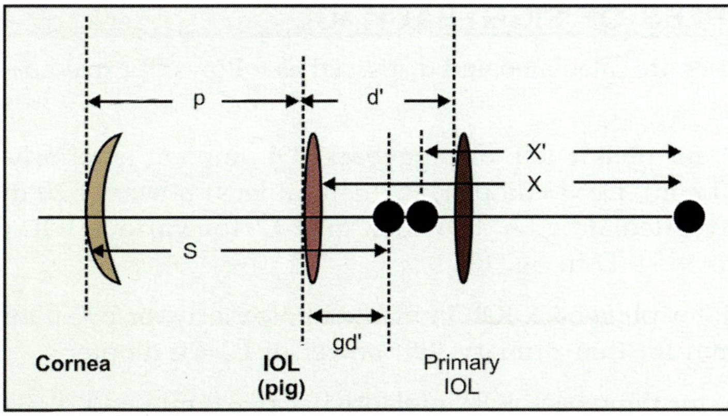

Fig. 6.3: A 3-optics system for piggyback IOL located at a distance of p (to the corneal front surface) and d' (to the primary IOL). Also shown is the effective ACD of the system, S=p+gd'

$$CF = [(1\text{-}b)^2 + a']Z^2 \quad (11.a)$$
$$a' = 2Z'[A/(1\text{-}A)]^2, \quad (11.b)$$

which is independent to P in the approximate formula when a′=0 and reduces to that of 2-optics ($CF=Z^2$), when d′=0 or Z′=1, a′=b=0.

The important feature of above analytic formulas, Eq.(10) and (11) are:

i. For small IOL separation (d′<1.5 mm) or posterior piggyback IOL, the small correction term, A in Eq.(10), may be ignored and the IOL power (P, for 3-optics) and for 2-optics (Po) are linearly related and their difference Delta=P-Po=b′/$(1\text{-}b)^2$ + 2bPo, with b′=2P′/Z+P2, which is independent to P and proportional to b (or d′).
ii. For larger d′>1.5 mm, the extra contribution (C′ term) in Eq.(10) is required, about 10% to 15% and cannot be ignored. Eq. (10) only suffers less than 5% error comparing to exact numerical results based on Eq.(9).
iii. As shown by Eq.(8), the effect of d′ is twofold: (a) shifted X′=X+gd′ and (b) Za=Z(1-A), where factor (a) is dominant, whereas factor (b) may be ignored for small d′<1.5 mm. These two factors are competing as seen by Eq.(9.c) resulting myopic and hyperopic shifted, respectively. Also note that the M function is the same as that of accommodating IOL defined as the power increase per 1.0 mm axial movement which is "equivalent" to the separation between the IOL and the natural lens (d′).
iv. In Eq.(11), the contribution of a′ to CF (about 2% to 8%) cannot be ignored (particularly when d′>1.5 mm and for minus IOL. The approximated Eq.(10) and (11) are more accurate for plus IOL than minus IOL.

EXAMPLES OF PIGGYBACK IOL

Three cases are calculated and discussed as follows (for fixed p+d′=6.0 mm):

Case (a): for phakic IOL or piggyback IOL implant anteriorly (with p=d′=3.0 mm), Dc=43 diopter, P2 (natural lens) power of 20 diopter. One may calculate g, A, b, which give C′ for various IOL power P=-5.0 to +15.0 D in Eq.(10).

Case (b): for piggyback IOL implanted posteriorly, or p=5.0 mm and d′=1.0 mm for thin primary IOL power of P2=20 diopter.

Case (c): for piggyback IOL implanted at p=3.0 mm and d′=3.0 mm.

The under- (or over-) estimated 2-optics IOL power defined by Delta=P-Po is shown as follow based on Eq.(10):

P		–5	–10	–15	+5	+10	+15
DELTA	(a)	1.8	1.7	1.8	–2.0	–2.1	–2.3
	(b)	3.8	3.5	3.9	–4.1	–4.3	–4.6
	(c)	5.5	6.3	8.1	–6.0	–6.2	–6.7

The above calculated results are shown in Figure 6.4 for minus IOL cases. The role of the cornea IOL separation (p) on Delta is shown in Figure 6.5 for P = –10 and +10 D. As one may see that Delta is a strong decreasing function of p, or increasing function of d′ since p+d′=6.0 mm (fixed) in the calculations.

THE CONVERSION FUNCTION FOR THREE-OPTICS

Unlike the 2-optics system, the CF for 3-optics given by Eq.(11) also depends on the initial value of the IOL-power (Pin) shown as follows:

	Pin	–5	–10	+5	+10
CF	(a)	98	104	98	96%
	(b)	96	100	95	94%
	(c)	106	126	93	92%

In comparison, the CF(2-optics)= (81.6, 76, 70, 65)% for Pin=(3, 4, 5, 6) mm, for corneal power of 43 D and they are independent to the IOL power.

COMPARING LIN AND HOLLADAY FORMULAS

The conversion from spectacle power (Ds) to IOL power (P), defined by TF=P/Ds=1/[D′/P)(Ds/D′)], or TF=1/(CF)(CFs), where CF=(D′/P) is defined as the conversion from IOL power to the refractive error

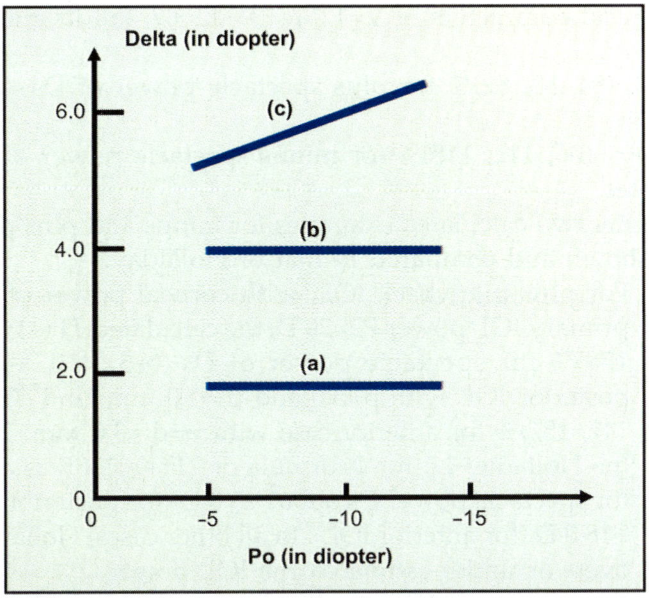

Fig. 6.4: Comparison of the under-corrected 2-optics IOL power (w.r.t. 3-optics) Delta for minus IOL implanted: (a) posteriorly (p=5.0 mm), (b) at p=4.0 mm and (c) anteriorly (p=3.0 mm)

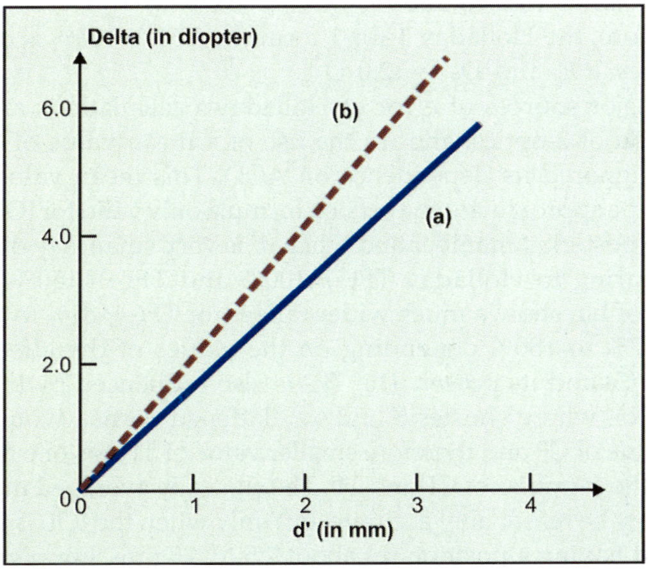

Fig. 6.5: Delta vs piggyback IOL position (away from the primary IOL by d'=6.0-p) for (a) plus (+10.0) and (b) minus (-10.0) power

on the corneal plane (D′) which is further converted to the spectacle power (Ds) given by

$$CFs=Ds/D'=1-0.012Ds. \qquad (12)$$

For typical parameters of V=12, fc=31, f2=62, (all in mm), Eq.(12) gives:

CFs(+)=(94, 88, 82)% for plus spectacle power of Ds=(5, 10, 15) diopter.

CFs(–)= (106, 112, 118)% for minus spectacle power of (–5, –10, –15) diopter.

Following two calculated examples for minus and plus piggyback IOL are shown and compared to that of Holladay.

Case (1). For plus piggyback IOL, with corneal power of Dc=43D, primary IOL power P2=20 D, the calculated TF(+)=(157, 166, 178)% for spectacle power of Ds=(+5, +10, +15) D for posterior IOL with p=5.0 and d′=1.0 mm; and TF(+)=(137, 147, 157)% for anterior case with p=d′=3.0 mm. Therefore, the Holladay 1.5-for-1 formula or TF(+)=150% is only good for spectacle power Ds about +3.0 D (for posterior IOL) and +18.0 D (for anterior IOL). In all other cases, Holladay either over- or under-estimated the IOL power.

Case (2). For piggyback IOL (p=d′=3.0 mm), TF(–)=(118, 112, 81)%; and TF(–)=(138, 130, 124)% for posterior (d′=1.0 mm), for Ds=(–5, –10, –15) D. In other cases, Holladay underestimated about 10% to 38%.

Therefore, the Holladay 1-for-1 formulas TF(–)=100% is only good for anterior IOL and Ds= –12.0 D.

The major sources of error of Holladay's calculations are: (a) the assumption of 2-optics, and (b) the use of a mean value of CF about 80% and ignored its dependence on ACD. This mean value method provides the approximate conversion formula only valid for IOL implanted in the posterior chamber and when d′ is very small, say d′<0.2 mm.

Comparing to Holladay TF(–)=100% and TF(+)=150%, the new formulas of Lin show a much wider ranges for TF(–)=81% to 138% and TF(+)=137% to 180% depending on the values of the effective IOL positions (S) and its power. The TFs is also influenced by the corneal power (Dc), where shorter S and/or flattened cornea would have a higher value of CF and therefore smaller value of TFs, as one may easily see from the formulas of CF and TF. The clinically averaged mean value for TFs may be reasonably accurate, but only when the IOL is anteriorly implanted having a position (p) about 2.5 to 3.5 mm. For personalized TFs, one requires the individual value of p, S, and the power of Dc, Ds and P related by Lin's new formulas shown by Eq.(11).

CONCLUSION

The commonly accepted formulas of TF(–)=100% (1-for-1) and TF(+)=150% (1.5-for-1) in converting the spectacle power to IOL power based on classical Vergence formulas could result in significant errors in IOL power calculations. Information on the individual power of cornea and primary IOL are also required to avoid errors using averaged CF values. In addition, the phakic or piggyback IOL power requires an adjusting factor of Delta = (1.8 to 2.3) diopter for posterior-IOL, and (5.5 to 8.0) for anterior IOL when the conventional 2-optics formulas are used.

Applications of the above described new formulas for the calculations of the efficiency of accommodating IOL may be found in other Chapters by Lin in this book.

APPENDIX (3-OPTICS FORMULAS)

IOL in Phakic Eye

Conventional classical IOL formulas are all based on a 2-optics system which is valid only for aphakic-IOL and for thin optics. For phakic-IOL or piggyback-IOL, a 3-optics system is required. The 3-optics system may be reduced to an effective 2-optics by considering the natural lens and IOL as a sub system (SS) which is further coupled to the cornea and treated as an effective 2-optics, the SS and the cornea. By Gaussian optics, the effective focal length (EFL) of the IOL and natural lens sub-system (SS) is given as (referred to Fig. 6.2)

$$1/f = 1/f2 + Z'/f1, \qquad \text{(A.1)}$$
$$Z' = 1 - d'/f2,$$

where f1 and f2 are the EFL of the IOL and natural lens; d' is the effective IOL position (away from the natural lens first principal plane location Q1) and given by d'=d+2.4 mm, where d is the IOL position and 2.4 mm is a shifted effective position due to the thickness (about 4.0 mm) of the natural lens. The EFL of the reduced 2-optic system consisting of cornea and SS is then given by

$$1/F = 1/fc + Za/f \qquad \text{(A.2)}$$
$$Za = 1 - S/fc,$$

where the effective distance between the cornea and SS (shown by the distance between Q1 and Q3 in Figure 6.2) may be calculated from S=p+gd', where g is a geometry factor given by

$$g = f/f2 = 1/[1 + Z'(f2/f1)] \qquad \text{(A.3)}$$

It can be readily seen that the 3-optics phakic eye reduces to a 2-optics aphakic eye when the natural lens is removed, or when f2 goes to infinite and g=0, f=f1. Eq.(2) becomes a simple cornea-IOL 2-optics system (or an aphakic IOL) which has the same format as that of cornea-natural lens system. By separating all the IOL power dependence term in Eq.(2), or a de-coupling of the f1-dependence of the second principle plane with others, one may obtain Eq.(6).

Piggyback IOL

It should be noted that the above method may be easily applied to the 3-optics system of piggyback IOL (in pseudophakia) by replacing the natural lens with the primary IOL which may be assumed to be a thin lens such that d'=d, without the extra term of 2.4 mm due to the thick natural lens. As shown in Figure 6.3, the emmetropic (De=0) IOL power may be given by a revised Eq.(5.a) as follows

$$Z'P = 1336/X' - 1336/Y' \qquad \text{(A.4)}$$
$$X' = X - gd',$$
$$Y' = fc - S,$$
$$S = p + gd',$$
$$Za = 1 - S/fc,$$

which shows the revised parameters of X', Y', S and Za shifted by the separation (d') between piggyback and primary IOL, and reduces to Eq. (5.a) when d'=0, S=1, Z'=g=1.

REFERENCES

1. Shammas HJ. Intraocular lens power calculations. Thorofare NJ: SLACK. 2004; pp 7-24; 59-61; 64-5.
2. Holladay JT. Optics and intraocular lens power calculation for phakic intraocular lenses. In Horden DR, Lindstrom RL, Davis EA, (eds): Phakic Intraocular Lenses: Principles and Practice. Thorofare NJ:SLACK. 2004; pp 37-44.
3. Lin, JT. Unified refractive-state analysis for customized vision correction. J Refract Surg 2004; 20(3), 398-400.
4. Lin, JT. New formulas comparing accommodation in human lens and intraocular lens. J Refract Surg 2005; 21(2): 200-1.
5. Lin, JT. A generalized refractive state theory and effective eye model. Chin J Optom & Ophthal 2005; 7(1):1-6.
6. Lin, JT. Analysis of refractive state ratios and the onset of myopia. Ophthal Physiol Opt 2005;26(1):97-105.
7. Lin, JT. Update on IOL power calculation formulas. In Garg A, Lin JT, (Eds): "Mastering Intraocular Lenses[IOLs]: Principles, Techniques and Innovations", New Delhi: Japypee Brothers, 2006; Chapter 3:pp 17-29.
8. Lin, JT. The new IOL formulas based on Gaussian optics. In: Garg A, Lin JT, (Eds): "Mastering Intraocular Lenses[IOLs]: Principles, Techniques and Innovations", New Delhi: Japypee Brothers, 2006; Chapter 6: pp 56-65.

CHAPTER

7

JT Lin (USA)

Error Factors in IOL Power Calculations

INTRODUCTION

Recent advances such as partial coherent interfermetry (PCI, or so called IOLMaster) and the advanced image devices called Orbscan have improved the accuracy of ocular biometry, particularly for eyes after cataracts or refractive surgeries. However, errors in the prediction of IOL power still exist in almost all methods, in which some of the error factors are intrinsic either clinically or theoretically. The existing methods (except Haigis' and Lin's) of IOL power calculation are all based on the mean-zero-error (MZE) concept, where the empirically fit parameters (such as ELP, estimated lens position) are defined by regression formulas with one-constant optimization.

Improvement of accuracy was developed by 3-constant optimization proposed by Olsen and Haigis. However, errors of IOL power are inevitable when the MZE methods are applied to individual eyes. The current MZE methods had personalized the following factors for improved accuracy.

- Axial length (L)
- Corneal power (based on keratometry reading)
- Corneal height (H) natural lens thickness (T)
- Anterior chamber depth (ACD).

Modern formulas of Olson predicted the postoperative ACD by a regression formula consisting of the preoperative parameters of (L, H, T, ACD). Haigis proposed the optical ACD given by the solution of a quadratic equation based on Colenbrander formula and the use of 3-constant for optimization which extended the valid range of axial length for both short and long eyes.

In Lin's S-formula, a geometry factor was introduced to further personalize the IOL types, where the effects of IOL thickness and configuration are included. Lin also presented the Gaussian optics formula for the true corneal power such that the intrinsic errors existing in all keratometry-based formulas may be eliminated by personalizing the posterior surface radius of the cornea, particularly for eyes after refractive surgery.

Based on Olsen's 500 patients study, the total error of IOL power is contributed to 3 major components: 54% to axial length errors, 38% to errors in the ACD estimation, and 8% to corneal power errors. With the optimized ACD calculation (e.g. the Binkhorst I formula), the predicted ACD (postoperative) may be reduced to half. However, for eyes after refractive surgeries, the errors due to postoperative corneal power may increase.

Most of the reported studies about the errors of IOL power due to the factors described above are limited to estimated, or qualitative discussion and lack of specifics on individual eyes.

SUMMARY AND NOTATIONS

This Chapter will present formulas and examples for in-depth guidance and quantitative discussion on IOL power errors (E) resulting from each or combined factors of the following:

1. True corneal power (Dc)
   Each 1.0 diopter error in corneal power will cause about 1.2 to 1.5 diopter in IOL power error (defined as E) depending on IOL positions. It is more sensitive for anterior implanted IOL. In addition, each 1.0 diopter error in K-reading will result in E = (1.3 to 1.7) diopter.
2. Estimated lens position (ELP) or effective ACD
   Each 1.0 mm error of ELP (or ACD) may result in E=(0.5 to 2.5) diopter.
3. Axial length (L) or vitreous depth (X)
   Each 1.0 mm error of L or X may result in E=(1.5 to 2.7) diopter, in which shorter eyes and/or steeper cornea is more sensitive to the errors.
4. Manufacturer labeling error or surgeon's implant error
   Depending on IOL types and thickness, E=(0.5 to 3.5) diopter may occur and the higher the IOL power, the higher the error will be. It also has a greater error effects in IOLs having smaller ACD.
5. Error from formulas used
   IOL power error of E= (0.5 to 2.5) diopter may result from eyes having abnormal axial length or posterior corneal surface, where the mean-zero-method based on K-reading of most of the existing formulas fail. Gaussian optics formulas based on true and personalized corneal power should be used to minimize these errors.

Notations

In the following discussion, we will use the definition below:

E: error of IOL power (P) defined as E = –dP (IOL power change)
E>0 (for resultant myopia) or (a plus-IOL power is underestimated), or (a minus-IOL power is overestimated)
E<0 (for resultant hyperopia) or (plus-P is overestimated)

dQ: error (or amount change) of the ocular parameters (assuming dQ>0)

M: IOL error per 1.0 mm (or 1.0 diopter) change/error of Q

Therefore E = –M(dQ), with Q=(L, X, ELP, ACD, Dc, gT):

The sign of E depends on the sign of –M since dQ is defined as positive. For example, in a hyperopia, plus-IOL implant an overestimated corneal power (dDc>0) will result in an underestimated IOL power (P), or E = dP<0; and vice versa.

The IOL power error analysis will be based on the following formulas derived from Gaussian optics by Lin (see also Table 7.1):

- The Z^2-formula (for dDc)
- The M1-formula (for dS)
- The M2-formula (for dL)
- The g-formula (for IOL geometry).

CORNEAL POWER ERRORS

The intrinsic errors of all the kerotometry-based (K-based) formulas resulted from the use of a mean, constant value for the corneal posterior surface (radius r2) or its power C. In Lin's Gaussian optics formula, personalized posterior surface power C=41/r2 is used such that the personalized true corneal power is given by

$$Dc = 1.117\ K - 41/r2, \qquad (1)$$

where K=337.5/r1 is the keratometry power as usual defined by the corneal anterior surface radius (r1). The conventional mean-value methods assumed C=5.5 (or mean r2=7.45 mm by Maloney), C=6.1 (or mean r2=6.7 mm by Koch), C=6.8 (or mean r2=6.03 mm by Shammas) all suffer from error of the true corneal power when it is applied to individual corneas having r2 deviating from the assumed mean values. For example, the error of corneal power of the mean-value method (or the K-based method) is given by dDc=41/r2-6.31 (with mean-r2=6.5 mm). Therefore dDc=(1.9, 1.14, 0.52, –0.45, –1.19) diopter for individual r2=(5.0, 5.5, 6.0, 7.0, 8.0) mm. These errors of -1.19 to +1.9 diopter in estimating the post-LASIK or post-cataract corneal power are inevitable in all the mean-r2 (or K-reading) based formulas.

By Lin's Z^2 formula, which converts the IOL power change (or error E) to the system power (or corneal power) change, defined by a conversion function CF=dDc/E. By defining Mc=1/CF, the IOL power error caused by the corneal power error (dDc) is then given by the Lin's Z^2 formula

$$E = Mc(dDc), \qquad (2.a)$$
$$Mc = 1\ /\ [(1\text{-}kE)Z^2], \qquad (2.b)$$
$$Z = 1 - S(Dc/1336). \qquad (2.c)$$

One may easily calculate the IOL power error (for a given corneal power Dc=43 diopter) as follows: E=1.27 (dDc) for an anterior chamber implant IOL with S=3.5 mm; and E=1.42 (dDc) for a posterior chamber IOL with S=5.0 mm, where the effective ACD is defined as S=ELP (or

ACD) for thin IOL; and S = ELP + gT, for a thick IOL having a geometry factor correction gT about 0.2 to 0.5 mm, for thickness T = 0.5 mm. Greater details of g-factor is presented in other Chapters of this book by Lin.

Therefore, depending on the IOL position S=(3.0 to 6.0) mm, each 1.0 diopter error of corneal power results in an IOL power error of E=(1.2 to 1.5) diopter.

The corneal power errors caused by the use of mean-r2, about (–0.45 to +1.9) diopter result in E=(–1.69 to +2.7) diopter, that is, a myopic error of 1.69 D (for individual r2=8.0 mm) or a hyperopic error of 2.7 D (for r2=5.0 mm) when the conventional mean-r2 method is used (with mean-r2=6.5 mm), in a plus-IOL implant.

Other corneal power error may result from the change of the ratio (r1/r2) after a refractive surgery. If one uses the pre-LASIK K-reading (or r1) and a mean-r2, more errors will be created by the combined approximation.

It should be noted that each 1.0 diopter error in K-reading (either preop or postop) will result in an IOL power error of E=1.117/CF=1.117Mc which is about 1.3 to 1.7 diopter depending on IOL position(ACD) and corneal power. However, it is much more sensitive to ACD value than corneal power. For example, E=1.36 (dDc) diopter for Dc = 38 diopter; and E=1.42 (dDc) for Dc=43 diopter for a given ACD (or S)=5.0 mm. In comparison, for a given Dc=43 diopter, E = (1.23, 1.32, 1.42, 1.54) (dDc), for ACD = (3, 4, 5, 6) mm.

IOL POSITION ERROR

The predicted IOL position may be defined by ELP (or postop ACD) or S (the effective optical ACD), where S = ELP for thin lens, and S = ELP + gT for thick lens, the geometry factor (g) proposed by Lin is defined by g=1/(1+Z'P1/P2) with Z'=1-T(P2/1336) determined by the thickness (T) of the IOL and its configuration defined by its front and back surface power ratio P1/P2. For thin IOL the axial length L = ELP (or S)+X, with X being the vitreous cavity length. Therefore, for a fixed L, the change of S will also result in a change in X, that is dS = –dX (for dL=0). The IOL power error could be the combined error from both dS and dX even the axial length L is accurately measured.

Given a fixed L, the IOL power error caused by the error (or change of S and X may be calculated by Lin's M1 formula (for the single-optics IOL case),

$$E = -M1(dS), \qquad (3)$$

$$M1 = (Z/1336)(PDc)(2+PZ/Dc),$$

which is proportional to the product of the IOL power (P) and the corneal power (Dc). Alternatively, M1 may be expressed by the vitreous cavity length (X)

$$M1 = (Z2/1336)\ P\ [2/X - P/1336], \quad (4)$$

which shows that the error (E) is more sensitive to short eyes (or smaller X).

Example 1, for a given corneal power Dc=43 D and L=23.8 mm, with adjusted S and X to meet the emmetropia, Eq.(3) gives

M1=(1.08, 1.14, 1.2, 1.29, 1.36) (diopter/mm)

for IOL power of P=(15.3, 16.6, 18, 20, 22) D,

which shows the increasing of M1 as P increases. It also shows M1 per 1.0 diopter of IOL power M1 is about 0.068.

Example 2, for fixed Dc=43 D and S=5.0 mm

M1 = (0.56, 0.82, 1.22, 1.87) (D/mm), for

X = (22, 21, 19, 17) mm

and P is adjusted for higher value accordingly to the emmetropia condition. It shows that shorter eye has larger M1 and higher IOL power error than a long eye.

Therefore, depending on the IOL power, S, X and Dc, E has a wide range of 0.5 to 2.5 diopter for per 1.0 mm error of S, or IOL position. Note that the M function is defined as an absolute value or $M>0$, therefore $E<0$ for $dS>0$ based on Eq.(3), this is the case that a plus IOL power is underestimated and results in a myopia due to the overestimation of S (or ACD).

AXIAL LENGTH ERROR

As discussed earlier, L=S+X, therefore for a fixed ACD (or S), the error of L is due to the error of X (or dL=dX) and the associated IOL power error may be expressed by Lin's M2-formula (for emmetropic state)

$$E = -M2(dL), \quad (5)$$

$$M2 = 1336/(XZ)^2, \text{ or}$$

$$M2 = 1336/F^2,$$

$$1/F = (Dc + ZP)/1336$$

Above formulas show that E is proportional to the IOL power (P), but inverse proportionally to X (or axial length L). That is, IOL power errors are more sensitive to short eyes and it is higher for higher P. For example, for fixed corneal power of Dc = 43 D and S = 5.0 mm, Z = 0.839, M2 = (1.66, 1.98, 2.68) (D/mm) for IOL power of P = (5, 10, 20) D. Therefore, the IOL error rate function M2 due to per 1.0 mm error of axial length (or strictly speaking, X) is about 1.5 times of M1 (due to error of S or ACD).

It should be noted that if both S and X have errors, the total IOL power error is given by

$$E = (M1 + M2)(dS) + M2(dX). \quad (6)$$

For the special case of $dX = -dS$, E becomes $E = M1(dS)$ or Eq.(3); and Eq.(6) reduces to Eq.(5) when $dS=0$, as one should expect.

MIS-LABELING ERROR

For thick IOL, the effective (or optical) ACD (defined as "S") is shifted by the first principal plane location of the IOL and is given by the geometry-factor defined earlier

$$S = ACD + gT, \quad (7)$$
$$g = 1 / (1+Z'P1/P2)$$

Example 1, for an IOL having a thickness T = 0.5 mm and a biconvex structure having front and back surface power of (P1, P2) = (+5, +10) D, g = 0.666, gives gT = 0.33 mm; whereas a mis-labeling (or surgeon's mis-implant) with a reverse structure of (P1, P2) = (+10, +5) D, g = 0.333, gives gT = 0.167 mm which causes a S value difference of about 0.16 mm, or IOL power error of E = –0.16 (M1) which is about (0.1 to 0.4) diopters, for M1 = (0.5 to 2.5) (D/mm).

Example 2, for a convex-plano IOL (P1, P2) = (+10.0, 0) D, gT = 0 (for the convex surface facing the cornea). A mis-implant of the plano surface facing the cornea with g = 1.0 will result in gT = 0.5 mm, or

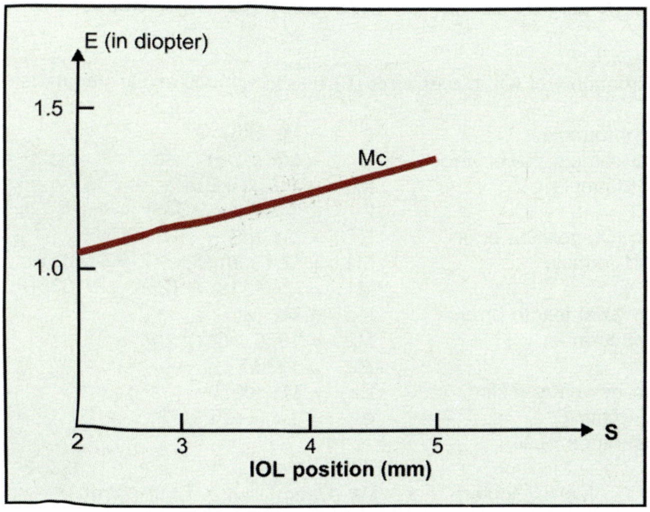

Fig. 7.1: IOL power error (E) versus IOL position (S) for 1.0 diopter error of corneal power

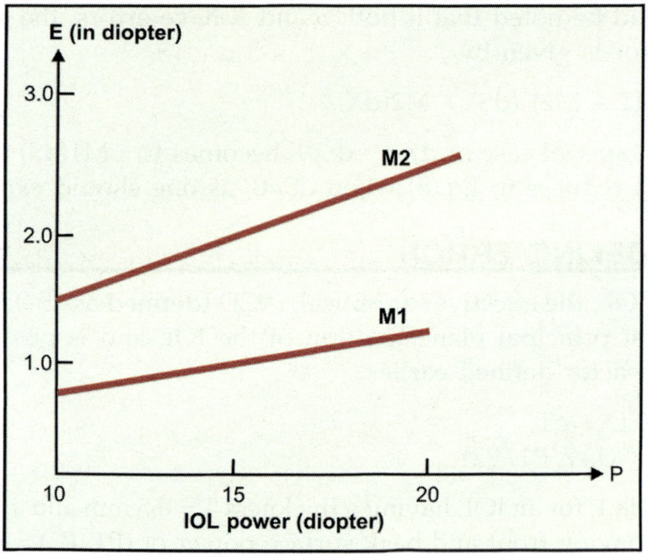

Fig. 7.2: IOL power error (E) for 1.0 mm error of ACD and axial length (L), given by curves M1 and M2, respectively

the S value increases by 0.5 mm. The associated IOL power error is E = –0.5 (M1), or about –0.25 to –1.25 diopter.

Example 3, for a convex-concave IOL with (P1, P2) = (+20, -10) D, gT = –0.5 mm. A mis-labeling or mis-implant of reversed direction with (P1, P2) = (–10, +20) D, having g=+2.0 and gT = +1.0 mm (noting that gT changes from – to +). Substantial errors in IOL power E = –1.5 (M1), or about –0.75 to –3.75 diopter may occur.

Table 7.1: Summary of IOL power error (E) due to various ocular parameter errors (dQ)

General formula	E	= Mj (dQ)
Due to corneal power error	E	= Mc (dDc)
The Z^2-formula	Mc	= 1 / [(1-kE)Z^2],
	Z	= 1 – S(Dc/1336).
Due to IOL-position error	E	= M1 (dS)
The M1-formula	M1	= (Z/1336)(PDc)(2+PZ/Dc), *or*
	M1	= (Z^2/1336) P [2/X – P/1336]
Due to axial length error	E	= M2 (dL)
The M2-formula	M2	= 1336 / $(XZ)^2$, or
	M2	= 1336/F^2
Due to geometry factor	E	= M1 (dg)T
The g-formula	g	= 1 / (1+Z'P1/P2)
Typical range of Mj		

Mj	Mc (D/diopter)	M1 (D/mm)	M2 (D/mm)
Range	(1.2 to 1.5)	(0.5 to 2.5)	(1.5 to 2.7)

CONCLUSION

As summarized in Table 7.1, the IOL power error (E) associates to the error of the corneal power (Dc), axial length (L, or X), ACD (or S) and mis-labeling (by the g-factor) may be expressed by analytic formulas, the Lin's M1, M2, g and Z^2-formula. Depending on IOL and ocular conditions, these calculated error functions have a wide range of value, covering most of the reported clinical data. However, most of the existing analysis assumed a mean value without specifying the ocular conditions. Finally, it should be noted that the discussions of this Chapter are based on 2-optics aphakic system. For 3-optics phakic IOL or piggyback IOL, the errors (E) caused by dX and dS would be about 10% to 25% smaller in the 3-optics system. The error caused by corneal power error may be also reduced by about 5 to 10% (Figs 7.1 and 7.2). Greater details of 3-optics system will be presented in other Chapter of this book.

BIBLIOGRAPHY

1. Atchison DA. Optical design of intraocular lens. I. On-axis performance. Optom Vis Science, 1989;66:492-506.
2. Ho A, Manns F, Pham T, et al. Predicting the performance of accommodating intraocular lens using ray tracing. J Cataract Refract Surg 2006;32:129-36.
3. Landenbucher A, Reese S, Jakob C, Seize B. Pseudophakic accommodation with translation lenses-dual optic vs. mono-optic. Ophthalmic Physiol Opt 2004:24:450-7.
4. Langenbucher A, Nguyen NX, Sertz B, Gusek-Schneider GC, Kuchle M. Measurement of accommodation after implantation of an accommodating posterior chamber intraocular lens. J Cataract Refract Surg 2003; 29:677-85.
5. Lin JT. Accommodating IOL: efficiency and optimal design. In Garg A, Lin JT (Eds): Mastering IOLs: Principles and Innovations. Jaypee Brothers Med Pub: New Delhi, India, 2006.
6. Lin JT. Unified formulas for phakic-aphakic IOL and spectacle-cornea power conversion. J Refract Surg 2006;22:(in press).
7. Lin, JT. New formulas comparing accommodation in human lens and intraocular lens. J Refract Surg 2005; 21:200-1.
8. Lin, JT. Unified refractive-state analysis for customized vision correction. J Refract Surg 2004; 20: 398-400.
9. Mcleod SD, Portney V, Ting A. A dual optic accommodating fordable intraocular lens. Br J Ophthalmol 2003;87:1083-5.
10. Nawa Y, Ueda T, Nakatsuka M, et al. Accommodation obtained per 1.0 mm forward movement of a posterior chamber intraocular lens. J Cataract Refract Surg 2003;29:2069-72.
11. Wang XJ, Jin CP, Wang QM. Aberration with IOLs based on different optical design. Chinese J Optom & Ophthal (in Chinese). 2003;5:209-11.

CHAPTER

8

JT Lin (USA)

Key Factors Determining the Estimated IOL Position

INTRODUCTION

In the early formulas, the estimated lens position (ELP), also known as the postoperative anterior chamber depth (ACDpost), is assumed as a constant. The modern formulas allow the dependence of ELP on many factors including: keratometry, axial length, horizontal white-to-white corneal height, corneal curvatures, IOL lens thickness, natural lens thickness, preoperative ACD, patient's age and preoperative refraction. Furthermore, the ELP is not only governed by the preoperative-ACD, but also by the placement of the IOL, whether it is in the anterior chamber, iris-supported, or in the posterior chamber (in the sulcus or in the capsular bag). For thick IOL, the ELP also needs modification to include the effects due to different types of IOL, or its configurations. The conventional ELP formulas assuming thin-IOL could not tell the difference for IOL types which require a geometry factor (g) to be introduced in this Chapter.

This Chapter will discuss the above issues and compare different formulas to correlate four parameters: the ELP, the A-constant, the surgeon's factor and the effective (or optical) ACD for IOL implanted in different positions and for both aphakic and phakic eyes. Comments on the existing formulas based on thin-lens in 2-optics system will be presented by new formulas for thick-lens in 3-optics system.

APHAKIC VERSUS PHAKIC IOL

As shown in Figure 8.1 A to E, various IOL implants in phakic and aphakic eyes for both thin and thick lens are defined by the following parameters:

ELP: Separation between the corneal front surface (N1) and IOL front surface (N2), ELP=ACD in aphakic IOL of Figure 8.1A.

- p: Separation between N2 and N3 (natural lens front surface), see Figure 8.1B.
- Q1: First principal plane position (PP) of the IOL-natural lens subsystem.
- Q2: First PP position of a thick IOL, see Figure 8.1D.
- Q3: Second PP of thick IOL.
- Q4: First PP of a thick natural lens.
- Q5: Second PP position of a thick natural lens, see Figure 8.1E.
- S: Effective (or optical) IOL position (or the effective ACD).

By above definition, the S is related to ELP and the effective focal length (EFL) of the corneal (fc), IOL (f1) and natural lens or primary IOL (f2) by equations shown in Table 8.1.

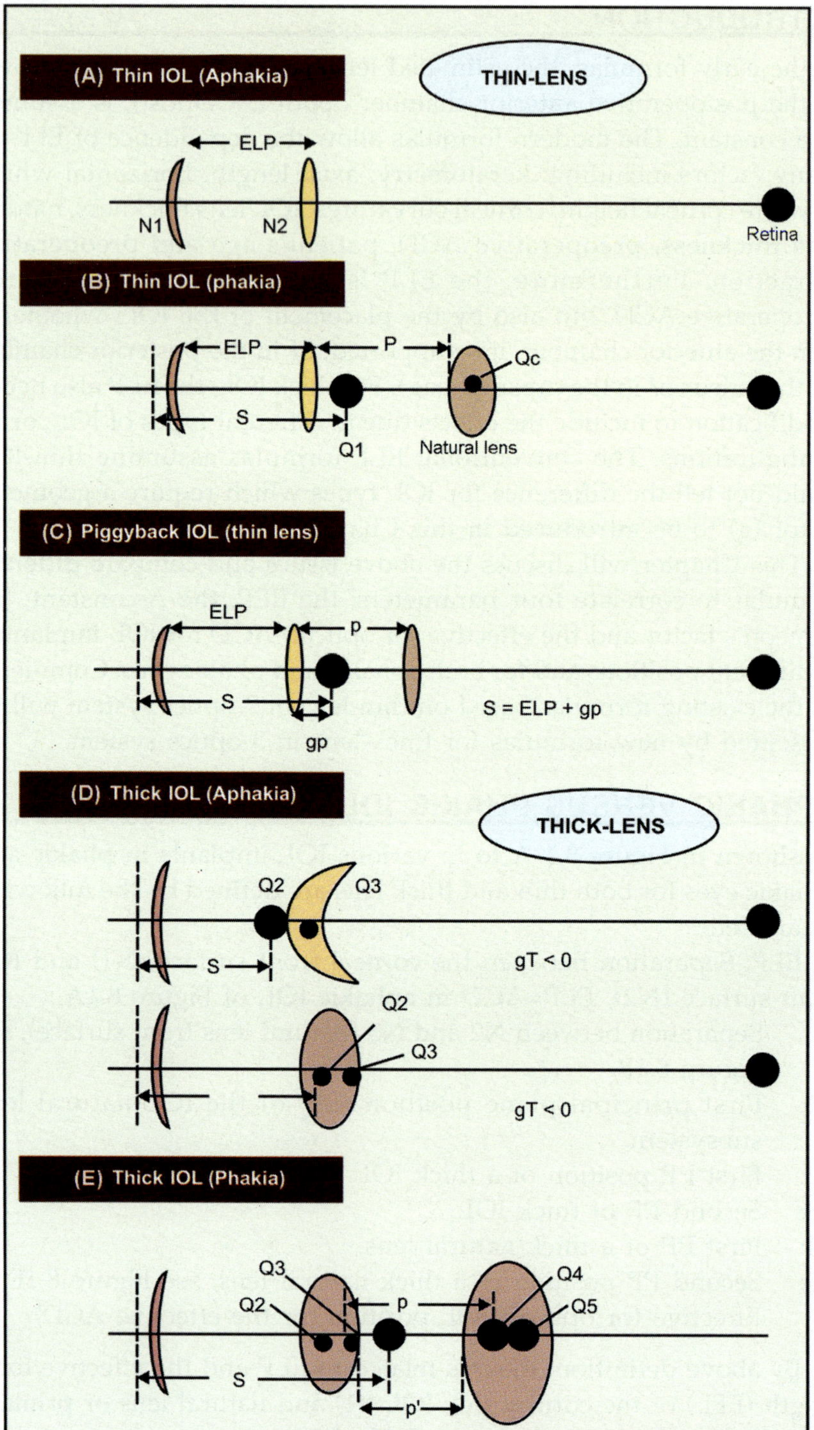

Fig. 8.1: Schematics for IOL implant in aphakic and phakic eyes

Table 8.1: The Lin's S formulas for effective (optical) IOL position (S) for various implants in phakia and aphakia (refer to Fig. 8.1).

	Implant types	*Relationship of S and ELP*
(a)	Thin IOL in aphakia	S=ELP=ACD
(b)	Thin IOL in phakia	S=ELP+gp' where g=f/f2=1[1+Z2(f2/f1)], p'=p+2.4 mm, Z2=1-p'/f2
(c)	Thin piggyback IOL	S=ELP+gp
(c)	Thick IOL in aphakia	S=ELP+g'T, where T=IOL thickness
(d)	Thick IOL in phakia	S=ELP+gp', where p'=p+g'T+2.4 mm

geometry factor g=1/(1+Z2P1/P2), g'=1/(1+Z2'P1'/P2')
(P1, P2) = (IOL power, natural lens power) in case (b)
= (piggyback, primary IOL) power in case (c) and (e)
(P1', P2') = (front, back) surface IOL power in case (d) and (e)

It should be noted that the effective or optical ACD (defined as S) is not directed related to the preoperative-ACD. It is governed by the postoperative-ACD, the IOL physical position and IOL types (in the case of thick IOL). Furthermore, it is also determined by the power of the natural lens (in the case of phakic eye) and the primary IOL (in the case of piggyback IOL in aphakic eye).

The new parameter "S" may be rigorously derived from Gaussian optics. Formulas shown in Table 8.1 may be further revised by adding 0.05 mm to the ELP to count for the second PP contribution of a thick-cornea (assumed to be 0.5 mm). The effect of retinal thickness about 0.18 mm (for a typical axial length of 23.5 mm) may be also added to ELP. That is the revised ELP becomes ELP'=ELP+(0.05+0.18) or about 0.23 mm longer than the conventional value which ignores the thickness of the corneal and retina. The ELP or ACD in this Chapter is defined from the front corneal surface to the front IOL surface, that is, the corneal thickness is included. This definition is consistent with the anatomical ACD defined by Holladay.

Greater details based on Figure 8.1 are shown as follows:

Case (a): S=ELP (thin IOL)=ACD for IOL in aphakia (see Fig. 8.1.A)

Case (b): S=ELP+gp' (in thick natural lens) for IOL in phakia (see Figure 8.1A and B).

where the S is shifted by the first principal plane (FPP) position at Q1 which may be calculated by the geometry factor defined by

$$g = f/f2 = 1[1+Z2(f2/f1)]$$
$$= 1/[1+Z2(P1/P2)],$$

where P1 and P2 being the power of IOL and natural lens; f being the EFL of the IOL natural lens given by $1/f=1/f1+Z1/f2$ or $1/f2 + Z^2/f1$; and $Z1=1-p'/f1$, $Z2=1-p/f2$; p is given by $p'=p+2.4$ mm, where 2.4

mm is the position of natural lens FPP, for a typical thickness of 4.0 mm. For example, for an IOL power of +10.0 D (or f1=133.6 mm) and natural lens of +15.0 D (or f2=1336/15=89.1 mm) and p=1.0 mm, Z1=1–3.4/133.6=0.974, f=54.4 mm. Therefore, gp'=0.61x3.4=2.07 mm, and S=ELP+2.07 mm, which is shifted to a larger value than ELP and can not be neglected for a typical value of ELP=(2.0 to 3.0) mm.

Case (c): the piggyback IOL (see Fig. 8.1.C).

where the primary IOL could be a thin or thick IOL. For thin IOL case, S=ELP+gp, with g=f/f2, similar to case (b), which is defined by the EFL (or power) of both piggyback (f1) and primary IOL (f2). For example, for primary IOL power of 20 D (or f2=1336/20=66.8 mm) and piggyback IOL power of -5.0 D (or f1=–267.2 mm), and separated by p=1.0 mm, one may calculate Z1=1+1.0/267.2=1.0037 and f=88.9 mm. Therefore, gp=1.33 mm which is smaller than the gp'=2.07 mm in case (b), because the natural lens thickness of 4.0 mm is greater than p=1.0 mm. For thick IOL, the S should be farther shifted by gT, with T being the IOL thickness as shown in the following case.

Case (d): thick IOL in phakia with two configurations (see Fig. 8.1.D).

For the convex-concave IOL, the FPP is left-shifted (shown by position of Q2) in contrast to that of biconvex IOL having Q2 right-shifted. For example, in convex-concave IOL having front and back surface radius of (R1, R2)=(66.8, 133.6) mm or power of (P1, P2)=(+20, –10) D, and IOL thickness of T=0.5 mm, we may calculate the geometry factor g which may be approximated by g=1/(1+P1/P2) for small T with Z2=1-T/f2=1.0, we obtain g=–1.0, therefore S=ELP–0.5 mm. In comparison, for a biconvex IOL having the same total power (P1+P2)of +10.0 D, we obtain g=+0.5 and S=ELP+0.25 mm. The smaller S value in convex-concave would require a smaller IOL power at a given refraction error than that of biconvex.

The shifted value gT could be neglected only for thin IOL, or T<0.2 mm; or when ELP>>gT in posterior chamber case with ELP about 4.0 to 5.5 mm. For anterior chamber IOL with ELP about 3.0 mm, the shifted amount may contribute about 8% to 15% and cannot be ignored.

Case (e): thick IOL in phakic eye (see Fig. 8.1.E).

where the effects from the shift from PP of both elements should be included and p is defined by the distance between the two second PPs position, or Q3 and Q4. Typical value is p'=p+g'T+2.4 mm, with g factor of the IOL g'=1/[1+Z2(P1'/P2')], Z2=1-T(P2/1336), where P1' and P2' are the front and back surface power of the thick IOL; and S=ELP+gp', where the g-factor for the IOL natural lens system g=f/f2 (similar to case b).

Table 8.2: Typical values of ELP, A-constant and surgeon's factor(s) for different IOL implants

IOL Implant	*ELP (mm)*	*A-Constant*	*s-factor*
Anterior chamber lens	2.8 – 3.1	115.0 – 115.3	–0.7 to –0.4
Iris-supported lens	3.3 – 3.5	115.5 – 115.7	–0.1 to +0.1
Posterior chamber lens			
in the sulcus	3.7 – 4.1	115.9 – 117.2	+0.1 to +0.7
in the bag	4.3 – 5.1	117.5 – 118.8	+0.9 to +1.6

Table 8.3: Lens constant conversion table*

A-constant	ELP	s-factor
114	2.63	–1.04
115	3.21	–0.48
116	3.80	0.03
117	4.38	0.66
118	4.97	1.22
119	5.55	1.79

* based on the relationships:
ELP=0.5836A-63.896 s-factor=0.5663A-65.6

THE ESTIMATED LENS POSITION (ELP)

As shown in Table 8.2, the ELP value (or ACD) depends on the IOL implant positions. Also shown are the corresponding values for the A-constant and the surgeon's factor(s) defined by Holladay. Table 8.3 shows some typical values of these 3 parameters. By knowing the ELP (or ACD), A-constant or surgeon's s-factor, the corresponding effective (optical) ACD (or S) may be calculated based on formulas shown in Table 8.1 given by S=ELP+gT (or gp).

NONLINEAR GAUSSIAN FORMULA

The Classical Formula

The IOL power may be calculated from the classical Vergence formulas developed by Fyodorov (1975), Colenbrander (1973), van der Heijde (1976) or Binkhorst (1975) given by a general format of

$$P = 1336/(L-C) - 1336/(y-C), \quad (1)$$
$$Y = 1336/(Kc+E),$$

where Kc is the corneal power measured by keratometer and E is the remaining refractive error, and C=ELP. The above formula for ametropic case was also used by Hoffer (1981) and more recently by Haigis (2003), where the original formula of Colenbrander or van der Heijde (for the emmetropic case with E=0) was revised to y for the ametropia. Unlike the new formula of Lin (to be shown below) which is rigorously derived from Gaussian optics, the above classical formula was "phenomenally" formatted by replacing Kc by y to count for the effect of remaining refractive error (E). This procedure is accurate under the assumption that the refractive error (E) may be added to the corneal power with a 100% conversion factor (CF). However, Lin had recently shown that CF is not 100%. It could range from 98 to 102% depending on the initial refractive error. Therefore, Eq.(1) is not exact and may have error about 2 to 4% comparing to the more accurate Gaussian optics modern formula of Lin.

The Modern Formula

The modern Z^2 formula of Lin (2005) derived from Gaussian optics is given by

$$P = 1336/(L\text{-}S) - 1336/(f1\text{-}S) - qE, \quad (2)$$

where f1 is the corneal focal length related to its true power (Dc) by f1=1336/Dc, and $g=(1+kP)/Z^2$ is the nonlinear term with Z=1-S/f1. Lin's formula is derived from the decoupling of the second principal plane contribution up to the second-order approximation.

Eq.(1) and (2) are identical for emmetropic case, or when E=0, except Lin used the effective ACD instead of the C=ELP in the classical formula. For ametropic case, the y term in Eq.(1) may be approximated to obtain a similar format as Eq.(2). Furthermore, Eq.(1) may be derived from the original Colenbrander formula (for E=0) by replacing 1336/Kc by the y term to include the effect of E, noting that y reduces to 1336/Kc when E=0.

It may be easily seen that both Eq.(1) and (2) give a quadratic equation for S (or ELP), therefore, S (or ELP) is a nonlinear function of (P, E, L, Dc).

Haigis proposed the optical ACD (or S) based on thin IOL implanted in 2-optics "aphakic" eye, where the effects of IOL thickness (T), the geometry factor (g) and the roles of the natural lens power (in phakic eye), or the primary IOL (in piggyback IOL) are ignored. The new formula of Lin based on the effective ACD (S) including all these factors, therefore representing a unified formula for aphakic, phakic and pseudophakic eyes and for thin, thick IOL in all styles (configurations) as shown by two geometry factors, g' for thick IOL and g for subsystem.

Eq.(1) and (2) are for 2-optics system. In 3-optics system such as case (b) IOL in phakia and case (c) piggyback IOL, a revised equation is needed as follows:

$$(Z1)P'(3\text{-optics}) = P(2\text{-optics}) - D2\text{-}(q'\text{-}q)E, \quad (3)$$

where Z1=1-p/f1, p being the separation between IOL and natural lens (in phakia case), or primary IOL (in the case of piggyback IOL) having the EFL of f1 and f2, and power of P and D2, respectively. The effective ACD(S) is further shifted to S′=S+0.5fcp′/f2 and Z also changed to Z′=1-S′/fc which defines the new q′. Therefore the P′(3-optics) IOL power reduces to P(2-optics) when f2 is infinity (or zero-power of natural lens or primary IOL). For finite f2, the effects of f2 about 10 to 20% cannot be ignored. Greater details of 3-optics formulas may be found in other Chapters of Lin in this book.

TRIPLE OPTIMIZATION

As proposed by Olson and Haigis, the postoperative ACD (or ELP) may be predicted from the preoperative (or mean) ACD by optimizing the regressions constants for zero mean predicted refractive error. Olson used the measured ACDpre whereas Haigis also proposed the effective (or optical) ACD derived from a quadratic equation based on the classical formula of Colenbrander, but assumed thin IOL and 2-optics system. In Lin's new formula, the following improvements are proposed:

- The ACDpre is revised by extra-terms of g′T to include the effects of IOL types, its thickness and configuration
- The ELP is shifted by the geometry factor gp to include the effects due to the presence of the natural lens (a 3-optics system of IOL in phakia) and/or primary IOL (for piggyback IOL case)
- The true corneal power (Dc) is used, rather than the keratometry-based corneal power (Kc) which ignores the effect due to individual back surface of the cornea.

  That is, the corneal power if given by

  Lin's formula:

  $$Dc = 1.117K - 41/r2 \quad (4)$$

  K-based formula:

  $$Kc = 1.114K - C \quad (5)$$

  where r2 is the posterior surface radius of the cornea, K is the portoperative keratometry power. In the K-based equation, the corneal power (Kc) is approximated by a mean constant C=5.5 (Malony), 6.1 (Koch) or 6.8 (Shammas). In Lin's equation, a personalized term 41/r2 is used.

NONLINER OPTIMIZATION

In the one-constant optimization method, the axial length (L) dependence curve of the ACD (or ELP) is fit for a mean zero error (MZE) prediction error by a parallel shift of the curve. Therefore its validation is limited to certain range of L. For example, Holladay (I) good for medium long eyes (24.5 to 26.0 mm), SRK/T good for very long eyes (>26.0 mm) and Hoffer's good for short eyes (<22.0 mm). The 3-cosntant optimization allows a non linear shift of the fitting curve, such that a wide range of axial length may be covered. As pointed out by Haigis, in the classical, one-constant optimization, a mean zero-error (MZE) might be due to the balanced errors at short and long eyes. Therefore the ACD-L curves based on MZE may still suffer significant errors when it is applied to individual eyes or different IOL types. The new formulas of Lin resolve these problems by introducing the geometry factor (g and g′) in the effective ACD (S) and by the use of true corneal power shown by Eq.(4).

For the 2-optics case, Eq.(1) may be used to solve for S (or ELP) based on a quadratic equation.

Furthermore, the S may be calculated from the Lin's Z^2 formula which converts the IOL power (P) to the refractive error correction on corneal plane (E),

$$E'-E = Z^2P, \; Z = 1-S/fc, \qquad (6)$$

where E′ and E are the pre-IOL refractive error and the remaining error (on corneal plane, not spectacle plane), respectively. Therefore, by knowing the IOL power, the refractive error and the corneal power (Dc), the predicted S (or ACDpost) for emmetropia (E=0) may be calculated by

$$S = (1336/Dc)[1-(E'/P)^{1/2}]. \qquad (7)$$

For example, given Dc=43 D, to correct an error of E′=+10.0 D, if the predicted IOL power P=+14.0 D, then the predicted postoperative ACD, or S should be 4.81 mm. It should be noted that above formula allows us to calculate S for given (Dc, E′, P) or to calculate P given (S, Dc, E′) without the knowledge of the axial length (L). Holladay II formula also allows the calculation of P without knowing L, however, he only presented the numerical method based on Colenbrander formula. The Lin Z^2 formula presents the simple analytic expression between S and P, rather than solving the complex quadratic equation or Haigis 3-constant equation.

Greater details about the calculations of IOL power in 3-optics system will be presented in other Chapters of Lin in this Book.

CONCLUSION

The conventional ELP may be revised to include the IOL types by a geometry factor (g′) in thick IOL case, but in aphakic 2-optics system. For piggyback IOL or IOL implant in phakic eye, a 3-optics system is needed, where the effective ACD (S) is further influenced by the power and location of the primary IOL or natural lens where a second

Table 8.4: Formulas for postoperative estimated IOL position (ELP) and effective/ optical ACD (S) and validity range of axial length (L)

Formula	*L (in mm)*	*Features*
(1) SRK/T	> 26.0	ELP = H + ACD-3.336
(2) Holladay(I)	24-26	ELP = a–ACD + Surgeon factor
(3) Hoffer Q	<22.0	ELP = p–ACD - adjusted constant
(4) Olson	22-28	ELP = ACDmean + 0.12H + 0.33ACDpre +0.3T+0.1L-5.18
(5) Haigis	all L	S = a + bACD + cL
(6) Lin	all L, all IOL types	S = a + bACD + cL + g'T +gp'

where:

H = corneal height;
ACD = anterior chamber depth
p-ACD = personalized-ACD;
a-ACD = anatomical-ACD;
(a, b, c) = 3 optimized constants for ACD, L, P;
g'T = geometry factor x IOL thickness (T)
gp = subsystem g-factor x separation (p)
p-ACD = 0.58375 (A-cosntant) – 63.896

geometry factor (g) is also needed. For accurate personalized IOL power prediction, accurate S and true corneal power based on personalized corneal back surface radius would be required, in addition to the empirically predicted ELP.

BIBLIOGRAPHY

1. Fyodorov SN, Galin MA, Linksz A. Calculation of the optical power intraocular lens. Invest Ophthalmol 1975;14:625-8.
2. Hill WE. Choosing the right formula. www.doctor-hill.com. (2003).
3. Holladay JT. Optics and intraocular lens power calculation for phakic intraocular lenses. In Horden DR (Ed).
4. Holladay JT. Refractive power calculation for intraocular lenses in the phakic eye. Am J Ophthalmol 1993;116:63-6.
5. Lin JT. Accommodating IOL: efficiency and optimal design. In Gag A, Lin JT (Eds). Mastering IOLs: Principles and Innovations. Jaypee Brothers Med. Pub. Delhi: India, 2006.
6. Lin JT. Analysis of refractive state theory and the onset of myopia. Ophthal Physiol Opt 2006;26:97-105.
7. Lin JT. Unified formulas for phakic-aphakic and spectacle-cornea power conversion. J Refract Surg 2006;22: (in press).
8. Lin JT. Unifired refractive-state analysis for customized vision correction. J Refract Surg 2004;20:398-400.
9. Olson T, Corydon L, Gimbel H. Intraocular lens power calculation with an improved anterior chamber depth prediction algorithm. J Cataract Refract Surg 1995;21:313-9.
10. Sanders DR, Retzlaff J, Kraff MC. Comparison of empirically derived and theoretical aphakic refraction formulas. Arch Ophthal 1983;10:965-7.
11. Sanders DR, Retzlaff J, Kraff MC. Comparison of the SRKII formulas and the other second generation formulas. J Cataract Refract Surg 1988;14:136-41.
12. Shamms HJ. Intraocular lens power calculations. Thorofare NJ: Slack;2004.
13. van der Heijde GL. The optical correction of unilateral aphakia. Trans Amer Academy Ophthalmol Otolarynogol 1976;81:80-8.

CHAPTER 9

JT Lin (USA)

IOL Power Calculations for Children after Cataract Surgery

INTRODUCTION

It was known that pediatric eyes after cataract/IOL surgery would suffer significant myopia progress due to the continuing axial growth of the eye if the IOL power is not adjusted for compensation. Based on Lin's double-rate theory,[1,2] the myopia power developed (age-dependence) may be calculated (predicted). This will allow us to better adjust the implanted IOL power by both age and individual ocular growth rates for a true customized IOL power, comparing to the mean value method of Wilson et al.[3,4] This Chapter presents customized IOL power for pseudophakic eye of pediatric patients and includes the following subjects by new formulas developed by the author.

- The Lin's double-rate theory for phakic eye after cataract surgery, in which the axial growth rate (N) and the refractive power change rate (M) are introduced for age 0 to 6
- The age-dependent refractive power of pseudophakic eye after an IOL is implanted
- Re-adjustment of the adjusted mean value IOL power based on the surgery age and the ocular condition (corneal and IOL power and the axial length) at the time of IOL implantation
- Factors which affect the IOL power adjustment.

REFRACTION POWER OF APHAKIC EYES

The refractive error (De), which is age dependent for pediatric eyes, in general, should be defined by the 4 growth factors due to the change of the anterior (S), posterior (X) chamber depth and the cornea (P') and lens (P) power. In the following, two age stages will be discussed:

1. Age 3 and up, where corneal and lens power remain at their stable values and only X and S change.
2. Age 0 to 3, where all 4 factors (X, S, P', P) change.

Age 3 and Up

For a comprehensive modeling (for age 3 and up), the corneal and lens power may be assumed to be constants (or having a neglectible change); therefore, the De value at any age A is mainly governed by the growth of S and X (or axial length L=S+X). Based on Lin's double-rate theory, it is given by:

$$De = Do - \int (m1)N1dA - \int (m2)N2dA, \quad (1.a)$$

$$= Do\text{-}G1\text{-}G2. \quad (1.b)$$

$$m2 = Pt^2/1336, \quad (1.c)$$

$$m1 = P'^2/1336, \quad (1.d)$$

where the change rates due to the growth of S and X given by m1 and m2 are defined by m1=–dDe/dS and m2=–dDe/dX; N1=dS/dA, N2=dX/dA are the age growth rates of the effective anterior and posterior chamber, which define the axial length change dL=dS+dX. The initial refractive Do is defined at the age when the pediatric cataract/IOL surgery is conducted. The total power Pt = P′ + ZP.

It should be noted that m2 in general is larger than m1 related by

$$m2 = (Pt/P')^2(m1), \quad (2)$$

that is, square ratio of the total power (Pt) and cornea power (P′) which has the stable state typical ratio about $(60/43)^2$=1.95 that is, m2 is about twice of m1. However, at the early stage, this ratio is higher due to the high Pt (about 70 diopter). In general, m2 and m1 are age dependent to be shown later. Furthermore, for typical growth rates of N1=0.2N2, one may approximate that dS=0.2dX during the infant stage (A<3 years) and dS=0 after age 3.

By further assuming typical stable corneal power P′=43 diopter and lens power P=21 diopter, one may calculate m1=1.39 (D/mm) and m2=2.7 (D/mm) and the power change due to dS and dX in Eq.(1) for age change from Ao to A is calculated as follows:

$$G1 = 1.39\,(N1)(A\text{-}Ao), \quad (3.a)$$

$$G2 = 2.7\,(N2)(A\text{-}Ao), \quad (3.b)$$

supposing that m1, m2, N1 and N2 are constant rates in a linear growth theory.

Age 0 to 3

For aphakic eyes, the age dependent natural lens (P), or its change dP, and axial length (L) had been reported.[6] By further assuming the corneal power change (dP′) from 45 D (at A=0) to 43 D (at A=3), one may obtain the age dependence for the total power (Pt) and the correspondent m2 values which further allow us to calculate the age dependent refractive power change dDe=De-Do given by

$$dDe = -m2(dL) + dP' + B(dP) \quad (4)$$

Example of age-dependent ocular parameters is shown as follow (for age 0 to 6 year):

A	0	0.5	1.0	2.0	3.0	6.0
P	35	31	28	26	24	22
Pt	73	69	66	64	60	60
m2	4.0	3.6	3.3	3.1	2.9	2.7
L	17	19	20.5	21.5	22.5	23.5
dDe	0	–4.9	–6.7	–7.6	–9.4	–11.0

The units of above: A (in year), L (in mm), P, Pt and dDe (in diopters)

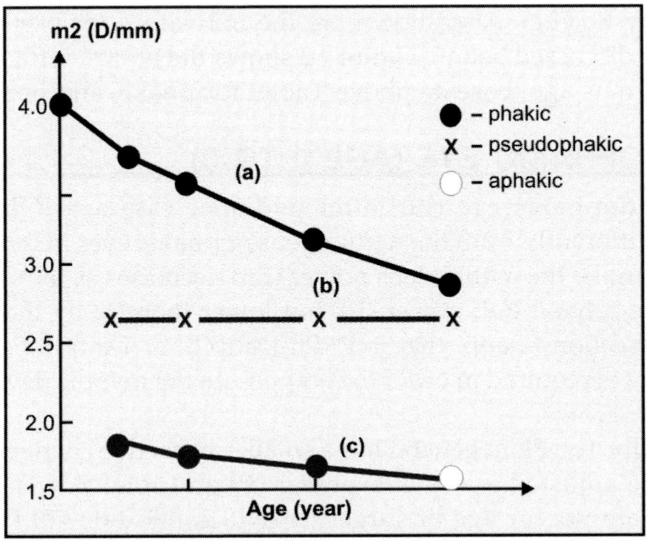

Fig. 9.1: The refractive rate function (m2) for: (a) typical phakic eyes (age 0 to 3 years); (b) pseudophakic pediatric eye after cataract/ IOL surgery at age Ao=(0.5, 1, 2, 3) years; and (c) aphakic with the natural lens removed

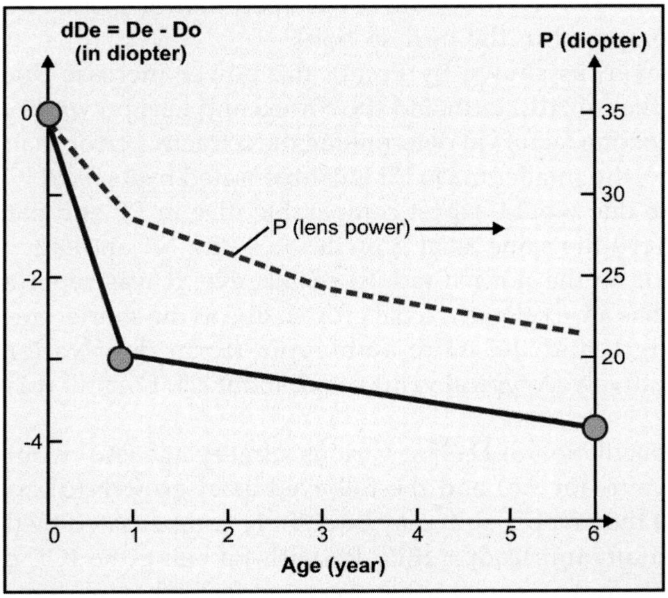

Fig. 9.2: The refractive power change (dDe) for a normal phakic eye governed by the competing between the axial growth and the decrease of the natural lens power (P) and corneal power

In above Table, I had used B=0.65 as a typical conversion for the lens power change. The age-dependence of m2 are shown in Figure 9.1, where the decrease of m2 is the result of total power decrease defined by Eq.(1.c). Also shown are the m2 values for pseudophakic eyes to be discussed below. Figure 9.2 shows the typical refractive error change versus age (base on above Table) for phakic and normal eyes.

PSEUDOPHAKIC EYE (AGE 0 TO 3)

The pseudophakic eye (PE) after pediatric cataract/IOL surgery behaves differently from the natural lens of phakic eyes in two aspects:

First, unlike the natural lens power (Pn) decreases as the eye grows, the PE has a fixed IOL power (P), but lower than Pn by the adjusted under-correction (Dadj), that is P=Pn-Dadj/B, or Dadj=B(Pn-P). This adjustment is required in order to compensate the myopic development as the eye grows.

Secondly, the PE in general has a smaller refractive change rate (m2) due to the adjusted lower IOL power (P) and total power (Pt).

For example, for age of surgery Ao=(0.2, 0.5, 1.0, 3.0) (year) and the adjusted power of Dadj=(+9, +7, +6, +4) D, respectively, one may calculate the total power Pt = 60 D and the corresponding rates, by Eq.(1.c), m2 = 2.7 (D/mm), which are higher than the values of aphakic eye (1.38 to 1.7) (D/mm), but lower than that of phakic normal eye (to be compared in the next section).

However, as shown by Eq.(4), the power increase due to axial growth, the (m2 dL) term and the cornea and lens power decrease are two competing factors in determining the refractive error change (dDe). Therefore, the smaller m2 in PE is compensated by its fixed IOL power. Therefore one would expect comparable dDe in PE and natural eyes if they have the same axial growth rates (the N1 and N2 values). In comparing to the normal (adult) phakic eye, it was reported [3,4] that aphakia has an accelerated axial growth due to the shorter preoperative axial length and the more amblyopia (form deprivation effects) postoperatively. A typical value of m2 about 2.5 (D/mm) was reported in PE.

The calculation of Dadj at various surgery age (Ao) would require the m2 value (at Ao) and the followed axial growth (dL, or dX+dS) such that the myopia-shift may be entirely compensated by the under-corrected amount Dadj = B(Po-P), with Po being the IOL power for plano (at age Ao), and B is a conversion factor having typical values of B=0.7 and 0.816 for S=5.0 and 3.0 mm, respectively.

THE LIN'S DOUBLE RATE THEORY (M AND N)

If one ignores the growth of anterior chamber (dS) and assumes that the posterior vitreous is the dominant factor for axial growth, or dL=dX, the Lin's double rate theory becomes dDe/dA = –MN, with M = –dDe/

dL and N = dL/dA. The total power (Pt) of normal phakic eye is about (depending on age) 60 (adult) to 72 (infant) diopter, whereas aphakic eye Pt = P′ (corneal power) = (43 to 45) D since the natural lens is removed and P=0. Pseudophakic eye (after the under-correction adjustment) has a typical Pt about 58 D, therefore, it has a lower M than that of normal (phakic) eye, but higher than aphakia. However, it was known that the aphakia has larger axial growth rate (N) than normal eye and pseudophakia due to its more amblyopia form deprivation which acclerates the axial growth. Therefore, the net "refractive growth" (dDe) governed by (MN) is still faster in aphakia than pseudophakia or phakia, in which dDe is partially reduced by the nature lens power decrease.

Comparisons of M and N are shown as follows in which M is calculated by Eq.(1.c) with Pt = P′ + ZP, where P=0 (in aphakia) and the Pt of pseudophakia is adjusted for under-correction IOL-power. For phakia, dDe is revised to dDe=-(MN)dA + B(dP) where dP is the lens power increase and B is a conversion factor.

	Phakia (normal eye)	*Pseudo-phakia**	*Aphakia*
Age (year)	0-5	0-5	0-5
Pt (diopter)	72-60	about 58	45-43
M (D.mm)	3.9-2.7	about 2.5	1.7-1.4
N (mm/year)	4.0-0.2	3.0-0.2	4.0-2.0
dDe (diopter)	–2.0 to –4.0	–3.0 to –12.0	–8.0 to –12.0
P (lens)	35-20	about 20*	0

* Pseudophakic IOL power adjusted (under-corrected) for a stable total power (Pt) to compensate the myopia progress due to axial growth

Definitions

M: Refractive change (decrease) per 1.0 mm growth of axial length (D/mm)

N: Axial growth per year (mm/year)

dDe: Refractive change due to emmetropization.

CUSTOMIZED IOL POWER

As discussed earlier, the refractive error (De) is governed by the product of (m1N1) and (m2N2), or by both of the refractive rate function (mj) and the axial length growth rates (Nj) which must be personalized, particularly for those eyes having the (mjNj) values deviating too much from the typical values of m1=0.5 m2, N1=0.2 N2, and m2=2.7 (D/mm), N2=0.3 (mm/year).

As illustrated in Figure 9.3, the Lin's double rate growth theory provides two situations (a) for fixed Nj, higher mj develops higher

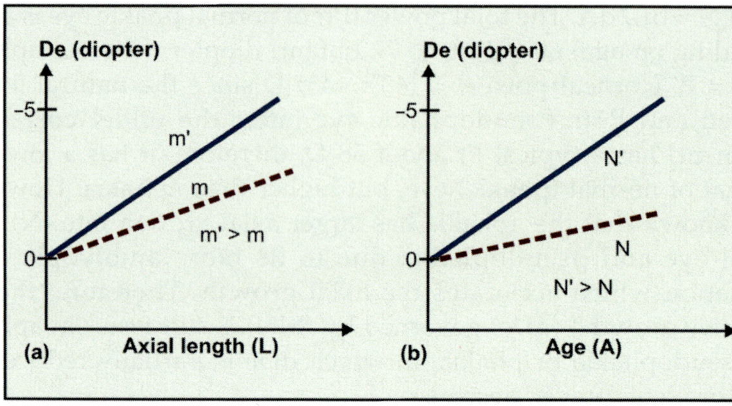

Fig. 9.3: Myopia power (De) progress versus age (A) in Lin's double rate theory for two cases: (a) fixed axial growth rate N=dL/dA (mm/year), comparing high and low. m = –dDe/dL (diopter/mm); (b) fixed m, and comparing high and low N.

myopia progress; and (b) for fixed mj, higher Nj results higher myopia. Therefore, the adjusted under-corrected IOL power, P=Po-Dadj, should be customized accordingly, where Po is the IOL power for emmetropia.

For example, for different vitreous cavity length X=(16, 18, 20) mm, one may use the emmetropic-state condition Pt=1336/(X/Z) to find m2=(3.4, 2.7, 2.2) (D/mm), respectively, for a typical value of Z=0.806. Therefore, for given axial growth rates of N1 and N2, short vitreous cavity eyes (or smaller X) having a higher (about 25%) m2 values would suffer greater myopia. In comparison, longer X (or L, say X=20 mm) having a smaller m2 would have a narrower range of myopia progress and can be easily adjusted. Furthermore, as shown in Figure 9.1 and Eq. (1.c), m2 is proportional to the square of the total power Pt, or the implanted IOL power which is age (Ao) dependent.

On the other hand, for a fixed mj rates, the higher Nj rates (with N2>0.4 mm/yr) would also suffer greater myopia and more difficult to be adjusted. Therefore, a true customized IOL power should be adjusted not just by the age of surgery (Ao) (proposed by Wilson et al [5]), but also by the individual rates (mj)(Nj), to be discussed further.

The Adjusted IOL Power

The age-adjusted De of Wilson et al is shown in Table 9.1 for various age when the cataract surgery is performed (Ao).

Table 9.1: The adjusted mean power (Wilson et al, 2005) at age of surgery (Ao)

Ao (year)	0.1	0.2	0.4	1-2	2-4	4	5	6	7-10	10-14	>14
Dadj (Wilson)	+12	+9	+8	+6	+5	+4	+3	+2	+15-1.0	+0.5	plano

According to Lin's formula, Dadj = B(Po-P), with Po being the IOL-power for plano (at age Ao), and B is a conversion factor having typical values of B=0.7 and 0.816 for S=5.0 and 3.0 mm, respectively.

According to Lin's double rate theory, the above mean Dadj should be further revised by 5% to 15% lower or higher for lower mN and higher mN which should be estimated pre-operatively. The new adjusted De should count for (mN) value deviating up to 50% of the mean (typical) values of (m2N2)=2.7 x 0.3 = 0.8 (D/year) and (m1N1)=1.39 x 0.03 = 0.03 (D/year), for dS=0.1dX, or N1=0.1N2 (for age 0 to 3) and dS=0 (for age 3 and up).

It was reported by Vasavada for the rate of axial growth after congenital cataract surgery [5] depends on the age at surgery (Ao). The 5-year average growth of axial length (dL) is reported as: dL=4.04 mm (for Ao<1 year); 1.07 mm (for Ao=1 to 3 years); 0.97 mm (for Ao=3 to 10 years).

In above examples, the mean N2=(4.0, 1.0, 0.3) (mm/yr), respectively, for various As ranges if one ignores the contribution from N1. Therefore, the corresponding myopia induced due to dL is given by De= –M(dL)= –(9.0, 4.0, 1.5) diopter, respectively, for a mean M=2.8 (D/mm), where M=m2 when dL=dX (with dS=0).Based on these data, the IOL power should be adjusted by –De to compensate the myopic-shift after cataract/IOL. These reported values, however, are only good for average over the studied subjects. For individual eyes, these adjustment should also consider the personalized values of M and N. It should be noted that M (or m2) is proportional to the square of the total power of the pseudophakic which decreases by age as shown in Figure 9.1.

ADJUSTED FACTORS

Depending on the environment factors such as nearwork of the patient, the personalized Dadj for teenagers (A=10 to 18) may be pre-estimated based on the historical values for age between 10 and 12 years. In other words, the above Table for Dadj (for age 6 to 14) should be further adjusted for eyes with abnormal axial growth rate due to nearwork.

Other factors impacting the Dadj are summarized as follows (see also Fig. 9.4):

a. Genetic factor: Abnormal axial growth rate of (N1, N2) may occur for children having myopic parent (one or both). Greater Dadj than the mean value shown in Table 9.1 are needed.
b. IOL power (Po) for emmetropia at surgery age (Ao): For the same age child but having different Po, a higher Po would result in higher value of m2, as shown by Eq. (1.c). Therefore, the myopic progress would be more for the same axial growth rate (N). The mean Dadj in Table 9.1 should be revised based on the following (Fig. 9.5).

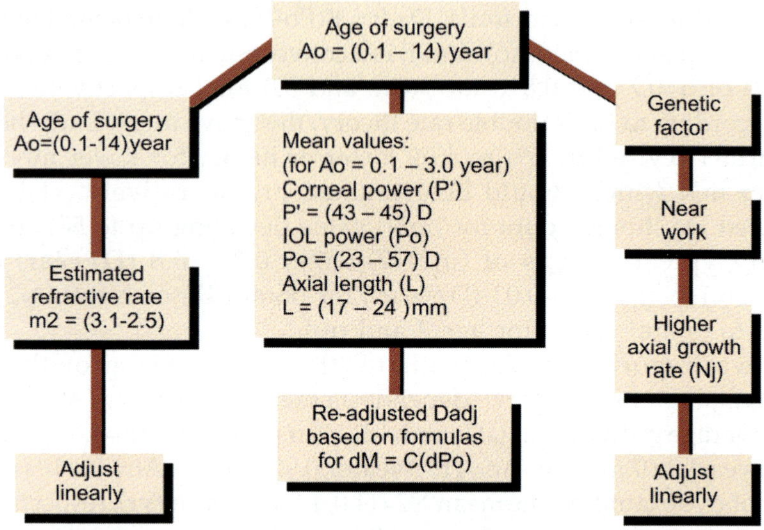

Fig. 9.4: Flow chart of factors for the adjusted IOL power calculation (Dadj) shown in Table 9.1 (see also text)

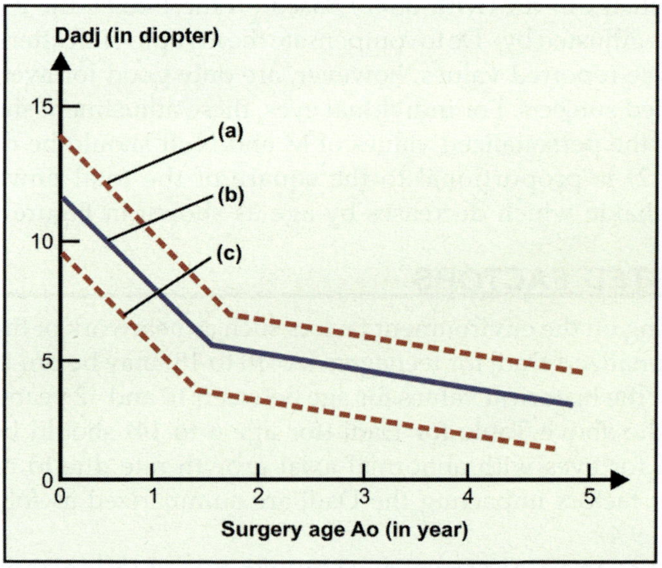

Fig. 9.5: The adjusted IOL power (Dadj) versus cataract surgery age (Ao) for emmetropic IOL power (Po) being higher than equal to, or lower than the mean value, shown by curve (a), (b) and (c), respectively

For a posterior implanted IOL (with S=5.0 mm), the typical parameters for (L, X, P', Po) meeting the emmetropic condition are shown as follows:

A (year)	L	X	P'	Po
0	17	12	45	57
1-2	19	14	44	43
3-6	21	16	43	32
>10	24	19	43	23

For individual ocular parameters (or IOL power needed for emmetropia) deviated from the above "mean" values, the adjustment of Dadj may be calculated based on the following situations.

a. For same P′, but different Po due to different X:

$$dM = (2Z^2/X)(dPo) = C(dPo), \quad (5.a)$$
$$dPo = Po'\text{-}Po, \quad (5.b)$$

which gives C = (0.07-0.12) for A = (0-14) year (for S=5.0 mm, Z=0.7). For example, for Po changes from 40 to 50 D, a change of dM=(0.7-1.2) (D/mm) corresponding to the increase of about (1.0-1.8) D of Dadj is needed, (for axial growth (dl) of 1.5 mm).

b. For same X, but Po changes due to different P′:

$$dM = -(2ZS/X2)(dP') = C'(dP'), \quad (6)$$

which gives C′ = (0.02-0.06) for A = (0-14) years. For example, corneal power change of dP′ = B(dPo) = 8.4 D, for IOL power change of dPo=10 D, and dM=(0.17-0.5), or dDadj=(0.26-0.8) D is needed (for dl=1.5 mm) which is less sensitive to case (i).

c. Corneal power (P′): The role of P′ on m2 is calculated as follows: (for fixed IOL power, P=30 D), m2=(3, 3.46, 3.9), for P′=(39, 43, 47). That is, a change of 10% of P′ results in about 12% to 13% change of m2.

d. Implant position of IOL. The IOL power for emmetropia (Po) is governed by the effective anterior chamber depth (S), axial length (L) and corneal power (P′) by

$$Po = 1336\ /\ (L\text{-}S)\text{-}1336\ /\ (1336/P'\text{-}S). \quad (7)$$

For example, L=23 mm and P′=43 D, Po=(19, 23) D, respectively, for anterior implanted IOL (such as in the ciliary suleus) with S=3.0 mm, and for posterior IOL (in lens capsular bag) with S=5.0 mm. Therefore, the m2 value is about 46% higher in posterior IOL which also requires a higher Dadj accordingly.

e. Secondary IOL power, P(2), may be calculated by a new formula of Lin which does not require the knowledge of axial length and is given by

$$P(2)=(Ppre\text{-}P'')/B, \quad (8)$$

where Ppre is the pre-IOL refractive error and P″ is the residual error, B is a conversion factor given by $B=Z^2$, with Z=1-S(P′/1336), P′ being the corneal power. For example, for P′=43 D, B=(0.82, 0.7), for S=(3, 5) mm, respectively, depending on the secondary IOL position.

f. For early age stage (0 to about 2 year), the rate function of the anterior chamber depth (m1) is proportional to the corneal power square, shown by Eq.(1.d). Therefore, steeper cornea results in a higher myopic progress due to the growth of S, the same trend as that of steep lens (or higher IOL-power), and a higher Dadj is needed. Figure 9.4 summarizes the above adjustment factors for revised Dadj accordingly.

Comparing to the Wilson's Dadj (which is only valid for average population), the Dadj (new) of Lin is customized based on the estimated preoperative rates functions m and N which, in general, are age dependent.

CONCLUSION

The myopic-shift after pediatric cataract surgery may be compensated by a new adjusted IOL power which is age-dependent and governed by rate functions (mj and Nj, with j=1,2). In comparison to the mean-value method of Wilson et al, the Lin's new Dadj is personalized by the measured (or estimated) pre-operative mj and Nj which may deviate from their mean (typical) values. Greater details for the discussion of Lin's double rate theory was published elsewhere.[2]

REFERENCES

1. Lin JT, The new IOL formulas based on Gaussian optics. In Garg A and Lin JT (Ed), Mastering IOLs: Principles and Innovations. New Delhi: Jaypee Brothers, 2006:Chapter 6; 56-65.
2. Lin JT. Analysis of refractive state ratios and the onset of myopia. Ophthal Physiol Opt 2006;26:97-105.
3. Wilson ME, Trivedi RH. Eye growth after pediatric cataract surgery. Am J Ophthalmol. 2004;38:1039-1040.
4. Trivedi RH, Wilson ME. Intraocular lens power calculation for children. In Garg A et al, (ed); Mastering the Techniques of IOL Power Calculations. Jaypee Brothers: New Delhi, 2005; 98-108.
5. Vasavada AR, Raj SM, Nihalani B. Rate of axial growth after congenital cataract surgery. Am J Ophthalmol. 2004;138:915-24.
6. Gordon LA, Donzis PB. Refractive development of the human eye. Arch Ophthalmol 1985;103:785-9.

CHAPTER

10

JT Lin (USA)

The Mathematical Handbook for IOLs

INTRODUCTION

The classical[1] formula based on 2-optics aphakic eye has been used for decades without revision. Phakic and piggyback IOLs are 3-optics system and should not be treated as 2-optics system which totally ignores the impact of the natural lens or the primary IOL. Furthermore, the existing formulas of Holladay[2] show the 1-for-1 for minus spectacle converted to IOL power and the 1.5-for-1 for plus spectacle. The new formulas of this Chapter will demonstrate that Holladay's formulas are valid only for certain spectacle powers and cannot apply to all IOL power ranges. Accommodative IOLs could be 2-optics or 3-optics system depending on if the natural lens is absent or not. For dual-optics IOL implanted in aphakic eye, the system is 3-optics. Figure 10.1 shows various configurations in both 2-optics and 3-optics (Table 10.1).

In this Chapter, the mathematical formulas and examples for the following areas would be covered:

- Gaussian optics for IOL in aphakic eye (a simple 2-optics system)
- IOL in phakic eye (a 3-optics system)
- Piggyback IOL Power in 3-optics system
- New formulas converting spectacle power to IOL power
- Design of aspherical IOLs
- Age-dependent IOL for pediatric eyes.

Table 10.1: Corneal power (Dc) calculation after refractive surgery

(1) Clinical-history method	Dc = Kpre-RC, RC = refractive correction of LASIK
(2) Contact lens method	Dc = B+P+Rw-Rno B = base curve; P = power of CL Rw = refractive error; Rno = bare refraction
(3) Shammas method	Dc = 1.114 Kpost – 6.8
(4) Maloney topography method	Dc = 1.114 Ktopo – 5.5
(5) Koch method	Dc = 1.114 Ktopo – 6.1
(6) Shammas refraction method	Dc = (1.114 Kpost – 6.8) – 0.23 (RC)
(7) Hoffer mean-value method	Dc = 337.5 (1/r1 + 1/r2)/2
(8) Lin gaussian-optics (I)	Dc = 1.117 Kpost – 41/r2
(II)	Dc = (377/r1)[1 – 0.109 (r1/r2)]

where:
r1 = cornea front surface radius (postop)
r2 = cornea back surface radius (postop)
Kpost = postoperative keratometry
Kpre = preoperative keratometry

IOL POWER IN APHAKIA (2-OPTICS)

The IOL power (P) required to correct refractive error of an aphakic eye (2-optic system) after cataract surgery (Table 10.2).

$$P = 1336(1/X - 1/Y) - qDe, \quad (1.a)$$

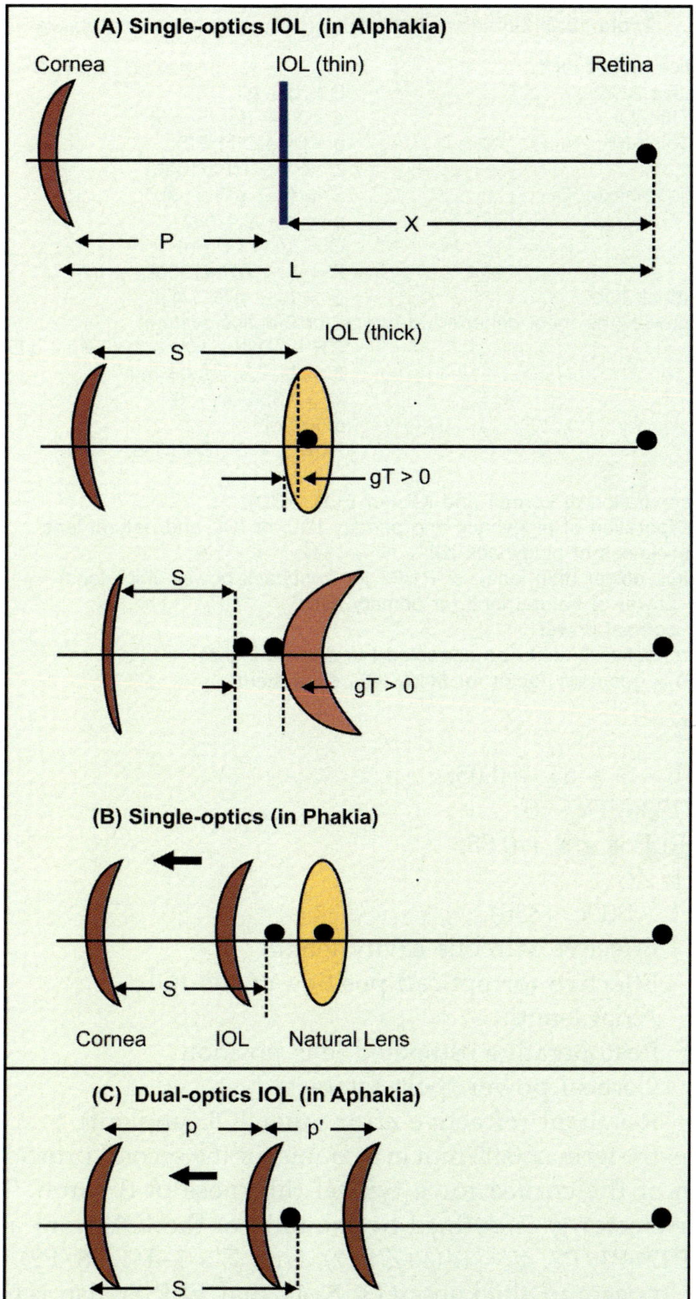

Fig. 10.1: Schematics of single-optics and dual-optics AIOL in aphakic and phakic eye

Table 10.2: Lin's formula for IOL power in aphakia and phakia

(A) 2-optics aphakia/IOL	
Effective ACD:	S = d + gT
Thin-IOL:	d = ELP (for T = 0)
Thick-IOL:	g =1/(1+Z"P1/P2)
	Z" = 1 – T(P2/1336)
(B) 3-optics phakia/IOL	S' = (d + gT) + Gp'
	p' = p + 2.4 mm
	G = 1/(1+Z'P/Pn)
	Z' = 1 - p'(Pn/1336)
(C) piggyback IOL	S' = (d + gT) + g'p'
(D) IOL power (the most generalized format for 3-optics system)	
	Z'P = 1336 [1/X' – 1/Y']-Pn - q'E
	X' = L – S – 0.05 mm
	Y' = 1336/Dc – S
	$q' = 1Z1^2$
	Z1 = 1 – S' (Dc/1336)

where:

d = separation of cornea and IOL (or ELP, ACD).
p = separation of piggyback and primary IOL, or IOL and natural lens
T = thickness of piggyback IOL
P = IOL power (thin lens), or P1/P2 for front/back power (thick lens)
Pn = power of natural lens (or primary IOL)
Dc = corneal power
E = refractive error to be corrected (on corneal plane)
(g, G) = geometry factor for (thick IOL, subsystem)

$$X = L - S + aT + 0.05, \quad (1.b)$$
$$Y = 1336/Dc - S, \quad (1.c)$$
$$S = ELP + g'T + 0.05, \quad (1.d)$$
$$q = 1/Z^2, \quad (1.e)$$
$$Z = 1 - S(Dc/1336). \quad (1.f)$$

X: Effective vitreous cavity length
S: Effective (or optical) position of the IOL
L: Axial length
ELP: Postoperative estimated lens position
Dc: Corneal power (post-cataract)
De: Resultant refractive error (after IOL implant).

The extra-term of 0.05 mm in S counts for the second principal plane position of the cornea for a typical thickness of 0.5 mm. The IOL geometry factor g′ is defined by the ratio of the IOL front and back power P12=P1/P2, g′ = 1/(1+Z′P12), with Z′= 1–T(1336/P2) to count for IOL types and thickness (T). Note that ELP is also referred as anterior chamber depth (ACD) which is defined, in this Chapter, as the distance between the front vertex surface of the cornea and the IOL: another small term in X, aT (with a=0.045) may be ignored for typical T<1.0 mm.

The above new formula reduces to the existing formula under the following special cases.

a. Reduced to Colenbrander formula when De=0 (emmetropic state) and when S=ELP=constant, ignoring the IOL configuration (g'T=0).
b. Reduced to Hoffer formula when S=ELP=constant.
c. Reduced to Haigis formula when g'T=0.

CONVERSION FUNCTION

The conversion function (CF) defines the ratio of system refractive error change and IOL power change, CF=dDe/dP, may be derived by taking the derivative of Eq. (1) to obtain

$$CF = (1+kdP)Z^2, \quad (2.a)$$
$$Z = 1 - S(Dc/1336), \quad (2.b)$$

where k=S/1336 is a nonlinear term. For corneal power Dc=43 diopter and ignoring the nonlinear term d(dP), CF vs. S is shown below.

S (mm)	2.0	3.0	4.0	5.0	6.0
CF(%)	87.6	81.6	75.9	70.4	65.1

Above example shows that IOL implanted anteriorly (with S=3.0 mm) is more efficient than that of posterior IOL (with S=5.0 mm).

Conversion to Spectacle Power

Conversion function between the spectacle power (Ds) and power on the corneal plane (Dc) defined by

$$CFs = Ds/Dc$$
$$= 1 - V(Ds/1000), \quad (3.a)$$
$$Dc = Ds/(1\text{-}0.012Ds), \quad (3.b)$$

For typical vertex V=12 mm, one may calculate CFs at various spectacle powers as follows.

a. plus-power

Ds	+5	+10	+15	+20
CFs(%)	94	98	82	76

b. minus-power

Ds	-5	–10	–15	–20
CF(%)	106	112	118	124

IOL Power (P) vs Spectacle Power (Ds)

The combined conversion function defined by the ratio of

$$TF = P/Ds = 1/[Dc/P)(Ds/Dc)] \\ = 1/[(CF)(CFs)] \quad (4)$$

Examples are shown as follows:

a. For anterior IOL (with S=3.0 mm), CF=81.6%

Ds(+/–)	5	10	15	20
TF(+)	130	139	149	161%
TF(–)	116	109	104	99%

b. For posterior IOL (S=5.0 mm), CF=70.4%

Ds(+/–)	5	10	15	20
TF(+)	151	161	173	187%
TF(–)	134	127	120	115%

c. For posterior IOL (S=6.0 mm), CF=65.1%

Ds(+/–)	5	10	15	20
TF(+)	163	174	187	202%
TF(–)	145	137	130	124%

THREE-OPTICS IOL SYSTEM

The earlier formulas for 2-optics system are only good for aphakic eye with the absence of natural lens. For phakic eye and piggyback IOL 3-optics systems involved two major factors must be included in the new formula: (i) the shifted effective ACD, S=p+gd′, and (ii) the shifted vitreous cavity length X′=X-gd′, due to the separation (d) between the IOL and the natural lens, or piggyback and primary IOL.

Phakic IOL

For IOL implanted in phakic eye (3-optics system, Lin, 2006)

$$Z'P = 1336(1/X' - 1/Y') - P2, \quad (5)$$
$$X' = X - gd'$$
$$Y' = 1336/Dc - S$$
$$S = p + gd'$$
$$g = 1 / [1+Z' (P/P2)]$$
$$Z' = 1 - d'(P2/1336),$$

where Dc and P2 are the EFL of the cornea and the natural lens (NL) which separate with the IOL (power P) by a distance of p and d, respectively. Above 3-optics formula reduces to that of 2-optics under the limiting case of when (i) P2=0 (absence of NL), or (ii) d′=0, such that Z′=1 and Z1=Z.

Table 10.3: Piggyback IOL power (P) formulas for residual ametropia error

(1) Sanders and Kraff (1980) based on empirical data of over 2500 IOL lens	P = E/0.67=1.49 E
(2) Feiz and Mannis (2001)	P = E/0.7 = 1.43E
(3) Holladay II (1993) based on Hoffer (1981), Colenbrander (1973)	P = (IOL)1- (IOL)2 (IOL)j = 1336/[1336/Kj-ELP] Kj (j=1,2), for pre- and postop corneal power
for plus IOL,	P(+) =1.5E,
for minus IOL,	P(–) = 1.0E;
E is the postop refractive error at spectacle plane.	
(4) Shammas (2001) where a = 0.03 for plus IOL, a = 0.04 for minus IOL. A = A-constant = (ACD+63.896)/0.5836	P = (E/a)/(138.3-A)-0.5
(5) Gills (1996) only for hyperopic correction	P(+) =1.4E+1.0
(6) Lin (2006) The Z^2-formula (3-optics)* for both plus and minus IOL.	P = Ec/(CF) = (1.3 to 1.6) Ec CF = (1-kE)(Ec/Z) [$(1-B)^2$ + C']Z^2 Z =1-S(Dc/1336) B = 1-d'(Pn/1336) Typical value: CF = (0.65 to -0.75)

* For simplified 2-optics system, d'=0 and B=1.
where:
Dc is the corneal power and k is a nonlinear term (k about 0.03).
S is the effective (optical) lens position, S=ELP+gT+ Gp'
E(Ec) is the refractive error on the spectacle (corneal) plane and may be related by another conversion factor Ec=E/Zs^2, with Zs=1-0.012E

Piggyback IOL

Analytic format of Eq.(5) (within 2% accuracy comparing to the exact numerical solution) for the piggyback IOL power (required for emmetropia)

$$P = (Po + C)/(1 - A)^2, \quad (6)$$
$$C = [(2Dc/Z)/(1\text{-}A) + P2]B,$$
$$B = d'(P2/1336),$$
$$A = DcB/(ZPt)$$
$$Pt = Z'P + P2$$
$$Z = 1\text{-}p(Dc/1336)$$

where Dc is the corneal power, P2 is the primary IOL power; Po is the piggyback IOL power for 2-optics limit, or when d'=0, that is, the 3-optics formula P reduces to the 2-optics value Po when the piggyback IOL is virtually contacted to the primary IOL (Table 10.3).

Conversion Function (CF)

To correct a refractive error (on corneal plane) of De, the piggyback IOL power may also be calculated by the 3-optics conversion function (CF)

$$CF' = (dDe/dP) = [(1-B)^2 + C']Z^2 \quad (7.a)$$
$$C' = 2Z'[A/(1-A)]^2 \quad (7.b)$$

which may be combined with the spectacle power conversion function CFs=1-0.012Ds to obtain the TF'=(P/Ds)=1/(CF')(CFs), similar to that of 2-optics, noting that CF'(3-optics) reduces to CF(2-optics)=Z^2 when d'=0, or B=C'=0.

Example 1

For 3 cases (a), (b), (c) of d'=1.0, 2.0 and 3.0 mm, respectively, are shown as follows (for Pc=43 diopter):

DS		–5	–10	–15	+5	+10	+15
CFS		1.06	1.12	1.18	0.94	0.88	0.82
TF'	(A)	1.38	1.30	1.24	1.55	1.66	1.78
	(B)	1.26	1.20	1.14	1.48	1.58	1.70
	(C)	1.18	1.12	0.81	1.37	1.47	1.57

Results of above are shown in Figure 10.4. It shows that at the Holladay formulas

TF(–)=100% is a mean value good for d'=3.0 mm and Ds=-15 D (with mean

CF'=0.8); and TF(+)=150% good for d'=3.0 mm and Ds=+15 D.

Example 2

For P2=20 diopter, P may be calculated for given Po (in the above 3 cases of d'=(1.0, 2.0, 3.0) mm

Po		–5	–10	+5	+10
P	(a)	–3.3	–8.4	+ 7.1	+12.2
	(b)	–1.5	–6.9	+ 9.1	+14.4
	(c)	–0.2	–5.3	+11.2	+16.7

The difference Delta = P–Po are shown in Figures 10.2 and 10.3.

Note that the case (c) with d'=p=3.0 mm also applies to phakic-IOL where the primary IOL becomes natural lens (Fig. 10.4 and Table 10.4).

ACCOMMODATIVE IOL

Accommodating IOLs (AIOL) including single-optics and two-optics configurations have been designed and analyzed by many researchers.[1-11] The accommodation rate (M) defined by the accommodation amplitude per 1.0 mm of the IOL axial movement has been studied both analytically

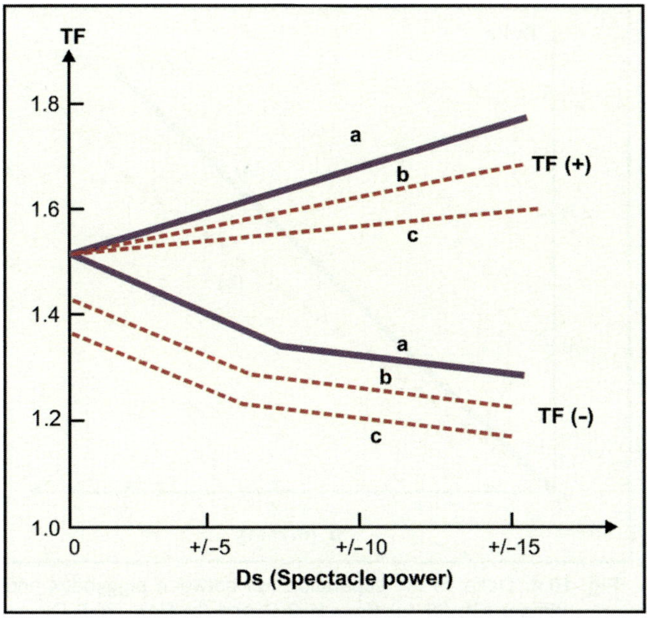

Fig. 10.2: The conversion function (CF) for plus and minus IOL in 3-optics system for 3 cases: (a) d'=1.0, (b) d'=2.0, (c) d'=3.0

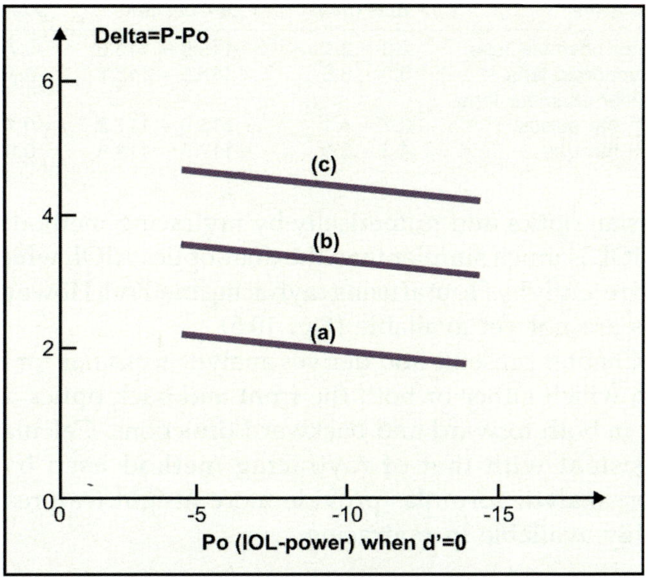

Fig. 10.3: The power difference Delta=P–Po, where 3-optics IOL power (P) is higher than 2-optics (Po)

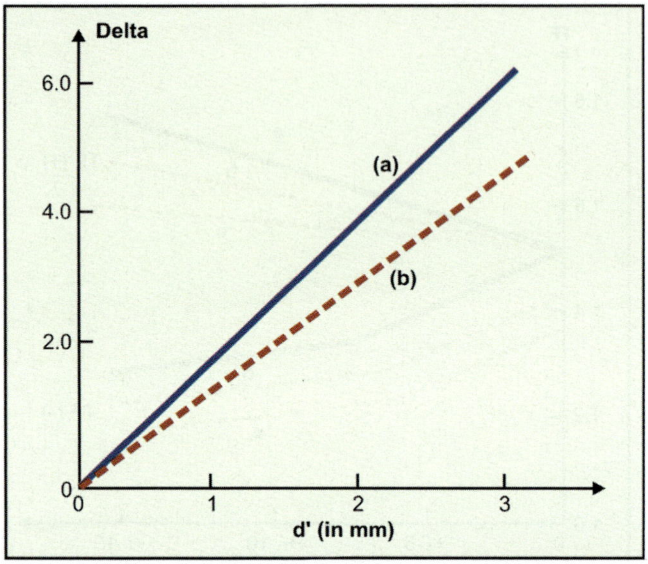

Fig. 10.4: Delta vs the separation (d') between piggyback and primary IOL for (a) Po=+10.0 D and (b) Po=−10.0 D

Table 10.4: Typical values of ELP, A-constant and surgeon's factor (s) for different IOL implants

IOL Implant	*ELP (mm)*	*A-Constant*	*s-factor*
Anterior chamber lens	2.8 – 3.1	115.0 – 115.3	–0.7 to –0.4
Iris-supported lens	3.3 – 3.5	115.5 – 115.7	–0.1 to +0.1
Posterior chamber lens			
in the sulcus	3.7 – 4.1	115.9 – 117.2	+0.1 to +0.7
in the bag	4.3 – 5.1	117.5 – 118.8	+0.9 to +1.6

by Gaussian optics and numerically by raytracing method.[2,3,5] Single-optics AIOL is much simpler than the dual-optics AIOL which has been analyzed recently by Ho et al using raytracing method. However, analytic formulas are not yet available (Fig. 10.5).

This Chapter presents and derives analytic formulas for dual-optics AIOL, in which either or both the front and back optics are allowed to move in both forward and backward directions. Calculated results are consistent with that of raytracing method used by Ho et al. However, analytic formulas provide more insight features which are not readily available in raytracing.

Two-optics Formulas (Lin, 2005)

The accommodation amplitude (A)

$$A = M(dS), \quad (8.a)$$

$$M = (Z^2P)(2/X - P/1336), \quad (8.b)$$

$$Z = 1 - S(Dc/1336), \quad (8.c)$$

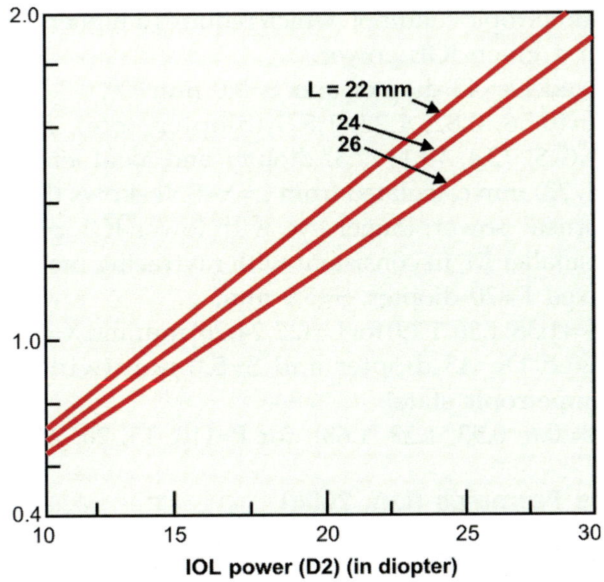

Fig. 10.5: Accommodation rate M (per 1.0 mm of forward movement) versus IOL power at various axial length L=(22, 24, 26) mm

where the rate function M (in diopter/mm) is governed by four parameters the corneal power Dc, the IOL power P, X and S as defined earlier. Note that A>0 (for near vision accommodation) when dS>0 defined by a movement toward the cornea. The values of M ranging (0.5 to 1.9) depends on ocular conditions. Examples are shown as follows:

Case (1): Fixed X=18.8 mm and S=5.0 mm, (or L=X+S=23.8 mm). M = (1.1, 1.29, 1.45, 1.62) (diopter/mm) for corneal power of Dc = (45, 43, 41, 39) diopter and the required IOL power for emmetropia P=(17, 20, 22.4, 25.6) diopter. It shows that higher IOL power, in general, produces higher accommodation for a given amount of anterior movement (dS).

Case (2): Fixed corneal power Dc=43 diopter and axial length L=23.8 mm.
M = (1.08, 1.14, 1.2, 1.29, 1.36) (diopter/mm), for S=(2.0, 3.0, 4.0, 5.0, 6.0) mm. It shows that M is an increasing function of the IOL position, where X decreases when S increases for a fixed axial length L=X+S.

Case (3): Fixed IOL power P=20 diopter and L=23.8 mm.
M=(1.36, 1.34, 1.32, 1.29, 1.25) (diopter/mm), for S=(2, 3, 4, 5, 6) mm.
The decrease of M for larger S is the net result of the competing factors from the decrease of X=L–S, and the

emmetropic condition which requires a higher corneal power for a given IOL power.

Case (4): Fixed Dc=43 diopter and S=5.0 mm
M=(0.56, 0.82, 1.22, 1.87) (diopter/mm), for IOLpower P=(9.5, 12.4, 19.1, 27.3) diopter and axial length L=(27, 26, 24, 22) mm calculated from L=X+S. It shows that, for a given corneal power, longer eye with lower IOL power result in a smaller M, in consistent with raytracing method of Nawa.

Case (5): Fixed P=20 diopter, S=5.0 mm.
M=(1.38, 1.26, 1.19) for L=(22, 24, 26) mm and X=(17, 19, 21) mm.

Case (6): Fixed Dc=43 diopter and S=5.0 mm (with L varies for emmetropic state).
M=(0.6, 0.93, 1.29, 1.68), for P=(10, 15, 20, 25) diopters.

Three-optics Formulas (Lin, 2006)

Mobile Front-optics Case

As shown in Figure 10.6, a doublet IOL (dual-optics) consists of 2 optics separated by p′, where the front optic separates from the corneal vertex surface by a distance p.

$$M = Z\,(D_1/1336)(2Dc+ZD_1)\text{- Delta}, \quad (9.a)$$
$$\text{Delta} = Z^2(D_1D_2/1336), \quad (9.b)$$
$$Z = 1\text{-}S(Dc/1336), \quad (9.c)$$

where S (in the unit of mm) being the effective anterior chamber depth (ACD) of the IOL; D_1, D_2 and Dc are, respectively, the front and back IOL power and corneal power.

The accommodation rate (M function) is almost linearly proportional to the moving front IOL power (D_1). M is positive for positive-power moving optics, that is an increase of p′ (or dp′>0 and dp<0) or a forward movement to the cornea is needed in order to have increasing accommodation (or myopic shift) for near vision of a presbyopia. These features are consistent with the numerical raytracing method of Rana et al and Ho et al.

Example 1

M is a decreasing function of S, or the corneal IOL separation (p). For example, given Dc=43 diopter, p′=1.0 mm, and the configuration with (D_1, D_2)=(+30, –10) diopter, g=–0.5, M=(2.39, 2.35, 2.29), for p=(2.5, 3.0, 3.5) mm or S=(2.0, 2.5, 3.0) mm, respectively.

Example 2

A positive-power would have a greater M (absolute value) than that of negative-power moving optics. For example, Dc=43 D, S=3.5 mm,

Z_2=1.0 and Z=0.887; the calculated M=+0.99 (D/mm) for D_1=+15 D and M=-0.724 (D/mm) for D_1=-15 D, which is about 27% smaller (comparing the absolute values). This novel feature is consistent with that of Ho et al using raytracing method.

Example 3

For a given IOL total power of $Dt=D_1+Z_1D_2$, with $Z_1=1-p'(D_1/1336)$, the M value for front positive and back-negative IOL is always larger than that of both optics are positive. This feature may be readily observed by re-expressing the moving front-optics power $D_1=Dt-ZD_2$ has a higher value when D2<0.

Mobile Back-optics Case

By symmetry feature of the dual-optics IOL, Lin (2006) also derived the case for mobile-back (with immobile-front) to obtain

$$M' = Z(D_2/1336)(2Dc+ZD_2) - \text{Delta}. \tag{10}$$

Similar to the mobile front-optics, the M′ value is proportional to the power of the mobile optics and slightly influenced by the immobile optics, via the Delta term.

Both Optics Mobile

In order to have a "positive" accommodation (for myopic shift), forward movement (toward the cornea) is needed if the moving optics has a positive power. In contrast, a backward movement is needed for a negative power moving optics. Therefore cancellation effect may occur when both optics having opposite-power are moving in the same directions or 2 optics having the same power sign but moving in the opposite directions. The actual amount of each components, M and M′, shall depend on the structure and implant configuration of the IOL, where contraction of the ciliary body results the direction and amount of each movement. Furthermore, one may also expect a small contribution from the non-linear coupling effect of M and M′, when both optics are allowed to shift in either direction. Therefore, the total (net) amount of accommodation (A) may be expressed as follows, in general,

$$A = M(dS1) + M'(dS2), \tag{11.a}$$

$$= A1 + A2 \tag{11.b}$$

where dS1 and dS2 are the movement amount (including directions) of the front and back optics, respectively. Cancellation occurs when A1 and A2 have opposite signs. Figure 10.6 shows the possible combinations for various IOL configuration. Because the sign of M and

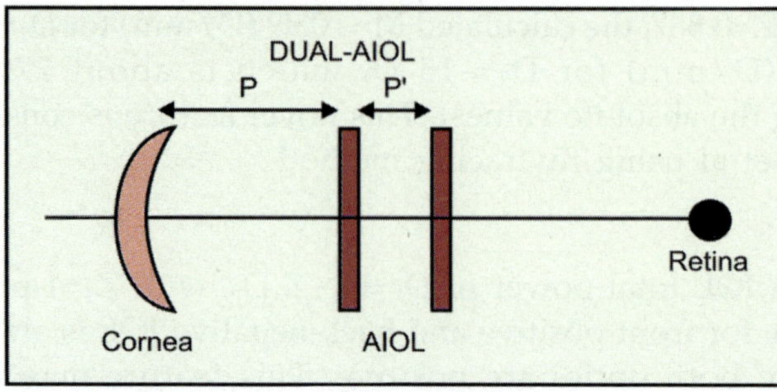

Fig. 10.6: Dual-optics AIOL (showing separations of p and p' (see text)

M′ are defined as the same as the power of the moving optics, one also needs to defined dS>0 for forward movement (toward the cornea), and dS<0 for backward (toward the retina) movement.

Analytic formulas are presented for dual-optics AIOL which could have the front or back-optics being the mobile element or both. The important features of the accommodation rate function (M) include:

- M is proportional to the moving optics power (including the sign)
- Positive accommodation amplitude, A=A1+A2, requires combination of plus-power optics moving forward to the cornea and minus-power optics moving backward to the retina (Fig. 10.7A)
- Convex-concave or bi-convex configuration for both front and back optics having positive power offers maximal A when both are moving forward to the cornea (Fig. 10.7B).

Dual-optics AIOL provides higher accommodation rates (M) than the 2-optics via optical configurations. However, the combined surface aberration (SA) to compensate the balanced SA of cornea and natural

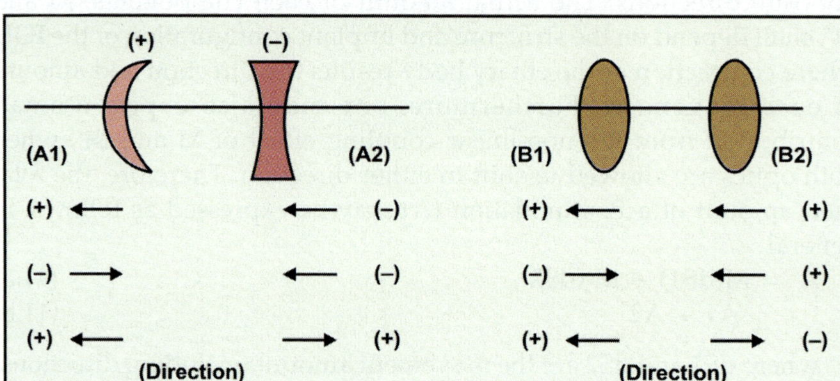

Fig. 10.7: Dual-optics accommodating IOL, where (←, →) stands for movement direction of (forward, backward) w.r.t the cornea position; (+, -) stands for (positive, negative) accommodation amplitude

lens for minimal high-order SA should also be considered in the IOL design.

DESIGN OF ASPHERICAL IOLs

It was known that the spherical aberration (SA) increases (or decreases) after myopic (or hyperopic) LASIK due to the increase (or decrease) of the corneal front surface asphericity (Q) or the shape factor (P=Q+1).

Similar to the LASIK procedure which induces a positive SA, larger population of cataracts surgery patients show an increase of positive SA. Therefore, optimized aspheric IOLs to minimize the cataract-induced SA and desired for best image quality. Most population have eyes with a positive SA (or Q<0) and about 10% of the population has negative SA, therefore most of the customized IOL would require a negative SA to minimize the remaining SA after the compensation from the natural lens which has a negative SA in general.

In addition, the aged-reduced positive SA must be also included as one of the factors to be considered. It was known that the natural crystalline lens has a SA of –25 μm, 0 and +25 μm at age 20, 40 and 60, although cornea SA remains constant throughout the whole life. When the positive SA increases in the eye, the presence of glare and night halos also increase. It was proposed that aging causes a gradient refractive index in the lens and causes a change from negative to positive SA of the lens over time. Therefore, as the eye ages, the combined positive SA of cornea and lens increase.

The need of customized IOL is to cause a perfect compensation of the positive SA of a prolate-cornea (with Q<0) by the implanted aspheric IOL having a negative SA of the cataract patients. However, an opposite strategy will be needed for the 10% abnormal patients having negative SA after cataracts. Furthermore, for IOL implanted to phakic eyes or piggyback IOL, the strategy for minimum SA or coma should base on a 3-optics system, in which the system is rather complex and requires minimal calculations.

The formula in aspherical IOL using Coddington shape factor for minimum spherical aberration (SA) and coma are shown in Table 10.5.

IOL FOR PEDIATRIC EYES

For pediatric eyes after cataract surgery, age-dependent adjustment of IOL power is needed (Table 10.6). See also Table 10.7 for related formulas.

Table 10.5: Formulas for spherical aberration (W) and Coddington shape factor (S)

W(total)	=	W(cornea) + W"(IOL)
S(lens)	=	(1+X)/(1-X),
S'(cornea)	=	(1+aX')/(1-aX'),
SM	=	$1(N^2 - 1)/(N + 2)$,
S*	=	-1/[1-PR/(n"' – 1.226)].

where
X = surface radius ratio (R'/R)
N = refractive indes ratio of IOL (n"') and humours (1.336)
SM = condition of S for minimum SA
P = IOL power with front surface radius R and index (n"')

Table 10.6. The adjusted mean power (Wilson et al, 2005) at age of surgery (Ao).

Ao (year)	0.1	0.2	0.4	1-2	2-4	4	5	6	7-10	10-14	>14
Dadj (Wilson)	+12	+9	+8	+6	+5	+4	+3	+2	+15-1.0	+0.5	plano

Table 10.7: The age-dependent refractive error given by Lin's double rate theory

dDe	= –(MN)(A' – A)
M	$= (P' + ZP)^2/1336$

where:
dA = (A' – A) is the age change from A to A'
dL = the axial length growth (in mm)
N = (dL/dA) = axial length growth rate per year (mm/year)
dDe = the refractive error increase due to axial growth after cataract surgery
M = (dDe/dL) = refractive change rate per 1.0 mm change of axial length (D/mm)
P and P' = power of the IOL and the cornea, respectively

CONCLUSION

For optimal design of aspherical IOLs, the minimum spherical aberration (SA) and coma of the whole eye may be achieved by minimum summation of the 3-optics, the cornea (W>0), the natural lens (W'<0) and the IOL (W"<0) such that W(total) is minimum. The Coddington shape factor (S) and the surface radius ratio (X) provide

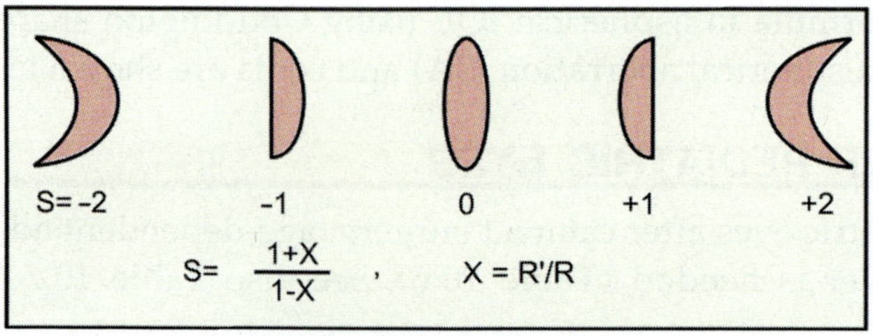

Fig. 10.8: Coddington shape factor (S) for various IOL configurations

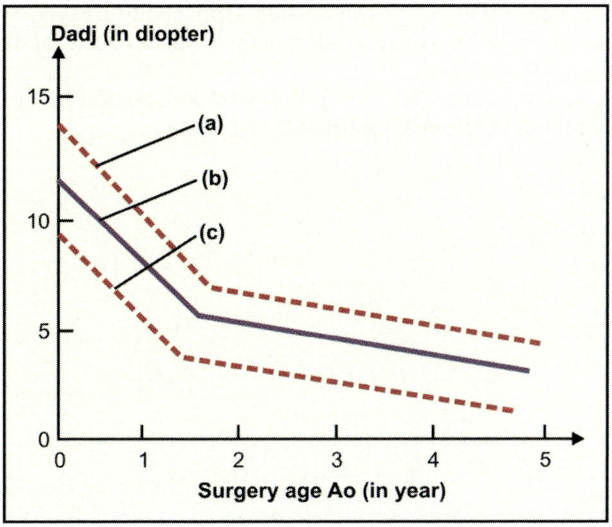

Fig. 10.9: The adjusted IOL power (Dadj) versus cataract surgery age (Ao) for emmetropic IOL power (Po) being higher than equal to, or lower than the mean value, shown by curve (a), (b) and (c), respectively

comprehensive and analytical formulas which are consistent to the numerical results of Want et al and Atchison (Figs 10.8 and 10.9).

REFERENCES

1. Shammas HJ. Intraocular lens power calculations. Thorofare NJ: SLACK. 2004; pp 7-24; 59-61; 64-5.
2. Holladay JT. Optics and intraocular lens power calculation for phakic intraocular lenses. In Horden DR, Lindstrom RL. Davis EA, (Eds): Phakic Intraocular Lenses: Principles and Practice. Thorofare NJ:SLACK. 2004; pp. 37-44.
3. Lin, JT. Unified refractive-state analysis for customized vision correction. J Refract Surg 2004; 20(3), 398-400.
4. Lin JT. The generalized refractive state theory and effective eye model. Chinese J Optom & Ophthal 2005;7:1-6.
5. Lin JT. New formulas comparing accommodation in human lens and intraocular lens. J Refract Surg 2005; 21(2): 200-21.
6. Lin JT. A generalized refractive state theory and effective eye model. Chin J Optom & Ophthal 2005; 7(1):1-6.
7. Lin JT. Analysis of refractive state ratios and the onset of myopia. Ophthal Physiol Opt. 2005;26(1):97-105.
8. Lin JT. Update on IOL power calculation formulas. In Garg A, Lin JT, (Eds): "Mastering Intraocular Lenses[IOLs]: Principles, Techniques and Innovations", New Delhi: Japypee Brothers, 2006; Chapter 3.pp 17-29.
9. Lin JT. The new IOL formulas based on Gaussian optics. In Garg A, Lin JT, Eds: "Mastering Intraocular Lenses[IOLs]: Principles, Techniques and Innovations", New Delhi: Japypee Brothers, 2006; Chapter 6: pp 56-65.
10. Atchison DA. Design of aspherical IOLs. Ophthal Physiol Opt 1991;11:137-46.

11. Pedrotti LS, Pedrotti FL. Optics and vision. Upper Saddle River, NJ 1998;122-41.
12. Smith G et al. The spherical aberration of the crystalline lens of the human eye. Vision Res, 2001;41:235-43.
13. Wang XJ, Jin CP, Wang QM. Aberration with IOLs based on different optical designs. Chinese J Optom & Ophthal 2003;5:209-11.

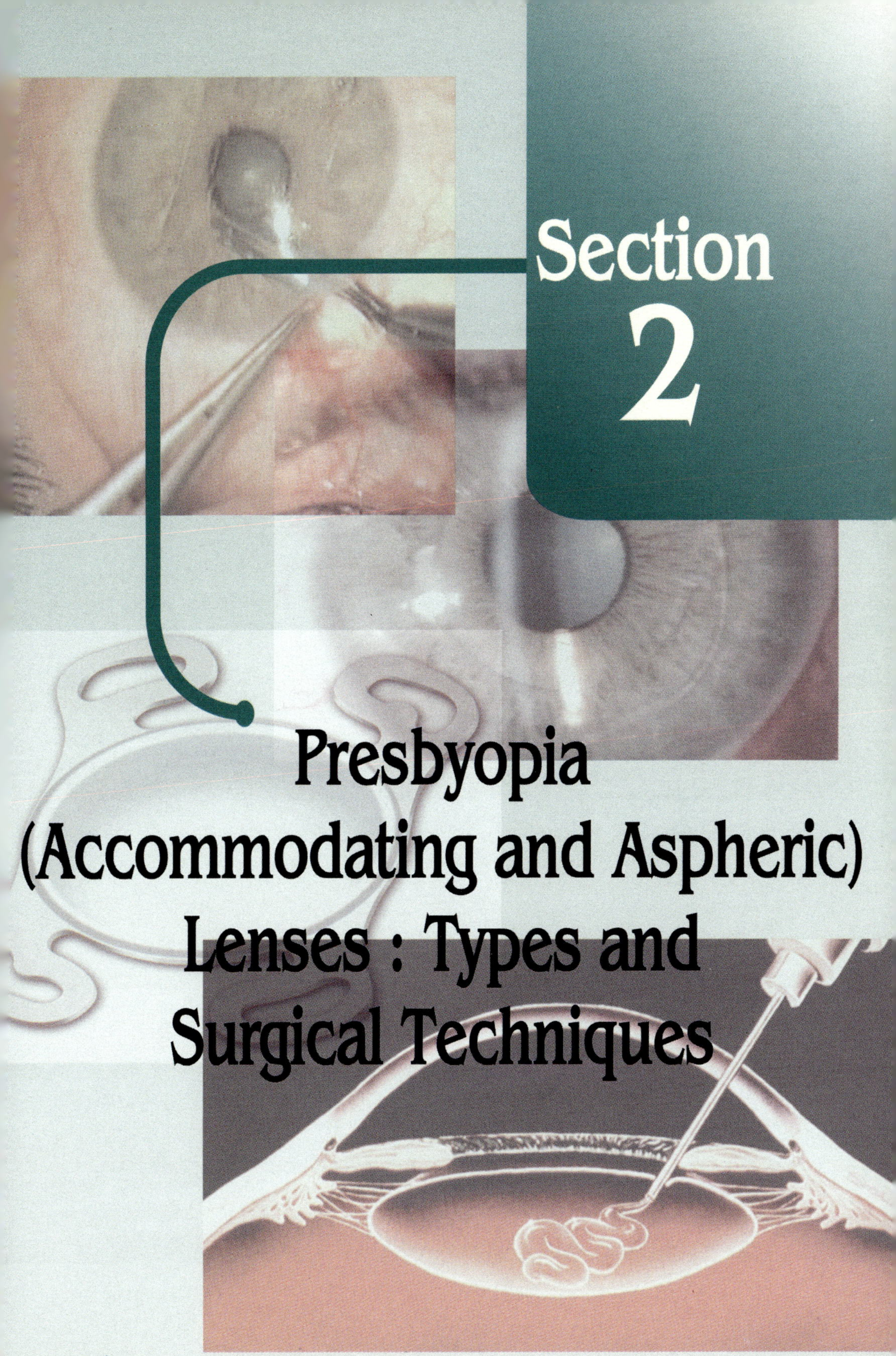

Section 2

Presbyopia (Accommodating and Aspheric) Lenses : Types and Surgical Techniques

CHAPTER

11

Ashok Garg (India)

Pearls of Presbyopic Lens Surgery

INTRODUCTION

Tremendous advances have taken place in modern refractive surgery specially in last one decade. In addition to correct myopia, hyperopia, astigmatism, refractive surgeon have got breakthrough to correct last obstacle presbyopia. There is sizable population of presbyopic patients throughout the world with increased life expectancy. Such patients are never satisfied with presbyopic glasses which they have to wear with frustation. New refractive technologies for presbyopia correction has certainly changed the situation.

PRELEX (Presbyopic Lens Exchange) is a procedure used to correct presbyopia for patients over the age of 45 who want to reduce their dependence on reading glasses. Using the same procedure that has been used for millions of patients undergoing cataract surgery, the PRELEX procedure involves removing the eye's natural lens and replacing it with an artificial lens implant. With the PRELEX procedure, multifocal intraocular lenses are used that allow the eye to focus for distance and NEAR–unlike other methods of refractive surgery which alter the shape of the cornea.

Although the PRELEX and cataract procedures are the same, the reasons for performing the surgery differ. While cataract surgery is done to remove a patient's cloudy lens; PRELEX is used to correct presbyopia and distance vision thereby reducing a person's dependence on glasses or contact lenses.

INDICATIONS FOR PRELEX

- Patients with very high levels of nearsightedness or farsightedness
- Patients who wish to eliminate their dependence on bifocals or reading glasses
- Patients who have corneas that are too thin for LASIK
- Patients who may be showing signs (even without symptoms) of developing cataracts.

PRELEX ADVANTAGES

- Recovery of unaided distance vision (no glasses needed for driving in over 99% of patients)
- Recovery of near vision in PRELEX patients with multifocal lens (no glasses needed for reading in over 80% of patients)
- Prevention of cataracts: With PRELEX surgery, the risk of developing a cataract (or clouding of the lens) in the eye is completely eliminated (Cataract surgery is required in over half the population by age 80 and occurs at a significantly younger age in patients with large refractive errors)

- FDA data shows that following PRELEX surgery with the Multifocal intraocular lens :
  - 80% of patients never wore glasses
  - 17% of patients sometimes wore glasses.

Ophthalmologists use the very latest, state-of-the-art lenses and techniques for PRELEX surgery. Refractive Surgeons are currently using the Alcon Acrysof ReSTOR intraocular lens, as clinic studiers have shown it to be the most effective lens for the correction of presbyopia, with over 80% of patients no longer requiring glasses following surgery.

Alcon's ReSTOR Intraocular Lens (IOL) Allowing PRELEX Patients to See Both Near and Far without Reading Glasses !

Refractive Surgeons currently uses Alcon's ReSTOR Intraocular Lens (IOL) for PRELEX. This lens can substantially rerstore a patient's ability to see both near and distant objects without the aid of reading glasses or bifocals. The ReSTOR´lens is used for PRELEX, Refractifve Lens Exchange (RLE) and cataract patients.

The Benefits of the ReSTOR Lens

- Quality vision at various distances, allowing patients to see both near and far without the use of reading glasses or bifocals
- A greater number of patients are candidates for this type of lens than for most other lenses
- In IOL clinical trials, the ReSTOR provides the highest level of spectacle freedom to date
- Works with pupil to provide quality range of vision in all lighting situations.

Multifocal synthetic lenses, which are implanted into the eye, provide relief for presbyopia at the same time as for nearsightedness or for farsightedness. Thus, the goal of multifocal synthetic lenses is to provide freedom from needing eyeglasses or contact lenses.

Module of Multifocal Lenses

Multifocal synthetic lenses such as the ReZoom Multifocal lens have several points of refraction, hence the term "multifocal". There are two main refractive points, namely the refractive point for close-up vision and the refractive point for distance vision. In order to achieve this goal, multifocal synthetic lenses are made from several individual lenses. Multifocal synthetic lens, which is constructed from several rings with different refractive powers. Because of the distribution of incoming light to various refractive points, multifocal intraocular lenses allow focused vision at all distances, ideally without the need for any eyeglasses.

Unfortunately, however, this comfort has its price : the distribution of light to several refractive points results in a certain loss of contrast. This means that at every point of refraction the image is not seen as sharply as with eyeglasses for that specific distance, but therefore eyeglasses are no longer needed.

Multifocal synthetic lens implants are a replacement of the eye's natural lens. First, an incision of only 3 mm is placed at the periphery of the cornea, and the eye's natural lens is aspirated by ultrasound through this incision. Then the multifocal lens is folded and placed into the eye. Once in the eye, it unfolds and takes the place of the eye's normal lens. This surgery is also performed routinely for the correction of opaque lenses, the so-called cataract. Hence, this surgery technique is very reliable and proven.

The implant of a multifocal synthetic lens is an outpatient procedure. Usually, it is only necessary to anesthetize the eye drops. Surgery is performed on each eye individually, with an interval of approximately 1 week between operations. On the day of surgery, a bandage is provided for your eye. Your vision is already improved one day after surgery, although final stability is only obtained approximately 8 to 12 weeks after surgery.

Multifocal synthetic lenses are most often used for the correction of nearsightedness and farsightedness together with existing presbyopia. They can also be used for presbyopia alone, if so desire to be free from using reading glasses. The severity of refractive error, the diameter of the pupil, the thickness of the cornea as well as other parameters have to be taken into consideration.

Contraindications for Multifocal Lenses

Generally, patients with chronic and progressive disorders of the eye such as glaucoma and certain retinal disorders as well as patients younger than 18 years old should not have multifocal synthetic lenses. Also, patients, who like to wear eyeglasses should not receive this treatment.

Multifocal synthetic lenses cannot offer the same image quality that can be reached with the eye's natural lens and an additional correction with eyeglasses. The purpose of the multifocal synthetic lens is rather to enable reasonably sharp vision at both far and near distances without the need for additional correction with eyeglasses, and in that sense it is superior to the natural lens of the eye at an advanced age.

FUTURE PROSPECTS

Presbyopic lens exchange is in its infancy but will likely take off when new lens options become available. The dual-optic accommodating IOL (Synchrony, Visiogen) is one of the pseudophakic presbyopic options in development. The lens can be implanted through a 2.5 mm incision and offers very good near vision, he added.

The NuLens Accommodating IOL (NuLens Ltd.) provides accommodation by changing its true power within the eye. The lens is designed with a small chamber of silicone gel and a posterior piston with an aperture in its center that allows the gel to bulge relative to the forces generated by accommodation.

This powerful technology allows a range of 10 D of accommodation and is about ready to enter clinical trials.

The Light Adjustable Lens (Calhoun Vision) is another unique option in development, which will allow for customized correction using light-sensitive material. The curvature of the lens can be altered using a laser.

With this technology, it will be possible to get precise correction of sphere, cylinder, and spherical aberration.

CHAPTER

12

JT Lin (USA)

The Principles of Accommodative IOLs

INTRODUCTION

Analytic formulas for accommodating intraocular lens with forward movement pseudoaccommodation (or apparent accommodation) in various intraocular lenses (IOLs) has been reported including 1CU lens (Human Optics, Inc.), AT-45 lens (C&C Vision) and MA30 lens (Eyeonics Vision, Inc.).[1-4] The preoperative and postoperative corneal power (or keratometry) or the estimated lens position (ELP), are believed to be the important factors in comparing the outcomes of different IOLs. The accommodation (A) per 1.0 mm anterior movement (defined as M) was measured [3-5] to be about M=(0.9 – 1.9) (diopter/ mm) and calculated by Nawa et al [6] to be (0.8-2.3) (diopter/mm) by ray tracing method.

It was known that widely scattered values of M may result from various ocular conditions such as corneal power, IOL power and axial length. These features are explored by numerical calculations based on a ray-tracing equation, where the roles of each of the ocular parameters have not been fully explored.

This chapter will cover the following subjects:

- Accommodation of single and dual-optics IOL (in aphakia)
- Accommodation of single-optics IOL (in phakia)
- Design aspects for maximal efficiency and minimal spherical aberration.

Analytic formulas for M in single-optics IOL will be derived (in the Appendix) to demonstrate explicitly the parameters determining M. These include the corneal and IOL power, the IOL postoperative effective position (S), the effective vitreous cavity length (X), axial length (L) and the remaining refractive error. For example, M should be determined by X and S, rather than the axial length alone, where M varies even for the same axial length. Six different ocular situations showing the roles of each of the parameters will be discussed.

CATEGORIES OF AIOL

As shown in Figure 12.1A, the accommodation of a single-optics accommodating IOL (AIOL) in aphakic eye (without the natural lens) may be achieved by the forward movement of the optics, and L=S+X, where S=p (position of the IOL) for thin-lens and S=p+gT, for thick-lens to include the geometry factor (g) and its thickness. Note that gT>0 for biconvex and gT<0 for convex-concave, and gT=0 for convex-plano. Figure 12.1B shows the 3-optics system where the AIOL is implanted in a phakic eye.

Figure 12.1C shows the dual-optics AIOL in which the accommodation may be achieved by the forward (or backward)

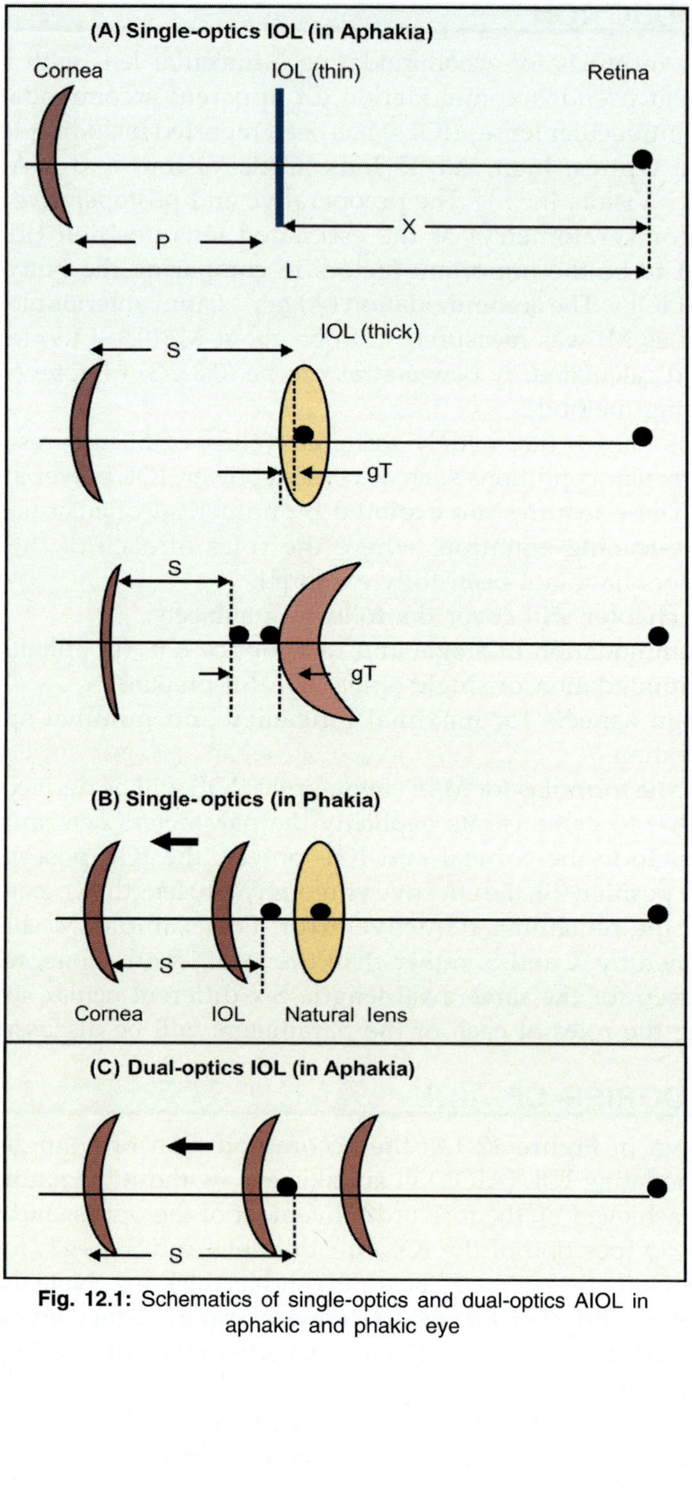

Fig. 12.1: Schematics of single-optics and dual-optics AIOL in aphakic and phakic eye

movement of the front (or back) optics. The net result depending on various situations that either front or back or both optics may be mobile, while the other optics could be immobile determined by the ciliary-body contraction on the AIOL and its configurations. Dual-optics AIOL is much more complex than the single-optics and will be presented in other Chapter of this book.[12]

THE BASIC PRINCIPLES

Single-optics IOL (Fig. 12.2)

By the definition of M = -dDe/dS (in diopter/mm), the accommodation amplitude (A) per mm axial movement of the lens is given by (see Appendix for derivation).

$$A = -M(dS), \quad (1)$$
$$M = M2\text{-}M1, \quad (2)$$
$$M2 = 1336/F^2, \quad (3.a)$$
$$M1 = 1336/fc^2, \quad (3.b)$$

The first term (m2) is attributed to the myopic-shift due to the increase of dX and the second term (m1) is the associate hyperopic-shift due to the forward movement of S and the backward-shift of SPP defined in Eq.(2).

As shown by Figure 12.2, positive accommodation (with A>0) due to lens axial forward movement (dX>0 and dS<0) may be expressed by 3 components:

a. Myopic-shift due to dX>0, increase of vitreous cavity length (X).
b. Myopic-shift due to the effective power (1336/F) increase when S decreases (or dS<0) since d(1/F) = -dS/(fcf2), d(1/F)>0 when dS<0.
c. Hyperopic-shift due to the back-shift of the second principal plane (SSP) resulting from the decrease of (SF).

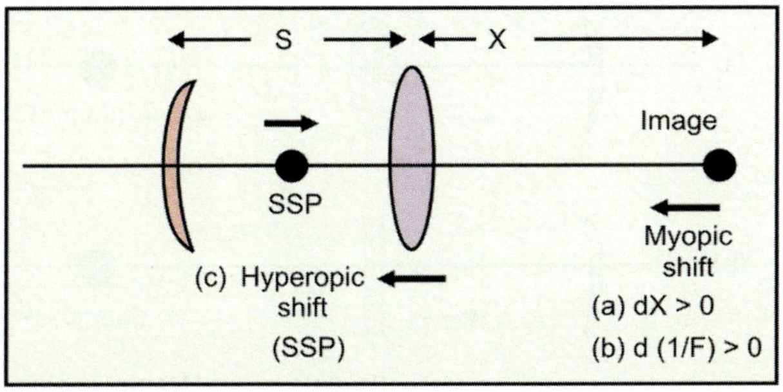

Fig. 12.2: The basics of accommodation (3-component analysis) due to axial movement in a positive-power IOL, where SSP is the position of second principal plane

Component (a) gives M2, and (b) + (c) give a net hyperopic shift given by M1. Typically, the contribution percentage of each component is: (b)=33%(a), and (c) = –80% (a). Therefore the net A = (1+0.33-0.80)(a) = 0.53(a). For example, for F=22 mm, fc=31 mm, f2=62 mm, (a)=M2=2.76, (b)=0.92, and (c)=-2.1, therefore A=1.58 (diopter). Some of the published articles had wrongly assumed that A mainly attribute from d(1/F). Furthermore, the contribution from the SSP-shift, about 33% of (a), could not be ignored.

Comparison of positive and negative A (for a plus IOL):

	dS	*dX*	*axial movement*
A>0	<0	>0	forward (to cornea)
A<0	>0	<0	backward (to retina)

For minus IOL, above signs are reversed as shown in Figure 12.3.

Eq.(3) may be re-expressed by cornea (P′) and lens (P) power as follows:

$$M = (Z/1336)P[2P'+ZP], \quad (4.a)$$

$$= (Z^2P)(2/X - P/1336), \quad (4.b)$$

Above Lin's M-formula provides the following features. M is proportional to the lens (or IOL) power for a given corneal power (P′) and axial lens (L) or S and X, since L=S+X+aT-0.13 mm. The accommodation amplitude (A) defined by A = –M(dS) could be positive or negative depending on the IOL is a positive (P>0) or negative (P<0) lens, where I define dS<0 for forward movement (toward the cornea) and dS>0 for backward movement. Greater detail of dual-optics IOL is shown in a separate Chapter of Lin in this book.

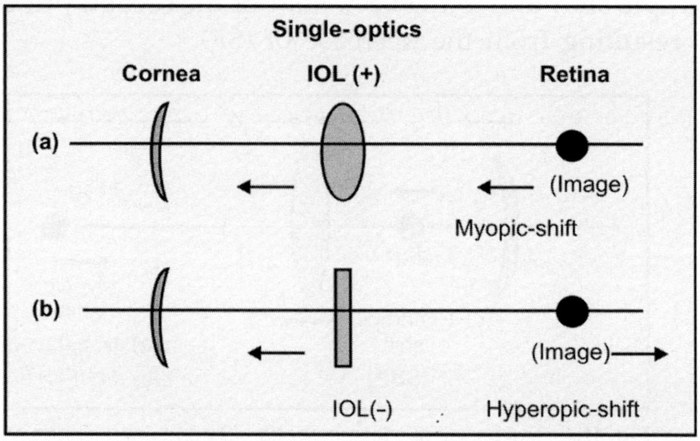

Fig. 12.3: Schematics of image shift caused by the axial forward movement of a positive lens (a) and negative lens (b) in single optics IOL (aphakic eye)

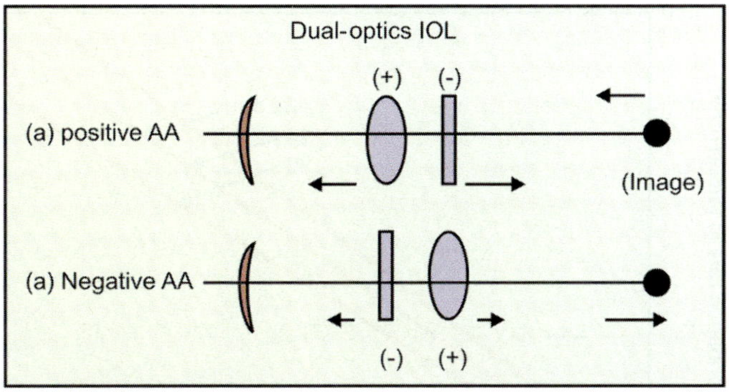

Fig. 12.4: Image shift caused by a dual-optics IOL for (a) positive-negative pair, and (b) negative-positive pair

Dual-optics IOL (refer to Fig. 12.4)

Above single-optics IOL formula of Eq.(3) may be generalized to a dual-optics IOL having a front and back optics power of P1 and P2. The A for dual-optics IOL is then attributed to both movements of the dual optics and given by

$$A = M1(dS1) + M2(dS2), \quad (5.a)$$
$$Mj\ (j=1,2) = (Z/1336)Pj[2P'+ZPj]. \quad (5.b)$$

As shown by Figure 12.2A, a positive A may be achieved for presbyopia eyes after cataract surgery. In contrast, shown by Figure 12.2B, a negative A is required for pediatric eyes in order to compensate (accommodate) the myopic-shift due to the axial elongation of the pseudophakic eye (after IOL implant). In Eq.(5), I had re-defined dSj>0 for forward movement.

DISCUSSION OF SINGLE-OPTICS IOL

There are six possible combinations shown as follows if only two parameters are measured or given and the other two are calculated: measured (X, S) with calculated (D_1, D_2); measured (X, D_1) with calculated (D_2, S); measured (X, D_2) with calculated (X, D_1); measured (D_1, S) with calculated (D_2, X); measured (D_2, S) with calculated (D_1, X); and measured (D_1, D_2) with calculated (X, S). Various examples based on the above combinations are discussed as follows:

Case (1): Fixed X=18.8 mm and S=5.0 mm, (or L=X+S=23.8 mm).

M = (1.1, 1.29, 1.45, 1.62) (diopter/mm) for corneal power of D_1 = (45, 43, 41, 39) diopter and the required IOL-power for emmetropia D_2=(17, 20, 22.4, 25.6) diopter calculated from Eq.(2). These calculated data show that IOL with a higher power, in general, produces higher accommodation for a

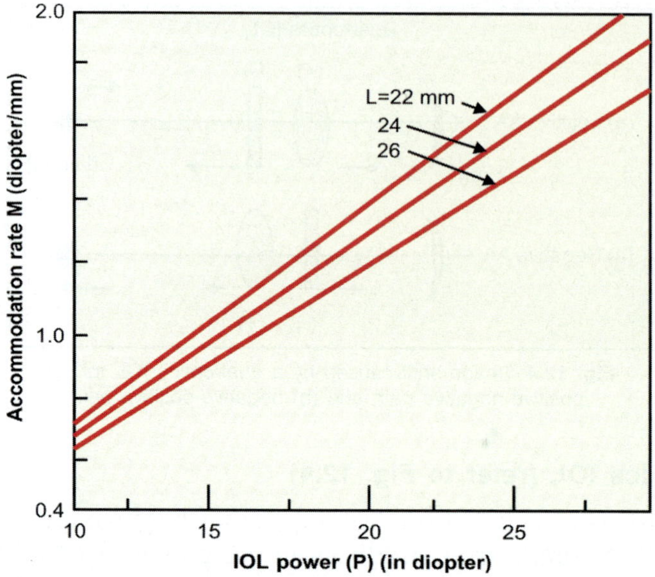

Fig. 12.5: Accommodation rate M (per 1.0 mm of forward movement) versus IOL power at various axial length L=(22, 24, 26) mm

given amount of anterior movement (dS), in consistent with the measured [1] and calculated values using a ray tracing method[6] (Fig. 12.5).

Case (2): Fixed corneal power D_1=43 diopter and axial length L=23.8 mm. M = (1.08, 1.14, 1.2, 1.29, 1.36) (diopter/mm), for S=(2.0, 3.0, 4.0, 5.0, 6.0) mm. These values show that M is an increasing function of the IOL position, where X decreases when S increases for a fixed axial length L=X+S (Fig. 12.6, curve B).

Case (3): Fixed IOL power D_2=20 diopter and L=23.8 mm. M=(1.36, 1.34, 1.32, 1.29, 1.25) (diopter/mm), for S=(2, 3, 4, 5, 6) mm. The decrease of M for larger S is the net result of the competing factors from the decrease of X=L- S, and the emmetropic condition which requires a higher corneal power for a given IOL power (Fig. 12.6, curve A).

Case (4): Fixed P′=43 diopter and S=5.0 mm M=(0.56, 0.82, 1.22, 1.87) (diopter/mm), for IOL power D_2=(9.5, 12.4, 19.1, 27.3) diopter and axial length L=(27, 26, 24, 22) mm calculated from L=X+S. This example shows that, for a given corneal power, longer eye with lower IOL power result in a smaller M, in consistent with that of Nawa[6] (Fig. 12.7, curve B).

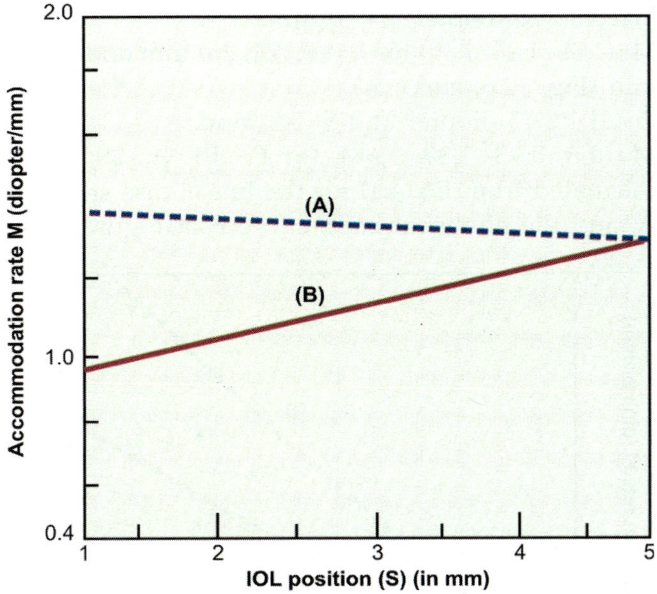

Fig. 12.6: M versus IOL position (S) for: (A) fixed IOL power at 20 diopter, and (B) fixed corneal power at 43 diopter, for a fixed axial length L=23.8 mm in both cases

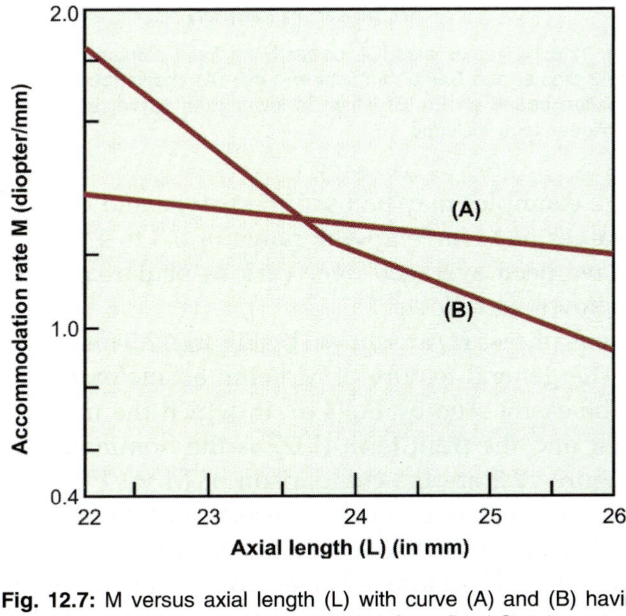

Fig. 12.7: M versus axial length (L) with curve (A) and (B) having the same conditions as Figure 12.5, but for a fixed S=5.0 mm, and L and X change

Case (5): Fixed P=20 diopter, S=5.0 mm.
M=(1.38, 1.26, 1.19) for L=(22, 24, 26) mm and X=(17, 19, 21) mm (Fig. 12.6, curve A).

Case (6): Fixed P′=43 diopter and S=5.0 mm.
M=(0.6, 0.93, 1.29, 1.68), for P=(10, 15, 20, 25) diopters, calculated from Eq.(4.a) for the linear case shown by curve A, and the nonlinear case, curve B in Figure 12.8.

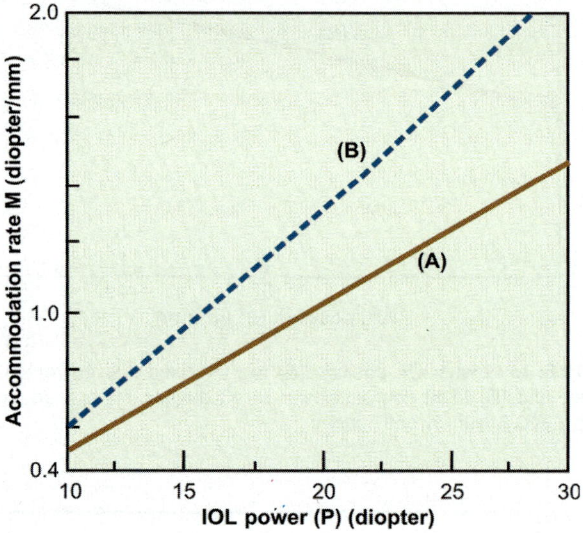

Fig. 12.8: M versus plus IOL power P for fixed corneal power at 43 diopter and S=5.0 mm, where curve (A) shows the linear function based on Eq.(3) which is lower than curve (B) with nonlinear term included

The above examples may be used to analyze and explain why the measured values of M have a wide range of 0.8 to 1.9 (diopter/mm) even they have been averaged over various ocular conditions. More details are shown as follows.

Calculations of case (1) are shown by Figure 12.5 for the role of IOL-power (P). The general feature of M being an increasing function of P may also be easily seen by Eq.(4.b), in which the minus term – P/1336 is minor and the front term $(P)Z^2$ is the dominating term. Also shown in Figure 12.2 are the comparison of M vs. P for axial length L=(22, 24, 26) mm, where longer eyes results in smaller M for a given P′, P and S. This may be realized by Eq.(4.b) showing M is proportional to 2/X, and X=L-S. Therefore a longer eye results in a smaller M. In addition, for a given axial length, steep corneas normally require a lower IOL power to achieve the emmetropic state, De=0 in Eq.(1), which also obtain a lower accommodate rate than that of a flat-cornea with high-power IOL. This trend is consistent with that of Nawa et al using lengthy numerical calculation which is readily available from Eq.(4.b).

Figure 12.6 shows the results for Cases (2) and (3) which have opposite trends when S increases. This feature may be further analyzed as follows. Case (2) shown by Curve (B) of Figure 12.5 indicates that given the same axial length and corneal power, posterior chamber implant (such as 1CU) is more efficient than that of anterior implant (such as AT-45), because higher IOL power is needed for larger S to achieve an emmetropia. In contrast, Case (3) shown by Curve (A) with a fixed IOL power and L, larger S requires smaller X and higher corneal power (P′) to meet the emmetropic condition.

Calculations based on parameters of Case (3) show a net increase of M, in contrast to Case (2), when S increases. These features were not explored in the ray-tracing method of Nawa et al. Furthermore, the statement made by these authors that longer eye with lower IOL-power results in higher M is only partially correct. As shown in this study, Cases (2) and (3), and Eq.(4.b), M is governed by the combined function of $Z^2(P)/X$, rather than their absolute values. As shown in the above example, M may be a decreasing or increasing function of S or X even for the same axial length (L). The role of axial length should be broken down by L=S+X to separate the roles of S and X as shown by Cases (2), (3) and (6).The roles of S, X and L were not differentiated in the calculations of Nawa et al. In other words, a longer eye does not necessarily result in a higher M which is also subject to the relative value of S and X.

Results of Cases (4) and (5) are shown by Curves (B) and (A) of Figure 12.7 and demonstrate that M is a decreasing function of L in both Cases, because X is an increasing function of L when S is fixed, and larger X results in a smaller M as shown by Eq.(4.b). The calculated values in Case (4) with M=(0.56-1.87) (D/mm) for L=(27-22) mm are consistent with that of Nawa, M=(0.8-1.9) (D/mm), where the small difference is due to the difference in corneal power chosen. The measured data of 0.9 and 2.02 (D/mm) for axial length of 21 and 25.8 mm also showed the similar trend, although their values are higher due to higher IOL powers are used.

Figure 12.7 (Curve B) shows that M is a strongly decreasing function of L (from 1.87 to 0.82) in Case (4) with a fixed corneal power and various IOL powers, in comparing to a weak dependence of L in Case (5) (Curve A) with a fixed IOL power and various corneal powers. In other words, M has a stronger dependence on IOL power than on corneal power.

Figure 12.8 shows the nonlinear behavior of M versus P (about 1% higher per diopter) as shown in Case (6). This nonlinear feature resulted from the second term of Eq. (3) was not shown by Nawa et al using a ray tracing method.

As shown in the Appendix, M, in general, is a function of six parameters (De, P′, P, S, X, L), where De is the refractive error after IOL implant (if any) and may contribute about 6% (for De=10.0 diopter) of the value of M at emmetropic state. The M value for ametropic state (post-IOL) may be calculated by adding an extra term of 2(1/X – 1/f2)De to Eq.(4.b). This ametropic term contributes about 0.06 (diopter/mm) for each diopter of De to the M value at emmetropic state.

THREE-OPTICS SYSTEM (IN PHAKIA)

The 3-optics IOL system include: (a) single-optics IOL in phakia, (b) piggyback IOL, and (c) dual-optics IOL in aphakia. Case (c) for dual-optics IOL is much more complex due to the variety of configurations and the movement dynamics of each optics which will be presented in a separate Chapter by Lin in this book. We shall now present the formulas for Cases (a) and (b).

Using Gaussian optics, Lin had derived the formula for the dual-optics accommodating IOL which may also apply to the single-optics IOL in phakic eye by replacing the back-optics of the dual-optics-IOL as the natural lens (for phakic IOL) or the primary IOL (for piggyback IOL). The M function of 2-optics system shown by Eq. (1) or (3) is revised as follows for a 3-optics phakic IOL (Lin, 2007)

$$M' = (f/f2)M - \text{Delta}, \quad (6.a)$$
$$\text{Delta} = 1336Z^2/(f2f3), \quad (6.b)$$

where f2 and f3 are the EFL of the IOL and the natural lens (NL), respectively and 1/f=1/f2+Z′/f3, with Z′=1-p′/f3, p′=p+2.4 mm. Above formula reduces to the 2-optics (M) when f3=infinity (or aphakic eye) and f=f2, Delta=0. The second term, Delta, is a reduction factor of M due to the presence of the NL. The configuration factor G=f/f2 may be re-expressed as

$$G = 1/[1+Z'(Pn/Pi)] \quad (7)$$

where Pn and Pi are the NL power and IOL power, respectively.

M′ may be further expressed as the power of the cornea (P′), Pn and Pi as follows:

$$M' = (Z/1336)Pi\ (2\ P'+Z'ZPi), \quad (8.a)$$
$$Z' = 1-p'/f3,\ Z = 1-S'/f1, \quad (8.b)$$
$$S' = S+gp',\ g=1/[1+Z'(Pi/Pn)]. \quad (8.c)$$

where $p'=p+2.4$ mm in phakic IOL and S=ELP is the position of the IOL (thin lens) or S=ELP+g'T (for thick lens), where g' is a geometry factor of the IOL having a thickness T and front and back surface power ratio of D12, $g'=1/(1+D12)$.

Eq. (6) may also be derived from the IOL power (Pi) of phakic 3-optics system given by (Lin, 2007)

$$Pi = (Pio + C)/Z', \quad (9.a)$$
$$C = (pGM')/Z^2, \quad (9.b)$$

and by using the conversion factor $CF=dDe/(Z'Pi-Pio)=Z^2$, where dDe is the system power change (or accommodation A) due to the axial movement (from p=0 to p). Pi and Pio are the IOL power for emmetropia at p and at p=0.

Comparing M' of Eq.(6) for IOL in phakic eye with Eq.(4) for the aphakia M, one may easily conclude the following:

1. For a given IOL power, M' in phakia is always smaller than that of the aphakia (M) by a reduction factor determined by Z and $Z'=1-p'/f3$, in which $Z'<1$, even the IOL closely contacts to the natural lens since $p'=2.4$ mm when p=0. In contrast, for a piggyback IOL contacts to a thin primary IOL $p'=0$, $Z'=1.0$ and $S'=S$, that is, no reduction effect from the primary IOL when p=0.
2. The new parameter $S'=S+gp'$ is further shifted due to the effective separation of the IOL and natural lens by $p'=p+2.4$ mm, and also affected by a geometry factor defined by the ratio of the IOL and natural lens power (Pi/Pn).
3. Eq.(6) for IOL in phakia may apply to piggyback IOL by redefining p' being their separation (assuming both are thin lens) and Pn being the power of the primary IOL.

Example 1

For an anterior IOL implanted in phakic eye having a corneal power P'=43 D and natural lens power of Pn=21.5 D, ACD=2.0 mm and p=2.0 mm, or $p'=p+2.4=4.4$ mm. The calculated $Z'=0.93$ (or a 7% reduction) and g=(0.82, 0.7, 0.61) for IOL power of Pi=(5, 10, 15) D. The calculated phakic IOL M'=(0.275, 0.59, 0.93), respectively, which are about 10% to 15% lower than the aphakia value of M=(0.32, 0.67, 1.05) (D/mm).

Example 2

Same as above, but for posterior IOL of ACD=4.0 mm, p=0, p'=2.4 mm, the calculated $Z'=0.96$ (or a 4% reduction) and g is about the same as above. Therefore M'=(0.25, 0.48, 0.69) versus M=(0.295, 0.62, 0.97) (D/mm), a reduction of about 8 to 29% in phakia IOL comparing to aphakia. Comparing to Example 1 (anterior IOL), the posterior IOL has higher reduction factor.

Example 3

For piggyback IOL separated from the primary IOL by p′. For ACD+p′=6.4 mm, the M′ value will be the same as that of Example 1 and 2. However, for smaller ACD+p′=4.0 mm, with ACD=3.0 and p′=1.0 mm, and a smaller Pn=15.0 D for Pi=+5.0 D, the calculated Z′=0.989 (reduction only about 1%), g=0.752, S′=4.0+0.752 x 1=4.752, Z=0.847. Therefore M′=0.286 of piggyback IOL versus M=0.306 (D/mm) for IOL in aphakia. These M′ and M values are approximately, except the nonlinear second-term (Delta) in Eq.(6), proportional to the piggyback IOL power. Therefore one shall expect M′=(0.57, 0.86, 1.14) (D/mm) for higher IOL power of Pi=(10, 15, 20) D, since M′ is insensitive to the primary IOL power (Pn).

OPTIMAL IOL DESIGN

Surface aberration including spherical aberration (SA) and coma have been reported by Wang et al [13] for various configurations with front and back surface radius of (in mm) (R1, R2) = (a) (15.4 – 15.4), (b) (7.29, infinity), (c) (infinity, -7.29), (d) (51.6, -9.1), (e) (9.1, -51.6), (f) (-55.3, -6.8), etc. Their calculations concluded that cases (b) convex-plano and (e) (bi-CX) have the smallest SA, whereas (e) and (a) have the smallest coma. Therefore, case (a), (b) and (e) configurations are the preferred IOL structure for minimal surface aberrations.

However, as reported by Atchison,[14] the optimal IOL design is that the negative SA of the cornea asphericity could be balanced by the positive SA from the IOL (and/or the natural lens). For corneal asphericity (Q) about –0.2 to –0.5 for most population, the optimal IOL form is close to convex-plano with the more-curved surface facing the cornea. This feature may be analyzed by Coddington shape factor (R) defined by the radius of the front and back surface, R1 and R2,

$$R = (R1 + R2) / (R1 - R2). \tag{10}$$

where R>1, for meniscus (or convex-concave) with more curved surface facing cornea; R=–1, for plano-convex; R=+1 for convex-plano; R>–1 for biconvex and R=0 for equi-convex. According to Smith and Liu, the optimal value of R=+1.1 or a convex-concave IOL (with convex facing cornea) in order to produce positive SA and balance the negative corneal SA for minimal overall SA of the eye. Based on the Gaussian formula of M′ and M, the convex-concave configuration also provides higher accommodation rate.

CONCLUSION

By Gaussian optics, the accommodation rate (diopter/mm) function (M) may be derived analytically for both aphakia and phakia IOL and piggyback IOL. The M value is determined by the combined factor of the products of ZPiPc(2+Z′ZPi/Pc) shown by Eq.(3). Following features of AIOL may be summarized:

- M is proportional to the product of Z and the IOL (Pi) and corneal power (Pc) and extra nonlinear term Z′ZPi/Pc which is influenced by the power of the natural lens (for the case of phakic IOL), or by the primary IOL power (for the case of piggyback IOL) by Z′ and S′=S=gp′
- The Z′ reduction term is a function of the IOL and natural lens (or primary IOL) separation and their power, Z′=1-p′(Pn/1336), having a value of about 0.96 to 0.98
- The effective ACD (S) is shifted to S′=S+gp′, where g is a geometry factor given by g=1/(1+Z′Pi/Pn) about 0.6 to 0.82
- The M′ function (for phakia) is about 10 to 30% lower than M (for aphakia)
- The general trend is that higher M or M′ for eyes with shorter axial length (L or X), flatter cornea or smaller ACD (or S) and for high IOL power
- IOL with convex-concave structure has a higher M′ and may achieve lower surface aberration of the eye comparing to other structures.

Above features are for single-optics IOL in phakia or aphakia, or piggyback IOL. For dual-optics IOL accommodation, see other Chapter of Lin in this book.

APPENDIX (SINGLE-OPTICS IOL)

By Gaussian optics theory,[8] the refractive error (De) after an IOL is implanted in an aphakic eye (a two-optics system) may be described by [9,10]

$$De = 1336[1/(L-L2) - 1/F], \quad \text{(A-1)}$$

where L is the axial length, L2 is the position of the second principal plane and F is the effective focal length (EFL) of the cornea IOL system related to the EFL of the cornea (f1) and IOL (f2) by

$$1/F = 1/f1 + Z/f2, \quad \text{(A-2)}$$

where Z=1-S/f1, S being the effective anterior chamber depth of the IOL which equals to the postoperative estimated lens position (ELP) when a thin IOL lens is assumed. Using the relation of L2=S(1-F/f1) (for thin lens) [8,10] and substituting Eq.(A-2) to (A-1), one obtains

$$qDe = 1336/X - P'/Z - P, \quad \text{(A-3)}$$
$$q = 1/Z^2, \quad \text{(A-4)}$$

where the effective vitreous length defined by X=L-S, and P′ and De are the power of the cornea and lens, respectively.

To formulate the accommodation amplitude (A) per 1.0 mm forward movement of a single-optics IOL, I define a rate function M=–dDe/dS=A/dS, which may be obtained by taking the derivative of Eq.(A-3) with respect to X (or S)

$$dDe = -M(dS), \quad \text{(A-5)}$$
$$M = M1 - M2, \quad \text{(A-6.a)}$$
$$M1 = 1336(1+dS/X)(Z/X)^2, \quad \text{(A-6.b)}$$
$$M2 = 1336/f1^2, \quad \text{(A-6.c)}$$

where the high-order term dS/X contributing about 5% for dS=1.0 mm since X is about 18 mm. In deriving above formulas, I had also used dX=dL-dS=-dS, since dL=0, that is axial length remains the same when the IOL is anterior shifted; and dZ=-dS/f1.

At emmetropic state (De=0), Eq.(A-3) gives the formula for IOL power

$$P = 1336/X - P'/Z, \quad \text{(A-7)}$$

which may be used to eliminate the second term in Eq.(A-6) since P′=1336/f1 and to obtain a more practical formula for M as shown in Eq.(1.b), where I also used the relationship of F=X/Z for emmetropic state in deriving Eq.(1.b) in which the high-order terms of (A-6) are neglected. Eq.(A-7) may be compared with the classical vergence formula of Heijde [11] by relating X=L-ELP and corneal power by the keratometric power (K). It was known that error occurs in using K for cornea power, therefore Eq.(A-7) is more accurate than all the classical vergence formulas which have been used in combining with the modern formulas for ELP.

The approximated Eq.(A-3) is derived by decoupling the second principal plane position P2=SF/f1 from L2=S-P2. Alternatively, one may use the following equation for exact numerical calculation for both De and M

$$De = 1336/(X+P2) - 1336/F, \quad \text{(A-8)}$$

which is just a rearrangement of Eq.(A-1) without using the decoupling approximation. Above equation also allows us to check the accuracy of the analytic approximate formulas of Eq.(1). For example, for P= 20.0 diopter with a fixed P′=43 diopter, S=5.0 mm and L=23.7 mm, M=1.30 (diopter/mm) calculated from the exact Eq.(A-3) in comparing to M=1.298 calculated from analytic formula, Eq.(1), which is only about 0.15% error.

Alternatively, one may also derive Eq.(A-6) by taking the derivative of Eq.(A-1) and using the relationship of Eq.(A-2). A third method is to take the Taylor second-order expansion of De in Eq.(A-7) or (A-8) with respect to the change of X. For example, $1/(X+dX)=1/X-(dX/X^2)[1-dX/X]$. All the above described three different methods lead to the same formula of (A-6) and justify the derivation of M.

Above formulas are for 2-optics system. Much complex algebra is involved in 3-optics system for thin IOL in phakic eye or dual-optics IOL in aphakia. The detailed derivation will be shown in a separate Chapter of Lin in this book.

REFERENCES

1. Langenbucher A, Nguyen NX, Sertz B, Gusek-Schneider GC, Kuchle M. Measurement of accommodation after implantation of an accommodating posterior chamber intraocular lens. J Cataract Refract Surg 2003; 29:677-85.
2. Cumming JS, Slade SG, Chayet A. Clinical evaluation of the model AT-45 silicone accommodating intraocular lens. Ophthalmology 2001; 108:2005-9.
3. Koeppl C, Findl O, Kriechbaum K, et al. Change in IOL position and capsular bag size with an angulated intraocular lens early after cataract surgery. J Cataract Refract Surg 2005;31:348-53.
4. Stachs O, Schneider H, Steve J, Guthoff R. Potentially accommodating intraocular lenses-an in vitro and in vivo study using three-dimensional high-frequency ultrasound. J Refract Surg 2005; 21: 37-45.
5. Holladay JT, Chandler TY, et al. Refractive power calculation for the phakic eye. Am J Ophthalmol 1993;116:63-6.
6. Nawa Y, Ueda T, Nakatsuka M et al. Accommodation obtained per 1.0 mm forward movement of a posterior chamber intraocular lens. J Cataract Refract Surg 2003;29:2069-72.
7. Lin JT. The roles of corneal power and anterior chamber depth on the accommodation of aphakic intraocular lenses. J Refract Surg 2005;21:765-66.
8. Pedrotti Ls, Pedrotti FL. Optics and Vision. Upper Saddle River NJ; 1998:74-8.
9. Lin, JT. Analysis of refractive state theory and the onset of myopia. Ophthal Physiol Opt 2006; 26:97-105.
10. Lin, JT. The generalized refractive state theory and effective eye model. Chin J Opt & Ophth 2005;7:1-6.
11. van de Heijde GL. The optical correction of unilateral aphakia. Trans Am Academy Ophthal Otolaryngol 1976; 81: 80-8.
12. Lin JT. Analysis of dual optics accommodating IOL. In: Garg A, Lin JT (Eds): Mastering Intraocular Lenses (IOLs): Principles, Technologies and Innovations. New Delhi: Jaypee Brothers Med Pub 2006;Chapter 48, 434-9.
13. Wang XJ, Jin CP, Wang QM. Aberration with IOLs based on different optical design. Chinese J Optom & Ophthal (in Chinese) 2003;5:209-11.
14. Atchison DA. Optical design of intraocular lens. I. On-axis performance. Optom Vis Science 1989;66:492-506.

CHAPTER

13

Oliver Stachs (Germany)

Analysis of Intraocular Behavior of Accommodative Intraocular Lenses

ABSTRACT

The fundamental idea of some approaches to achieve potentially accommodating intraocular lenses is to allow an axial displacement of the IOL optic. The currently commercial available accommodative implants are designed to convey ciliary muscle activity via the haptic into an optic shift of the optic. The aim of this contribution is the evaluation of haptic geometry based on a three-dimensional reconstruction of single section, ultrasound biomicroscopic data sets. To simulate accommodation, a test chamber using an artificial capsular bag and a stretching device was developed. The haptic regions of the Accommodative 1CU and the CrystaLens AT-45 were scanned in the simulation model during different accommodative (stretched) states. These *in vitro* results were correlated and used to describe the *in vivo* condition in patients with these implants in different accommodative states.

INTRODUCTION

Accommodation is the ability of the eye to project a focused image, positioned at varying distances from near to far, on to the retina. The physiological decrease in accommodation with age (presbyopia) is caused by a decrease in the elasticity of the crystalline lens, an equatorial diameter change of the lens, alterations in the elastic properties of Bruch's membrane, and atrophy of the ciliary muscle [Kaufman 1992]. After cataract surgery and because the implanted intraocular lens optic cannot change its position and/or shape, pseudophakic patients cannot accommodate. However, as a result of a number of factors (e.g. pupil size, myopic astigmatism, etc), some patients may have an increased depth of focus, called pseudoaccommodation. To date, lens-based pseudophakic accommodation has only been achieved by multifocal IOLs and by an axial shift of the IOL optic. Other surgical techniques like lens refilling with a inflatable endocapsular balloon or flexible gel are in early experimental stages. Additionally varying outcomes have been reported: scleral expansion surgery, zonal refractive keratectomy and decentred LASIK.

The shift of the IOL optic occurs when the ciliary muscle contracts and induces a change in haptic configuration. Recently, several attempts using different designs [Hara 1990, Hardman 1990, Cumming 1996, Legeais 1999, Küchle 2002, Sarfarazi 2003] have been made to achieve pseudophakic accommodation. The basic approach to achieve potentially accommodating IOLs is to allow an axial displacement of the IOL optic. Quantification of axial IOL movements induced by accommodation in humans has been performed with ultrasound [Hardman 1990, Nakazawa 1984, Ravalico 1990, Gandolfi 2003] and with the highest resolution by using dual-beam partial coherence interferometry [Findl 1998, Findl 2003, Findl 2003a, Findl 2003b, Findl 2004]. In terms of understanding the principle of so-called accommodative IOLs, high frequency ultrasound [Pavlin 1995] is the only tool available to visualize the IOL haptic geometry hidden behind the iris diaphragm. Unfortunately, high frequency sonographic image analysis can be difficult if information from only one plane is available. This contribution is based mainly on two publications in Journal of Refractive Surgery [Stachs 2005, Stachs 2006] and presents the three-dimensional ultrasound evaluation of pharmacological-induced haptic changes and accommodative response in patients with the AT-45 and 1CU implant.

THREE-DIMENSIONAL ULTRASOUND BIOMICROSCOPY

It has long been appreciated that three-dimensional (3D) ultrasonic images can be produced from an ordered series of scan planes. This technique was first applied to the anterior segment of the eye by Iezzi et al. [Iezzi 1996] and required considerable effort and ingenuity with regard to apparatus [Reinstein 1997, Coleman 1998, Cusumano 1998]. Iezzi et al. used a scanning control arm for a continuous z movement and stored the data on videotape for subsequent digitalization. Silverman et al. [Silverman 2001] characterized the ciliary body including the state of the ciliary processes of rabbits and normal human subjects using 3D high-resolution ultrasound. There the scanning system consists of two orthogonal linear stages with a computer-controlled stepping motor.

In author's laboratory a simple and low-cost extension of the commercial Ultrasound Biomicroscope Model 840 (Humphrey Instruments, Carl Zeiss Group) into a userfriendly 3D- ultrasonic imaging system was developed. Here 3D data sets consist of Bscan stacks of in-parallel planes with a defined distance between them. Patients were scanned with the ultrasound probe coupled to the eye with Methocel (Ciba Vision) and a normal saline water bath. The examiner positioned the transducer in the center of the ocular segment of interest using standard B-mode. For 3D imaging the computer-controlled scanning system moved the transducer perpendicular (z-direction) to the B-scan plane (xy-plane) over the area being scanned. For this motion an additional miniature skid was mounted on the original linear motor of the UBM scanning device where the ultrasound transducer is attached. Because of its weight it is not possible to attach also the drive of this skid. Therefore the skid is powered from an external stepping motor via a Bowden wire. The video signal of the ultrasound unit is digitized using a frame-grabber board (HaSoTec, Germany) synchronized with the z motion control system. That means during image capturing the z movement is stopped and the image plane is exactly perpendicular to the z-axis. 10 s acquisition time with a scanning range of 2.5 mm was used for all subjects, which is thought to be the maximum considering patient and examiner movements. Thus, all 3D scans have the same sampling density. The original UBM raw data (256 scan lines x 1024 samples per line, 256- level grayscale) pictured on the UBM display with 880x440 pixels were converted into 440x440 pixels (256-level gray-scale) during capturing by the frame grabber. No degradation of the image quality is observable and the influence of the conversion is negligible compared with the movement artefacts and contour finding. The motion control and data acquisition system is connected with an SGI workstation via a local area network for 3D reconstruction using AMIRA (TGS, San Diego, CA, USA). This commercial volume rendering software package provides an interactive environment allowing features such as volume orientation for viewing planes and 3D perspectives, segmentation and determination of distances and surfaces. The feature of model building allows outlining of anatomic structures in space and can be used for volume measurements.

An example for 3D imaging is given in Figure 13.1 showing the anterior segment with ciliary body. There are some publications about *ex vitro* and *in vivo* applications of these instruments [Stachs 2005, Stachs 2002, Kirchhoff 2001, Stachs 2005a, Stachs 2006]. The investigations are mainly focused on accommodation studies and the evaluation of so-called accommodative lenses.

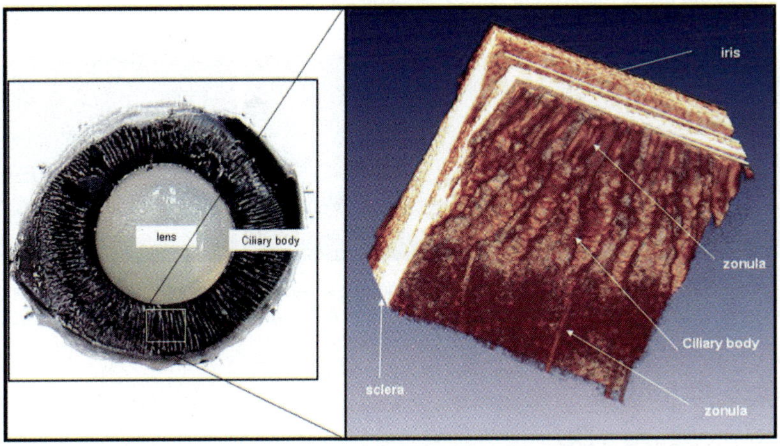

Fig. 13.1 3D reconstruction of the human ciliary body (anterior segment viewed from behind)

STRETCHING DEVICE FOR IN VITRO EXPERIMENTS

To simulate accommodation, a test chamber using an artificial capsular bag and a stretching device was developed [Stachs 2005]. For analysis of the IOL performance, the artificial capsular bag was mounted in a simulation device. The arms of the fixture clamp the bag around its periphery at eight points. Rotation of the inner ring stretches or relaxes the bag (Fig. 13.2). Inner ring rotation is accomplished by a stepping motor driving a worm gear. The amount of stretching correlates with the rotation of the inner ring. The entire arrangement is submerged in water for sonographic imaging. The haptic regions of the accommodative 1CU and the CrystaLens AT-45 were scanned in the simulation model during different accommodative (stretched) states (Fig. 13. 3). These *in vitro* results were correlated and used to describe the *in vivo* condition in patients with accommodative implants.

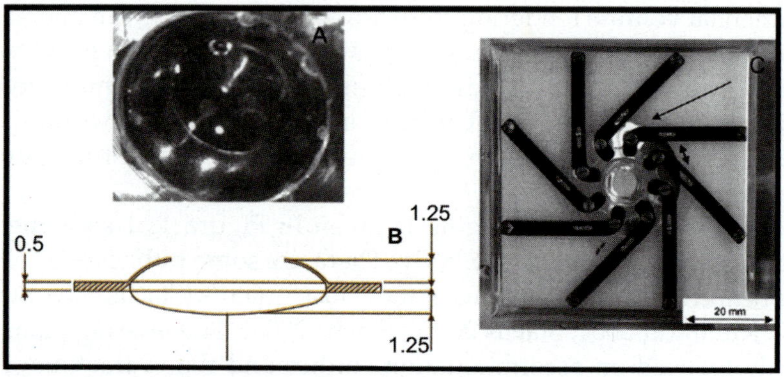

Figs 13.2A to C: Artificial capsular bag and (C) stretching device for accommodation simulation. The rotation of the inner ring with pins (marked in C) shifts the arms and stretches or relaxes the bag to simulate the force effects of the ciliary muscle. The 1CU IOL is implanted (Stachs 2005)

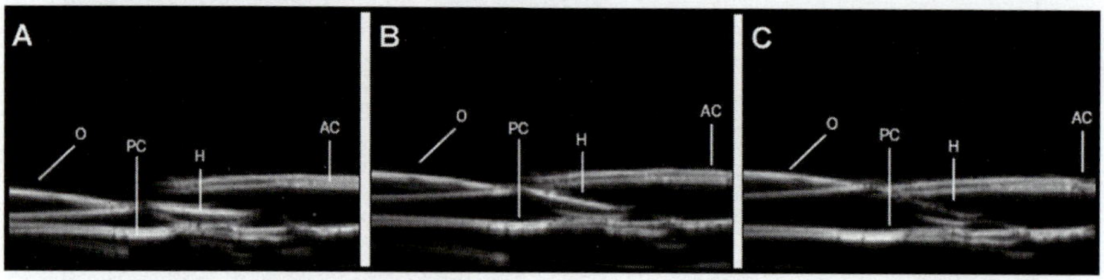

Figs 13.3 A to C: B-scan series exemplifying the stretching experiment. Abbreviations: O = optic, PC = posterior capsule, H = haptic, AC = anterior capsule (Stachs 2005)

In Vitro Findings

Accommodative 1CU

The posterior chamber lens 1CU was examined. Theoretically, a contraction of the ciliary muscle, thus a relaxation of the zonules, leads to a relaxation of the capsular bag. The haptics turn and produce an anterior axial shift according to the modified force ratio in the haptic region. Our simulation experiments show a similar effect during capsular bag relaxation. A 0.5 mm change in r was used for maximal relaxation/stretching. With this unphysiological and unexpected amount of relaxation in humans, a 0.36 mm anterior shift was observed for the 1CU caused by a haptic 10.4° angulation change. Using a 50-year lens and the linear regression of Strenk for the ciliary body displacement, a 0.25 mm ciliary body displacement can be assumed. A 0.28 mm anterior IOL shift and an angulation change of 4.3° was observed. For this lens, the theoretically predicted 30° haptic angulation change for 1 mm axial shift could not be achieved (Figs 13.4 and 13.5).

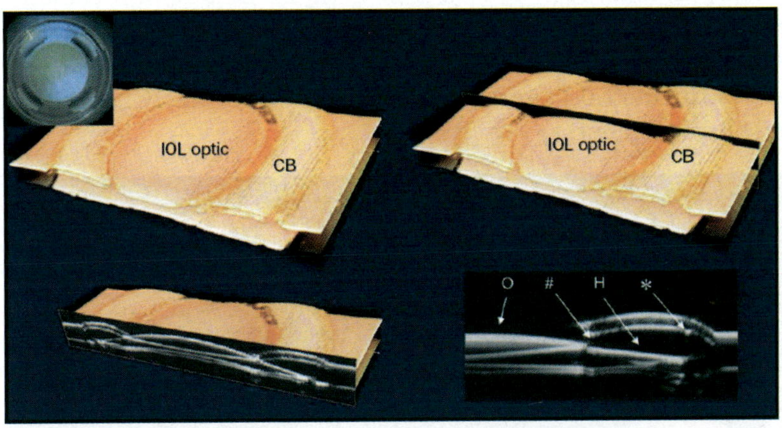

Fig. 13.4: Photograph and three-dimensional ultrasound biomicroscopy image and B-scan of the 1CU in the artificial silicone capsular bag (CB). Abbreviations: O = optic, # = fulcrum, H = haptic, and * = haptic ridge (Stachs 2005)

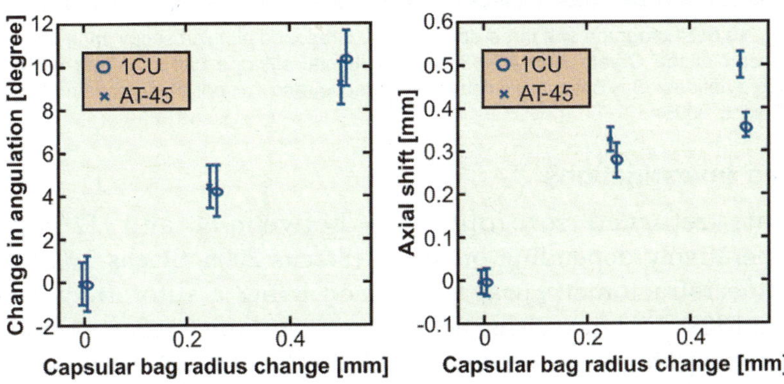

Fig. 13.5: Change in angulation (left) and axial IOL movement (right) by lens type showing the effect of equatorial stretching respectively relaxing (Stachs 2005)

CrystaLens AT-45

The three-dimensional reconstruction and the interactive selection of sections across the haptic as well as a photographic image are shown in Figure 13.6. In this example, the optic and the haptic can be differentiated. The echo patterns are caused by the polyimide construction of the plate haptic. The posterior lens surface can be imaged, whereas this interface cannot always be seen under different scanning directions. The point # acts as the fulcrum and is used as the center of rotation for angulation determination. In the *in vitro* model, a maximal forward shift of 0.50 mm (9.3° haptic angulation change) for the AT-45 lens was observed using the maximal radius change of 0.5 mm. For 0.25-mm radius change as the expected value for the 50-year lens, an axial shift of 0.33 mm with 4.5° angulation change was found. In our model, equatorial changes can be simulated, but vitreous pressure variations cannot be simulated. Regarding the axial shift, the AT-45 performed 0.14 mm better compared to the 1CU for 0.5 mm radial displacement.

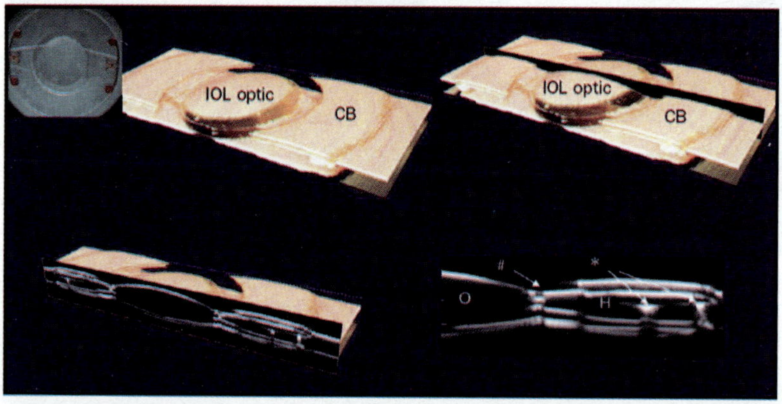

Fig. 13.6: Photograph and three-dimensional ultrasound biomicroscopy image and B-scan of the CrystaLens AT-45 in the artificial silicone capsular bag (CB). Abbreviations: O = optic, # = fulcrum, H = haptic, and * = polyimide construction (Stachs 2005)

In Vivo Investigations

Patients returned for follow-up between 4 and 12 weeks postoperatively depending on study [Stachs 2005, Stachs 2006]. The objective refractometry was performed using a autorefractometer (Canon RK3). Distance visual acuity was determined using a standard Snellen projector system (Optostar IR-2000; Schwind, Kleinostheim, Germany). Near reading vision was determined using Birkhäuser reading charts (Scalae Typographicae Birkhaeuseri, Birkhäuser Verlag) and an illumination of 70 cd/m^2. After determining best and uncorrected far vision, near vision without additional near/distance correction and with the addition of +1.0, +2.0, +3.0, and +3.5 sphere, was determined. Visual acuity values were expressed in decimal values and logMAR. Details can be seen in [Stachs 2005, Stachs 2006]. An in-house three-dimensional ultrasound biomicroscope (UBM) was used to evaluate IOL placement and haptic confi guration in patients with the AT-45 implant. The principles of the UBM and three-dimensional UBM have been described in detail elsewhere. The three-dimensional reconstruction was performed using Amira software (TGS, San Diego, Calif). Building three-dimensional constructs allows outlining of anatomical structures in space and can be used for oblique reconstructions. In addition, the software package ImageJ (National Institutes of Health, Bethesda, Md) and MatLab (The MathWorks Inc.) were used for the evaluation of haptic configurations and axial changes in IOL position.

Three-dimensional UBM measurements were carried out after pharmacologically induced accommodation (two drops of pilocarpine 2% administrated in 5-minute intervals) or disaccommodation (two drops of cyclopentolate 1% administrated in 5-minute intervals) on 2 consecutive days 4 weeks after surgery. The ciliary body regions of four patients were scanned 30 minutes after pharmacological treatment. The three dimensional volumes were then used to identify the tangential plane of the IOL haptic; an oblique reconstruction is possible to perform the biometric measurements. The center of rotation was placed at the fulcrum and the angle between the IOL optic and haptic was measured using the anterior IOL interface. Positive values in angulation represent an anterior vaulting, and negative values represent a posterior vaulting. Changes in haptic angulation and the IOL shift were analyzed (mean and standard deviation) using five B-scans for each accommodative state and for all patients. Positive values for change in anterior chamber depth represent a forward shift of the IOL.

Accommodation Stimulus

Pilocarpine application is an objective way of stimulating accommodation as it requires no participation from the patient. Topical application of pilocarpine is advised and commonly used to stimulate accommodation. Variability in accommodation amplitudes is partially due to the capability and attendance of volunteers to accommodate to various kinds of stimuli. Using pilocarpine, this subjective component to accommodation is eliminated; however, the role of pilocarpine must be discussed. Abramson et al [Abramson 1973] measured the accommodation effect in human individuals using A-scan ultrasound. They determined a greater increase in axial lens diameter after pilocarpine application than is possible with stimulus-driven accommodation. Thus, topical application of pilocarpine may produce overstimulation of the ciliary muscle. These early results are consistent with the findings of Findl [Findl 2004] and Köppl et al [Köppl 2003] who used dual-beam partial coherence interferometry. These studies have shown a difference in lens movement between pilocarpine-induced and stimulus-driven ciliary muscle contraction. Pilocarpine acts "physiologically" in young phakics and as a superstimulus in presbyopic phakics and pseudophakes. Therefore, IOL movement and angulation change data may be overestimated when using pilocarpine.

Accommodative 1CU

Figure 13.7 shows a three-dimensional reconstruction and the image analysis of a 1CU haptic region. Changes in angulation and "ACD by four different individuals show the effect of cyclopentolate and pilocarpine 4 months postoperatively (Fig. 13.8). In disaccommodation, a haptic angulation between 2° and 4° caused by capsular bag shrinkage and secondary cataract formation is visible. This could mean that a

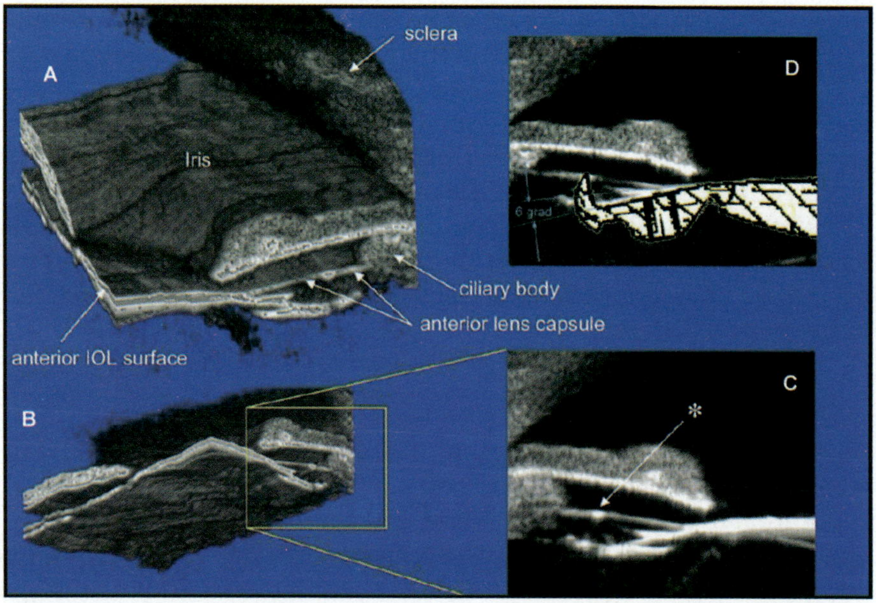

Fig. 13.7: (A,B) Three-dimensional reconstruction and (C, D) image analysis (with design drawing) of the 1CU haptic region in a 75-year-old patient 4 months postoperatively (disaccommodation). A 6° haptic angulation compared with the relaxed IOL condition is observed (Stachs 2005)

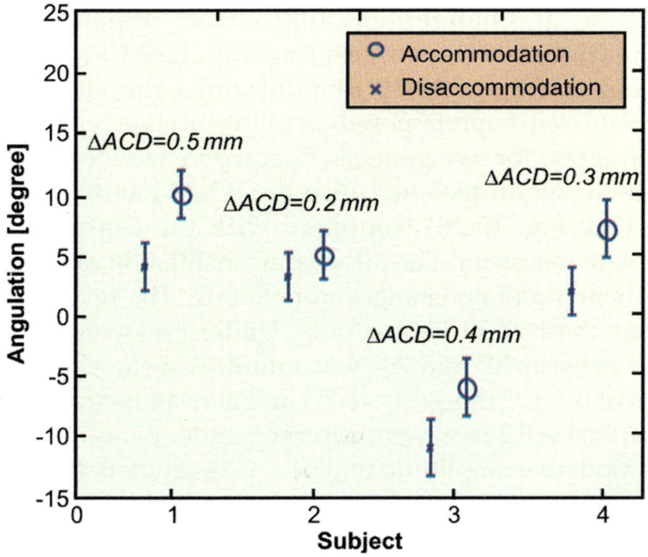

Fig. 13.8: Angulation and anterior chamber depth (ΔACD) by subject (implant 1CU) showing the effect of cyclopentolate and pilocarpine (Δ = angle of difference to the relaxed haptic configuration, o = change under pilocarpine treatment; mean ± standard deviation). Positive values for ΔACD represent a forward shift of the IOL under pilocarpine (Stachs 2005)

haptic angulation is already present in the disaccommodated state. In the cases studied, pilocarpine induced an additional angulation variation between 5° and 10° for the 1CU IOL, which causes a change in anterior chamber depth between 0.2 and 0.5 mm. Using Gullstrand's eye model, this 0.2 mm forward movement results in a refraction change <0.38 D (0.95 D for 0.5 mm of movement), depending on exact IOL position. These findings are in agreement with the results of Findl et al [Findl 2003, 2004]. Using partial coherence interferometry, Findl et al found a moderate forward movement under pilocarpine with induced mean accommodative amplitude of 0.50 D. These mechanical performance of the does not appear to provide the range of accommodation necessary for close work.

CrystaLens AT-45

The echo characteristics of the AT-45 seen in Figure 13.6 were used to describe the *in vivo* situation in four patients with accommodative implants 4 weeks after surgery. Figure 13.9 shows the haptic region of a 71-year-old woman after pilocarpine instillation. A haptic angulation of 33° (uncorrected 190°) compared with the relaxed IOL haptic (0°, uncorrected 157°) is seen in this case. For a descriptive visualization of changes in angulation depending on the accommodation state, corresponding UBM sections were superimposed. Figure 13.10 demonstrates the situation under cyclopentolate (red) superimposed on a UBM section under pilocarpine stimulation (grey) for two patients. Pilocarpine induced an additional angulation change in patient 1 (See Fig. 13.2A) and no changes for patient 2 (See Fig. 13.2B) compared with the configuration after cyclopentolate treatment. The pilocarpine instillation causes a forward shift in patient 1 and no changes in patient 2. The results of the four eyes are summarized in Figure 13.11. Under cyclopentolate, a haptic angulation between10° and 26° was found. A mean change in haptic angulation of 3.3 3.3° (range: 0° to 7°) and a mean forward shift of 0.13 mm (range: 0.06 to 0.2 mm) were observed under pilocarpine treatment. An accommodative amplitude of 0.44 ± 0.24 diopters (D) (range: 0.25 to 0.75 D) was found in the four eyes using a Hartinger coincidence refractometer.

For the AT-45, the proposed mechanism is that accommodation restoration occurs through the ciliary muscle activity. The manufacturer has developed the lens to provide good vision at all distances by moving backward and forward along the optical axis of the eye in response to pressure changes in the vitreous and anterior chamber. In the cases studied, pilocarpine induced an angulation change between 0° and 7° (mean 3.3±3.3°) compared with the situation under cyclopentolate. The angulation change causes a change in anterior chamber depth between 0.06 and 0.2 mm (mean 0.13±0.08 mm). Using Gullstrand's eye model and a 20.0 D IOL placed in the bag, the observed maximal 0.2 mm forward movement results in a refraction change 0.4 D, depending on the exact IOL position. The cases studied showed a maximal accommodation response of mean 0.44 ± 0.24 D (range: 0.25 to 0.75 D) measured by a Hartinger coincidence refractometer. This value is slightly larger than the calculated values using Gullstrand's eye model, possibly caused by individual pseudoaccomodative effects (e.g. pupil size, myopic astigmatism, etc).

Pilocarpine-induced ciliary muscle contraction caused a slight change in haptic angulation and an anterior shift of the AT-45 in these four eyes. This slight change in angulation and the anterior shift resulted in an accommodative amplitude between 0.25 and 0.75 D. Therefore, in these four eyes, the AT-45 did not seem to provide the range of accommodation necessary for close work. We expect that capsular fibrosis and capsular bag shrinkage result in a hardening of the haptic and optic in the capsule, resulting in further decrease of the accommodative performance later postoperatively.

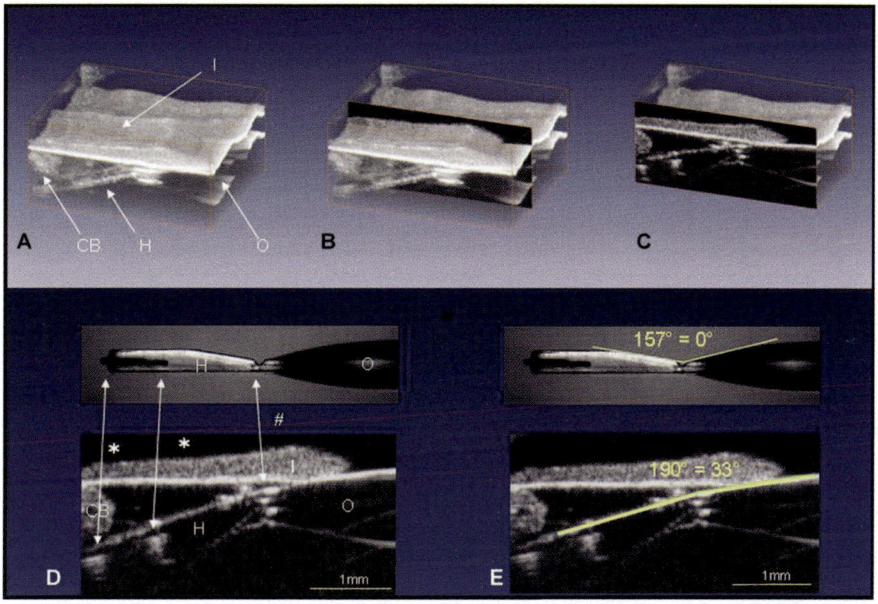

Figs 13.9: A to E: (A-C) Three-dimensional reconstruction and (D) image analysis of the AT-45 haptic region (patient 1: 71-year-old woman, 4 weeks after surgery, pilocarpineinduced accommodation). The fulcrum is marked (#). The optic (O) and haptic (H) are well differentiated, whereas the echo pattern (*) is caused by the polyimide construction of the AT-45 plate haptic. The 157° angle for the relaxed haptic configuration was set to zero for angulation change determination. A haptic angulation of 33° (uncorrected 190°) compared with the relaxed IOL haptic is observed. O = optic, H = haptic, * = polyimide construction, # = fulcrum, I = iris, CB = ciliary body (Stachs 2006)

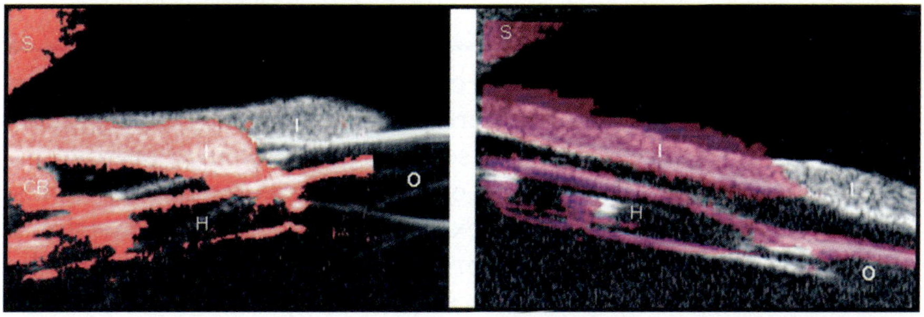

Fig. 13.10: Superimposed UBM sections showing the effect of cyclopentolate and pilocarpine in two patients—A) patient 1, 71-year-old woman and B) patient 2, 77- year-old woman. The disaccommodated state after cyclopentolate treatment (red) and under pilocarpine stimulation (grey) is shown. S = sclera, I = iris, CB = ciliary body, H = haptic, O = optic (Stachs 2006)

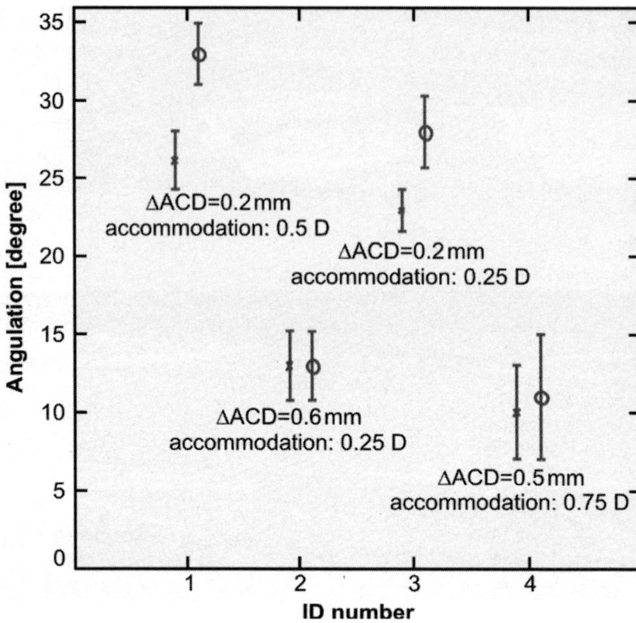

Fig. 13.11: Change in angulation (°) and anterior chamber depth (ACD) [mm] as well as accommodation amplitude (D) in all patients showing the effect of cyclopentolate (cross) and pilocarpine (circle). Positive values for change in anterior chamber depth represent a forward shift of the IOL. Positive values in angulation represent an anterior vaulting (Stachs 2006)

CONCLUSION

One of the challenging tasks of the cataract surgery is the conservation or restoring the accommodative performance in pseudophakic patient. Various attempts have been made so solve the problem of presbyopia. One example is the development of so-called accommodative IOL's. The *in vitro* simulation device examined with three-dimensional ultrasound biomicroscopy provided information on the accommodative performance of these potentially accommodative IOL designs. Using three-dimensional ultrasound biomicroscopy, corresponding changes in haptic angulation during pharmacological induced accommodation were observed. Pilocarpine-induced ciliary muscle contraction caused a change in haptic angulation and an anterior shift of the investigated IOL's, which resulted in approximately an estimated accommodative amplitude between 0.40 and 0.95 D (1CU) as well as 0.25 and 0.75 (AT-45). The mechanical performance of the investigated IOL's *in vitro* and in the eyes studied does not appear to provide the range of accommodation necessary for close work.

BIBLIOGRAPHY

1. Abramson DH, Franzen LA, Coleman DJ. Pilocarpine in the presbyope. Demonstration of an effect on the anterior chamber and lens thickness. Arch Ophthalmol 1973;89:100-2.
2. Coleman D, Silverman R., Daly S., Advances in ophthalmic ultrasound. Radiol Clin North Am, 1998; 36: p. 1073-82.
3. Cumming JS, Kammann J. Experience with an accommodating IOL. J Cataract Refract Surg 1996;22:1001.
4. Cusumano A, Coleman D, Silverman R, Reinstein D, Rondeau M, Ursea B, Daly S. Three-dimensional ultrasound imaging – clinical applications. Ophthalmology 1998; 105: p. 300-6.
5. Findl O, Drexler W, Menapace R, Bobr B, Bittermann S, Vass C, Rainer G, Hitzenberger CK, Fercher AF. Accurate determination of effective lens position and lens-capsule distance with 4 intraocular lenses. J Cataract Refract Surg 1998;24:1094-98.
6. Findl O, Kriechbaum K, Köppl C, Menapace R, Drexler W. Laser interferometric measurements of IOL movement with accommodating IOLs. Proceedings of the American Society of Cataract and Refractive Surgery annual meeting; 2003; 12-16, San Francisco, Calif. Abstract #94.
7. Findl O, Kiss B, Petternel V, Menapace R, Georgopoulos M, Rainer G and Drexler W. Intraocular lens movement caused by ciliary muscle contraction; Journal Cataract Refract Surg 29. 2003b; 669-76.
8. Findl O, Menapace R, Kriechbaum K, Koeppel C, Drexler W. Laser interferometric measurements of movement of an "accommodating" IOL. In: Guthoff R, Ludwig K, eds. Current Aspects in Accommodation II. Heidelberg, Germany: Kaden, 2003c; 211-21.
9. Findl O, Kiss B, Petternel V, Menapace R, Georgopoulos M, Rainer G, Drexler W. Intraocular lens movement caused by ciliary muscle contraction. J Cataract Refract Surg 2003d;29:669-76.
10. Findl O, et al. Laserinterferometric assessment of pilocarpine-induced movement of an accommodating intraocular lens: a randomized trial. Ophthalmology 2004;111(8):1515-21.
11. Findl O. Accommodative intraocular lens: funktionelle Ergebnisse. Klin Monatsbl Augenheilkd 2004b;221(Suppl):36.
12. Gandolfi SA, Marchini G, Tosi R, Mora P, Pedrotti E, Sartori P, Manzotti F. UBM changes during accommodation in eyes implanted with Crystalens AT45 and 1CU IOL. A pilot study. Invest Ophthalmol Vis Sci. 2003;44:E- abstract 252.
13. Hara T, Hara T, Yasuda A, Yamada Y. Accommodative intraocular lens with spring action, I design and placement in an excised animal eye. Ophthalmic Surg 1990;21:128-33.
14. Hardman Lea SJ, Rubinstein MP, Snead MP, Haworth SM. Pseudophakic accommodation. A study of the stability of capsular bag supported, one piece, rigid tripod, or soft fl exible implants. Br J Ophthalmol 1990;74:22-25.
15. Iezzi R, Rosen R, Tello C, Liebmann J, Walsh F, Ritch R. Personal computer-based Three-dimensional ultrasound biomicroscopy of the anterior segment. Arch Ophthalmol, 1996; 114: p. 520-24.
16. Kirchhoff A, Stachs O, Guthoff R. Three-dimensional ultrasound findings of the posterior iris region. Graefes Archive for Clinical and Experimental Ophthalmology 2001;239(12):968-71.

17. Kaufman PL. Accommodation and presbyopia: neuromuscular and biophysical aspects. In: Hart WM Jr, ed. Adlers Physiology of the eye. Clinical Application. (9th edn) St Louis, Mo: Mosby; 1992;391-411.
18. Köppl C, Findl O, Kriechbaum K, Dexler W. Comparison of pilocarpine-induced and stimulus-driven accommodation in phakic eyes. Proceedings of the XXI Congress of the European Society of Cataract and Refractive Surgery; 2003; 6-10, Munich, Germany.
19. Küchle M, Nguyen NX, Langenbucher A, Gusek-Schneider GC, Seitz B, Hanna KD. Implantation of a new accommodative posterior chamber intraocular lens. J Refract Surg 2002;18:208-16.
20. Langenbucher A, Huber S, Nguyen NX, Seitz B, Gusek- Schneider GC, Kuchle M. Measurement of accommodation after implantation of an accommodating posterior chamber intraocular lens. J Cataract Refract Surg 2003;29:677-85.
21. Legeais JM, Werner L, Werner L, Abenhaim A, Renard G. Pseudo-accommodation: BioComFold versus a foldable silicone intraocular lens. J Cataract Refract Surg 1999;25:262-67.
22. Nakazawa M, Ohtsuki K. Apparent accommodation pseudophakic eyes after implantation of posterior chamber intraocular lenses: optical analysis. Invest Ophthalmol Vis Sci. 1984;25:1458-60.
23. Pavlin CJ, Foster FS. Ultrasound Biomicroscopy of the eye. New York, NY: Springer; 1995.
24. Ravalico G, Baccara F. Apparent accommodation in pseudophakic eyes. Acta Ophthalmol 1990;68:604-6.
25. Reinstein D, Raevsky T, Coleman D. Improved system for ultrasonic imaging and biometry. J Ultrasound Med 1997; 16: p. 117-24.
26. Sarfarazi FM. Optical and mechanical design for human implantation of the Sarfarazi Elliptical Accommodation IOL. Proceedings of the American Society of Cataract and Refractive Surgery annual meeting; 2003;12-16; San Francisco, Calif. Abstract #738.
27. Silverman R, Lizzi F, Ursea B, Rondeau M, Eldeen N, Kaliscz A, Lloyd H, Coleman D. High-resolution ultrsonic imaging and characterization of the ciliary body. Invest Ophthalmol Vis Sci, 2001. 42: p. 885-94.
28. Stachs O, Martin H, Kirchhoff A, Stave J, Terwee T, Guthoff R. Monitoring accommodative ciliary muscle function using three-dimensional ultrasound. Graefes Arch Clin Exp Ophthalmol 2002;240:906-12.
29. Stachs O, Schneider H, Stave J, Guthoff R. Potentially accommodating intraocular lenses—an *in vitro* and *in vivo* study using three-dimensional high-frequency ultrasound. J Refract Surg 2005;21(1):37-45.
30. Stachs O, Martin H, Behrend D, Schmitz K P, Guthoff R. Three-dimensional ultrasound biomicroscopy, environmental and conventional scanning electron microscopy investigations of the human zonula ciliaris for numerical modelling of accommodation. Graefe's Arch Clin Exp Ophthalmol 2005a; 5: p. epub ahead of print.
31. Stachs O, Schneider H, Beck R, Guthoff R. Pharmacological-induced haptic changes and the accommodative performance in patients with the AT-45 accommodative IOL. J Refract Surg 2006;22(2):145-50.

CHAPTER

14

JT Lin (USA)

Accommodative IOLs: Efficiency and Optimal Designs

INTRODUCTION

Analytic formulas for accommodating intraocular lens with forward movement pseudo-accommodation (or apparent accommodation) in various intraocular lenses (IOLs) has been reported including 1CU lens (Human Optics, Inc.), AT-45 lens (C&C Vision) and MA30 lens (Eyeonics Vision, Inc.).[1-4] The preoperative and postoperative corneal power (or keratometry) or the estimated lens position (ELP), are believed to be the important factors in comparing the outcomes of different IOLs. The accommodation (A) per 1.0 mm anterior movement (defined as M) was measured [3-5] to be about M=(0.9 – 1.9) (diopter/mm) and calculated by Nawa et al [6] to be (0.8-2.3) (diopter/mm) by ray tracing method.

As reported by Nawa et al that widely scattered values of M may result from various ocular conditions such as corneal power, IOL power and axial length. These features are explored by numerical calculations based on a ray-tracing equation, where the roles of each of the ocular parameters have not been fully explored.

In this Chapter, analytic formulas for M in single-optics IOL will be derived (in the Appendix) to demonstrate explicitly the parameters determining M. These include the corneal (D_1) and IOL power (D_2), the IOL postoperative effective position (S), the effective vitreous cavity length (X), axial length (L) and the remaining refractive error. For example, M should be determined by X and S, rather than the axial length alone, where M varies even for the same axial length. Six different ocular situations showing the roles of each of the parameters will be discussed. This Chapter will cover the following subjects:

1. Accommodation in single optics IOL (in aphakia)
2. Accommodation in two optics IOL (in phakia)
3. Design aspects for maximal efficiency and minimal spherical aberration.

As shown in Figure 14.1A, the accommodation of a single-optics accommodating IOL (AIOL) in aphakic eye (without the natural lens) may be achieved by the forward movement of the optics, and L=S+X, where S=p (position of the IOL) for thin-lens and S=p+gT, for thick-lens to include the geometry factor (g) and its thickness. Note that gT>0 for biconvex and gT<0 for convex-concave, and gT=0 for convex-plano. Figure 14.1B shows the 3-optics system where the AIOL is implanted in a phakic eye.

Figure 14.1C shows the dual optics AIOL in which the accommodation may be achieved by the forward (or backward) movement of the front (or back) optics. The net result depending on various situations that either front or back or both optics may be mobile,

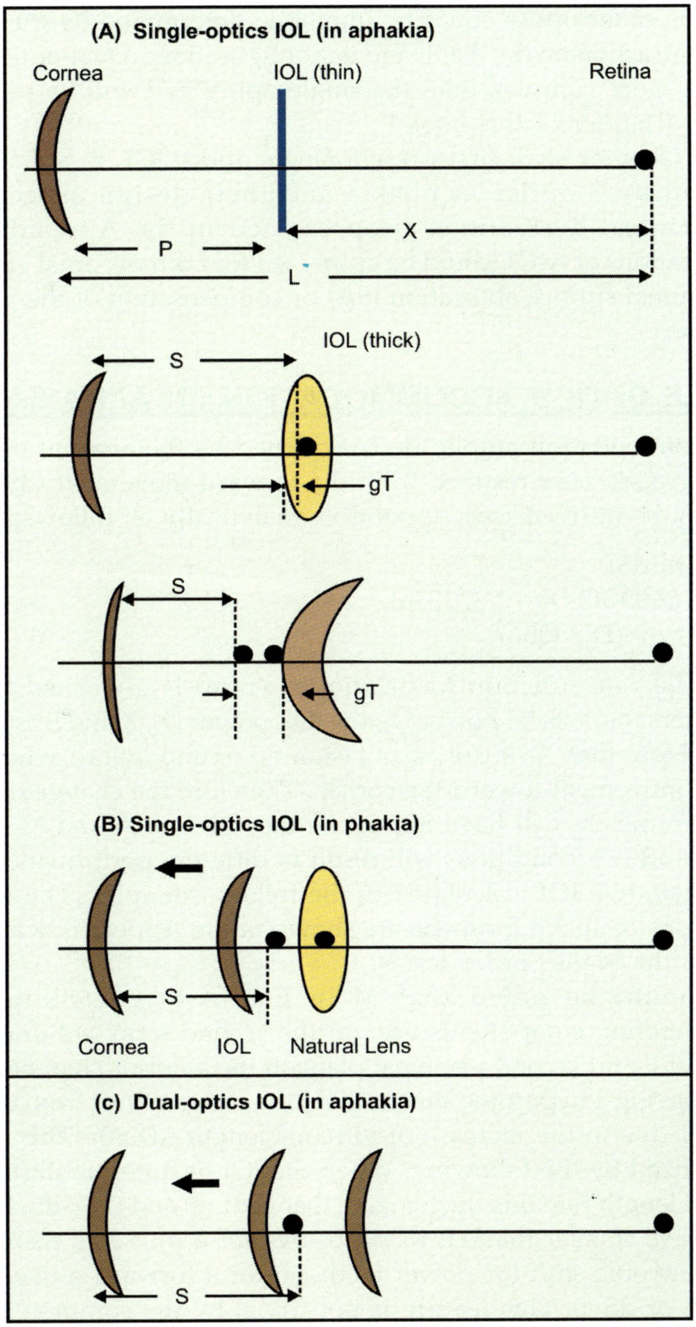

Fig. 14.1: Schematics of single-optics and dual-optics AIOL in aphakic and phakic eye

while the other optics could be immobile determined by the ciliary-body contraction on the AIOL and its configurations. Dual-optics AIOL is much more complex than the single-optics and will be presented in other Chapter of this book.[12]

This Chapter shall first present single-optics IOL in aphakia and followed by 3-optics in phakia and their design aspects. The mathematical derivations are presented in the Appendix. The configurations of AIOL could be optimized for both maximal efficiency and minimal surface aberration (SA) or compensation of the SA from the cornea.

SINGLE-OPTICS ACCOMMODATION (IN APHAKIA)

The accommodation amplitude (A) defined by the amount of power increase to see near resulted from the forward movement (dS) of the IOL may be derived (see Appendix) analytically as follows

$$A = M(dS), \quad (1.a)$$
$$M = (Z^2D_2)(2/X - D_2/1336), \quad (1.b)$$
$$Z = 1 - S(D_1/1336), \quad (1.c)$$

where the rate function M (in diopter/mm) is governed by four parameters the corneal power D_1, the IOL power D_2, X and S as defined earlier. Note that A>0 (for near vision accommodation) when dS>0 defined movement toward the cornea. Therefore the change of any of these parameters will have impact on the value of A and M.Various corneal and IOL conditions will result in different performance of the accommodative IOL calculated in the follow examples. The detailed derivations of above formulas are shown in the Appendix which also includes the higher order terms.

It should be noted that M in Eq. (A-6) contribute from two competing components are: (a) the second-term M2 due to the change of F and second principal plane in the anterior chamber depth (dS<0) having a hyperopic shift, and (b) the myopic-shift from the first-term M1 due to the increase of vitreous length (dX>0). This may be also realized by the following. When the IOL is anterior shifted with the axial length remains unchanged, that is dL=0 and dX=-dS. Because F is always smaller than f1, M is positive for a plus IOL resulting in a "net" myopic shift (or power increase) for a forward movement of the IOL, or dS<0. This feature is not trivial by the common concept that forward movement causing a myopic shift. Formulas of this study show that the myopic shift is a net result from the hyperopic shift from dS<0, and the larger myopic shift from dX>0. Above discussion is for a plus IOL case. For a minus IOL, a reverse process is needed for myopic-shift, that is when dS>0, or a backward movement toward the retina.

The above formulas show that A and M is governed by the correlation between each of the four ocular parameters (D_1, D_2, X, S) rather than their absolute magnitudes. These correlations are further defined by the emmetropic condition of

$$D_2 = 1336/X - D_1/Z. \tag{2}$$

Using Eq.(2) to eliminate X of Eq. (1.b), one may obtain an alternative expression of M

$$M=(Z/1336)D_2(2D_1+ZD_2). \tag{3}$$

The above formula shows that M is proportional to the product of Z and the IOL and corneal power. It also has a nonlinear term, the second term proportional to the IOL power. In comparison, Eq.(1) shows that M is a decreasing function of X (or axial length L=X+S). Eq.(3) also shows higher M for positive IOL (contributed from the second term, whereas M (absolute value) is lower for minus IOL, or when $D_2<0$.

There are six possible combinations shown as follows if only two parameters are measured or given and the other two are calculated: measured (X, S) with calculated (D_1, D_2); measured (X, D_1) with calculated (D_2, S); measured (X, D_2) with calculated (X, D_1); measured (D_1, S) with calculated (D_2, X); measured (D_2, S) with calculated (D_1, X); and measured (D_1, D_2) with calculated (X, S). Various examples based on the above combinations are discussed as follows.

Case (1): Fixed X=18.8 mm and S=5.0 mm, (or L=X+S=23.8 mm).

M = (1.1, 1.29, 1.45, 1.62) (diopter/mm) for corneal power of D_1 = (45, 43, 41, 39) diopter and the required IOL power for emmetropia D_2=(17, 20, 22.4, 25.6) diopter calculated from Eq.(2). These calculated data show that IOL with a higher power, in general, produces higher accommodation for a given amount of anterior movement (dS), in consistent with the measured [1] and calculated values using a ray tracing method[6] (Fig. 14.2).

Case (2): Fixed corneal power D_1=43 diopter and axial length L=23.8 mm.

M = (1.08, 1.14, 1.2, 1.29, 1.36) (diopter/mm), for S=(2.0, 3.0, 4.0, 5.0, 6.0) mm. These values show that M is an increasing function of the IOL position, where X decreases when S increases for a fixed axial length L=X+S. (Fig. 14.3, Curve B).

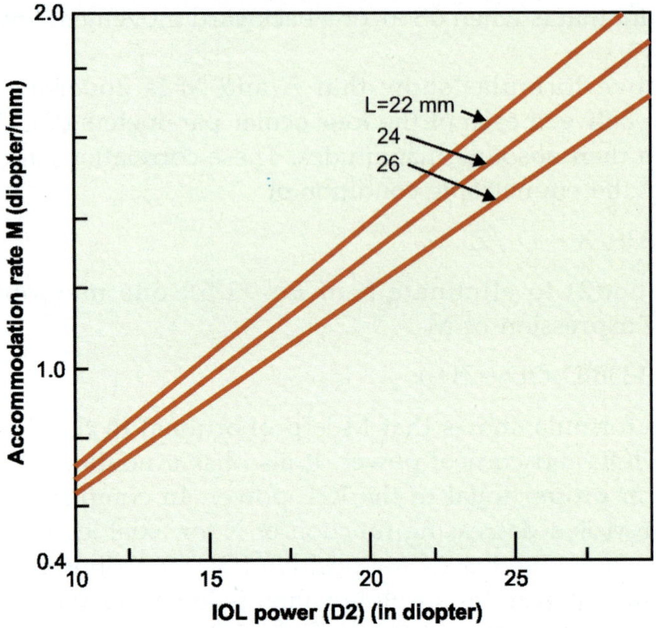

Fig. 14.2: Accommodation rate M (per 1.0 mm of forward movement) versus IOL-power at various axial length L=(22, 24, 26) mm

Case (3): Fixed IOL power D_2=20 diopter and L=23.8 mm.
M=(1.36, 1.34, 1.32, 1.29, 1.25) (diopter/mm), for S=(2, 3, 4, 5, 6) mm.
The decrease of M for larger S is the net result of the competing factors from the decrease of X=L–S, and the emmetropic condition which requires a higher corneal power for a given IOL power (Fig. 14.3, curve A).

Case (4): Fixed D_1=43 diopter and S=5.0 mm
M=(0.56, 0.82, 1.22, 1.87) (diopter/mm), for IOL power D_2=(9.5, 12.4, 19.1, 27.3) diopter and axial length L=(27, 26, 24, 22) mm calculated from L=X+S. This example shows that, for a given corneal power, longer eye with lower IOL power result in a smaller M, in consistent with that of Nawa[6] (Fig. 14.4, curve B).

Case (5): Fixed D_2=20 diopter, S=5.0 mm.
M=(1.38, 1.26, 1.19) for L=(22, 24, 26) mm and X=(17, 19, 21) mm. (Fig. 14.3, curve A).

Case (6): Fixed D_1=43 diopter and S=5.0 mm.
M=(0.6, 0.93, 1.29, 1.68), for D_2=(10, 15, 20, 25) diopters, calculated from Eq.(3) for the linear case, curve (A) and the nonlinear case, curve (B) in Figure 14.5.

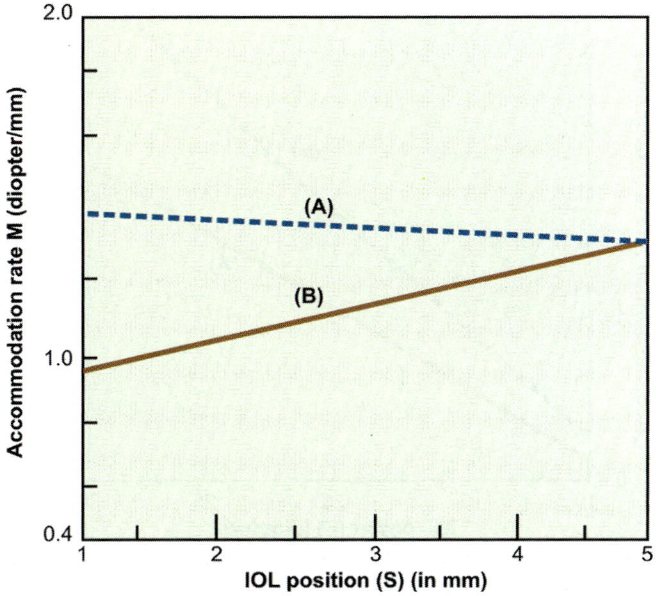

Fig. 14.3: M versus IOL position (S) for: (A) fixed IOL power at 20 diopter, and (B) fixed corneal power at 43 diopter, for a fixed axial length L=23.8 mm in both cases

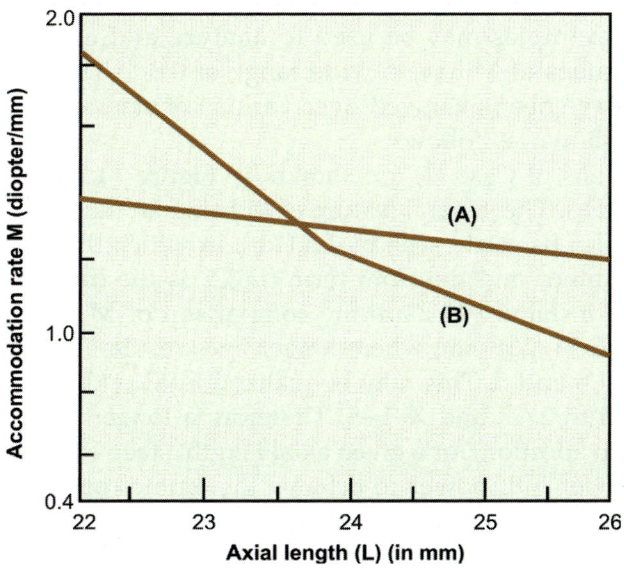

Fig. 14.4: M versus axial length (L) with curve (A) and (B) having the same conditions as Figure 14.2, but for a fixed S=5.0 mm, and L and X change

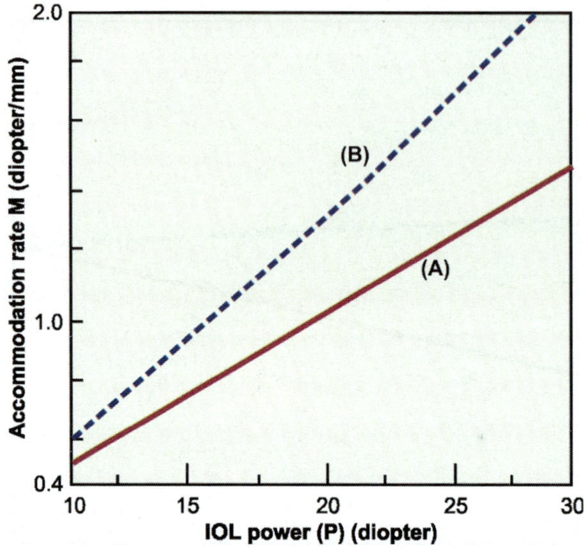

Fig. 14.5: M versus plus IOL power D_2 for fixed corneal power at 43 diopter and S=5.0 mm, where curve (A) shows the linear function based on Eq.(3) which is lower than curve (B) with nonlinear term included

DISCUSSIONS OF APHAKIC-IOL

The above examples may be used to analyze and explain why the measured values of M have a wide range of 0.8 to 1.9 (diopter/mm) even they have been averaged over various ocular conditions. More details are shown as follows.

Calculations of Case (1) are shown by Figure 14.2 for the role of IOL power (D_2). The general feature of M being an increasing function of D_2 may also be easily seen by Eq.(1.b), in which the minus term $-D_2/1336$ is minor and the front term $(D_2)Z^2$ is the dominating term. Also shown in Figure 14.2 are the comparison of M vs. D_2 for axial length L=(22, 24, 26) mm, where longer eyes results in smaller M for a given D_1, D_2 and S. This may be realized by Eq.(1.b) showing M is proportional to 2/X, and X=L–S. Therefore a longer eye results in a smaller M. In addition, for a given axial length, steep corneas normally require a lower IOL power to achieve the emmetropic Eq.(2) which also obtain a lower accommodate rate than that of a flat-cornea with high-power IOL. This trend is consistent with that of Nawa et al using lengthy numerical calculation which is readily available from Eq.(1.b).

Figure 14.3 shows the results for Case (2) and (3) which have opposite trends when S increases. This feature may be further analyzed as follows. Case (2) shown by curve (B) of Figure 14.2 indicates that given the same axial length and corneal power, posterior chamber implant (such as 1CU) is more efficient than that of anterior implant (such as AT-45), because higher IOL power is needed for larger S to achieve an emmetropia. In contrast, Case (3) shown by curve (A) with a fixed IOL power and L, larger S requires smaller X and higher corneal power (D_1) to meet the emmetropic condition, Eq.(2).

Calculations based on parameters of Case (3) show a net increase of M, in contrast to Case (2), when S increases. These features were not explored in the ray-tracing method of Nawa et al. Furthermore, the statement made by these authors that longer eye with lower IOL power results in higher M is only partially correct. As shown in this study, Case (2) and (3), and Eq.(1.b), M is governed by the combined function of $Z^2(D_2)/X$, rather than their absolute values. As shown in the above example, M may be a decreasing or increasing function of S or X even for the same axial length (L). The role of axial length should be broken down by L=S+X to separate the roles of S and X as shown by Case (2), (3) and (6).The roles of S, X and L were not differentiated in the calculations of Nawa et al. In other words, a longer eye does not necessarily result in a higher M which is also subject to the relative value of S and X.

Results of Case (4) and (5) are shown by curves (B) and (A) of Figure 14.4 and demonstrate that M is a decreasing function of L in both Cases, because X is an increasing function of L when S is fixed, and larger X results in a smaller M as shown by Eq.(1.b). The calculated values in Case (4) with M=(0.56–1.87) (D/mm) for L=(27-22) mm are consistent with that of Nawa, M=(0.8-1.9) (D/mm), where the small difference is due to the difference in corneal power chosen. The measured data of 0.9 and 2.02 (D/mm) for axial length of 21 and 25.8 mm also showed the similar trend, although their values are higher due to higher IOL powers are used.

Figure 14.4 (curve-B) shows that M is a strongly decreasing function of L (from 1.87 to 0.82) in Case (4) with a fixed corneal power and various IOL powers, in comparing to a weak dependence of L in Case (5) (curve A) with a fixed IOL power and various corneal powers. In other words, M has a stronger dependence on IOL power than on corneal-power.

Figure 14.5 shows the nonlinear behavior of M versus D_2 (about 1% higher per diopter) as shown in Case (6). This nonlinear feature resulted from the second term of Eq. (3) was not shown by Nawa et al using a ray tracing method.

As shown in the Appendix, M, in general, is a function of six parameters (De, D_1, D_2, S, X, L), where De is the refractive error after IOL implant (if any) and may contribute about 6% (for De=10.0 diopter) of the value of M at emmetropic state. The M value for ametropic state (post IOL) may be calculated by adding an extra term of 2(1/X – 1/f2) De to Eq.(1.b) derived from Eq.(A-6) by using Eq.(A-3) to eliminate f1. This ametropic term contributes about 0.06 (diopter/mm) for each diopter of De to the M value at emmetropic state.

THREE-OPTICS ACCOMMODATION (IN PHAKIA)

The 3-optics IOL system include: (a) single-optics IOL in phakia, (b) piggyback IOL, and (c) dual-optics IOL in aphakia. Case (c) for dual-optics IOL is much more complex due to the variety of configurations and the movement dynamics of each optics which will be presented in a separate chapter by Lin in this book. We shall now present the formulas for case (a) and (b).

Using Gaussian optics, Lin had derived the formula for the dual-optics accommodating IOL which may also apply to the single-optics IOL in phakic eye by replacing the back-optics of the dual-optics IOL as the natural lens (for phakic IOL) or the primary-IOL (for piggyback IOL). The M function of 2-optics system shown by Eq. (1) or (3) is revised as follows for a 3-optics phakic IOL

$$M' = (f/f_2)M - \text{Delta}, \quad (4.a)$$
$$\text{Delta} = Z^2/(f_2 f_3), \quad (4.b)$$

where f_2 and f_3 are the EFL of the IOL and the natural lens (NL), respectively and $1/f=1/f_2+Z''/f_3$, with $Z''=1-p'/f_2$, $p'=p+2.4$ mm. Above formula reduces to the 2-optics (M) when f3=infinity (or aphakic eye) and $f=f_2$, Delta=0. The second term, Delta, is a reduction factor of M due to the presence of the NL. The configuration factor $G=f/f_2$ may be re-expressed as

$$G = 1/[1+Z''(Pn/Pi)]$$

where Pn and Pi are the NL power and IOL power, respectively.

M′ may be further expressed as the power of the cornea (Pc), Pn and Pi as follows

$$M' = (Z/1336)Pi\ (2Pc+Z'ZPi), \quad (5.a)$$
$$Z' = 1-p'/f3,\ Z = 1-S'/f1, \quad (5.b)$$
$$S' = S+gp',\ g=1/[1+Z'(Pi/Pn)]. \quad (5.c)$$

where p′=p+2.4 mm in phakic IOL and S=ELP is the position of the IOL (thin lens) or S=ELP+g′T (for thick lens), where g′ is a geometry factor of the IOL having a thickness T and front and back surface power ratio of D_{12}, $g'=1/(1+D_{12})$.

Comparing M′ of Eq.(4) for IOL in phakic eye with Eq.(4) for the aphakia M, one may easily conclude the following:

1. For a given IOL power, M′ in phakia is always smaller than that of the aphakia (M) by a reduction factor determined by Z and Z′=1–p′/f_3, in which Z′<1, even the IOL closely contacts to the natural lens since p′=2.4 mm when p=0. In contrast, for a piggyback IOL contacts to a thin primary IOL p′=0, Z′=1.0 and S′=S, that is, no reduction effect from the primary IOL when p=0.
2. The new parameter S′=S+gp′ is further shifted due to the effective separation of the IOL and natural lens by p′=p+2.4 mm, and also affected by a geometry factor defined by the ratio of the IOL and natural lens power (Pi/Pn).
3. Eq.(5) for IOL in phakia may apply to piggyback IOL by redefining p′ being their separation (assuming both are thin lens) and Pn being the power of the primary IOL.

Example 1

For an anterior IOL implanted in phakic eye having a corneal power Dc=43 D and natural lens power of Pn=21.5 D, ACD=2.0 mm and p=2.0 mm, or p′=p+2.4=4.4 mm. The calculated Z′=0.93 (or a 7% reduction) and g=(0.82, 0.7, 0.61) for IOL power of Pi=(5, 10, 15) D. The calculated phakic IOL M′=(0.275, 0.59, 0.93), respectively, which are about 10% to 15% lower than the aphakia value of M=(0.32, 0.67, 1.05) (D/mm).

Example 2

Same as above, but for posterior IOL of ACD=4.0 mm, p=0, p′=2.4 mm, the calculated Z′=0.96 (or a 4% reduction) and g is about the same as above. Therefore M′=(0.25, 0.48, 0.69) versus M=(0.295, 0.62, 0.97) (D/mm), a reduction of about 8% to 29% in phakia IOL comparing to aphakia. Comparing to Example 1 (anterior IOL), the posterior IOL has higher reduction factor.

Example 3

For piggyback IOL separated from the primary IOL by p′. For ACD+p′=6.4 mm, the M′ value will be the same as that of Example 1 and 2. However, for smaller ACD+p′=4.0 mm, with ACD=3.0 and p′=1.0 mm, and a smaller Pn=15.0 D for Pi=+5.0 D, the calculated Z′=0.989 (reduction only about 1%), g=0.752, S′=4.0+0.752 x 1=4.752, Z=0.847. Therefore M′=0.286 of piggyback IOL versus M=0.306 (D/mm) for IOL in aphakia. These M′ and M values are approximately, except the nonlinear second-term in Eq (3), proportional to the piggyback IOL power. Therefore one shall expect M′=(0.57, 0.86, 1.14) (D/mm) for higher IOL power of Pi=(10, 15, 20) D, since M′ is insensitive to the primary IOL power (Pn).

PHAKIC IOL AT EMMETROPIC STATE

The emmetropia condition, Eq.(2) for aphakia, becomes more complicated in a 3-optics phakia IOL as follows.

$$Pi = [1336/X' - Pc/Z - Pn]/Z', \quad (6)$$

which reduces to Eq.(2) when Pn (the power of natural lens or the primary IOL)=0, and Z′=1.0 (or p′=0) and S′=S, X′=L–S′=X, as one expects. Under the condition that the phakic IOL is very close to the natural lens, that is p=0 and p′=2.4 mm, Z′=1–p′(Pn/1336). The calculated Z′=(0.973, 0.964) for Pn=(15, 20) diopter. In comparison, for piggyback IOL contacted to the primary IOL, p′=p=0, Z′=1.0.

Therefore the M′, proportional to the IOL power (Pi), is now governed by more parameters than the aphakia (M) by the extra contribution or impact from Z′, S′ and Pn, where S′=S+gp′ also influenced by the geometry factor having a wide range of g=(0.6 to 0.82) for Pi=(+15 to +5) D.

Similar to the discussed case (1) to (6) for the aphakia IOL, one may also expect the following for the phakia IOL:

Case (a): For fixed axial length (L), X′ and S′

Eq.(6) shows that flatter cornea or natural lens (NL), or primary IOL (PIOL) with smaller Pc or Pn, would require higher IOL (or piggyback IOL) Pi, therefore M′ is proportionally larger. For example, for Pc=43 D, X′=16 mm, S′=6.0 mm and Z′=1.0, Z=0.806, Pi=(5, 10) D, for Pn=(25, 20) D, and the calculated M′=(0.28, 0.58) (D/mm), respectively based on Eq.(4).

Case (b): Same as (a) but fixed Pn=20 D

In this case Pi=(10, 15) D for corneal power Pc=(43, 38) D. Therefore Z=(0.806, 0.829) to obtain M′=(0.58, 0.85) (D/mm), which increases when corneal power decreases.

Case (c): For fixed Pc=43 D, Pn=20 D, S′=6.0 mm

Pi=(10, 22) D, for X′=(16, 14) mm, or L=(22, 24) mm, therefore M′=(0.58, 1.43) (D/mm) which is a decreasing function of axial length (L) or X′.

Above trends also apply to piggyback IOL by defining Pn as the primary IOL power. The above features in phakic IOL are similar to that of the aphakia, except all the M′ values are reduced by about 10 to 30%.

OPTIMAL IOL DESIGN

Surface aberration including spherical aberration (SA) and coma have been reported by Wang et al [13] for various configurations with front and back surface radius of (in mm) (R1, R2) = (a) (15.4 – 15.4), (b) (7.29, infinity), (c) (infinity, –7.29), (d) (51.6, –9.1), (e) (9.1, –51.6), (f) (–55.3, –6.8), etc. Their calculations concluded that cases (b) convex-plano and (e) (bi-CX) have the smallest SA, whereas (e) and (a) have the smallest coma. Therefore, case (a), (b) and (e) configurations are the preferred IOL structure for minimal surface aberrations.

However, as reported by Atchison,[14] the optimal IOL design is that the negative SA of the cornea asphericity could be balanced by the positive SA from the IOL (and/or the natural lens). For corneal asphericity (Q) about –0.2 to –0.5 for most population, the optimal IOL form is close to convex-plano with the more-curved surface facing the cornea. This feature may be analyzed by Coddington shape factor (X) defined by the radius of the front and back surface, R1 and R2,

$$X = (R1 + R2) / (R1 - R2). \qquad (7)$$

where X>1, for meniscus (or convex-concave) with more curved surface facing cornea; X=–1, for plano-convex; X=+1 for convex-plano; X>–1 for biconvex and X=0 for equi-convex. According to Smith and Liu, the optimal value of X=+1.1 or a convex-concave IOL (with convex facing cornea) in order to produce positive SA and balance the negative corneal SA for minimal overall SA of the eye. Based on the Gaussian formula of M′ and M, this convex-concave configuration also provides higher accommodation rate.

CONCLUSION

By Gaussian optics, the accommodation rate (diopter/mm) function (M) may be derived analytically for both aphakia and phakia IOL and piggyback IOL. The M value is determined by the combined factor of the products of ZPiPc(2+Z′ZPi/Pc) shown by Eq.(3). Following features of AIOL may be summarized:

- M is proportional to the product of Z and the IOL (Pi) and corneal power (Pc) and extra nonlinear term Z′Zpi/Pc which is influenced by the power of the natural lens (for the case of phakic IOL), or by the primary IOL power (for the case of piggyback IOL) by Z′ and S′=S=gp′;
- The Z′ reduction term is a function of the IOL and natural lens (or primary IOL) separation and their power, Z′=1–p′(Pn/1336), having a value of about 0.96 to 0.98.

- The effective ACD (S) is shifted to S′=S+gp′, where g is a geometry factor given by g=1/(1+Z′Pi/Pn) about 0.6 to 0.82.
- The M′ function (for phakia) is about 10 to 30% lower than M (for aphakia).
- The general trend is that higher M or M′ for eyes with shorter axial length (L or X), flatter cornea or smaller ACD (or S) and for high IOL power.
- IOL with convex-concave structure has a higher M′ and may achieve lower surface aberration of the eye comparing to other structures.

Above features are for single-optics IOL in phakia or aphakia, or piggyback IOL. For dual-optics IOL accommodation, see other Chapter of Lin this book.

APPENDIX

In the following, the formulas of Eq.(1) with additional nonlinear correction terms to account for the effects of remaining refractive error will be derived.

By Gaussian optics theory,[8] the refractive error (De) after an IOL is implanted in an aphakic eye may be described by [9,10]

$$De = 1336[1/(L\text{-}L2) - 1/F], \qquad \text{(A-1)}$$

where L is the axial length, L2 is the position of the second principal plane and F is the effective focal length (EFL) of the cornea-IOL system related to the EFL of the cornea (f_1) and IOL (f_2) by

$$1/F = 1/f_1 + Z/f_2, \qquad \text{(A-2)}$$

where $Z=1\text{-}S/f_1$, S being the effective anterior chamber depth of the IOL which equals to the postoperative estimated lens position (ELP) when a thin IOL lens is assumed. Using the relation of L2=S(1-F/f1) (for thin lens) [8,10] and substituting Eq.(A-2) to (A-1), one obtains

$$qDe = 1336/X - D_1/Z\text{-}\ D_2, \qquad \text{(A-3)}$$

$$q = (1+kDe)/Z^2, \qquad \text{(A-4)}$$

where the effective vitreous length defined by X=L-S, and k=SF/($1336Zf_1$) is a small nonlinear term[9] with a typical value of about $0.003D_1$ and De are the power of the cornea and lens, respectively.

To formulate the accommodation amplitude (A) per 1.0 mm forward movement of a single-optics IOL, I define a rate function M=-dDe/dS=A/dS, which may be obtained by taking the derivative of Eq.(A-3) with respect to X

$$dDe = \text{-}M(dS), \qquad \text{(A-5)}$$

$$M = M_1 - M_2 - (B_{-1})/(f_1f_2), \qquad \text{(A-6.a)}$$

$$M1 = 1336B(1+dS/X)(Z/X)^2, \quad \text{(A-6.b)}$$
$$M2 = 1336B/f_{12}, \quad \text{(A-6.c)}$$
$$B = 1 + 2FDin/1336. \quad \text{(A-6.d)}$$

where the high-order term dS/X contributing about 5% for dS=1.0 mm and the last term is the initial refractive error (Din) after the forward movement, about 0.02 (diopter/mm) for Din=1.0 diopter. In deriving above formulas, I had also used dX=dL–dS=–dS, since dL=0, that is axial length remains the same when the IOL is anterior shifted; and $dZ=-dS/f_1$. At emmetropic state (De=0), Eq.(A-3) gives the formula for IOL power

$$D_2 = 1336/X - D_1/Z, \quad \text{(A-7)}$$

which may be used to eliminate the second term in Eq.(A-6) since $D_1=1336/f_1$ and to obtain a more practical formula for M as shown in Eq.(1.b), where I also used the relationship of F=X/Z for emmetropic state in deriving Eq.(1.b) in which the high-order terms of (A-6) and the Din term are neglected. Eq.(A-7) may be compared with the classical vergence formula of Heijde [11] by relating X=L-ELP and corneal power by the keratometric power (K). It was known that error occurs in using K for cornea power, therefore Eq.(A-7) is more accurate than all the classical vergence formulas which have been used in combining with the modern formulas for ELP.

The approximate Eq.(A-3) is derived by decoupling the second principal plane position $P_2=SF/f_1$ from $L_2=S-P_2$. Alternatively, one may use the following equation for exact numerical calculation for both De and M

$$De = 1336/(X+P2) - 1336/F, \quad \text{(A-8)}$$

which is just a rearrangement of Eq.(A-1) without using the decoupling approximation. Above equation also allows us to check the accuracy of the analytic approximate formulas of Eq.(1). For example, for D_2= 20.0 diopter with a fixed D_1=43 diopter, S=5.0 mm and L=23.7 mm, M=1.30 (diopter/mm) calculated from the exact Eq.(A-3) in comparing to M=1.298 calculated from analytic formula, Eq.(1), which is only about 0.15% error.

Alternatively, one may also derive Eq.(A-6) by taking the derivative of Eq.(A-1) and using the relationship of Eq.(A-2). A third method is to take the Taylor second-order expansion of De in Eq.(A-7) or (A-8) with respect to the change of X. For example, $1/(X+dX)=1/X-(dX/X^2)[1-dX/X]$. All the above described three different methods lead to the same formula of (A-6) and justify the derivation of M.

REFERENCES

1. Langenbucher A, Nguyen NX, Sertz B, Gusek-Schneider GC, Kuchle M. Measurement of accommodation after implantation of an accommodating posterior chamber intraocular lens. J. Cataract Refract Surg 2003; 29:677-85.
2. Cumming JS, Slade SG, Chayet A. Clinical evaluation of the model AT-45 silicone accommodating intraocular lens. Ophthalmology 2001; 108:2005-9.
3. Koeppl C, Findl O, Kriechbaum K, et al. Change in IOL position and capsular bag size with an angulated intraocular lens early after cataract surgery. J. Cataract Refract Surg 2005;31:348-53.
4. Stachs O, Schneider H, Steve J, Guthoff R. Potentially accommodating intraocular lenses-an in vitro and in vivo study using three-dimensional high-frequency ultrasound. J Refract Surg 2005; 21: 37-45.
5. Holladay JT, Chandler TY, et al. Refractive power calculation for the phakic eye. Am J Ophthalmol 1993;116:63-6.
6. Nawa Y, Ueda T, Nakatsuka M, et al. Accommodation obtained per 1.0 mm forward movement of a posterior chamber intraocular lens. J Cataract Refract Surg 2003;29:2069-72.
7. Lin JT. The roles of corneal power and anterior chamber depth on the accommodation of aphakic intraocular lenses. J Refract Surg 2005;21: 765-6.
8. Pedrotti Ls, Pedrotti FL. Optics and Vision. Upper Saddle River; NJ; 1998:74-8.
9. Lin, JT. Analysis of refractive state theory and the onset of myopia. Ophthal Physiol Opt 2006; 26:97-105.
10. Lin, JT. The generalized refractive state theory and effective eye model. Chin J Opt. & Ophth 2005;7:1-6.
11. van de Heijde GL. The optical correction of unilateral aphakia. Trans Am Academy Ophthal Otolaryngol 1976; 81: 80-8.
12. Lin JT. Analysis of dual optics accommodating IOL. In: Garg A, Lin JT (Eds), Mastering IOLs: Innovations and Principles, Jaypee Brothers Med. Pub. New Delhi, India 2006.
13. Wang XJ, Jin CP, Wang QM. Aberration with IOLs based on different optical design. Chinese J Optom & Ophthal (in Chinese). 2003;5:209-11.
14. Atchison DA. Optical design of intraocular lens. I. On-axis performance. Optom Vis Science 1989;66:492-506.

CHAPTER

15

Yoshiaki Nawa (Japan)

Ray-tracing Analysis of Accommodating IOLs

INTRODUCTION

Accommodative intraocular lenses (IOLs) have recently entered the market. Forward movement of the IOLs is postulated to create most of the accommodation in eyes with such IOLs.[1-4]

For example, AT-45 R (C&C Vision, Aliso Viejo, California, USA) was reported to move forward by 0.7 mm.[5] ICU R (HumanOptics, Spardorfer, Erlangen, Germany) was reported to move forward by 0.78 mm.[6] Recently it has been reported that a double-optic IOL could obtain more accommodation than a single-optic.[7-9]

In this chapter, I describe

1. The method of calculating accommodation in eyes with accommodating single-optic IOLs using ray-tracing analysis.
2. Accommodation obtained per 1 mm forward movement IOL highly correlates with IOL power.
3. Methods to enhance the effect of accommodating IOLs; double-optic IOLs, and combination of corneal surgery and IOL.

THE METHOD OF CALCULATING ACCOMMODATION IN EYES WITH SINGLE-OPTIC ACCOMMODATING IOL

A ray-tracing analysis of pseudophakic eyes is obtained by analyzing each spherical surface of the eye.[10] The method is shown in the appendix 1. In this chapter the Computer Software Mathematica R (Wolfram, Champaign, Illinois, USA) was used to calculate refractions of the model eye used here.

We can analyze mutual relationship between several parameters of the eye using this equation as described in the past report.[4] Figure 15.1 shows an example that plotted the relationship between anterior chamber depth, axial length, and ocular refraction.

Here I investigated accommodation obtained per 1mm forward movement of IOL using a more detailed eye model than that used in the past report.[4] I varied anterior corneal radius of curvature of the cornea from 7.2 to 8.4 mm and axial length from 21 to 27 mm. Other parameters were assumed as follows: posterior radius of curvature of the cornea—6.8 mm; anterior radius of curvature of the cornea—7.7 mm; thickness of the cornea—0.5 mm; anterior chamber depth (posterior surface of cornea to anterior surface of IOL)—4.0 mm; IOL—MA30BA (10 - 30 D, Alcon Japan, Tokyo); refractive index of the cornea—1.376; refractive index of the anterior chamber and vitreous—1.336; anterior and posterior radius of curvature of IOL, IOL thickness, and refractive index of IOL—provided by the manufacturer.

The IOL power in each theoretical eye with different parameters (corneal radius of curvature and axial length) was selected for the

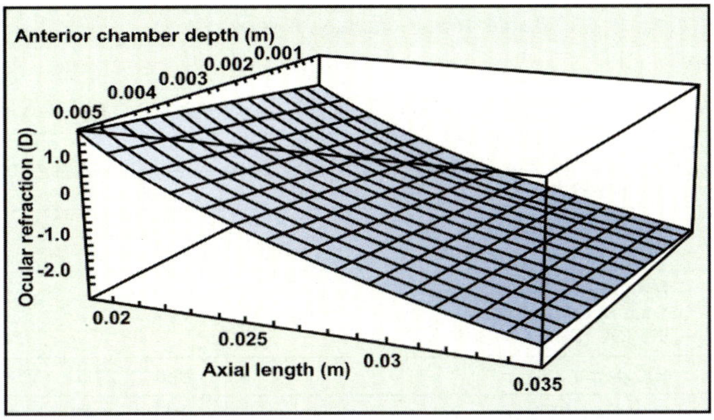

Fig. 15.1: The relationship between anterior chamber depth, axial length, and ocular refraction in a pseudophakic eye model. By using the equation of Appendix 1, we can analyze mutual relationships between several different parameters of the eye

refraction of the model eye to become the least minus power (nearest to emmetropia).

Then I plotted the relationship between the amount of myopic shift of the theoretical eye for a 1 mm forward movement of IOL, and axial length, corneal curvature, and IOL power. The summary of the analysis is shown in Table 15.1 and plotted in Figure 15.2. The analysis revealed that 0.65 to 2.07 diopter of accommodation was obtained per 1 mm forward movement of IOL, depending on corneal curvature, axial length, and IOL power.

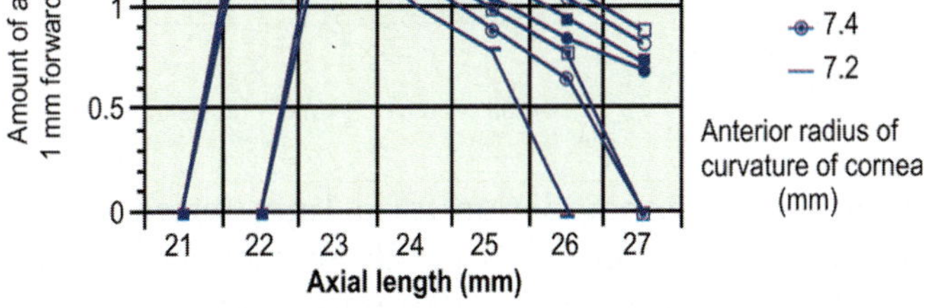

Fig. 15.2: The relationship between corneal curvature, axial length, and amount of accommodation for a 1 mm forward movement of IOL. Shorter eyes with high power IOLs can obtain more accommodation per 1 mm forward movement of IOL

Table 15.1: Summary of section 1

Anterior radius of curvature of cornea(mm)		8.4	8.2	8.0	7.8	7.6	7.4	7.2
Axial length (mm)								
21	IOL power (D)							29.0
	Predicted refraction (D)							-0.24
	Myopic shift for a 1mm movement of the IOL (D)							**2.07**
22	IOL power				29.0	27.5	25.5	23.5
	Predicted refraction				-0.14	-0.27	-0.15	-0.18
	Myopic shift for a 1mm movement of the IOL (D)				**2.00**	**1.90**	**1.80**	**1.68**
23	IOL power	29.0	27.5	26.0	24.5	22.5	21.0	19.0
	Predicted refraction	-0.26	-0.20	-0.26	-0.32	-0.10	-0.27	-0.27
	Myopic shift for a 1mm movement of the IOL (D)	**1.93**	**1.83**	**1.74**	**1.67**	**1.54**	**1.45**	**1.33**
24	IOL power	24.5	23.0	21.5	20.0	18.5	17.0	15.0
	Predicted refraction	-0.09	-0.01	-0.06	-0.09	-0.19	-0.35	-0.33
	Myopic shift for a 1mm movement of the IOL (D)	**1.59**	**1.50**	**1.39**	**1.32**	**1.24**	**1.14**	**1.00**
25	IOL power	21.0	19.5	18.0	16.5	15.0	13.5	11.5
	Predicted refraction	-0.25	-0.16	-0.20	-0.22	-0.30	-0.31	-0.29
	Myopic shift for a 1mm movement of the IOL (D)	1.33	1.21	1.14	1.04	0.98	0.89	0.78
26	IOL power	17.5	16.0	15.0	13.5	12.0	10.0	
	Predicted refraction	-0.13	-0.03	-0.40	-0.29	-0.36	-0.16	
	Myopic shift for a 1mm movement of the IOL (D)	**1.10**	**1.03**	**0.93**	**0.84**	**0.77**	**0.65**	
27	IOL power	14.5	13.5	12.0	10.5			
	Predicted refraction	-0.00	-0.24	-0.26	-0.27			
	Myopic shift for a 1mm movement of the IOL (D)	**0.88**	**0.81**	**0.73**	**0.69**			

The amount of accommodation for a 1mm forward movement of IOLs should be determined individually in each eye. Long eyes with small power IOLs will obtain a small myopic shift, and short eyes with high power IOLs will obtain a large myopic shift, for a 1 mm forward shift of accommodative IOLs.

This kind of analysis can be done for any type of single-optic IOLs.

ACCOMMODATION OBTAINED PER 1 MM FORWARD MOVEMENT IOL HIGHLY CORRELATES WITH IOL POWER

McLeod described that using the ray-tracing analysis the amount of accommodation for a 1mm forward movement of IOL was approximately (1/13) × IOL power[7]. I also evaluated the relationship.

Under the assumption of section 1, I analyzed and plotted the relationship between IOL power and accommodation per 1mm forward movement of IOL.

Figure 15.3 shows the relationship between the IOL power and the amount of accommodation for a 1 mm forward movement of IOL. These two parameters are highly correlated ($y = 0.0723x - 0.1159$, $R^2 = 0.9862$). It is similar to that shown by McLeod ($y = x/13$).[7] The difference may stem from the differences of assumed parameters.

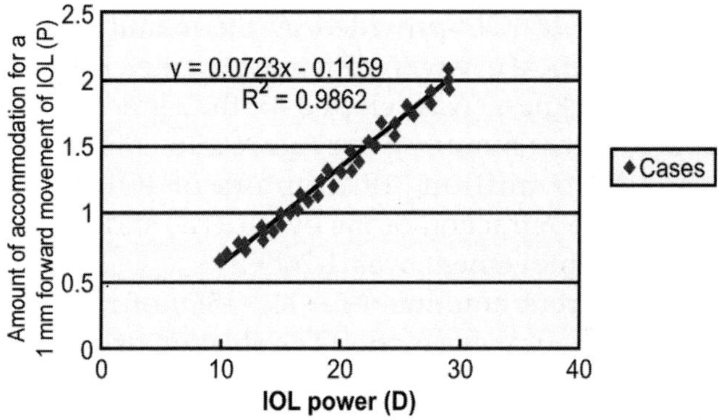

Fig. 15.3: The correlation between IOL power and amount of accommodation for a 1mm forward movement of IOL. They are highly correlated. Other models of single-optic IOLs show similar trends

METHODS TO ENHANCE THE EFFECT OF ACCOMMODATING IOLs; DOUBLE-OPTIC IOL, COMBINATION OF CORNEAL SURGERY AND IOL

To enhance the effect of accommodating IOLs, double-optic IOLs have been developed.[7-9]

Ray-tracing analysis of double-optic IOLs can be similarly done by inputting each parameter of spherical surfaces of the components of the eye and IOL into an equation of double-optic IOL. Appendix 2 shows an equation of double-optic IOL.

Ho[9] analyzed the accommodation performance of 14 design variations for 2 configurations of two-optic IOL. These represented 4 possible combinations (positive/negative, mobile/static, front/back element). Configurations with high positive-power front element returned the best amplitude of accommodation (up to approximately 3.0 D/mm when the front element power was +40D). This paper shows many good examples of ray-tracing analysis of two-optic IOLs.

Here I describe another possible method to enhance the effect of accommodating IOLs. As described above section 2, higher power IOLs are able to elicit more accommodation per 1 mm forward movement of IOL. Combined myopic PRK and IOL would increase IOL power.

I assumed as follows: anterior corneal radius of curvature of the cornea—7.7 mm; axial length—24 mm; posterior radius of curvature of the cornea—6.8 mm; thickness of the cornea—0.5 mm; anterior chamber depth (posterior surface of cornea to anterior surface of IOL)—4.0 mm; IOL: VA60BB (HOYA, Tokyo, Japan); refractive index of the cornea—1.376; refractive index of the anterior chamber and vitreous—1.336; anterior and posterior radius of curvature of IOL, IOL thickness, and refractive index of IOL: provided by the manufacturer. The IOL power in each theoretical eye with different parameters (corneal radius of curvature and thickness) was selected for the refraction of the model eye to become the least minus power (nearest to emmetropia). In this initially assumed condition, 19 diopters of IOL was the most appropriate with the refraction of the eye–0.21D, and accommodation per 1 mm forward movement was 1.26D.

Next, three different amounts (-5, -10, -15D) of myopic PRK was assumed in the theoretical eye model. The ablation depth was assumed to be 12 × x (micrometer). A maximum of 2.28D of accommodation was obtained when -15D of myopic PRK was performed with 39D of IOL implanted. Figure 15.4 shows the summary of the analysis. It revealed that a modest amount of accommodation could be obtained.

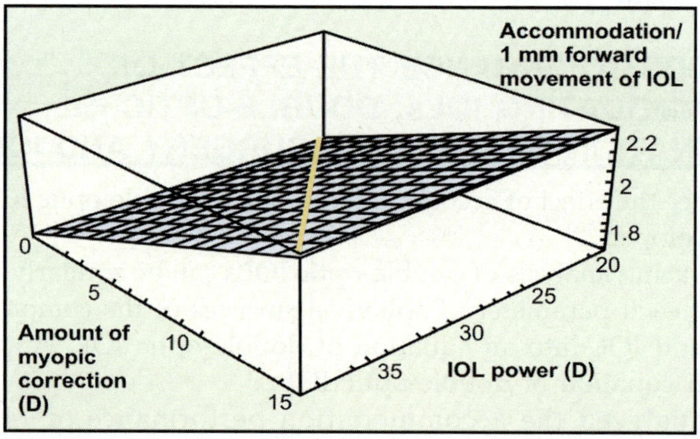

Fig. 15.4: The relationship between myopic correction, IOL power, and accommodation/1mm forward movement of IOL. Combination of myopic PRK and IOL implantation fairly enhance the effect of accommodating IOL

APPENDIX 1

Ray-tracing analysis of pseudophakic eyes

$$Rs= 1/[1/(1/\{1/[1/(1/\{1/[1/(1/t_5 -p_4) +t_4] -p_3\} +t_3) -p_2] +t_2\} -p_1) +v]$$

Rs: Refraction (diopters) in glasses; v: Vertex distance (meters); t: Corneal thickness (meters); ACD: Anterior chamber depth (meters); d: IOL thickness (meters); VIT: Length of vitreous space (meters); AXL: Axial length (meters); t*i*: Reduced vergence of t, ACD, IOL thickness, and VIT ($t_2= t/n_2$, $t_3= ACD/n_3$, $t_4= d/n_4$, $t_5= VIT/n_5$); p*i*: Refractive power of each interface (diopters); R_1: Anterior radius of curvature of cornea (meters); $P_1= (n_2-n_1)/ R_1$; R_2: Posterior radius of curvature of cornea (meters); $P_2= (n_3-n_2)/R_2$; R_3: Anterior radius of curvature of IOL (meters); $p_3= (n_4-n_3)/R_3$; R_4: Posterior radius of curvature of IOL (meters); $p_4= (n_5-n_4)/R_4$; VIT= AXL-t-ACD-d; n*i*: Refractive index of each tissue; 1: Air; 2: Cornea; 3: Anterior chamber; 4:IOL; 5:Vitreous

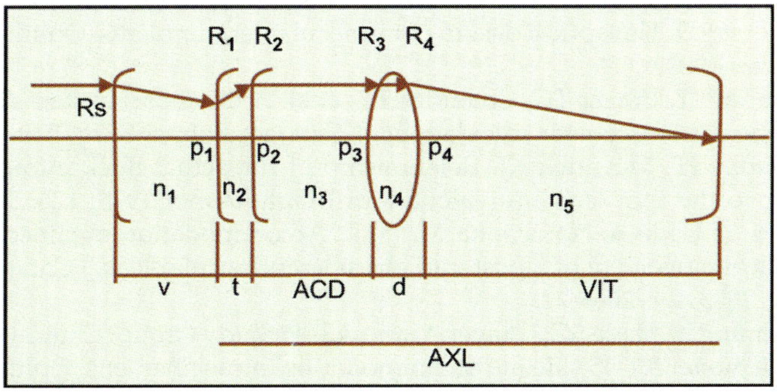

APPENDIX 2

Ray-tracing analysis of pseudophakic eyes with piggyback IOL or double-optic IOL.

$$Rs= 1/\{1/[1/(1/\{1/[1/(1/\{1/[1/(1/\{1/[1/(1/t_7 -p_6) +t_6] -p_5\} +t_5) -p_4] +t_4\} -p_3) +t_3] -p_2\} + t_2) -p_1] +v\}$$

Rs: Refraction (diopters) in glasses; v: Vertex distance (meters); t: Corneal thickness (meters); ACD: Anterior chamber depth (meters); d_1, d_2: IOL thickness (meters); x: Distance between IOLs (meters); VIT: Length of vitreous space (meters); AXL: Axial length (meters); t*i*: Reduced vergence of t, ACD, d_1, d_2, x, and VIT ($t_2= t/n_2$, $t_3= ACD/n_3$, $t_4= d1/n_4$, $t_5= x/n_5$, $t_6=d_2/n_6$, $t_7=VIT/n_7$); p*i*: Refractive power of each interface (diopters); R_1: Anterior radius of curvature of cornea (meters); $p_1= (n_2-n_1)/ R_1$; R_2: Posterior radius of curvature of cornea (meters); $p_2= (n_3-n_2)/R_2$; R_3: Anterior radius of curvature of IOL_1 (meters); $p_3= (n_4-n_3)/R_3$; R_4: Posterior radius of curvature of IOL_1

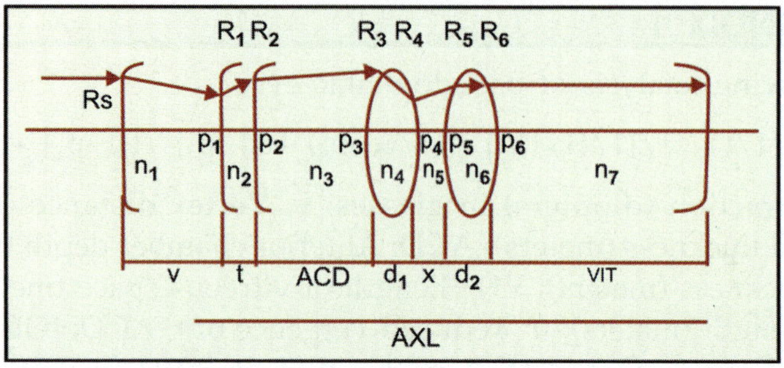

(meters); p_4= $(n_5$-$n_4)/R_4$; R_5: Anterior radius of curvature of IOL_2 (meters); p_5= $(n_6$-$n_5)/R_3$; R_6: Posterior radius of curvature of IOL_2 (meters); p_6= $(n_7$-$n_6)/R_6$;VIT= AXL-t-ACD-d_1-x-d_2; n*i*: Refractive index of each tissue; 1: Air; 2: Cornea; 3,5: Anterior chamber; 4,6:IOL; 7:Vitreous

REFERENCES

1. Binkorst RD. The optical design of intraocular lens implants. Ophthalmic Surg 1975;6: 17-31.
2. Holladay JT, Prager TC, Chandler TY, et al. A three-part system for refining intraocular lens power calculations. J Cataract Refract Surg 1988; 14: 17-24.
3. Holladay JT, Maverick KJ. Relationship of the actual thick intraocular lens optic to the thin lens equivalent. Am J Ophthalmol 1998; 126: 339-47.
4. Nawa Y, Ueda T, Nakatsuka M, et al. Accommodation obtained per 1mm forward movement of a posterior chamber intraocular lens. J Cataract Refract Surg 2003; 29: 2069-72.
5. Cumming JS, Slade SG, Chayet A, and AT-45 Study Group. Clinical evaluation of the model AT-45 silicone accommodating intraocular lens. Ophthalmology 2001; 108: 2005-10.
6. Langenbucher A, Huber S, Nguyen NX, et al. Measurement of accommodation after implantation of a new accommodative posterior chamber intraocular lens (1CU). J Cataract Refract Surg 2003;29: 677-85.
7. McLead SD, Portney V, Ting A. A dual optic accommodating foldable intraocular lens. Br J Ophthalmol 2003;87: 1083-85.
8. Langenbucher A, Reese S, Jakob C, et al. Pseudophakic accommodation with translation lenses-dual optic vs mono optic. Ophthalmoc Physiol Opt 2004;24: 450-57.
9. Ho A, Manns F, Pham T, et al. Predicting the preformance of accommodating intraocular lenses using ray tracing. J Cataract Refract Surg 2006;32: 129-36.
10. Horiuchi I, Akagi Y. A new theoretical formula for the intraocular lens power caliculation by the ray tracing method. J Jpn Ophthalmol Soc 2001;105: 619-27.

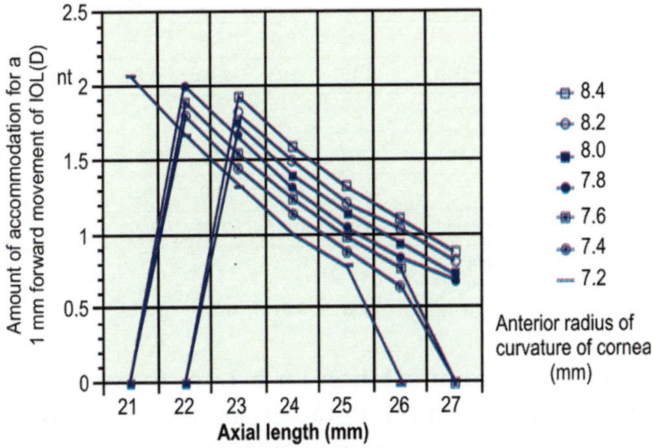

CHAPTER

16

GU Auffarth (Germany)

Dual Optics Accommodating IOLs

INTRODUCTION

The last step in successful cataract or lens removal surgery is the restoration of accommodation.[1,5,7] Several single-optic systems have been introduced on the market. In Germany the 1CU IOL manufactured by Humanoptics AG (Erlangen, Germany) came on the market as single optic IOL based on Patents by Hanna. Several studies in Europe have shown certain limitations for these IOLs based on the anterior shift principle. Those lenses need movements of around 1.5 to 2.5 mm to achieve 3 diopters of accommodation.[1-5, 7,8,10] Even though the lens showed satisfactory clinical results, the amount of accommodation measured never exceeded 0.75 to 1 diopter, indicating a big range of pseudoaccommodative parameters (such as residual refraction, myopia, astigmatism, pinhole effect of pupil, corneal refractive changes etc.). On the US-Market the Crystalens AT 45 was actually FDA approved and widely used. Apart from visual acuity results no objective means for accommodative measurements were presented in the peer reviewed literature. Studies in Europe by Findl. and coworkers indicate a similar performance of this sinfle optic IOL like the 1CU.[8] A dual-optic design offers potential advantages over single-optic designs in that less lens movement is necessary with the dual optic to achieve a certain amount of accommodation (Fig. 16.1).[3,5,7,9] For example, in order to achieve 2.0 D of pseudoaccommodation, a 22-D single-optic IOL would need to move forward 1.6 mm within the capsular bag. A dual-optic IOL with a +30-D front lens and a –8-D posterior lens (overall power = 22 D) would only require 0.8 mm of separation to achieve 2.0 D of power change (Fig. 16.1).

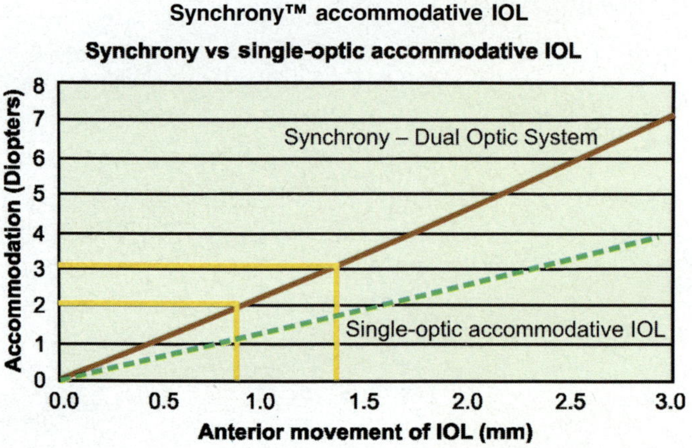

Fig. 16.1: Graphical illustration of the accommodative effect in relation to amount of optic shift of single and dual optic systems

Synchrony™ accommodative IOL: Dual Optic-IOL

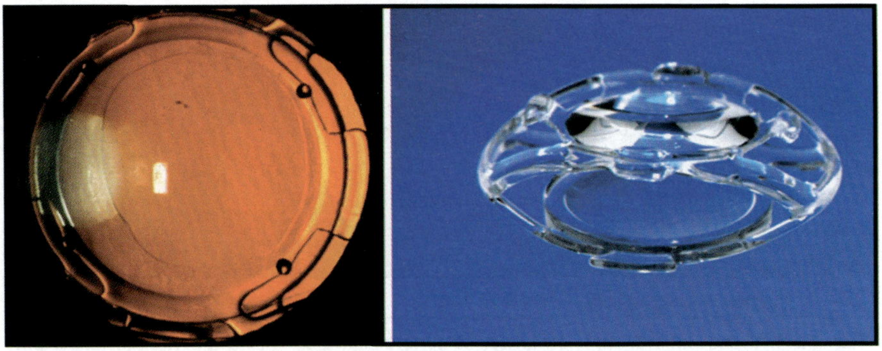

Fig. 16.2: Clinical retroillumination photograph and still picture of the synchrony IOL

Two dual optic IOLs are currently tested. The Sarfarazi Elliptical Accommodating IOL and the Visiogen Synchrony lens (Fig.16.2).[1-5,7-10,13] Both utilize a plus-powered biconvex front lens connected to a negatively powered concave-convex lens. During the accommodative effort the two lens components increase their distance from each other, resulting in increased effective power of the overall lens. The Sarfarazi IOL is now under evaluation by Bausch and Lomb.[13] No clinical data have been presented so far.

The Visiogen synchrony accommodative IOL consists of a high power (30 D) anterior optic and a variable minus power posterior optic (Fig. 16.2). It is made of silicone material. Implantation of the first

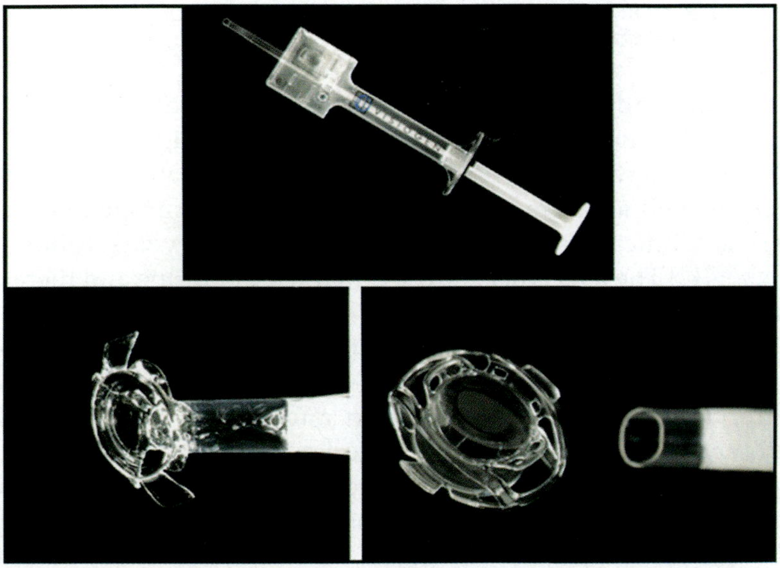

Fig. 16.3: Injector system for synchrony IOL

2 Years Follow-up: Synchrony™ accommodative IOL

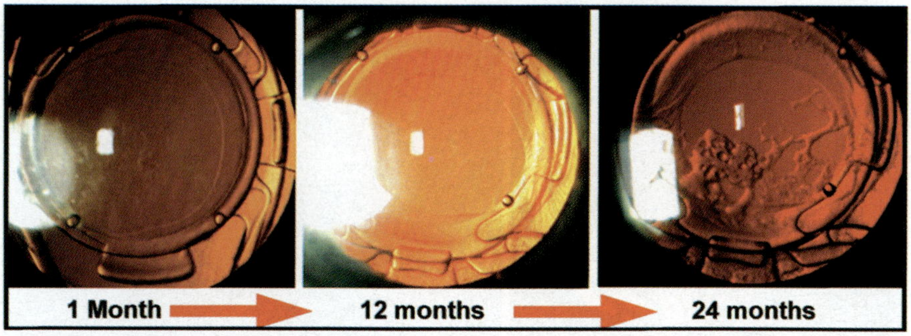

Fig. 16.4: Retroillumination photograph of synchrony IOLs with a 24 months follow-up. Only small amount of PCO, no ILO

2 Years Follow-up: Synchrony™ accommodative IOL

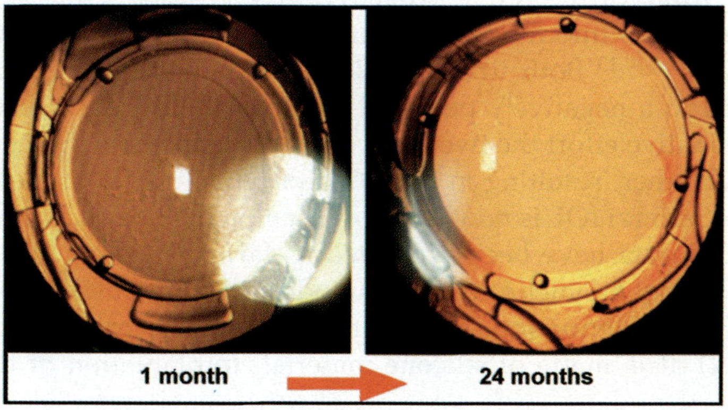

Fig. 16.5: Retroillumination photograph of synchrony IOLs with a 24 months follow-up. Only small amount of PCO, no ILO

generation models were done with folding forceps. The latest generation has now an injector for implantation (Fig.16.3).

The synchrony IOL as been extensively studies in laboratory (rabbit) models as well as in multicentre clinical trials in Europe and Latin America. Clinical data are available with a 3-4 years follow-up now.[1-5,7,9,11,12] The lens is also now CE-marked in Europe and therefore available for clinical use.

The first clinical generation of the Synchrony dual optic accommodative IOL showed over a 2-3 years follow-up period good functional results, stable refraction and low to mediocre PCO development (Figs 16.4 and 16.5). Interlenticular opacification (ILO) was the main concern regarding these dual-optic IOLs. To date, however, this has not been reported as a complication of these IOLs. Studies of the IOL in rabbits suggest that the design features of the Synchrony may help prevent posterior and anterior capsule fibrosis.

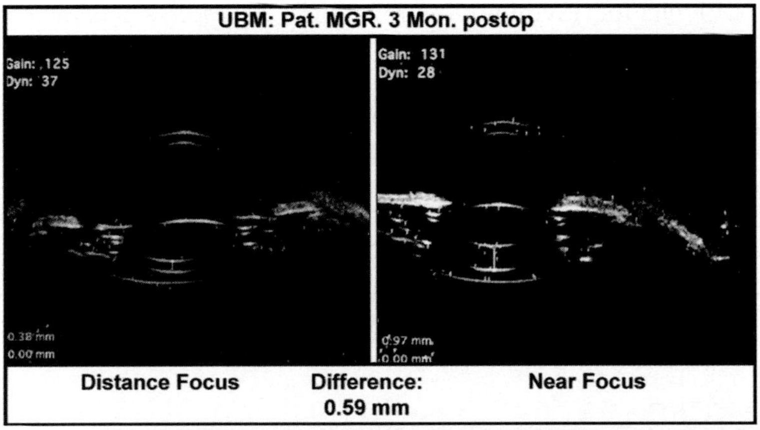

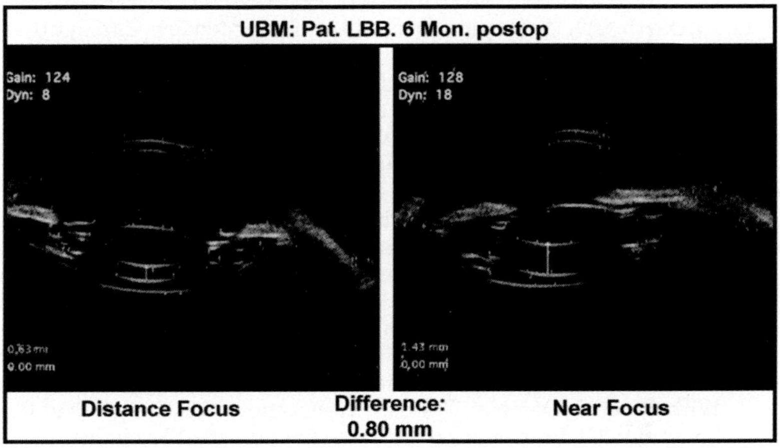

Figs 16.6 and 16.7: Ultrasound biomicroscopy of synchrony IOL indicating movement between lenses of 0.59 (Fig.16.6) and 0.80 mm (Fig. 16.7)

In another study in rabbits the incidence of ILO was zero, also indicating that the lens material (silicone) may prevent interlenticular lens epithelial cell migration.[11,12]

Ossma and Coworkers could demonstrate by ultrasound biomicroscopy movements between the two IOLs of up to 0.6 to 0.8 mm (Figs 16.6 and 16.7). The residual near addition to reach J1 was around 0.78 diopters and UDVA and UNVA was in all cases >20/40.[5,7]

Dick et al. and Auffarth et al presented similar results with the early Synchrony model.[3,5,7] In contrast to single optic designs the dual optic designs offer theoretically and practically the chance of a real accommodative effect. Several questions still need to be scientifically evaluated. The IOL calculation or in other words the exact location of the IOL inside the capsular bag is difficult to predict or to determine. The prevention of posterior capsule opacification (PCO) is still a longterm concern. New instruments such as the "perfect capsule" system by Milvella Inc. (Sydney, Australia) offer nowadays new means to target the elimination of lens epithelial cells (LEC).[6]

In summary the dual optic IOLs seem to be the most effective design or IOL type achieving a significant amount of accommodation. Other (new) concepts in accommodative IOLs include the Powervision Fluidvision IOL, which is capable of curvature changes to achieve accommodative changes or the smart lens, a lens refilling device consisting of a thermoplastic material.

New clinical studies especially with the now clinically approved Visiogen Synchrony IOL will show how successful these dual optic designs on the market will be.

REFERENCES

1. Auffarth GU. Accommodative intraocular lenses. Can synthetic lenses accommodate? Ophthalmologe 2002 Nov;99(11):809-10.
2. Auffarth GU, Martin M, Fuchs HA, Rabsilber TM, Becker KA, Schmack I. Validity of anterior chamber depth measurements for the evaluation of accommodation after implantation of an accommodative Humanoptics 1CU intraocular lens. Der Ophthalmologe 2002; 99; 815-19.
3. Auffarth GU, Reuland AJ, Entz BB, Holzer MP. First experiences with a dual optic accommodative IOL. In: Pham DT, Auffarth GU, Wirbelauer C, Demeler U (Eds): Transactions: 18. Congress of the German Society for IOL Implantation and Refractive Surgery, Biermann (Publ.), Cologne 2004; 285-88.
4. Auffarth GU, Schmidbauer J, Becker KA, Rabsilber TM, Apple DJ. Miyake-Apple video analysis of movement patterns of an accommodative intraocular lens implant. Der Ophthalmologe 2002; 99; 811-14.
5. Auffarth GU. Accommodative intraocular lenses. In: Pham DT, Auffarth GU, Wirbelauer C, Demeler U (Eds.): Transactions: 18. Congress of the German Society for IOL Implantation and Refractive Surgery, Biermann (Publ.), Cologne, 2004; 239-44.
6. Auffarth GU, Rabsilber TM, Reuland AJ. New methods for the prevention of posterior capsule opacification. Ophthalmologe 2005;102(6):579-86.
7. Dick HB. Accommodative intraocular lenses: Current status. Curr Opin Ophthalmol 2005;16(1):8-26.
8. Findl O, Kiss B, Petternel V, Menapace R, Georgopoulos M, Rainer G, Drexler W. Intraocular lens movement caused by ciliary muscle contraction.J Cataract Refract Surg 2003;29(4):669-76.
9. McLeod SD, Portney V, Ting A. A dual optic accommodating foldable intraocular lens. Br J Ophthalmol 2003;87(9):1083-5.
10. Vargas LG, Auffarth GU, Becker KA, Rabsilber TM, Holzer MP. Performance of the Accommodative 1 CU IOL in Relation with Capsulorhexis Size. J Cataract Refract Surg 2005; 31:363-68.
11. Werner L, Pandey SK, Izak AM, Vargas LG, Trivedi RH, Apple DJ, Mamalis N. Capsular bag opacification after experimental implantation of a new accommodating intraocular lens in rabbit eyes. J Cataract Refract Surg 2004; 30(5):1114-23.
12. Werner L, Mamalis N, Stevens S, Hunter B, Chew JJ, Vargas LG. Interlenticular opacification: dual-optic versus piggyback intraocular lenses. J Cataract Refract Surg 2006; 32(4):655-61.
13. Sarfarazi FM. Sarfarazi dual optic accommodative intraocular lens. Ophthalmol Clin North Am 2006; 19(1):125-8.

CHAPTER

17

JT Lin (USA)

High Efficiency Dual Optics Accommodating IOLs

INTRODUCTION

Accommodating IOLs (AIOLs) including single-optics and two-optics configurations have been designed and analyzed by many researchers.[1-11] The accommodation rate (M) defined by the accommodation amplitude per 1.0 mm of the IOL axial movement has been studied both analytically by Gaussian optics and numerically by raytracing method.[2,3,5] Single optics AIOL is much simpler than the dual optics AIOL which has been analyzed recently by Ho et al using raytracing method. However, analytic formulas are not yet available.

This Chapter presents and derives analytic formulas for dual optics AIOL, in which either or both the front and back optics are allowed to move in both forward and backward directions. Calculated results are consistent with that of raytracing method used by Ho et al. However, analytic formulas provide more insight features which are not readily available in raytracing. The dual-optics formulas may be also compared to the single optics AIOL in phakia or piggyback IOL which are presented by Lin in other Chapters of this book.

THE ACCOMMODATING RATE (M)

Mobile Front Optics Case

As shown in Figure 17.1A, a doublet IOL (dual optics) consists of 2 optics located at N2 and N3 and separated by p′, where the front optic separates from the corneal vertex surface by a distance p. As derived in the Appendix, the 3-optic system consisting of the cornea and the dual optics IOL may be reduced to an effective 2-optic system shown in Figure 17.1B by Gaussian optics and the system refractive error (De) is given by Lin's image equation.[9,11]

$$De = 1336[1/(X+P2)-1/F], \quad (1)$$

By taking the derivative of De with respective to the IOL front optic position (p), the accommodation rate (M), defined as the increase of system power due to per 1.0 mm forward movement of the front IOL (assuming the back optics is immobile), or $M = -dDe/dp$, may be derived (see Appendix) and expressed in an analytic format.

$$M = Z\,(D_1/1336)(2Dc+ZD_1), \quad (2.a)$$
$$Z = 1-S(Dc/1336), \quad (2.b)$$

where S (in the unit of mm) being the effective anterior chamber depth (ACD) of the IOL; D_1, D_2 and Dc are, respectively, the front and back IOL power and corneal power.

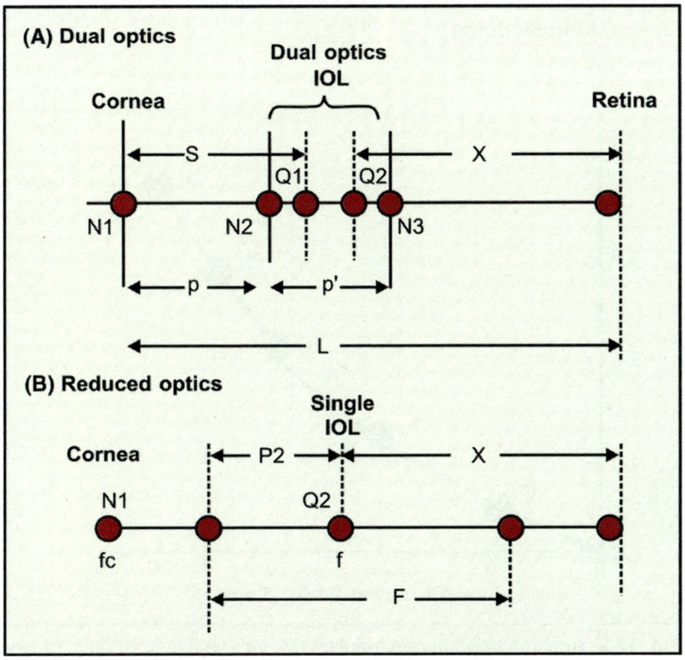

Fig. 17.1: Schematics for the 3-optics system, shown in (A) consisting of the cornea and 2-optics IOL separated by p and p'. Also shown are the principal plane locations of IOL (Q1 and Q2) and the second principal plane of the reduced 2-optics system (P2), effective focal length (F) and effective distance (S) shown in (B)

The validation of the analytic formula, Eq.(2), is checked by comparing to the exact numerical value of M by calculating the De in Eq.(1) for different IOL position (p) given by M = (0.59, 2.32, 2.94, 3.62) (diopter/mm) for the configurations of (a) to (e) defined earlier. These numerical data show that the error of analytic formula is about 1 to 3%. Comparing to the numerical raytracing results of Rana et al [2], the analytic results of this study are also within 5% in difference due to the choice of the effective ACD(S), corneal power and refractive index of the humors (1.333 in Rana vs. 1.336 of this study).

Validation of Eq.(2) may be also justified by the following special case. In the convex-plano configuration, D_2=0 and S=p, the 3-optics formula reduces to the formula for a 2-optics, cornea plus single IOL system or IOL implanted in an aphakic eye.[7,8]

Based on Eq.(2) and for typical IOL position of p=3.0 mm, p'=1.0 mm, corneal power Dc=43 diopter, the calculated values M=(0.57, 1.41, 2.35, 2.89, 3.65) (diopter/mm), respectively, for various IOL doublet configurations with (front, back) power, (D_1, D_2) equals: (a) (+10, +10), (b) (+20, 0), (c) (+30, –10), (d) (+35, –15) and (e) (+40, –20) diopters. The above 5 configurations have the same total IOL power of +20

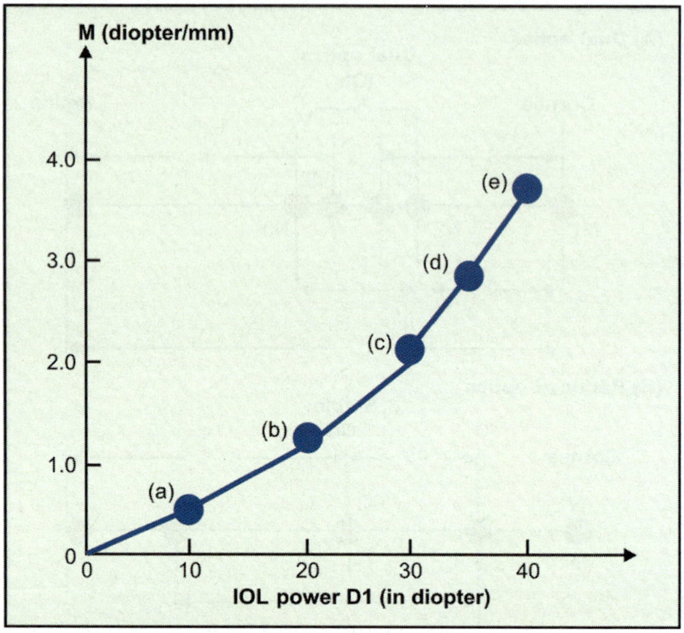

Fig. 17.2: Accommodation rate function (M) versus IOL front optic power (D1) for various configurations with a fixed IOL total power of 20 diopters

diopters but different in shapes of biconvex, convex-plano and convex-concave. The non-linearly increasing feature of M by the front-IOL power (D_1) is shown in Figure 17.2 for the plus front optics IOL which has a higher M value than that of the absolute value of M in minus front-optics IOL due to the cancellation of the second term in Eq.(2.a).

The following significant features of the dual optics accommodative IOL, which may not be readily available by numerical raytracing method, can be easily addressed based on the analytic formula of Eq.(2):

a. The accommodation rate (M function) is nonlinearly proportional to the moving front IOL power (D_1) as shown by Eq.(2). M is positive for positive-power moving optics, that is an increase of p' (or $dp'>0$ and $dp<0$) or a forward movement to the cornea is needed in order to have increasing accommodation (or myopic shift) for near vision of a presbyopia. These features are consistent with the numerical finding of Rana et al[2] and Ho et al.[5]
b. M is insensitive to the corneal power change due to the combined factor of ZDc, where $Z=1-S(Dc/1336)$ is a decreasing function of Dc and therefore cancellation occurs in M value when Dc increases. In contrast, M is a decreasing function of S, or the corneal IOL separation (p). For example, given Dc=43 diopters, p'=1.0 mm, and the configuration with (D_1, D_2)=(+30, –10) diopters, g=–0.5, M=(2.39,

2.35, 2.29), for p=(2.5, 3.0, 3.5) mm or S=(2.0, 2.5, 3.0) mm, respectively.

c. As shown by the second term of Eq.(2), cancellation occurs when $D_1<0$. Therefore, a positive-power would have a greater M (absolute value) than that of negative-power moving optics. For example, Dc=43 D, S=3.5 mm, $Z_2=1.0$ and Z=0.887; the calculated M=+0.99 (D/mm) for $D_1=+15$ D and M=–0.724 (D/mm) for $D_1=-15$ D, which is about 27% smaller (comparing the absolute values). This novel feature is consistent with that of Ho et al using raytracing method.

d. For a given IOL total power of $Dt=D_1+Z_1D_2$, with $Z_1=1-p'(D_1/1336)$, the M value for front positive and back-negative IOL is always larger than that of both optics are positive. This feature may be readily observed from Eq.(2) by re-expressing the moving front-optics power $D_1=Dt-ZD_2$ has a higher value when D2<0.

Mobile Back Optics Case

Eq.(2) is derived for the case that the forward moving element is the front optics of the dual optic IOL, where the back optics is static. In general, both optics may be mobile in practice. By symmetry feature of the dual optic IOL, one may also derive the case for mobile back (with immobile-front) to obtain (see Appendix).

$$M = Z(D_2/1336)(2Dc+ZD_2) - \text{Delta}. \tag{3}$$

Similar to the mobile front optics, the M′ value is proportional to the power of the mobile optics and slightly influenced by the immobile optics, via Z_1 and the third term of the formula which is absent in the front mobile case.

Both Optics Mobile

In order to have a "positive" accommodation (for myopic shift), forward movement (toward the cornea) is needed if the moving optics has a positive power. In contrast, a backward movement is needed for a negative power moving optics. Therefore cancellation effect may occur when both optics having opposite-power are moving in the same directions or 2 optics having the same power sign but moving in the opposite directions. The actual amount of each components, M and M′, shall depend on the structure and implant configuration of the IOL, where contraction of the ciliary body results the direction and amount of each movement. Furthermore, one may also expect a small contribution from the nonlinear coupling effect of M and M′, when both optics are allowed to shift in either direction. Therefore, the total (net) amount of accommodation (A) may be expressed as follows, in general,

$$A = M(dS1) + M'(dS2) + N(dS1)(dS2), \quad (4.a)$$
$$= A1 + A2 + A12 \quad (4.b)$$

where dS1 and dS2 are the movement amount (including directions) of the front and back optics, respectively, and N is a nonlinear coupling factor. Cancellation occurs when A1 and A2 have opposite signs. Figure 17.3 shows the possible combinations for various IOL configuration. Because we had defined the sign of M and M′ are the same as the power of the moving optics, we also need to defined dS>0 for forward movement (toward the cornea), and dS<0 for backward (toward the retina) movement.

PERFORMANCE AND CONFIGURATIONS

Definition

As shown in Figure 17.2, there are many possible combinations of front-back optics configurations and movement directions. They can be described by the following definition:

+ : For positive accommodation A (or myopic shift), A>0.
– : For negative accommodation A (or hyperopic shift), A<0.
← : Forward movement of the IOL (toward cornea) or dS>0.
→ : Backward movement of the IOL (away from cornea), or dS<0.
• : Static (immobile)
CX = convex, CA = concave

Example 1 (Fig. 17.3A)

For the (front, back) optics are CX-CA (with positive power) and CA-CX (with negative power), respectively. The movement direction, for example, (←, →) means (front optics move forward, back optics move backward); (+, +) means the resultant accommodations are both positive, and A1>0, A2>0; (←,•) means front-optics forward moving and back optics static and the result is given by (+, 0) for A1=positive, A2=0. By these definitions, the 8 possible cases are: (Fig. 17.3).

Moving direction	*Accommodation (A1, A2)*
(←, •)	(+, 0)
(→, •)	(–, 0)
(•, →)	(0, +)
(•, ←)	(0, –)
(→, →)	(–, +)
(→, ←)	(–, –)
(→, ←)	(+, +)*
(←, ←)	(+, –)

* case for both A1 and A2 are positive for maximal myopic accommodation

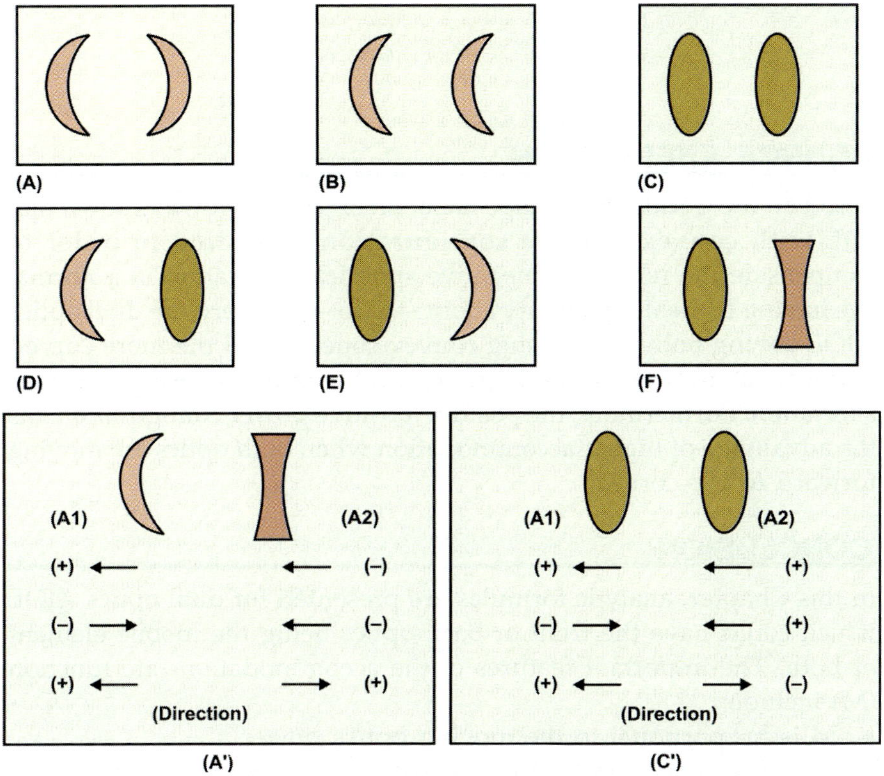

Fig. 17.3: Configurations and movement direction of various dual optics accommodating IOL, where (←, →,•) stands for movement direction of (forward, backward, immobile) w.r.t the cornea position; (+, –) stands for (positive, negative)

Example 2 (Figs 17.3B and C)

For (front, back) optics = (CX-CA, CX=CA) or both are bi-CX having positive power for both optics. The possible combinations are shown as follows:

Direction	(←, •)	(→, •)	(•, ←)	(•, →)	(←, ←)*	(?, →)	(→, ←)	(→, →)
(A1, A2)	(+, 0)	(–, 0)	(0, +)	(0, –)	(+, +)	(+, –)	(–, +)	(–, –)

* The optimal movement (both are forward) for maximal A = A1 + A2.

Maximal Accommodation

Among the above configurations and movement directions, the following cases produce maximal-myopic accommodation having both A1 and A2 are positive:

Power	*Direction*
(D1, D2)	(front, back)
(+, –)	(←, →)

(+, +)	(←, ←)
(–, +)	(→, ←)
(–, –)	(→, →)

SOURCE ABERRATION

Based on the Coddington shape factor analysis,[8,12,13] it was known that IOL with convex-concave configuration is desired in order to compensate the remaining negative spherical aberration in a normal eye having corneal asphericity about –0.2 to –0.6. Therefore dual optics AIOL having both optics being convex-concave and the more curved surfaces facing the cornea is preferred for minimal overall surface aberration. Furthermore, the positive-positive power configuration has the advantage of higher accommodation when both optics are moving forward to the cornea.

CONCLUSION

In this Chapter, analytic formulas are presented for dual optics AIOL which could have the front or back optics being the mobile element or both. The important features of the accommodation rate function (M) include:

- M is proportional to the moving optics power
- Positive accommodation amplitude, A=A1+A2, requires combination of plus power optics moving forward to the cornea and minus power optics moving backward to the retina
- Convex-concave or bi convex configuration for both front and back optics having positive power offers maximal A when both are moving forward to the cornea.

Dual optics AIOL provides higher accommodation rates (M) via optical configurations. However, the combined surface aberration (SA) to compensate the balanced SA of cornea and natural lens for minimal high order SA should also be considered in the IOL design.

APPENDIX: DERIVATION OF LIN'S M FORMULA

By Gaussian optics, [8,9] the effective focal length (EFL) of the dual optics IOL is given as

$$1/f = 1/f1 + Z'/f2,$$
$$Z' = 1 - p'/f1, \qquad \text{(A-1)}$$

where f1 and f2 are the EFL of the IOL and front and back optics separated by a distance p′ and related to their power by $f1=1336/D_1$, $f2=1336/D_2$, respectively; S is the effective anterior chamber depth

(ACD) as shown in Figure 17.1A. The EFL of the reduced 2-optic system consisting of cornea and IOL is then given by (refer to Fig. 17.1A)

$$1/F = 1/f + Z/fc, \quad \text{(A-2)}$$
$$Z = 1 - S/fc,$$

where the effective distance between the cornea and the front IOL optic (shown by the distance between N1 and Q1 in Fig. 17.1) may be calculated from S=p+gp′, p is the estimated IOL position (away from the corneal vertex surface) and g=1/(1+Z′f2/f1) is a geometry factor of the dual optics IOL. It can be readily seen that the 3-optics system reduces to a 2-optics system when f2 goes to infinite and f=f1. Eq.(A 2) becomes a simple cornea IOL 2-optics system (or a single optic aphakic IOL) which has the same format as that of cornea-natural lens system[10].

The refractive error of the reduced 2-optics system is given by[9-11] (for humors refractive index of 1.336).

$$De = 1336/(X+P2)-1336/F, \quad \text{(A-3)}$$

where the effective vitreous cavity depth (X) is related to the axial length by X=L–p–p′+p12 with p12=p′f/f1 being the IOL second principal plane position, or the distance between Q2 and N3 as shown in Figure 17.1A. In Figure 17.1B, P2=SF/f1 is the position of the system second principal plane. In this study, all the length parameters are in mm, except refractive power in diopter.

Case (1): Front Optics Mobile

To find the accommodation rate (M) defined by the accommodation amplitude (or system power increase) due to the forward movement of the front IOL (assume back optics is immobile), one may take the derivative of Eq.(A-3) with respective to the IOL front optic position (p), or M = –dDe/dp, to obtain

$$M = (1336a/F2)(dX+dP2)+1336d(1/F) \quad \text{(A-4)}$$

where a is a nonlinear term given by a=(1+FD in/1336) to count for the effect of the initial refractive error Din. dX and dP2 are derived from the earlier definitions as follows:

$$dX = -(f/f1)(1+p'f/f1f2)(dp), \quad \text{(A-5)}$$
$$dP2 = (F/fc)(dS) - (SF^2/fc)d(1/F), \quad \text{(A-6)}$$

where dS and d(1/F) may be further expressed as

$$dS = Gdp \quad \text{(A-7.a)}$$
$$d(1/F) = -dS/(ffc)+(Z/f1f2)dp, \quad \text{(A-7.b)}$$
$$G = 1-(f/f2)(1+p'f/f1f2). \quad \text{(A-7.c)}$$

In deriving Eq.(A-5) and (A-7), I had also used the basic relation that dp′=–dp to count for the fact that the forward movement of the front IOL causes a decrease of p and an increase of p′ given that p′+p=constant.

Substituting Eq.(A-5) to (A-7) to Eq.(A-4) and after lengthy but straightforward algebraic manipulation, I obtained the final analytic formula for M,

$$M = 1336[af/(f1F^2) - G(a/F-Z''/f)/fc\text{-}Z''Z/(f1f2)], \quad \text{(A-8)}$$

where Z″=1–aS/fc. Above formula may be further simplified by eliminating F by Eq.(A-2) and using the approximated value of a=1.0, ignoring the contribution from Din, if system is initially at emmetropic state; G=f/f1, ignoring the small term (less than 0.5%) of p′f/(f1f2) in Eq. (A-7.c) for typical value of p′=(0.5-1.0) mm; and for a fixed value of IOL effective power 1336/f =(10 to 25) diopters.

$$M = (f/f1)Mo - Delta, \quad \text{(A-9.a)}$$
$$Mo = 1336[1/F^2-1/fc^2], \quad \text{(A-9.b)}$$
$$Delta = Z^2/(f1f2). \quad \text{(A-9.c)}$$

The validation of the above analytic formulas may be justified by their special cases and comparison to the exact numerical results based on Eq.(A-3). See detailed discussion in the text. Above formula may be further expressed by the corneal power (Dc) and IOL front and back optic power D_1 and D_2 as shown in the text Eq.(2) for the emmetropic case a=1 and Z″=Z.

Case (2): Back Optics Mobile

Similar technique may be used to derive the rate function (M′) for the case that front optics is immobile and back-optics is mobile, where (A-5) and (A-7) change to

$$dX = (f/f1 - 1)(dp'), \quad \text{(A-10)}$$
$$dS = (f/f2)(dp'). \quad \text{(A-11)}$$

Therefore, one obtains M′, similar to Eq.(A-9),

$$M' = (f1/f2)\ Mo - Delta, \quad \text{(A-12)}$$

In terms of the IOL power and after some algebra, Eq.(A-12) gives Eq.(3) in the text. It should be noted that Eq.(A-4) and (A-12) are symmetry.

REFERENCES

1. Shammas HJ. Intraocular lens power calculations. Thorofare NJ, SLACK Inc., 2004.
2. Rana A, Miller D, Magnante P. Understanding the accommodating intraocular lens. J Cataract Refract Surg 2003;29:2284-7.
3. Nawa Y, Ueda T, Nakatsuka M, et al. Accommodation obtained per 1.0 mm forward movement of a posterior chamber intraocular lens. J Cataract Refract Surg 2003;29:2069-72.
4. Missotten T, Verkamme T, Blanckaert J, et al. Optical forumula to predict outcomes after implantation of accommodating intraocular lens. J Cataract Refract Surg 2004;30:2084-7.
5. Ho A, Manns F, Pham T et al, Predicting the performance of accommodating intraocular lens using ray tracing. J Cataract Refract Surg 2006;32:129-36.
6. Mcleod SD, Portney V, Ting A. A dual optic accommodating fordable intraocular lens. Br J Ophthalmol 2003;87:1083-5.
7. Landenbucher A, Reese S, Jakob C, Seize B. Pseudophakic accommodation with translation lenses-dual optic vs. mono optic. Ophthalmic Physiol Opt 2004:24:450-7.
8. Pedrotti LS, Pedrotti FL. Optics and Vision. Liper Saddle River, NJ, Prentice Hall 1998; 74-87; 92-5.
9. Lin, JT. Unified refractive-state analysis for customized vision correction. J Refract Surg 2004;20:398-400.
10. Lin, JT. New formulas comparing accommodation in human lens and intraocular lens. J Refract Surg 2005;21:200-1.
11. Lin, JT. Analysis of refractive state ratios and the onset of myopia. Ophthal Physiol Opt 2005;26:97-105.
12. Atchison DA. Optical design of intraocular lens. I. On-axis performance. Optom Vis Science 1989;66:492-506.
13. Wang XJ, Jin CP, Wang QM. Aberration with IOLs based on different optical design. Chinese J Optom & Ophthal (in Chinese) 2003;5:209-11.

CHAPTER

18

Georges Baikoff (France)

Presbyopia Correction with "Newlife" Multifocal Phakic Implant

INTRODUCTION

Correcting presbyopia is an essential challenge for refractive surgery. This particular type of surgery is not so much to do with restoring accommodation, but more a question of giving patients an opportunity of living without spectacles for distant and near vision. This opens the door to a number of compromises or alternatives to real accommodation surgery.

Presbyopia affects most people over the age of 45 and if we consider that in the United States 50% of the population is presbyopic,[1] through extrapolation, this represents several billion individuals throughout the world.

Considering the degree of ammetropia (high/low myopia, high/low hyperopia, emmetropia) several options are available. Unilateral myopisation (monovision) of the dominant eye or multifocal correction of either the cornea or crystalline lens, either by adding a new lens or exchanging the crystalline lens if it is still transparent.

A choice is therefore available to both surgeons and patients as not one of all these techniques provides the perfect solution and in the years to come, it is quite probable that several different but complementary solutions will be available. We decided to work on three possible options: the cornea, the crystalline lens and the sclera and will give the results we obtained following implantation of a bifocal lens for correcting both slight ametropia and an average presbyopia of + 2.50 D.

NEWLIFE BIFOCAL PHAKIC IMPLANT

The bifocal refractive phakic IOL is an anterior chamber angle-supported lens marketed under the trade name of NEWLIFE (**Ioltech**,).* The optic is of soft 28% hydrophilic acrylic, the haptic is of poly (methyl methacrylate) (PMMA), and the footplates at the extremities are of hydrophilic acrylic. The 5.5 mm diameter optic is divided into 3 zones: the center, which is for distance vision, the medium periphery which is for near vision; and the periphery which is for distance vision. The central zone diameter is 1.50 mm, and the near intermediate zone is 1.1 mm wide (Figs 18.1 and 18.2). The haptic is shaped like the number 2 and is available in overall diameters of 12.0 mm, 12.5 mm and 13.0 mm.

The IOL comes in powers between –5.00 D and +5.00 D for distant vision with a single addition of +2.50 D for near vision. This addition

---

* **Ioltech**, Avenue Paul Langevin, BP 5, 17053 La Rochelle, France, Tel + 33 5 4644 8550 ; Fax + 33 54 644 8560

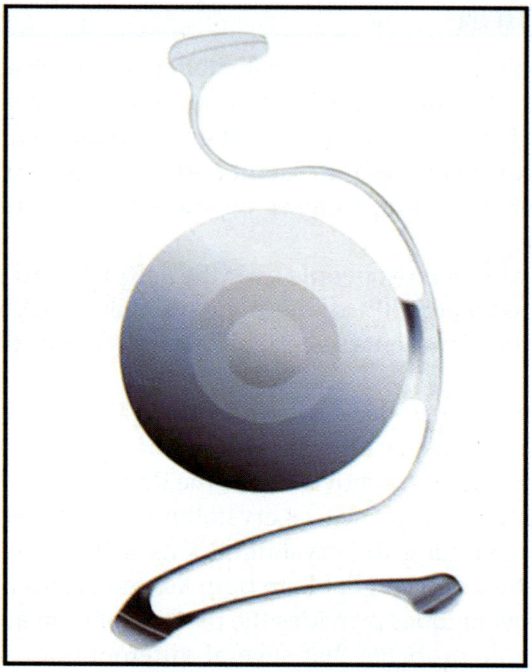

Fig. 18.1: Drawing of presbyopic anterior chamber implant

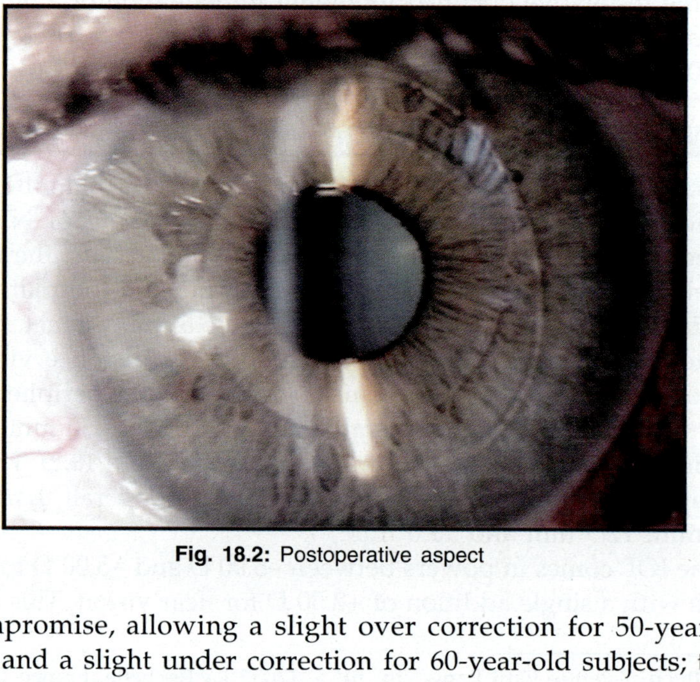

Fig. 18.2: Postoperative aspect

is a compromise, allowing a slight over correction for 50-year-old subjects and a slight under correction for 60-year-old subjects; these slight refractive inaccuracies will prove to be generally well accepted.

ANTERIOR CHAMBER DIMENSION

Internal Diameter

For all angle-supported implants, it is essential to carry out a precise evaluation of the internal diameter of the anterior chamber. We began by using the white-to-white method, then we used a PMMA graduated sizer which was inserted into the anterior chamber during surgery. In fact, all these measurements are relatively approximate and for an implant to remain stable in the anterior chamber, it must not only be adapted to the eye's largest diameter in order to avoid rotation but also as near as possible in size to this diameter so that there is no pressure on the iris which in the long run gives rise to pupil ovalisation.

These problems cannot be solved with the actual ultrasound A and B scan techniques. However, modern imaging techniques such as the ARTEMIS, ultrahigh frequency ultrasound equipment and the anterior segment OCT give more precise measurements of the anterior chamber's internal diameter. We were able to demonstrate *in vivo*, and this was confirmed by Liliana WERNER on cadaver eyes, that in 75% of cases, the anterior chamber's internal vertical diameter was bigger than the horizontal one. In daily practice, we therefore systematically preoperatively measure the anterior segment helping us in the choice of implant (Fig. 18.3).

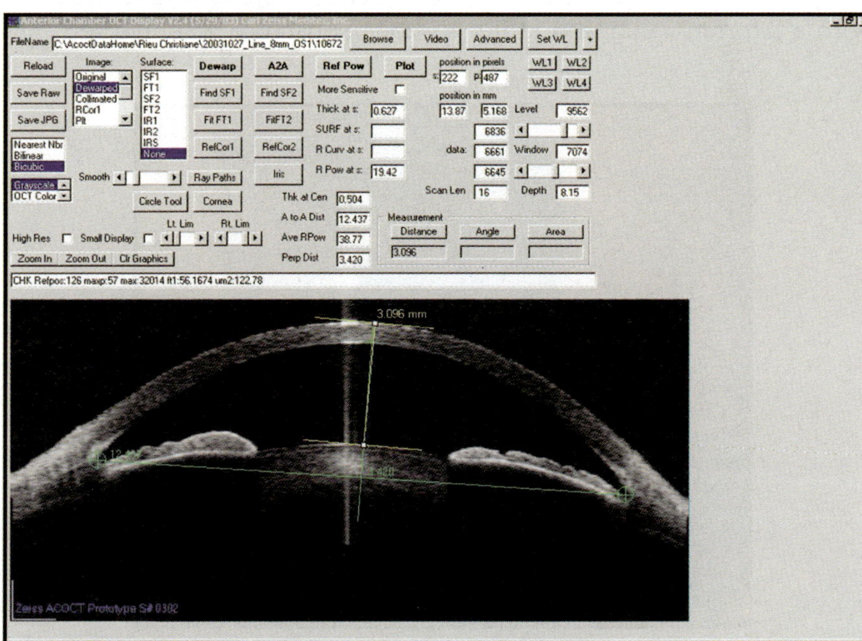

Fig. 18.3: AC measurements with the Visante™ OCT prototype

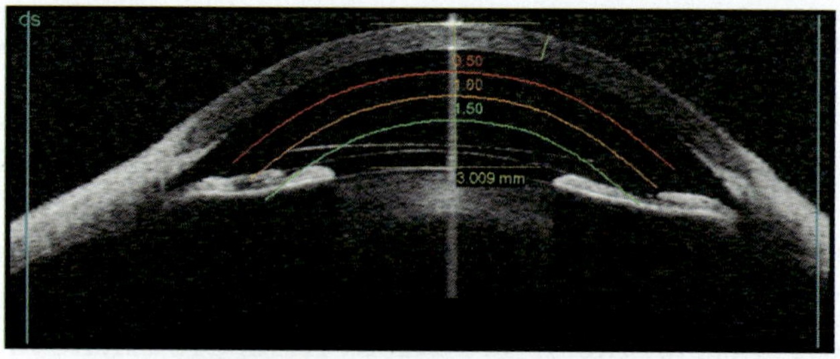

Fig. 18.4: Endothelial safety distances

Anterior Chamber Depth

Minimum anterior chamber depth must be equal to or above 3.1 mm (measured from the corneal epithelium to the anterior surface of the crystalline lens). This is of course a safety notion but does not in fact take into account the implant's vault (Fig. 18.4).

Surgical Techniques

Topical, local regional or general anesthesia was used based on the surgeon's or patient's choice. Surgery (Fig. 18.5) is relatively simple and consists in placing the lens, which is folded at the time of surgery, into the anterior segment of the eye in front of the iris.

A preoperative myosis is essential (preoperative installation of 2% pilocarpine drops). A corneal or corneoscleral incision is carried out with a 2.8 mm calibrated knife. Viscous substance was injected into

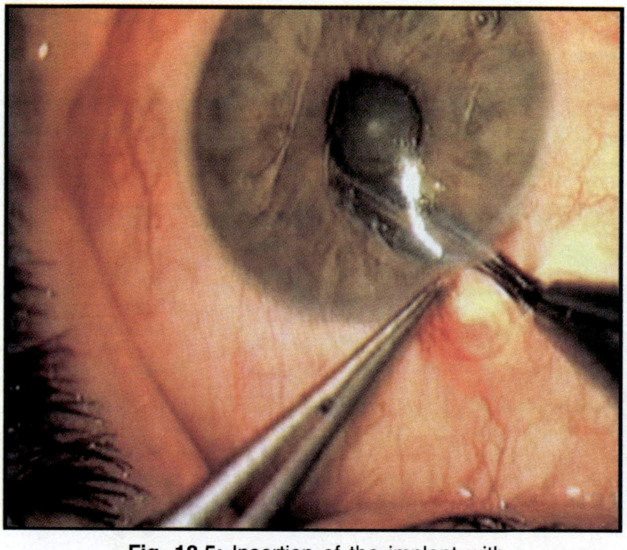

Fig. 18.5: Insertion of the implant with optic folded in three

the anterior chamber, two paracenteses were made at 3 and 9 o'clock to allow subsequent maneuvers in the anterior chamber.

The lens is folded into three with a special folder before being inserted. First, the two leading footplates are introduced into the anterior chamber followed by the optic and trailing haptic. Once the lens is in the anterior chamber, pressure on the forceps is gently released and the optic unfolds. When the lens is open in the anterior chamber and depending on the largest axis, the implant will be rotated to fit this axis. It is essential that all the viscous substance is removed at the end of surgery to avoid postoperative hypertonia with Urrets Zavalla syndrome (fixed dilated pupil). The viscous substance is replaced with BSS. No sutures are required with the self-sealing incision. An iridectomy is not routinely suggested because the optic is soft and the optic/haptic junction can act as a gentle hinge. If mechanical blockage of the pupil in the anterior chamber occured, the iris was pushed forward and the optic, which is soft, would in turn be pushed forward letting the aqueous humour escape through the pupil. In the event of an inflammatory pupil blockage, mydriatic therapy would be proposed first and if that failed, an iridectomy with the YAG laser was done. At the end of surgery, *500 mg of DIAMOX®* is systematically administered intravenously and a tablet of 250 mg DIAMOX is also prescribed on the first night after surgery. A one month antibiotic steroid eye-drop treatment is prescribed postoperatively.

Anatomical Exclusion Criteria

Only patients with normal anterior segments, normal endothelium cell counts, without ocular hypertonia or associated pathologies are considered. It is essential to have a clear crystalline lens and a normal macula.

Choice of Implant

To avoid rotation, the implant is placed along the axis of the anterior chamber's biggest diameter, which, in general is the vertical diameter. If for instance, the vertical diameter is the bigger diameter and the implant is placed on the horizontal diameter, this will lead to instability and a risk of the implant rotating. If the implant is well placed on the largest axis, there is no longer any risk of rotation.

Power of the Implant

Choice of the IOL optical power was based on distant refraction according to the HOLLADAY formula.[2] The IOL comes in powers between – 5.00 D and + 5.00 D. A single addition is available with this model (+ 2.50 D). All hyperopes between the age of 50 and 60 can be corrected in this way, knowing that the younger subjects will be slightly over corrected and the older subjects slightly under corrected. This under or over correction has no incidence on everyday life.

Any corneal astigmatism, (which alters the quality of the IOL), must be corrected beforehand either with laser or lasik in order to make the most of this multifocal implant.

RESULTS

Our initial study concerned 55 eyes of 33 patients: 21 women, 12 men, 29 right eyes, 26 left eyes. Preoperative refraction was between –5.00 D and +5.00 D. There were 9 myopic eyes and 46 emmetropic or hyperopic eyes. The anterior chamber was over 3.1 mm in almost all of the cases and the endothelial cell density equal to or above 2000 C/mm^2. Average age of patients was 54 ± 5.4 years (ranges between 45 and 70 years). The average follow-up was 42.6 weeks (ranges between 83 and 2 weeks).

Refraction

Mean preoperative refraction is + 1.8 D ± 1.3 D (ranges –2.75 D to + 5.00 D) Postoperative mean refraction is – 0.12 D ± 0.51 D (ranges –1.5 D to 1.25 D). There is therefore a very satisfactory precise refractive effect. Without going into detail, the first series of patients (Baikoff[3]) for whom we used the van der Heijde formula,[4] showed a higher rate of myopisation than the patients subsequently operated on using the more precise Holladay Refractive formula.[2]

On the diagrams showing the evolution of the results after one-year follow-up, refraction remains stable (Fig. 18.6).

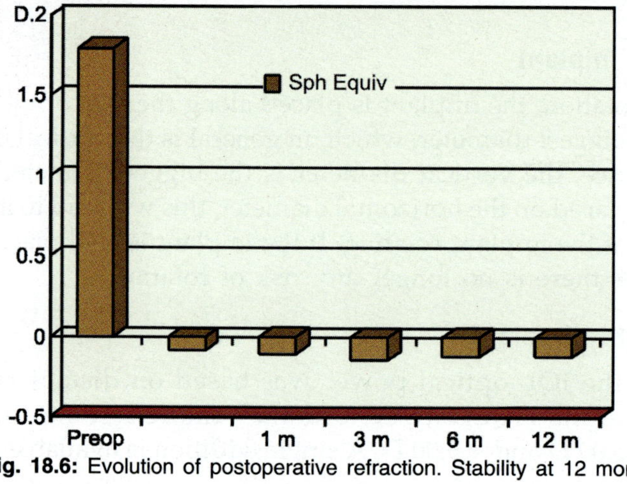

Fig. 18.6: Evolution of postoperative refraction. Stability at 12 months

Distant Visual Acuity

Uncorrected preoperative visual acuity was 0.41 ± 0.29 (decimal scale), and postoperative uncorrected visual acuity (UCVA) was 0.78 ± 0.20 (decimal scale). This uncorrected visual acuity (UCVA) result is equivalent to the other refractive surgery techniques where the mean result is around 0.8.[5-7] Preoperative best corrected visual acuity is 0.98 ± 0.02 and postoperatively best corrected visual acuity drops to 0.92 ± 0.09. This loss of visual acuity is the result of a drop in contrast sensitivity due to the multifocal lens. It is a well known fact that multifocal lenses reduce image lighting, decreasing contrast sensitivity and BCVA. This has been observed in pseudophakic IOLs.[8]

Near Visual Acuity

Before surgery, near BCVA is Parinaud 2.03 ± 0.1. Postoperative UCVA is Parinaud 2.3 ± 0.6 (ranges 2 to 3).

Efficacy and Safety Ratio

The optical and refractive target was obtained, as distant UCVA was satisfactory with an 94% safety ratio (Postoperative BCVA/ preoperative BCVA) and an 80% efficacy ratio. (Postoperative UCVA/ Preoperative BCVA). These results were slightly below those that we normally observe with refractive implants where the two factors are respectively between 120% and 140% and around 100%.[9-12] Finally, UCVA was satisfactory in most cases as 84% of eyes operated on obtained 0.6 or better for distant vision and Parinaud 3 or better for near vision both without correction. These figures correspond to a normally demanding population leading normal everyday lives.

ANATOMICAL RESULTS: INCIDENTS AND COMPLICATIONS

Loss of Visual Acuity

One patient showed a 3-line loss of BCVA three months after surgery of both eyes. Residual myopia existed but despite the correction of this myopia, the patient's visual acuity did not improve. The posterior pole was explored (angiography, OCT, Visual field, color vision) and was normal. Three or four months after surgery visual acuity returned to 1.0. This patient had PRK at a later date to correct her residual myopia with an excellent optical result.

A second patient found her visual acuity reduced to 0.5 and it was impossible to improve after surgery whereas preoperatively she had 0.8. In fact, this 70-year-old patient presented a moderate cataract.

The addition of a multifocal lens in front of a slightly opalescent crystalline lens leads to a very severe drop in visual acuity for two reasons: decrease in light transmission due to the incipient cataract, and a decrease in the lighting of the focused image. Infact, crystalline lens opalescence can reduce retinal illumination by 30% and the added effect of a multifocal lens is therefore particularly harmful. The implant was removed at the same time as cataract surgery was performed by phakoemulsification using the same 3.2 mm incision. A monofocal implant was inserted into the bag with excellent visual results and a postoperative corrected visual acuity of 1.0.

Loss of Contrast Sensitivity

Loss of contrast sensitivity was not studied objectively, and patients may be sensitive to it after surgery of the first eye as they can compare with the other non-operated eye. A slight greyish sensation is perceived. Once the second eye has been operated on, there is no element of comparison and the discomfort is better accepted. In mesopic vision, that is to say reading at night in dim light conditions, some patients occasionally wear additional glasses.

Reduction of Retinal Illumination

We have seen that the problem with multifocal lenses was a reduction of retinal illumination. One patient suffered from this problem because of an pre-existing crystalline lens pathology.

The problems we are faced with concern anatomical predispositions such as senile myosis. A study should be carried out to define the acceptable minimum pupil diameter for this type of implant.

Therefore, multifocal lenses must be contraindicated for patients with slight macular pathologies such as Drüsens or epithelium pigment disorders because they are particularly sensitive to reductions in retinal illumination.

Halos

One of the problems of multifocal lenses is the possibility of parasite optical side effects. We have mentioned before that multifocal lenses reduce contrast sensitivity, however, they also produce halos that are particularly disturbing in night vision. 18% of eyes and 24% of patients complained of halos, but these had no incidence on night driving except in two patients out of 33 (6%).

This high percentage of complaints concerning halos disappears in time because the brain adapts to this inconvenience. In the end, very few patients complained of this discomfort and in time none of them requested change or removal of the implant for this particular reason. Thanks to the Visante™ OCT pupil ovalizations have almost disappeared as the size of the implant is now correctly adapted to the largest axis which is generally the vertical one.

Pupil Ovalization

Ten percent of slight pupil ovalizations showed up under the slit lamp's intensive light. There were fewer under normal lighting. Generally, pupil ovalizations are the result of over sizing the implant.

Cataract

No implant-induced cataracts have been observed in this study to date.

Ocular Hypertonia

No ocular hypertonia induced by the implant has been observed in this series to date.

Endothelium

After a year, mean endothelial cell loss is below 5%. The results meet the FDA's guidelines (Fig. 18.7).

Explantations

4 explantations were carried out on patients who were disappointed with the results. One patient had excellent near and distant vision, 1.0 (decimal scale) and Parinaud 2 but was not satisfied with the intermediate vision. He therefore requested that the implant be removed.

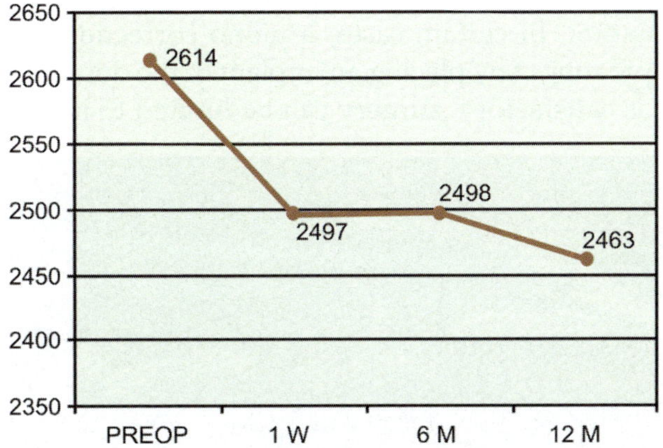

Fig. 18.7: Evolution of corneal endothelium at 1 year

Two explantations were suggested because of insufficient visual results. (cf. supra patient with cataract). One was due to unsolvable postoperative diplopia. In both cases, they recuperated their initial visual status.

Optical defects are inevitable with multifocal lenses; therefore, patient selection must be very strict. Patients too demanding and who think that they will recuperate the vision they had at the age of 20 must be excluded and before surgery, it is essential to provide precise information concerning the risks and drawbacks of this procedure.

SUMMARY

Since this preliminary study, we have continued to use this technique and to continue rigorous patient selection. The results are confirmed and more than 80% of the patients have an distant UCVA over 0.6D and Parinaud 3 or better for near vision also uncorrected . This means all the patients lead normal lives without glasses in diurnal conditions; only a few (less than 10%) need them in mesopic conditions, for instance to read at home in the evenings. In this series, everyday acts are done without glasses. Halos are generally well tolerated and the loss of contrast sensitivity is unavoidable. This technique can therefore be proposed but very strict inclusion criteria must be taken into account with regards to anatomy and psychology. This procedure can only be offered to patients with an anterior chamber depth equal to or above 3.0 mm, with an open angle, with a healthy endothelium and without anterior segment or retinal disorders (Fig. 18.8). Any astigmatism must be corrected either before or after implantation. Patients that are too demanding must be excluded as well as patients who, for professional reasons, have to drive at night. The interest of phakic implants is their reversibility, in our series we had no persistent pupillary ovalisation after explantation. In certain cases, a mono correction is possible on an emmetropic subject by placing an implant in the dominated eye only. If the result is satisfactory, surgery can be limited to just one eye, and

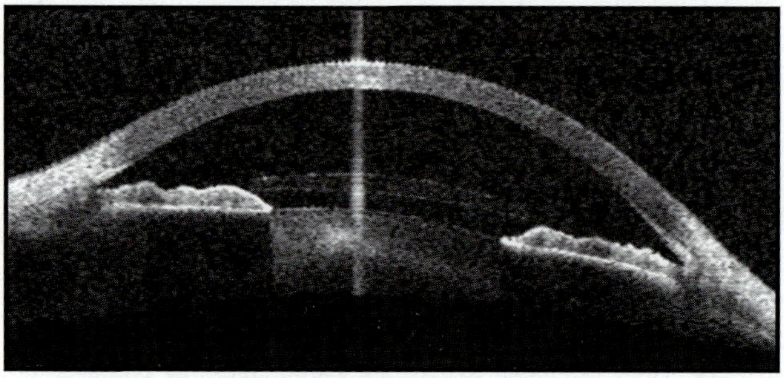

Fig. 18.8: Aspect of a NEWLIFE presbyopic IOL with the AC-OCT

surgery of the other eye proposed only if the patient wishes it. Experience has shown us that patients who had postoperative slightly hypermetropic refraction were more satisfied than patients slightly myopic. This had already been proved with multifocal pseudophakic implants (Steinert 13). However, to obtain a satisfied patient, it is important to explain that the correction of presbyopia with this multifocal implant for phakic eyes is a compromise between an excellent preoperative vision with glasses and a good postoperative vision without glasses.

NB: An important part of this article (text & illustrations) has already been published in the Journal of Cataract & Refractive Surgery 2004;30:1454-60 courtesy of Elsevier, Philadelphia USA.

REFERENCES

1. Lindström R. Correction of presbyopia with intraocular and intracorneal lenses Binkhorst Lecture. American Society of Refractive and Cataract meeting. San Francisco California, 12 april 2003.
2. Holladay JT. Refractive power calculations for intraocular lenses in the phakic eye.Am J Ophthalmol 1993; 116(1): 63-6.
3. Baïkoff G .Presbyopic Phakic Intraocular Lenses.In Agarwal A (Ed); Presbyopia: A Surgical Textbook Thorofare NJ Slack Inc 2002; pp 225-8.
4. Fechner PU,van der Heijde GL, Worst JGF.The correction of myopia by lens implantation into phakic eyes. Am J Ophthalmol 1989;107:659-63.
5. Sawelson H, Marks RG. Ten years refractive and visual results of radial keratotomy. Ophthalmology 1995;102:1892-1901.
6. Hersh PS, Stulting RD, Steinert RF, et al. Results of phase III Excimer laser photorefractive keratectomy for myopia. The Summit PRK study group. Ophthalmology 1997;104: 1535-53.
7. Davidorf JM, Zaldivar R, Oscherow S. Results and complications of laser in situ keratomileusis by experienced surgeons. J Refract Surg, 1998;14:114-22.
8. Monte-Mico R, Alio J. Distance and near contrast sensitivity function after multifocal intraocular lens implantation . J Cataract Refract Surg 2003; 29(4):703-11.
9. Perez-Santoja JJ,Alio Jl, Jimenez-Alfaro I,Zato MA. Surgical correction of severe myopia with an angle supported phakic intraocular lens. J Cataract Refrat Surg 2000;26(9):1288-302.
10. Baïkoff G, Arne JL, Bokobza Y, et al . Angle fixated anterior chamber phakic intraocular lens for myopia of –7 to –9 diopters . J Refract Surg 1998; 14:282-93.
11. Menezo JL,Avino JA,Cisneros A, et al. Iris claw phakic intraocular lens for high myopia. J Refract Surg 1997;13: 545-55.
12. Zaldivar R,Oscherow S,Ricur G.Implantable contact lens. In Clear Corneal Lens Surgery.Thorofare,NJ:SlackInc, 1999; pp 287-324.
13. Steinert RF, Aker BL, Trentacost DJ, et al. A prospective study of the AMO-Array zonal progressive multifocal silicone intraocular lens and a monofocal intraocular lens. Ophthalmology 199;106:1243-5.

CHAPTER

19

JT Lin (USA)

Presbyopia Corrections: Laser vs Nonlaser

INTRODUCTION

"Presbyopia" derived from the Greek word of "old eye" is an age-related loss of accommodation to see near, about 2.3 diopters per decade. Therefore presbyopia becomes common for age over 45.

Accommodation is the ability to focus on near objects through controlled changes in the shape and thickness of the crystalline lens and mediated by ciliary muscle contraction. To correct presbyopia, it is a fundamental necessity to understand how accommodation occurs and how it changes the optical and tissue parameters of an aged-eye. The effectiveness of ciliary body contraction for lens relaxation (or accommodation) may be influenced by the combined aging factors, including lens property changes (index, size, thickness and curvature), tissue elastic changes (in sclera and ciliary) and the zonular tension change. There have been controversy regarding the mechanisms of accommodation and the "true" restoring of accommodation after certain treatments, namely the debates between classical Helmholtz theory (1855) and the Schachar's hypothesis (1994), where the lens power increase for accommodation is the result of the increased curvature of either (i) the entire front surface (Helmholtz), or (ii) central portion of the front surface due to the decreased peripheral surface (Schachar). The Helmholtz theory has been better accepted and well supported by measurements than Schachar's.

In this Chapter, the following key issues (or systems) will be addressed:

- The mechanisms of presbyopia: conventional and new theories (hypothesis)
- Presbyopia treatments techniques: laser and non-laser methods (or systems)
- The two component theory for accommodation amplitude (the Lin's dynamic model)
- The pseudo-accommodation (bifocal reshaping by LASIK)
- New directions.

Presbyopia treatment using "monovision" thermal keratoplasty (such as LTK, DTK and CK) will be presented in other Chapter by Lin in this book.

THE AGE EFFECTS OF HUMAN EYES

Many theories have been proposed for the age-related loss of accommodation including :

a. Lens-based theories.
b. Geometric theories.

c. Lenticular theories; and
d. Multi-factor theory.

The factors, which may contribute to changes in overall refractive power, include the corneal shape and thickness, lens shape and thickness, anterior and vitreous chamber depth and globe axial length. The correlations between lens shape and lens placement (anterior chamber depth, lens thickness, and anterior segment length) was recently reported (Koretz et al 2001). The anterior chamber depth decreases, while lens thickness increases, with increasing age. However the sum of the two (anterior segment length) appeared to remain approximately constant with increasing age. The change in lens thickness with age was due almost entirely to an increase in anterior and posterior cortical thickness. This lens growth is due to the addition of lens fiber cells to the superficial cortex and the volume of the lens nucleus remains constant.

Fisher (1969) showed that the elasticity of the human lens capsule decreases with aging. He also showed that the human lens becomes increasingly resistant to the effects of stretching forces applied through the ciliary body/zonular complex. A geometric disorder attributed to changes in the size and volume of the lens and the angle of zonular insertion onto the lens was proposed by Koretz and Handelman (1988). Weale (1962) introduced a multifactorial basis for presbyopia in which the age-related loss of accommodation was attributed to decreased zonular tension resulting from the continuing growth of the lens, which changed the lens capsule and lens matrix elastic properties.

A change in the refractive index gradient of the lens cortex has been suggested (Koretz and Handelman, 1988: Pierscionek, 1993) to be a substantial factor contributing to the progression of presbyopia. Pierscionek and Weale (1995) proposed that because of the increased thickness of the lens and the anterior shift of the zonular attachments, presbyopia is a failure of the lens to be maintained in a flattened state. Cross-sectional studies of age-related changes in resting refraction show a drift toward hyperopia from about age 30 to 65 yeas and then a drift toward myopia after age 65 yr (Slataper, 1950; Saunders, 1981) attributed to growth and the forward movement of the lens.

Table 19.1 summarizes the possible aging-factor, which may cause the patient vision to be myopic or hyperopic shift (competing processes). It was found by Scheimpflug techniques, that lens thickness increased steadily and linearly with increasing age, whereas anterior chamber depth decreased linearly with aging. Lens paradox was reported by the radii curvature decreases of the lens by aging (Brown, 1974) and the anterior shift of the zonules (Farnsworth and Shyne, 1979).

Table 19.1: The aging effects of presbyopic eyes

Eye condition change due to aging	*Effects on vision or accommodation*
Eye axial length decrease	hyperopic (1)
Lens equivalent refractive index decrease	hyperopic (2)
Lens anterior radius decrease	myopic (2)
Lens cortex thickness increase	myopic (4)
Lens capsule rigidity	less accommodation (4)
Zonule-lens coupling weakness	less accommodation (5)
Anterior zonular shift	myopic (6)
Decrease of chamber depth	myopic
Decrease of globe-axial length	hyperopic
Gravitation effects	myopic
Sclera/ciliary muscle rigidity	less accommodation
Age-altered alpha crystalline sticky	reduced accommodation capacity
Accumulated accommodative efforts	reduced accommodation capacity (7)
Hyperope	less accommodation than myope (8)
UV radiation and high temperature	earlier onset of presbyopia (9)
Reduction of pupil diameter	smaller subjective accommodation (10)

Notes: (1) reduction of eye axial length by age was reported by Grosvenor (1987); (2) lens nucleus refractive index may increase with age, but the net equivalent index may decrease combining the effects of lens nucleus and lens capsule (Hemenger, 1995 and Doubbelman, 2001); (3) lens curvatures steepened with age causing myopic shift which may be counter balanced by the lens net index decrease, or hyperopic shift (Brown, 1974); (4) Koretz (1987); Lin and Kadambi (2002); (5) reported by Kaufman (1992); (6) reported by Fansworth (1979); (7) proposed by Pierscioneck (2000); (8) published by Lavinsky (1995); (9) reviewed by Bullimore and Gilmartin (2000); (10) reported by Miege (2000)

It should be noted that the "lens paradox" showing "myopic-shift' with ageing (due to lens curvature changes) may be counter-balanced by all those factors which may cause a hyper-shift including the decreases of lens equivalent index and globe axial length with age. We shall also note that the increase of lens power due to radii decrease is a weaker age-dependence that the of the equivalent refractive index change, therefore the "net effects" cause a "hyper-shift" by aging.

PRESBYOPIA TREATMENT TECHNIQUES

The effectiveness of ciliary body contraction for lens relaxation (or accommodation) may be reduced by the combined aging factors, including lens property changes (index, size, thickness and curvature), tissue elastic changes (in sclera and ciliary) and the zonular tension change. Therefore the treatment of presbyopia shall involve methods which may change one or more of these factors. Progressive addition spectacle lenses, monovision, bifocal or multifocal contact lenses, monovision, bifocal or multifocal corneal refractive surgery, multifocal and diffractive intraocular lenses (IOLs) and accommodative intraocular lenses have been used for the correction of presbyopic by changing the corneal refractive power.

Thornton, attempted to cause scleral expansion through the procedure of anterior ciliary sclerotomy (ACS) which was shown to have major regression due to the tissue healing postoperatively. Schachar has proposed a scleral expansion band (SEB) procedure with the help of scleral implants. Fukasaku, undertook anterior ciliary sclerotomy in combination with silicone implantation (SEP) wedged into the incision in the hope of achieving greater effect and greater stability. Fukasaku and Schachar believe that presbyopia is the result of crowding in the posterior chamber due to continuous growth of the lens throughout life. The SEP technique improved the 24-momth post-op regression from about 94% (in a simple ACS) to about 39% (in SEP) according to Fukasaku's report in the ESCRS meeting in 2001. Baikoff, used a technique to position the segments in front of the ciliary body in order to release the tension on the zonule and modify the shape of the crystalline lens.

The most recent method called Laser Presbyopia Treatment (LPT), proposed and patented by J T Lin, was to use an infrared or UV laser to ablate the sclera or ciliary-body tissue and increase its elastic properties exerting a positive effect on accommodation. Comparison of presbyopia correction methods and the mechanisms using scleral expansion band (SEB), anterior ciliary sclerotomy (ACS), silicon expansion plug (SEP), supraciliary segment implant (SCI) and laser presbyopia treatment (LPT) is listed in Table 19.2.

OTHER TECHNOLOGIES FOR PRESBYOPIA

Various strategies have been developed to treat presbyopia including:

- Discrete power change using multifocal spectacles or contact lenses
- Progressive aspheric spectacle lenses, contact lenses, IOLs
- Bifocal corneal reshaping using PRK or LASIK
- Monovision using LTK, DTK or CK
- Accommodative and pseudoaccommodative IOLs
- Lens refilling phaco-Ersatz (intracapsular-balloons)
- Phocamodulation: using Q-switch Nd:YAG laser to photodisrupt the crystalline lens to reduce lens volume or softened the lens nucleus.

The ideal technologies for presbyopia correction is one that would "restore" the accommodation function of the normal young eye. This includes SEB and LTP surgical procedures on the sclera. The other technologies using monovision or multifocal do not actually restore the accommodation via lens bulging and they are called "pseudo-accommodation" as shown in the following section.

Table 19.2: Comparison of presbyopia correction methods and the mechanisms

Methods	*Technique descriptions*	*Mechanisms*
SEB (1)	Scleral expansion band	Lens equatorial diameter expansion with increased zonules tension for accommodation
ACS (2)	Radial incision of sclera	Scleral tissue incision for the expansion of "crowding" chamber and lens
SEP (3)	Silicon expansion plugs	Same as ACS but with implant for reduced regression
SCI (4)	Band implanted in ciliary body	Based on Helmholtz theory that lens diameter decreases with zonules relaxation
LASA (5)	IR or UV laser sclera ablation	Based on 'Elastic theory" of Lin-Kadambi hypothesis, where the laser-ablated scleral gap is filled with sub conjunctival tissue with increased elasticity for effective accommodation. Regression caused by tissue healing is minimized by the laser "excision"
LATK (6)	Laser thermal keratoplasty	Thermal shrinkage deep into the choroids or ciliary body combined with LTK (DTK)
CK (7)	Conductive keratoplasty	Thermal reshaping of cornea by radio frequency wave (RF), monovision
DTK (8)	Thermal keratoplasty	Using diode laser (1.4-1.9 μm) for thermal reshaping of cornea, monovision
PLASIK (9)	Presby-LASIK	Using either central-myopia (CM) or peripheral myopia (PM) bifocal corneal reshaping
AIOL (10)	Accommodative IOL	Axial movement of implanted AIOL
Phaco (11)	Laser phaco	Femto second laser phacomodulation of crystal lens

Notes: (1) method first proposed by R. Schachar; (2) first proposed by Cramer in 1860, see also S. Thornton ; (3) first proposed by H. Fukasaku in Japan; (4) method proposed by G. Baikoff in France; (5) method proposed in 1998 and patented by J.T. Lin in 2001; (6) Lin, US pending patents, 2005.
Notations:
Scleral Expansion Band (SEB), Anterior Ciliary Sclerotomy (ACS),
Silicon Expansion plug (SEP), Supraciliary segment implant (SCI) and
Laser Presbyopia Treatment (LPT) which includes LASA, LACA and LATK.

THE MECHANISMS

Presbyopia, as traditionally accepted by the Helmholtz theory, is due to progressive weakening or atrophy of the ciliary muscles. However, Schachar hypothesized that the ciliary muscle does not really become weak but rather "functionally less efficient". This inefficiency, he proposes, can be attributed to a progressive increase in the diameter of the lens during middle-age which causes a "crowding effect". Consequently, the ciliary muscle is left with no space to contract.

Helmholtz's theory and Schachar's hypothesis explain how accommodation occurs in a normal person. Helmholtz says that the ciliary muscles contract which relaxes the zonules causing the lens capsule to become lax. The jelly like lens material hence bulges at the center. There is a decrease in the equatorial diameter in the process. Schachar, on the other hand, postulates that when the ciliary muscles contract the "equatorial" zonules tighten while the non-equatorial zonules relax. This has the effect similar to holding a balloon filled with water at its two poles and pulling it outward. The net result is a bulging in the center, i.e. an increase in the anterior-posterior diameter. The degenerative changes, which have been observed in the ciliary muscle of presbyopic eyes, he postulates, may be related to disuse atrophy and not suggestive of age-related atrophy.

Both theories agree that during accommodation the lens bulges in the center. So when the lens starts hardening as in cataract there will be a loss of accommodation due to inability of the lens to bulge in the center. But we are interested in the physiology of accommodation in the absence of lens hardening or cataract.

Comments on Schachar's theory, the concept of scleral expansion is under hot debate. Many studies have actually discounted Schachar hypothesis. Glasser and Mathews demonstrated a decrease in the equatorial diameter of the crystalline lens as an effect of scleral expansion. They also found no evidence of a dynamic change in power of presbyopic patients provide by Schachar.

Helmholtz stated that the ciliary muscle is relaxed when the eye is focused for distance. The relaxed ciliary muscle maintains the zonule under tension to flatten the crystalline lens for distance viewing. When the eye focuses on a near object, the ciliary muscle contracts and releases tension on the zonule. The release of zonular tension allows the crystalline lens to become more curved due to elastic forces in the lens. Fincham added additional experimental support to the accommodative theory of Helmholtz and also offered evidence that presbyopia was caused by the inability of the lens capsule to mold the hardened lens substance into the accommodated form. Fisher and Pau and Kranz supported Fincham's theory of presbyopia by showing that the lens hardens with age. In addition to the classical theories of accommodation and presbyopia that conflict with Schachar's ideas, there are additional reasons suggesting that further verification of the efficacy of scleral expansion surgery would be prudent. The reported evidence showing improvement in the human accommodative amplitude is based solely on subjective push-up measures (Yang GS, Yee RW, Cross WD, et al 1997).

Matthews found no evidence of a dynamic change in power of the eye, which is what accommodation is. Indeed, the methods employed are the best to objectively demonstrate whether accommodation is present. Accommodation is not simply the ability to see clearly at near.

By definition, accommodation is a change in the optical power of the eye. For example, a presbyope with a bifocal spectacle lens or a multifocal contact lens on the eye can see both at distance and at near, but this is by no means accommodation. Accommodation is a dynamic process. Mathews had suggested in EyeWorld (2001) that some of the improved reading ability demonstrated with subjective push-up testing might be a result of inadequate testing procedures. It may be due to some kinds of induced multifocality of the eye, either in the cornea or in the crystalline lens, as a consequence of these surgical procedures. Patients may be left with some kind of aberration, either astigmatism or higher-order aberrations of the eye, which allows them to have functional near and distance vision simultaneously. Heraldo stated that it is difficult to find a physiological explanation for how a surgical procedure done on one eye should restore accommodation in the contralateral eye.

THE LIN-KADAMBI HYPOTHESIS

Lin-Kadambi hypothesis attempts to explain the mechanism by which the procedure of LPT causes a positive effect on the range of accommodation. The immediate effect due to the scleral thinning is an increase in the elasticity of the scleral "ring" as a whole. The ciliary muscle that takes its attachment on the inner side of this more elastic scleral ring is now able to work more efficiently as it now works against less resistance. Myopic or hyperopic shift that has not been reported after LPT. Some studies seem to indicate a paradoxical increase in the scleral diameter. We are not convinced that there is any change in the scleral diameter as there has been no reported change in the distance refractive status after LPT. However, we do not rule out the possibility of this occurring in some cases. Perhaps incisions and excisions that go full thickness may tend to produce this effect.

Lin and Kadambi did not totally discount the existence of the phenomenon of "posterior chamber crowding". We believe that this phenomenon may exist in many cases but may not be directly related to the physiology of accommodation in all cases. After the LPT procedure the ablated scleral groove gets filled with subconjunctiva tissue. Although this tissue forms a good barrier to infection and adds some amount of lateral strength to the wound, it is our contention that the tissue is still "softer" and more elastic. We also believe that the increased radial elasticity of the scleral ring is preserved as a whole and hence the positive effect on accommodation retained. Under this scenario, it will not all be surprising if some regression of effect is observed. Clinically the regression has been reported as minimal over two years and more. We also believe that the "filing-in effect" of the scleral grooves by the subconjunctival tissue plays a role in preventing regression. In acceptance of the Lin-Kadambi hypothesis, it naturally follows that there should be an immediate maximal demonstrable improvement soon after the procedure or in the following days. This has been clinically observed (for a patient to see J3 even within 4 to 5 hours postoperatively). It takes a few days for the patient to subjectively demonstrate significant improvement.

ANALYSIS OF ACCOMMODATION

By the scanning microscopic studies of the zonular in human (Robert, 1979) the ciliary body moves forward and inward when its contracted and cause the bulging of the lens and a small displacement of the lens toward the cornea. Accommodation of the lens is accomplished by changing the thickness and curvature of the elastic lens capture. The elasticity is most likely in the lens capsule rather than in the interior portion of the lens. Due to the high water content, the lens is almost incompressible and the hard nucleus deeply buried in the soft cortex is unlikely to contribute to the observed elasticity of the lens. The equatorial diameter increases from an average of 5.8 mm in the newborn to around 9.0 mm in the adult. With the increase of lens cortex thickness (average of 1.0 mm), the radius of curvature of the anterior lens surfaces decreases with age of around 5 mm in average between age of 20 and 60, or about 1.5 mm decrease each 10-year.

In addition to the change of size of the aged lens, the aging of the lens is also associated with the changes at the molecular level, especially involving the lens protein, which is the major constituent of its dry weight. The protein molecular level at birth is that almost 95% of the lens structure protein is water soluble and converted to a non-soluble protein as aging proceeds. The changes in protein solubility result in a significant increase in light scattering and a decrease of its refractive index. The layers of the lens have a stepwise increase of refractive indices toward the interior. The refractive index for a young adult is about 1.37 in the cortex and rises to about 1.405 in the nucleus (Davson, 1969). The lens nucleus refractive index increases by age from 1.405 (at age 0) to 1.4125 (at age 60).

Koretz and Handelual (1988) proposed a theory for presbyopia. The found that the older the individual, the more curved the lens becomes for a given accommodative demand because the refractive index of the lens decreases with aging, related to the known shift in its protein from soluble to insoluble form. The image of a presbyopic eye hyper-shifted when the lens index decreased. They also found that the angle of zonular insertion should change with increasing lenticular size, weakening its effectiveness. As the lens increases in size with aging, the zonules come to exert a force that is tangential (or nearly so) to the surface of the lens so that zonular relaxation has less and less effect on the shape of the lens. In addition, the sclera tissue and ciliary body become more rigid in elder people than young people. The thickness of the lens capsule also increases with age but reducing its elasticity, in addition to the increase of its curvatures.

The effectiveness of ciliary body contraction for lens relaxation (or accommodation) is therefore reduced by age due to the combined effects of the above-mentioned aging factors, including lens property changes (index, size, thickness and curvature), tissue elastic changes (in sclera and ciliary) and the zonular tension change.

THE TWO COMPONENT THEORY

The von Helmholtz theory states accommodation is achieved by ciliary muscle contraction that causes zonules and lens relaxation. Lin proposed the two-component theory to analyze a true accommodation which excludes the myopic-shift caused by axial length elongation or corneal curvature change.

$$\begin{aligned} A &= A1 + A2 \\ &= CF(dP') - m(dS), \end{aligned}$$

where, CF is the conversion factor from lens power change (dP2) to system power change, m is a refractive rate function for 1.0 mm axial forward movement of the lens (dS). The CF is given by CF=[1–S(P/1336)], with S being the effective anterior chamber depth and P is the corneal power, and has a typical value of 0.65 mm and P=43 diopter.

We note dS<0 (anterior lens shift) will result higher accommodation (A), in addition to lens bulging, or decrease of lens radius of curvature (R1, R2).

For typical ocular parameters (in mm) R1 = (10-13), –R2 = (6-8), anterior chamber depth S = (3-4), cornea radius r1 = (7-8), r2=(6.5-7.0) and axial length L = (21-24), the calculated value for m=(1.1-1.5) (D/mm) which defines the contribution from lens anterior shift, A2= –mdS. Greater detail of the m-function may be found in book Chapters of Lin (2007) entitled: Accommodating IOLs.

One may also calculate the reported pseudoaccommodation caused by a myopic shift –2.6 diopters for an axial length increase 0.89 mm (with L=22.94 mm). However, Uozato(Uozato H, ARVO Meeting, 2003, Abstract.) measured a very small axial length elongation (mean of 0.06 mm) in true accommodation. Therefore our theory proposes lens relaxation (A1) and anterior shift (A2) to be the only two major components required.

Lin and Mallo reported laser sclera ablation (LASA) procedures for presbyopia patients (age 42-60, mean 53.2) where the laser ablated a portion of the scleral tissue outside the limbus to cause a mean true accommodation of 1.96 diopter, without myopic-shift induced pseudo-accommodation. This was justified by no change of the far vision or corneal topography in treated eyes or comparing the preoperative and postoperative kerometer-(K)readings. Lin proposed the two-component theory A=A1+A2=aA + bA, with a=(0.1-0.4) for old eyes (age 50-60) and a=(0.5-0.7) for young eye (age 40-49) where lens capsules are less rigid. For extremely rigid eyes, lens anterior shift, A2=-mdS, becomes the only contribution, but it is limited to about (1.0-1.5) diopters.

Based on above theory, accommodation is easier to achieve (for a given amount of ciliary body contraction) under the following initial ocular parameters: smaller radius of curvature of the lens or the cornea; shallower anterior chamber depth or shorter globe axial length; less rigid lens capsule and larger spacing between the lens edge and ciliary muscle. Furthermore, any power changes due to corneal surface change or axial length elongation should be excluded from the true accommodation amplitude which may be further justified by the amount of lens anterior shift and the lens radius of curvature (or thickness) changes.

The effectiveness of ciliary body contraction for lens relaxation (or accommodation) may be influenced by combined aging factors, including lens property changes (index, size, thickness and curvature), tissue elastic changes (in sclera and ciliary) and the zonular tension change. The methods using sclera expansion techniques (SEB, SEP, ACS, SCI) suffer from major regression due to tissue healing, whereas the laser method, LPT, showed a minimum regression even after 24 months follow-up. The fundamental difference between the mechanism behind LPT and those of non-laser method are presented by the Lin-Kadambi hypothesis proposing the increasing of elasticity of the sclear-cilairy units is achieved by subconjunctival tissue filling. This filling process also prevents the sclera tissue healing which closes the gap and leads regression.

PRESBYOPIA-LASIK (PSEUDOACCOMMODATION)

Bifocal corneal reshaping using laser in situ keratomileusis (LASIK) procedure to create either a central-myopia (CM) island or peripheral-myopia (PM) ring for near vision has been recently reported as an alternative for presbyopia treatment (Fig. 19.1). The intent of the

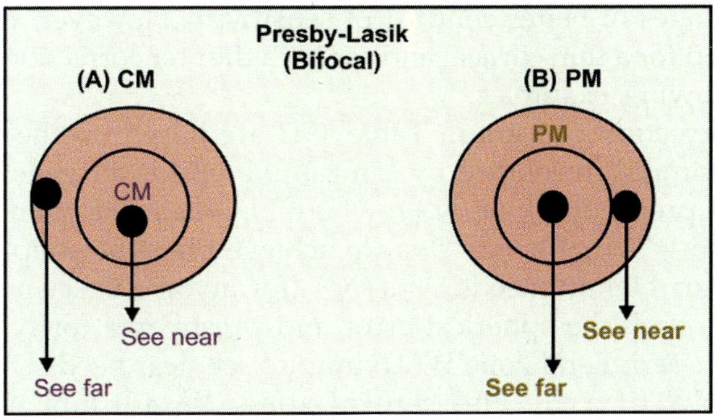

Fig. 19.1: Presbyopia-LASIK using bifocal corneal profile for (A) center-myopia (CM) and (B) peripheral myopia (PM)

presbyopic-LASIK procedure is to achieve a pseudo-accommodation versus the true-accommodation achieved by the modification of sclera or ciliary body. Combining with the conventional LASIK nomogram, bifocal reshaping may be used to treat presbyopic patients having myopia or hyperopia. A two-step procedure based on the linear superposition (LSP) (either subtraction or addition) of ablation profiles could simultaneously correct aged patents' far vision while creating a central or peripheral myopia for near vision. This Chapter will present formulas for LSP, the change corneal asphericity and compare two treatment strategies for presbyopic-LASIK.

Table 19.3 compares the strategies based on a center-myopia (CM) with peripheral for distance and on a peripheral-myopia (PM) with center for distance vision. The PM strategies used in Nidek system offer

Table 19.3: Strategies of presbyopia-LASIK using a center-myopia island (CM) or peripheral-myopia ring (PM) (see Fig. 19.1)

Preoperative cases	*Correction diopter (zone size, in mm)* *PM*	*CM*
(a) Plano NA* = +2.0 D	+2.0 (W = 7.0) –2.0 (W = 4.0)	+2.0 (W = 4.0) No W ring needed
(b) Hyperope +1.0 D NA = +3.0 D	+4.0 –3.0	+1.0 (W ring) +4.0 (W =4.0)
(c) Myope –2.0 D NA = +3.0 D	+3.0 –5.0	–2.0 +1.0
(d) Myope –4.0 D NA = +2.0 D	+2.0 –6.0	–4.0 –2.0

* NA stands for the near addition power of a presbyopic eye.

** Each treatment consists of two steps: a large (7.0 mm) followed by a small (4.0 mm) zone correction in PM; and a ring-zone W ring (4/7 mm) followed by a central zone W = 4.0 in CM the advantages of better contrast of sensitivity. However, CM would be preferred for a thin corneal and/or high diopter correction as shown in the following examples.

The correction powers in Table 19.3 are based on the following general formulas developed by Lin (unpublished) for general case of (spherical, presbyopia)=(a, NA), where NA=near addition.

a. For CM: W (ring) needs D=a (to achieve plano at peripheral) and W (center 4.0 mm) needs D'=a+NA (for myopia to see near) which corrects both the spherical error and presbyopia (or NA).
b. For PM: peripheral zone W(7.0 mm) to see near needs D=a+NA (if a>0), NA (if a<0); and central zone (W=4.0 mm to achieve plano)D'=NA (if a>0), (a-NA) (if a<0).

As shown in Table 19.3, case (c) as an example, the –2.0 D myopic presbyopia (with a near addition of +3.0 D) may be corrected by PM having two steps: first is to treat a larger zone of W=7.0 mm at +3.0D hyperopic correction and followed by a -5.0 D myopic for the inner zone of 4.0 mm. The LSP provides the center area +3.0–5.0 = –2.0 D myopic treatment for far vision, whereas the outer zone (ring) has a +3.0 D overcorrection for the presbyopic eye to see near. This PM method has a maximal ablation depth (MAD) about 3×7×7/3=49 μm. In comparison, the CM method in case (c) consists of correcting a ring-shape area (defined between 4 and 7 mm circle) by –2.0 D myopia which gives the outer ring (or peripheral) to see far. The second step of +1.0 D hyperopic treatment (with W=4.0 mm) adding to the preoperative -2.0 D myopia results a center-myopia of –3.0 D which corrects the presbyopia having a +3.0 D near addition. The MAD in this CM case is about 2×7×7/3=32.7 μm, or 25% less than PM (49 μm).

The above calculated MAD values demonstrated that CM always removes less corneal tissue (in both depth and volume) resulted from the lower diopter correction required. Furthermore, the procedure of CM is faster than PM since less corneal tissue is removed, while it suffers worse contrast than that of PM.

It should be noted that the preoperative asphericity (defined by Q) may not be perfectly preserved after the LSP, when D12=D1+D2 is a non-zero quantitative. Therefore the PM and CM post-LASIK profiles also have different Q values, in which the CM with smaller MAD also has the advantage of smaller postoperative spherical aberration (SA). This is based on the fact that SA increases after myopic correction and it is also proportional to the power of correction. The increase positive SA is resulted from the increase of Q (or the shape factor p=Q+1) in myopic correction, whereas decrease of SA resulted in hyperopic correction.

In conclusion, ametropic presbyopia may be treated via CM or PM strategy which may be analyzed by LSP theory. An improved ablation algorithm shall include the nonlinear terms and asphericity of the cornea which have been ignored in most systems using the spherical Munnerlyn formula.

COMBINE LASER AND MEDICINE

The "Lin-Kadambi" hypothesis proposed that after the LPT, the area of sclera ablated gets filled-in through the natural process of healing by "softer" subconjunctival tissue. The alteration in the elasticity of the tissue structure results in the ciliary body having to work against less resistance, a resistance initially caused by age-reduced rigidity of the sclera-ciliary-zonules complex. This leads to a greater relaxation of zonules and hence a greater central bulge of the crystalline lens for accommodation. This hypothesis may explain the minimal regression after LPT, however, can not explain some of the clinically reported cases with no accommodation effects after LPT.

For patients with "rigid" lens and/or ciliary body, the effectiveness of LPT may be very low due to the fact that the amount of ciliary-body contraction may not be sufficient to cause enough lens curvature change or anterior shift. Therefore, Lin proposed additional mechanism which uses pharmacological means to "trigger" or enhance the contraction effect after LPT for larger accommodation and/or for more stable postoperative results.

Pharmacological methods for the studies of the role of sympathetic innervations in accommodation in humans have been reported in several prior arts. Rosenfield reported a study using an alpha-adrenergic antagonist caused an average increase in accommodative amplitude of 1.5 D, which however only maintain for less than 2 hours (Rosenfiled M, The influence of alpha-adrenergic agents on tonic accommodation." Current Eye Research, 1990; 9(3): 267-72).

Nyberg reported the use of Timolol, a beta-adrenergic antagonist to cause a net increase in tonic accommodation in unfocused eyes of a group of subjects with a mean age of 23. This effect has not been demonstrated in presbyopic patients.

Eskridge reported a brief increase in the maximum accommodative response in a 36 year old subject treated with the parasympathomimetic drug eserine (Am J Optometry; 1972, pp. 632-35). A similar transient gain in accommodation was measured after treating subjects with the alpha-1 antagonist thymoxamine (Zetterstrom, Acta Ophthalmologica, 1987, 65:699-704). In a prior art of Neufeld (US Pat. 5,488,050), vision of a 50 years old presbyopia was improved after administration of the eye by a beta-adrenergic antagonists of Timolol. However the long term results and accommodation amplitude were not disclosed.

Recently, Nolan (US Pat. 6,273,092) reported the results of topical application of an acetylcholine esterase inhibitor to treat presbyopic patient. Acetylcholine esterase inhibitors such as (2-mercaptoethyl) trimethylammonium iodide O, O-diethyl phosphorothioate sold as Phospholine iodide and physostigmine (also known as eserine) sold as Antilirium are commercially available and currently used for glaucoma and accommodative esotropia at a standard concentration of 0.03% to 0.25%. Nolan proposed to use a much lower concentration of 0.0075% to 0.12% to treat presbyopia. This prior art can improve near vision without side effect such as blurring, loss of distant vision or induction of myopia, which however only provides transient gain of accommodation and only lasts for (5-7) days.

NEW DIRECTIONS

As shown in Table 19.4, presbyopia may be treated by (i) true accommodation (via lens bulging) or (ii) pseudoaccommodation via lens axial movement or bifocal corneal reshaping (Fig. 19.2). All of the existing methods (devices) suffer certain technical or clinical drawbacks. Some new directions for improvement are:

- Minimal invasive: SEB and LASA need surgical improvement to minimize bleeding and damage to the sclera
- Stability: CK and DTK are minimal invasive, but suffer major post-operative regression and only limit to low presbyopia. New laser source and fiber or conductive tips may be improved for better controlled temperature profile and deeper penetration
- New AIOL: To improve the efficiency of axial movement of the lens. Dual-optics AIOL proposed by Lin (US patent pending) is one example of new direction
- High-power: Higher accommodation (>4.0 D) may be achieved by combined procedures of LASIK, CK and AIOL.

Table 19.4: Comparing presbyopia correction by two methods (see Fig. 19.2)

(A) True accommodation (via lens bulging):
SEB, ACS, SEP, SCI, LASA, LATK

(B) Pseudo-accommodation via:

- AIOL-lens axial movement
- CK, DTK-monovision
- Presby-LASIK(bifocal)

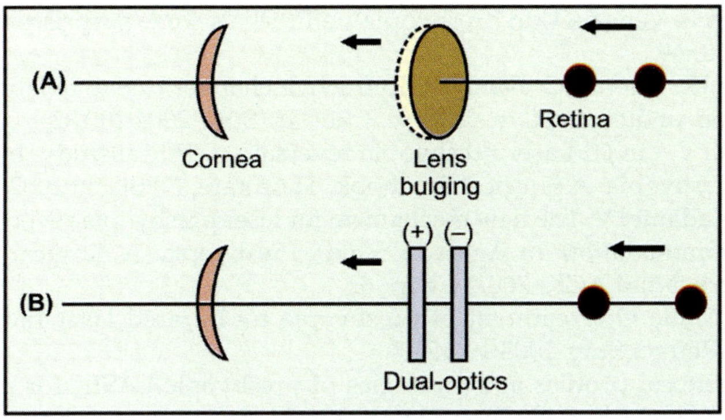

Fig. 19.2: Accommodation via (A) lens bulging, or (B) lens axial movement (dual optics AIOL)

CONCLUSION

Accommodation caused by a laser or non-laser techniques is a very complicated mechanism and can only be understood quantitatively by treating the eye as a "whole", where its refractive state is governed by many of the optical and tissue properties. Further studies, particularly the lenticular and ageing aspects, must be measured before a complete and accurate picture of the cause and correction of presbyopia can be addressed.

Both the SEB and LPT methods are still in clinical trials. Improvements on the surgical techniques (for minimal invasive), reduction of postoperative regression is the key issue for further studies for CK and DTK methods. The new directions listed earlier offer challenging opportunity for presbyopia treatments which are technically much behind the LASIK procedures for corneal reshaping.

BIBLIOGRAPHY

1. Atchison DA, Smith G, Optics of the human eye. Woburn, MA: Butterworth-Heinemann; 2000; pp 14-6, 143-7, 160-2.
2. Avalos G, Silva A. Presbyopia LASIK-the PMMA technique. In Agarwal A.(Edn): Presbyopia: A Surgical Textbook. Thorofare NJ: Slack; 2004; pp 139-46.
3. Cantu R, Rosales MA, Tepichin E, Curioca A, Montes V, Ramirez-Zavaleta G. Objective quality of vision in presbyopic and non-presbyopic patients after pseudo-accommodative advanced surface ablation. J Refract Surg 2005;21(Suppl): S603-5.
4. Fukasaku H. Anterior ciliary sclerotomy with silicon expansion plug implantation. In Agarwal S (Ed). Presbyopia: A Surgical Textbook. NJ Slack 2002; Chap. 13.
5. Guttman C. Editor, Study finds anterior ciliary sclerotomy may be ineffective. Ophthalmology Times; 2002;27(5):1.

6. Henahan S. Venezuelean presbyopia poll reveals some surprises. EyeWorld 2001;6(10):69.
7. Jimenez JR, Anera RG, Barco LJ. Refractive changes due to ablation parameters after photorefractive surgery. J Refract Surg 2004;20:182.
8. Kadambi V, Lin JT, Laser Presbyopia reversal—a clinical study, In: Agarwal S, ed. Presbyopia: A Surgical Textbook. Thorofare, NJ:Slack; 2002; Chap. 13.
9. Lin JT, Kadambi V, The new mechanism for laser presbyopia reversal (LAPR) and accommodation. In Agarwal S (ed): Presbyopia: A Surgical Textbook. Thorofare, NJ:SLACK; 2002; Chap. 6.
10. Lin JT, Mallo O. Treatment of presbyopia by infrared laser radial sclerotomy. J Refract Surg 2003;19:465-7.
11. Lin JT. Bifocal profiles and strategies of presbyopic-LASIK for pseudo accommodation. J Refract Surg 2006;22:736-8.
12. Lin JT. Prediction and control of corneal asphericity after refractive surgery. J Refract Surg 2006; 22:848-9.
13. Malecaze FL, Gazagne CS, Tarroux MC, Gorrand JM. Scleral expansion bands for presbyopia. Ophthalmology 2001; 108:2165-71.
14. Mathews S. Scleral expansion surgery does not restore accommodation in human presbyopia. Ophthalmology 1999;106:873-7.
15. Schachar R. The mechanism of accommodation and presbyopia: the scleral expansion band procedure. In: Agarwal S. (ed): Presbyopia: A Surgical Textbook. NJ Slack, 2002; Chap. 4.
16. Singh G, Chanlfin S. A complication of scleral expansion surgery for treatment of presbyopia. Am J Ophthalmol 2000;130:521-3.
17. Telando A. Pseudoaccommodative cornea: a new concept for correction of presbyopia. J Refract Surg 2004;20(Suppl.):S714-7.
18. Thornton S. Anterior ciliary sclerotomy, a procedure to reverse presbyopia. In: Sher N.A., Ed, Surgery for hyperopia and presbypopia. Williamas and Wilkins, MD (1997).
19. Von Helmholtz H. Handbuch der Physiologishen Optik. In Southall JPC (trans-ed) Helmholtz's Treatise on Physiological Optics. New York: Dover, 1962;143-72.

CHAPTER

20

JT Lin (USA)

Customized Aspherical IOLs

INTRODUCTION

It was known (Lin, 2006) that the spherical aberration (SA) increases (or decreases) after myopic (or hyperopic) LASIK due to the increase (or decrease) of the corneal front surface asphericity (Q) or the shape factor (P=Q+1). Similar to the LASIK procedure which induces a positive SA, larger population of cataracts surgery patients show an increase of positive SA. Therefore, optimized aspheric IOLs to minimize the cataract-induced SA are desired for best image quality. Most population have eyes with a positive SA (or Q<0) and about 10% of the population has negative SA, therefore most of the customized IOL would require a negative SA to minimize the remaining SA after the compensation from the natural lens which also has a negative SA in general.

In addition, the aged-induced positive SA must be also included as one of the factors of customized IOL to be considered. It was known that the natural crystalline lens has a SA of –25 μm, 0 and +25 μm at age 20, 40 and 60, although cornea SA remains constant throughout the whole life. When the positive SA increases in the eye, the presence of glare and night halos also increase. It was proposed that aging causes a gradient refractive index in the lens and causes a change from negative to positive SA of the lens over time. Therefore, as the eye ages, the combined positive SA of cornea and lens increase.

The need of customized IOL is to cause a perfect compensation of the positive SA of a prolate-cornea (with Q<0) by the implanted aspheric IOL having a negative SA. Furthermore, for IOL implanted to phakic eyes or piggyback-IOL, the strategy for minimum SA or coma should base on a 3-optics system, in which the system is rather complex and requires numerical method. This Chapter will present a comprehensive analysis without the use of numerical method.

This Chapter will cover the following subjects:

- Aspherical compensation in phakic IOL
- Coddington shape factor
- Comparison of various IOL configurations.

ASPHERICITY COMPENSATION

The total SA of a phakic eye after IOL implantation is a linear summation of the cornea, natural lens and IOL given by

$$W(\text{total}) = W(\text{cornea}) + W'(\text{natural lens}) + W''(\text{IOL}). \quad (1)$$

where W(cornea) is related to its asphericity (Q) by (Smith, 2002)

$$W(\text{cornea}) = (198.6 + 376\, Q)/R^3, \quad (2)$$

where W in ($\mu m/mm^4$) and R (in mm) is the cornea front surface radius. For R=7.7 mm and typical corneal Q-value of –0.2 to –0.5, W=(0.27 to 0.023); and the ideal corneal surface (when W=0) is given by Q*= –198.6/376 = –0.528. The typical W′(natural lens) values are –0.01 to –0.04 for natural lens Q″ of 0 to –1.0. Therefore, without the contribution from IOL, a positive W(total) is expected.

To achieve W(total)=0 post-IOL, one requires the IOL asphericity-induced SA to be negative such that

$$W''(IOL) = -[W(cornea) + W'(natural\ lens)] \quad (3)$$

The SA may be analyzed by a comprehensive theory based on the following Coddington shape factor rather than the numerical method of Atchison and Smith (1991) which was limited to aphakic eye (or the absence of natural lens) Table 20.1.

Table 20.1: Formulas for spherical aberration (W) and Coddington shape factor (S)

W (total)	=	W(cornea) + W″(IOL)
S (lens)	=	(1+X)/(1-X),
S ′(cornea)	=	(1+aX′)/(1-aX′),
SM	=	$2(N^2 - 1)/(N + 2)$,
X*	=	1-PR/1000(n‴ – 1.336).

where X = front and back surface radius ratio (R/R′) of IOL
N = refractive index ratio of IOL (n‴) and humours (1.336)
SM = condition of S for minimum SA
P = IOL power

CODDINGTON SHAPE FACTOR (S)

For an optical element having front and back surface radius of curvature of (R, R′), the Coddington shape factor (S) is defined by the degree of the "lens bending" (Pedrotti, 1998; Atchison, 1991) (Fig. 20.1).

$$S = (1+X)/(1-X), \quad (4)$$

where, S=R/R′ is the front and back surface radius ratio of the optics which is surrounded by the same media for both surface, such as natural lens or IOL inside the media of the humours (aqueous and vitreous of an eye).

However, for an optic surrounded by two different media, such as the cornea having front surface in air (with refractive index of no=1.0) and back surface in humours (with n′=1.336). The effective focal lens of the cornea with n=1.377 and front and back radius of (r, r′) is given by (Lin, 2005)

$$1/f' = (n-1.0)/(n'r) - (n-n')/(n'r') \quad (5)$$
$$= 0.282\ (1-ar/r')/r,\ (\text{with } a=0.109),$$

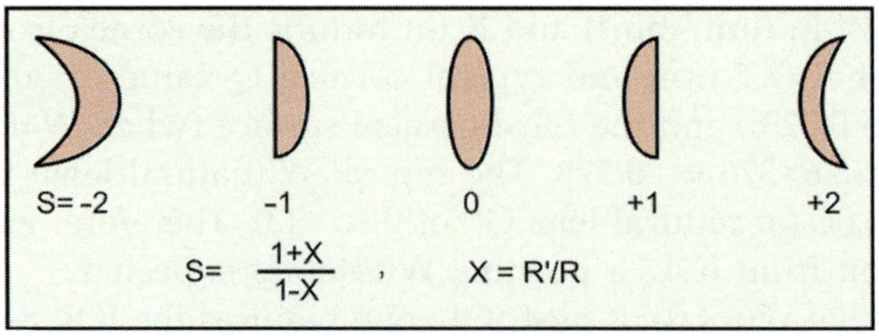

Fig. 20.1: Coddington shape factor (S)

comparing to that of the lens with n″=1.42 and radius (R, R′) of

$$1/f = [(n'' - n')/n'](1/R - 1/R'). \quad (6)$$

Therefore, the shape factor for the lens and cornea are given by

$$S\ (\text{lens}) = (1+X)/(1-X), \quad (7.a)$$
$$S'\ (\text{cornea}) = (1+aX')/(1-aX'), \quad (7.b)$$

where, a=0.109 defined by a=(n-n′)/(n-1.0). One may see that S′ reduces to S when a=1.0 (for optic in the same media). In above equation, X=R/R′ and X′=r/r′.

It was reported (Pedrotti and Pedrotti, 2000) the minimum spherical aberration (SA) is achieved when the shape factor is given by (for an infinity object)

$$SM = 2(N^2 - 1)/(N + 2), \quad (8)$$

which was only good for optics in air with N=n (the refractive index of the optics). For optics in non-air media such as human cornea and lens, Lin (unpublished) has derived the generalized N values of N=N′ = 1+(n-1)/n′ = 1.28 (for cornea) and N=n″/n′ = 1.06 (for lens). Using these values in Eq.(8), one readily obtains the shape factor for minimum SA for cornea (S1) and lens (S2) (for an infinity object) SM=S1=0.39 and SM=S2=0.085, respectively. Furthermore, one may also derive the condition for minimum coma given by S1'=0.44 and S2'=0.094. In the following discussion, I will use S1 and S2 since they are very close to the coma values.

For typical radius surface of cornea (r, r′)=(7.8, 6.5) mm and natural lens (R, R′)=(10, 6) mm, one may easily calculate, from Eq.(7), S (lens) = –0.25 and S′(cornea)=+1.3. The differences of these values and the idea values (for minimum SA and/or coma) are: d′ = S′ – S1 = +0.95 and d = S – S2 = -0.34. These positive (d′) and negative (d) values imply the positive and negative SA of typical cornea and lens surface, respectively since SA is proportional to d or d′.

Given the S1 and S2 for minimum SA, one may also calculate the associated front-back surface radius ratio X′= r/r′, X = R/R′ to be X′

= –4.0 and X = 1.18 which are far from the typical (actual) values of X′ = 1.2 and X = –1.65. Therefore, it may be concluded that the ideal surface of cornea or lens for minimum SA (or coma) could not be achieved simultaneously. In addition, these conditions are not what we desired. What we need is the minimum SA (or coma) for combined overall (whole eye), rather than just for cornea or lens (natural lens or IOL) separately.

Analytic relationship for the shape factor for the "system" of the whole eye having minimum SA or coma is quite complex and not yet available so far. However, the S1 and S2 give us the first order approximation condition defined by S* = d+d′ = (S+S′) – (S1+S2), with (S1+S2) = 0.39 + 0.085 = 0.48, to be minimum such that the combined 2-optics system has minimum SA and coma. This goal may be achieved by the followings:

1. Customized LASIK (Lin, 2006), where the post-LASIK corneal asphericity (Q″) becomes more prolate (or more negative) to better compensate (cancellation) the negative lens Sam W′(lens) < 0. In other words, the corneal shape factor (S′) decreases from its pre-LASIK value of about +1.3 (for r=7.8, r′=6.5 mm) to a smaller value (for example, +0.9) such that d′=0.9 – S1 = 0.9 – 0.39 = 0.61 and therefore S*=d′+d=0.61-0.34=0.27 which is smaller than the pre-LASIK value of S*=+0.95 – 0.34 = 0.61, and results in a reduced SA of the whole eye. Note that the absolute value of SA associated with S* is still unknown since we only know SA is proportional to S*.
2. Additional compensation from the phakic-IOL given by S*=d+d′+d″ (to be detailed as follows).

THE 3-OPTICS ASPHERICITY

The earlier 2-optics (cornea and natural lens) formula for S* may be extended for 3-optics system including the contribution from the implanted IOL as: S*=d+d′+d″, where d″=S″-S3, and S″ has the same formula as S in Eq.(7), but SM of Eq.(8) is revised by different refractive index of the IOL (n‴) having values of n‴ = (1.43, 1.49) in silicon and PMMA materials. The associated minimum SA shape factor SM=S3= (–0.1, –0.16), respectively. These examples show the strong dependence of S3 on the n‴ value. Therefore the design for optimal IOL should include the lens geometry (shape) and its refractive index. Given n″=1.43 and 1.49, one may calculate the minimum SA value from Eq.(8) S3= –0.1 and –0.16. Given the fixed corneal and natural lens value of (d+d′) = –0.35 + 0.95 = 0.6, one obtains the combined value of S*=d+d′+d″.

In general, the S*=0 condition gives us the IOL shape factor optimized to meet S″= S3–(d1+d2). Solving X in Eq.(7.a) for (d1+d2)=0.6, S3=0.1, S″= –0.5 (the case of n″=1.43) to obtain X*(optimal)= –(1–S″)/(1+S″)= –3.0; and X*= –2.57, for different IOL index of n″=1.49, S″= –0.44.

For a given IOL power of P=1000(n‴ – 1.336)(1/R – 1/R′), the optimal X* defined by X*=R/R′ is related to P by

$$X^* = 1-PR/1000(n''' - 1.336). \quad (9)$$

For example, for a plus IOL-power P= +10.0 D, n‴=1.43, X* = 1–0.01064R Therefore the case of X* = –3.0 gives R=37.6 mm and R′= –3R = –113 mm which is a "bi-convex" lens with the more curved surface facing cornea. For the case of X*= –2.57 (for n″=1.49), one obtains R=23.5 and R′=X*R= –70.5 mm.

Above examples are for (d+d′)=0.6. For (d+d′)=0.3, S″=0.1 – 0.3 = –0.2, X* (for n‴=1.43) = –1.5, one obtains the optimal IOL surface (R, R′)=(27.9, –83.7) mm. For larger (d+d′)=0.8, S″=0.1 – 0.8 = –0.7, X* = –5.66, and therefore (R, R′)=(6.26, –18.8) mm which is almost a convex-plano lens.

COMPARING WITH WANG RESULTS

Above new concept is based on the optimal compensation of SA among 3-optics (the cornea, natural lens and IOL) such that the combined system SA 9 and/or coma) is minimized. These criteria are different from the condition for "isolated" IOL consideration. For example, it was reported (Wang et al, 2003) that comparing the configurations of IOL surface (R, R′)= (a) (15.4, –15.4), (b) (7.3, infinity), (c) (infinity, –7.3), (d) (51.64, –9), (e) (+9, –51.64), (f) (6.8, 55) mm, they conclude the following:

i. For spherical aberration (SA): (b)< (e) < (f); and
ii. For coma: (e) < (a) < (b).

Therefore, configuration (b) convex-plano offers the lowest SA whereas (e) convex-concave offers the lowest coma and also low SA. These results are consistent with the analysis based on Coddington shape factor (S) and X*. However, the S and X* method offers analytic rather than numerical data of method of Wang's. In addition, the Wang's method is only good for isolated IOL and has ignored the influence from the individual corneal and natural lens contribution.

CONCLUSION

For optimal design of aspherical IOLs, the minimum spherical aberration (SA) and coma of the whole eye may be achieved by minimum summation of the 3-optics, the cornea (W>0), the natural lens (W′<0) and the IOL (W″<0) such that W(total) is minimum. The Coddington shape factor (S) and the surface radius ratio (X) provide comprehensive and analytical formulas which are consistent to the numerical results of Want et al and Atchison.

BIBLIOGRAPHY

1. Atchison DA. Design of aspherical IOLs. Ophthal Physiol Opt. 1991;11:137-46.
2. Lin JT. Prediction and control of corneal asphericity after refractive surgery. J Refract Surg 2006; 22:848-9.
3. Lin JT. The generalized refractive state theory and effective eye model. Chinese J Optom & Ophthal. 2005;7:1-6.
4. Pedrotti LS, Pedrotti FL. Optics and vision. Upper Saddle River, NJ. 1998;122-41.
5. Smith G, et al. The spherical aberration of the crystalline lens of the human eye. Vision Res. 2001;41:235-43.
6. Wang XJ, Jin CP, Wang QM. Aberration with IOLs based on different optical designs. Chinese J Optom & Ophthal. 2003;5:209-11.

CHAPTER

21

Sanjay Chaudhary (India)

Aberration Free IOLs (Aspheric IOLs)

INTRODUCTION

Conventional spherical IOLs (Clariflex, Acrysof, Akreos, etc) have a positive spherical aberration, which results in reduced contrast sensitivity under mesopic and scotopic conditions. Aspheric IOLs like the Tecnis (AMO), Acrysof IQ (Alcon) and Akreos AO (B&L) minimize the spherical aberration resulting in improved vision. A normal corneal spherical aberration is positive, i.e. +0.27 microns (μm) ± 0.02 μm. Tecnis has a negative spherical aberration of –0.27 μm, Acrysof IQ — 0.20 μm and Akreos AO — 0.0 μm (neutral). Following is a comparison of these three different lenses.

UNDERSTANDING SPHERICAL ABERRATION

A spherical aberration occurs when parallel rays of light do not focus on one point. The central bundle of rays may focus in front of or behind the focus of the peripheral bundle of rays. The refractive power in the periphery of the lens may either be too weak or (usually) too strong. When the peripheral rays of light focus in front of the central rays, it is called positive SA, and if they focus behind the central rays, it is called negative SA. The resulting image despite a SA might be clear, but it has less contrast than an ideal optic.

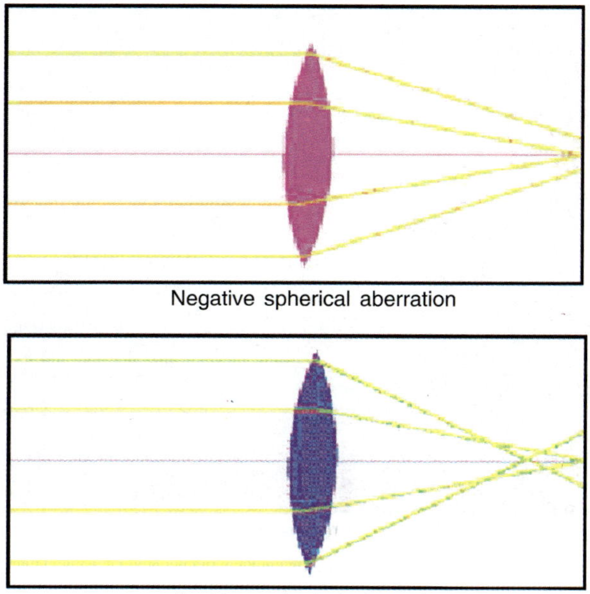

Negative spherical aberration

Positive spherical aberration

Fig. 21.1: Spherical aberration (SA) in a lens system

Spherical Aberrations in a Human Eye

The human cornea has a positive SA. This means that the light entering the eye from the peripheral parts of the cornea converge more to focus in front of the rays entering the central portion of the cornea. The SA of the cornea hardly changes during lifetime. In a 4 mm pupil, rays from the peripheral part of the cornea are obstructed and therefore the eye would manifest with very little SA. If the pupil dilates to 6 mm or more, the peripheral rays also reach a focus within the eye. Such an eye with a co-existing large quantum of SA would experience a loss of contrast.

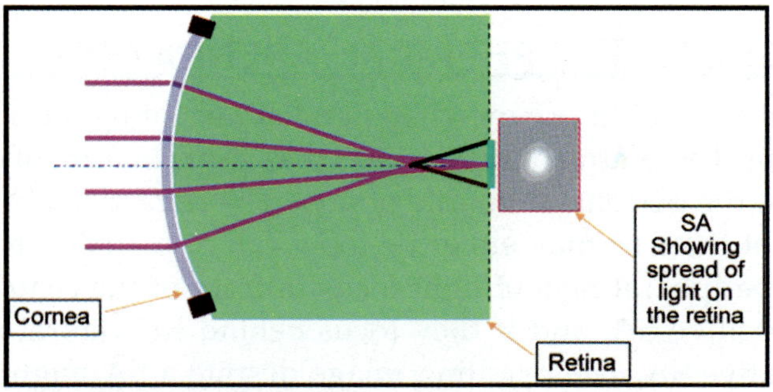

Fig. 21.2: Positive SA in a normal human cornea. Peripheral rays focus in front of retina

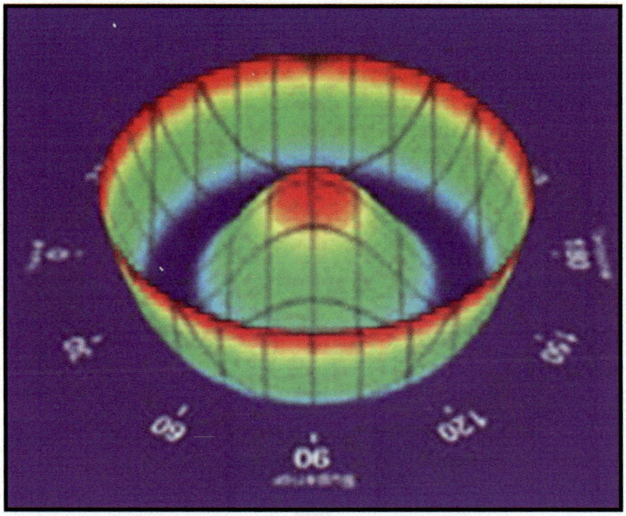

Fig. 21.3: 3 D representation of SA

In a Young Eye

The cornea of a young eye has a positive spherical aberration, which gets compensated by the negative spherical aberration of the crystalline lens. There is a young adult, the rays of light come to a point focus on the retina, and the contrast sensitivity is good.

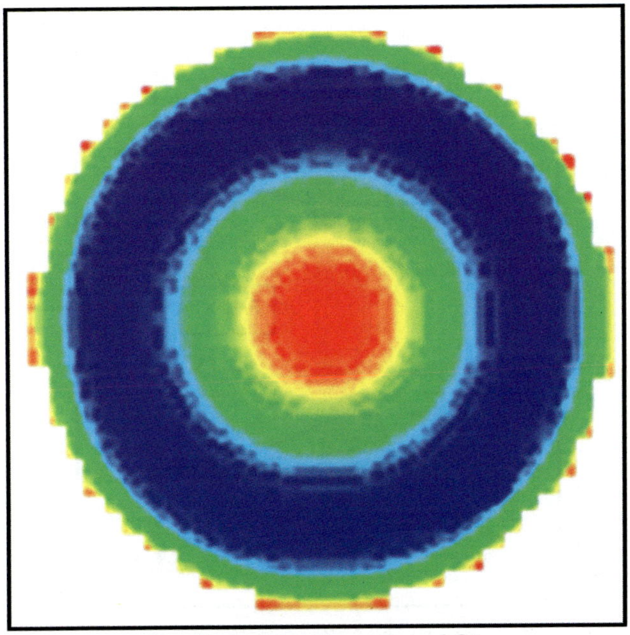

Fig. 21.4: 2 D color coding of SA

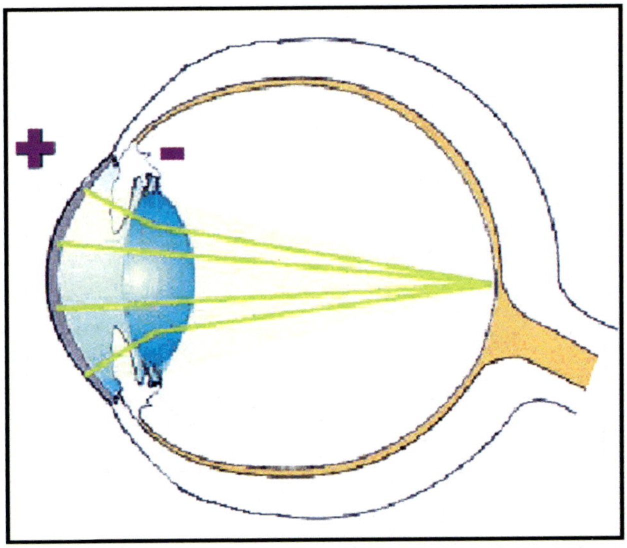

Fig. 21.5: Point focus on the retina as –ve SA of young lens neutralizes +ve SA of cornea

In the Elderly Eye

The lens is growing over a lifetime. In the process, it gets thicker. Its refractive index also increases. So from a negative SA, with age it develops a positive SA.

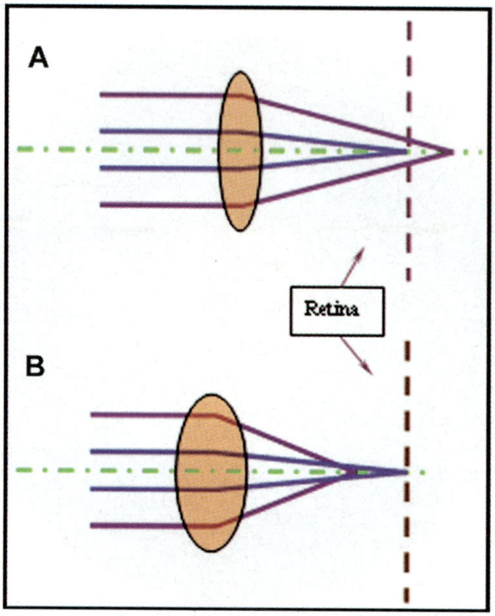

Figs 21.6A and B: (A) A young lens with a negative SA (B) An aging lens with a positive SA

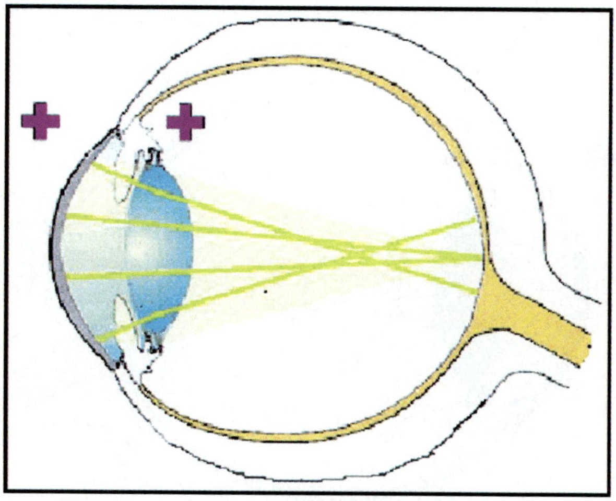

Fig. 21.7: +ve SA of an aging lens compounds the +ve SA on the cornea

In an elderly person, the cornea has a positive SA, and the crystalline lens also has a positive SA. The two lead to an even stronger effect, greatly increasing the overall SA and a marked decrease in contrast.

CONVENTIONAL SPHERICAL IOLs

They also have an inherent positive SA and therefore they also amplify the SA of a cornea.

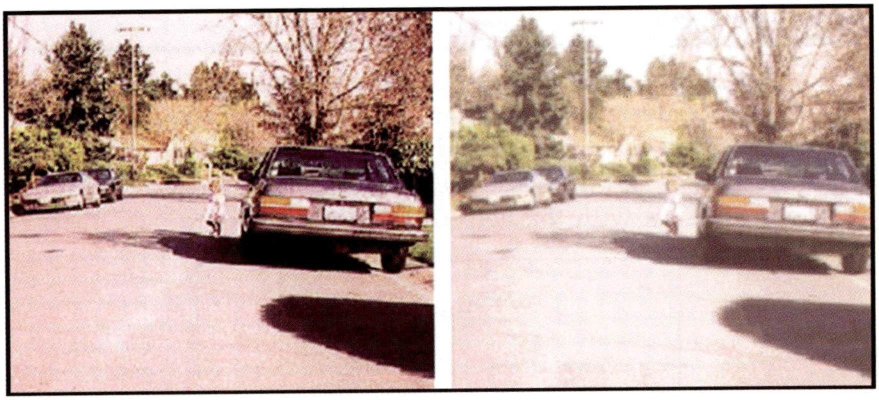

Fig. 21.8: Reduced contrast sensitivity during the day (Courtesy: AMO)

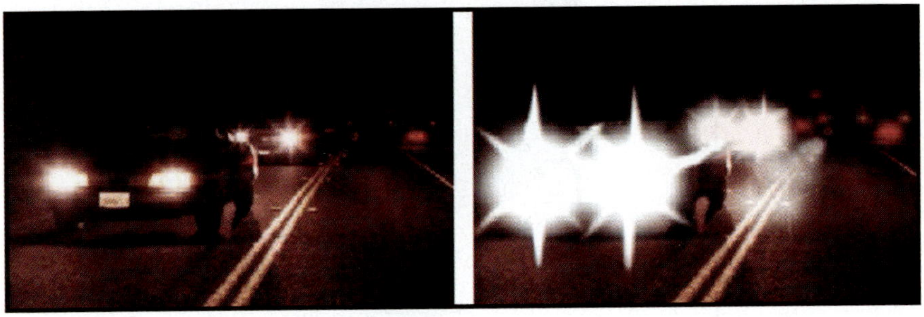

Fig. 21.9: Glare and halos at night (Courtesy: AMO)

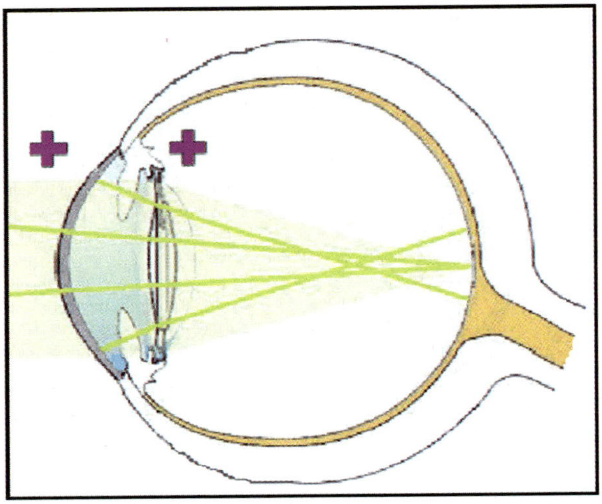

Fig. 21.10: +ve SA of conventional IOL add to SA of cornea

THE TECNIS LENS (AMO)

This is a multipiece second-generation silicon lens. It has a negative prolate surface designed on the anterior surface of the lens and has a SA of – 0.27 µm. It has a square edged optic design. It refractive index is 1.46 and an edge thickness is 0.50 mm. It can be injected through a 2.8 mm incision with the help of an injector system.

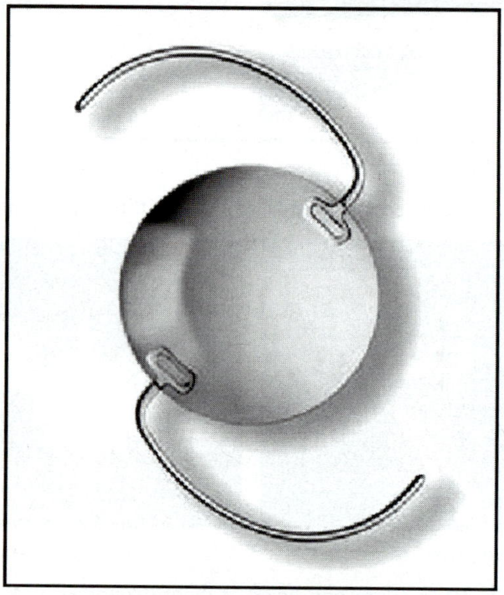

Fig. 21.11: The Tecnis lens

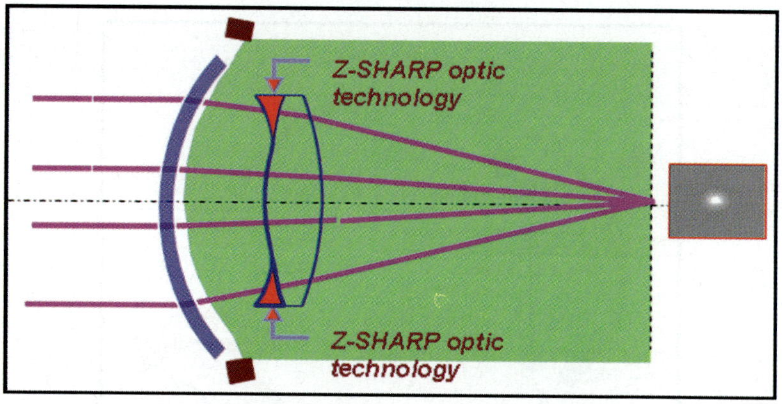

Fig. 21.12: The –ve SA on the anterior surface compensates for the +ve SA of cornea

Fitting Philosophy

The lens is designed to fully correct the +ve SA of the cornea thereby enhancing the contrast sensitivity to the maximum. The lens is based on the Z-sharp optic technology. The peripheral part of the anterior surface of the lens gets a more concave design and therefore neutralizes the positive SA of the peripheral cornea. Various studies have shown that the asphericity of the cornea is + 0.27 μm with a standard deviation of ± 0.02. This lens has a negative SA of –0.27 μm and targets to fully correct the total corneal SA of the eye.

THE ACRYSOF IQ (IMAGE QUALITY) (ALCON)

This lens is a single piece hydrophobic acrylic and is a blue light filtering lens (lens is impregnated with yellow chromophore). The asphericity is designed on the posterior surface of the lens by thinning the lens in the centre. The lens has a –ve SA of –0.20 μm. It has a refractive index of 1.55, an edge thickness of 0.21. It can be injected through a 2.8 mm incision with the injector system.

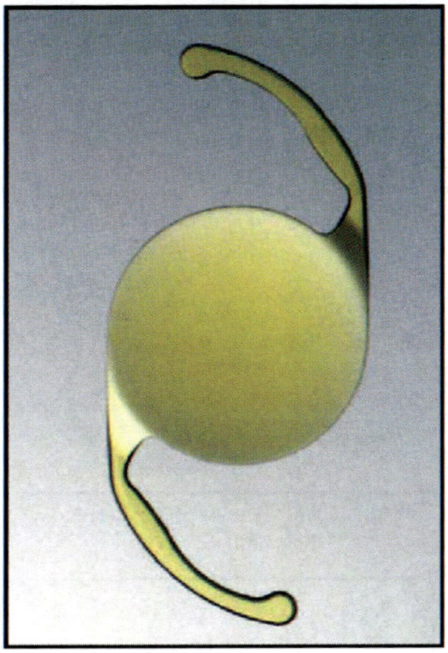

Fig. 21.13: The Acrysof IQ

Fitting Philosophy

Studies reveal that a normal vision is best when there is a residual positive SA of +0.1 μm in the optical system of the eye. This lens has a –ve SA of – 0.20 μm and after neutralizing the +ve SA of the cornea (SA of + 0.27 μm), there is still a residual +ve SA of +0.07 ± 0.02 μm.

Tanzer & Schallhorn reported that 338 Navy pilots had a mean positive spherical aberration of approximately 0.1 μm (6.0 mm pupil) (ASCRS Symposium, May 1-5, 2004, San Diego, CA). Levy *et al* (AJO, 2005) found that for 70 "supernormal" eyes with an UCVA = 20/15, the positive spherical aberration of the whole eye was 0.11 μm ± 0.077 μm, with a 6.0 mm pupil. These clinical observations suggest that preserving a moderate amount of positive spherical aberration may enhance the quality of vision in normal pseudophakic eyes.

AKREOS ADAPT AO (ADVANCED OPTIC) (BAUSCH & LOMB)

This is a single piece hydrophilic acrylic with a square edge. Its refractive index is 1.458 (hydrated). It has an anterior and posterior aspheric surface. It neither has a positive or a negative SA, i.e. a SA of ±0.00 μm. It therefore does not result in any aberration being introduced in the eye. It can be injected through a 3.0 m incision.

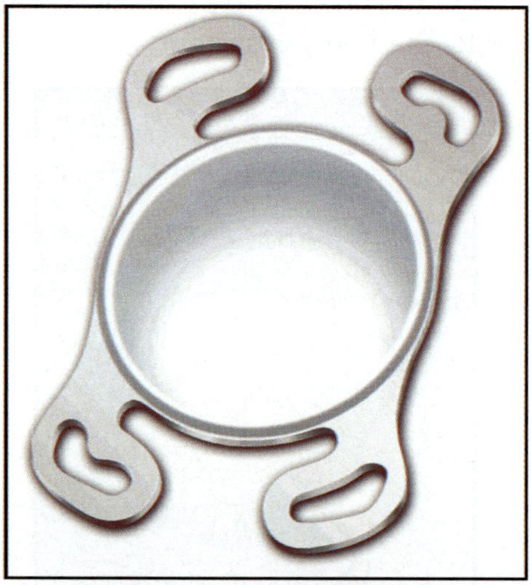

Fig. 21.14: The Akreos Adapt AO (Bausch & Lomb)

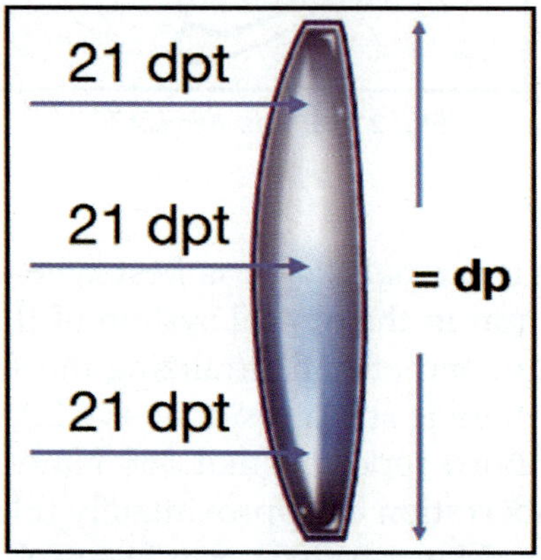

Fig. 21.15: Uniform power of the Akreos AO from centre to edge

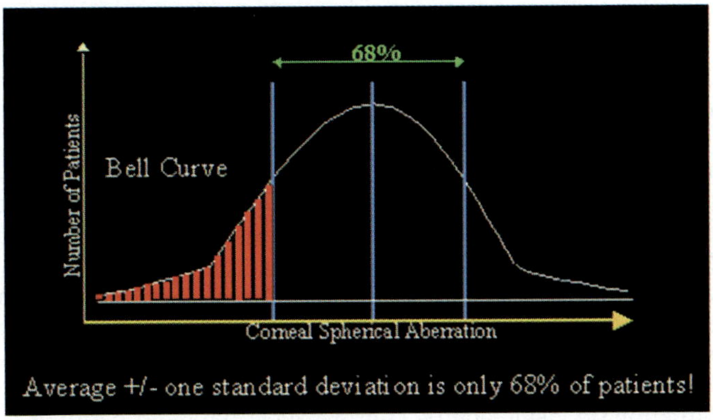

Fig. 21.16: Bell curve showing the variation in the corneal SA

Comparison of Aspheric IOLs		
6.0 mm pupil size	*Lens spherical aberration*	*Residual spherical aberration*
AcrySof IQ	– 0.20 mm	0.10 mm
Tecnis	– 0.27 mm	0.00 mm
Akreos AO	0.00 mm	0.27 mm

The lens has a uniform power from the centre to the edge. This gives the lens independence from the eye's optical alignment. Therefore the image quality is not disturbed even if the lens is slightly decentered.

Fitting Philosophy

The aberrations present in a human eye differ from person to person. Therefore an aspheric lens, which is aberration neutral, offers control of SA, which is independent of the patient's profile. This implies that the other lens manufacturers assume that the corneal SA is +0.27 ± 0.02 μm in all cases. Some studies show that the variation may be even more. Therefore, if the corneal +ve SA were less than the amount assumed, these lenses would result in an overall –ve SA that is worse. The best situation would be not to have a +ve SA of a conventional lens, and at the same time avoid disturbing the SA of the cornea. This opinion is supported by the Bell curve which shows that only 68 % of the human cornea's fall in the bracket of a standard +ve SA.

BIBLIOGRAPHY

1. Aggarwal A, Khurana A K, Nada M. Contrast sensitivity function in pseudophakic eyes and phakics. Acta Ophthalmol Scand 1999; 77: 441-4.
2. Altmann GE, Nichamin LD, Lane SS, Pepose JS. Optical performance of three intraocular lens designs in the presence of decentration. J Cat Refract Surg 2005;31: 574–85.

3. Atchison D A. Third order aberrations of pseudophakic. Ophthal Physiol Opt 1989;9:205-11.
4. Barbero S, Marcos S, Jiminez-Alfaro I. Optical aberrations of intraocular lenses measured in vivo and in vitro. J Opt Soc Am A 2003;20: 1841-51.
5. Erie JC, Bandhuuer MH, McLaren JW. Analysis of postoperative glare and intraocular lens design. J Cat Refract Surg 2001;27: 614-21.
6. Holladay J T, Piers P A , Koranyl G, et al. A new intraocular lens design to reduce spherical aberration of pseudophakic eyes. J of Refractive Surg 2002;18:683-91.
7. Lopez-Gil N, Howland H C, Howland B, et al. Generation of third order spherical and coma aberrations by use of radially symmetrical fourth order lenses. J Opt Soc Am A 1998;15:2563-71.
8. NIO Y-K, Jansonius N M, Geraghty E, et al. Effect of intraocular lens implantation on visual acuity, contrast sensitivity and depth of focus. J Cat Refract Surg 2003; 29: 2073-81.
9. Wang L, Dai E, Koch DD, Nathoo A. Optical aberrations of the human anterior cornea. J Cat Refract Surg 2003;29: 1514-21.

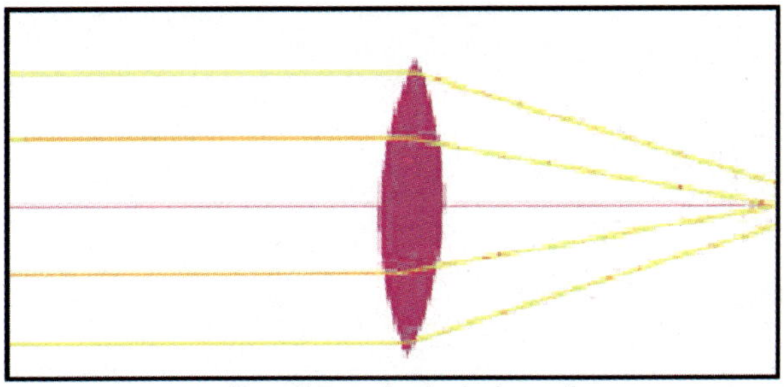

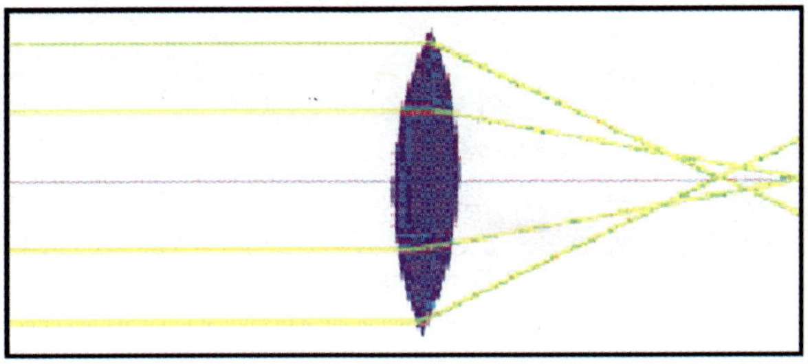

CHAPTER

22

Okihiro Nishi, Kayo Nishi,
Yutaro Nishi, Shiao Chang, (Japan)

Capsular Bag Refilling Using Capsulotomy: Capturing Intraocular Lens

INTRODUCTION

Refilling the lens capsule with an injectable material, while preserving capsular integrity including zonules and ciliary muscles, offer a potential to restore ocular accommodation[1,2] (Fig. 22.1). The greatest technical challenge in this procedure was primarily preventing the leakage of injectable IOLs.[3-6]

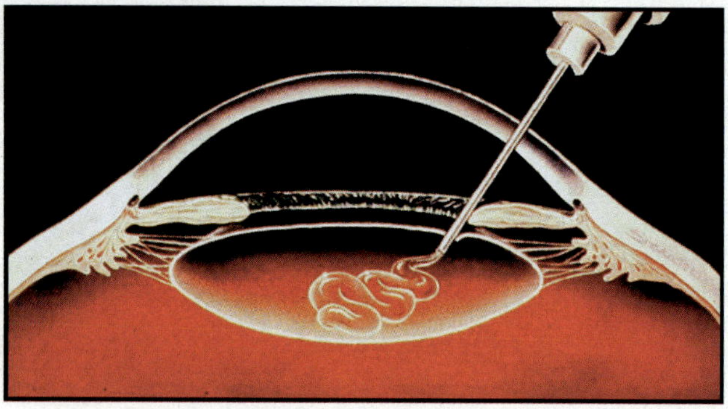

Fig. 22.1: Schematic illustration of the lens refilling procedure (Courtesy: DJ Apple)

To prevent leakage, we developed a silicone plug to seal the capsular opening[7,8] (Fig. 22.2). We could confirm some accommodation in the young macaca monkies. Figure 22.3 shows the Scheimpflug photographies of the eye of a monkey before and after surgery, showing evidence of some accommodation being obtained. After application of 4% pilocarpine, there is thickening of the lens with steepening of the anterior capsule and shallowing of the anterior chamber, both before and after surgery, although the findings were much less marked after surgery.

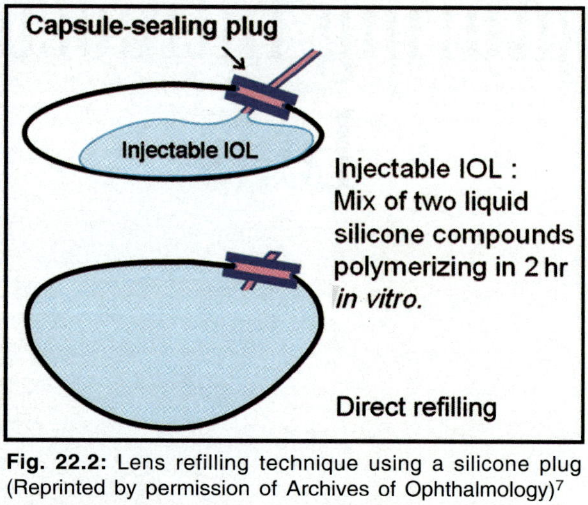

Fig. 22.2: Lens refilling technique using a silicone plug (Reprinted by permission of Archives of Ophthalmology)[7]

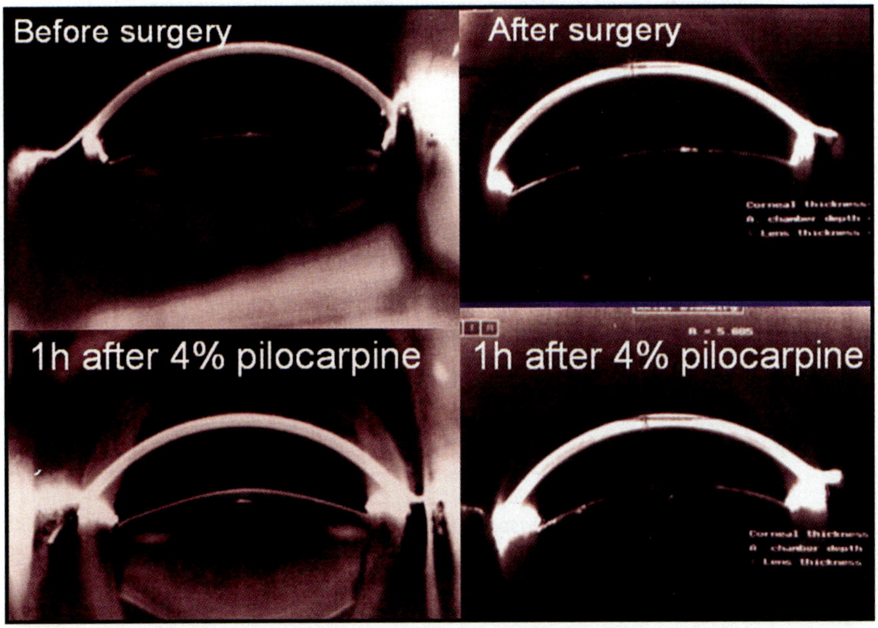

Fig. 22.3: Scheimpflug photographs of a monkey eye before and after refilling the lens capsule. Note that there was thickening of the lens with steepening of the anterior capsule and shallowing of the anterior chamber. After surgery (right), there were similar findings, though less remarkable. Note also that there were discontinuous zones in the lens before surgery, while the refilled lens was optically empty due to the silicone compound

From these experiments, we have concluded that refilling the lens capsule is technically quite feasible. It is suggested that the procedure may restore ocular accommodation in humans. However, there are some essential problems to overcome: refining and simplifying the technique; prevention of anterior capsule opacification (ACO) and posterior capsule opacification (PCO); reducing surgically-induced astigmatism because the unilateral CCC, though tiny, caused a great astigmatism (unpublished data).

Here, I will demonstrate a completely new concept and novel lens refilling procedure that may solve these problems. We had this concept already in 1989[9] and resumed the technique, because endocapsular balloon technique and the capsular plug technique will not be supposed to be applied clinically, and the technique will solve the problems mentioned above.

REFILLING THE LENS CAPSULE WITH CAPSULOTOMY-CAPTURING INTRAOCULAR LENS

IOL

The IOL shape is similar to that of a conventional IOL, but the optic has small narrow grooves over its entire circumference (Fig. 22. 4). The

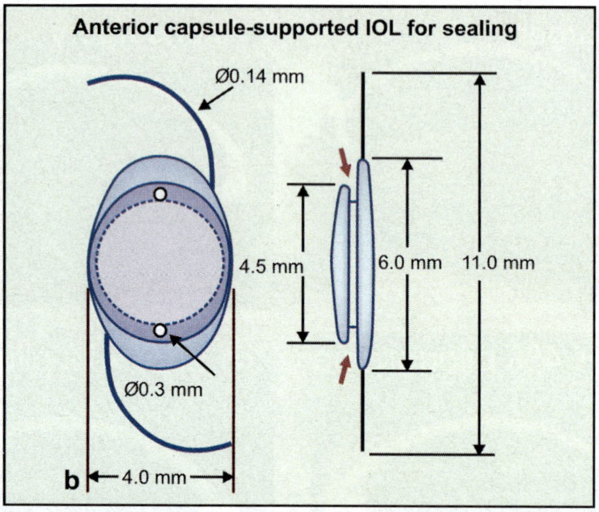

Fig. 22.4: Anterior capsule-supported IOL for sealing CCC. The arrows show the small narrow, grooves at the optic (Reprinted by permission of Graefe's Archives of Clinical and Experimental Ophthalmology)[9]

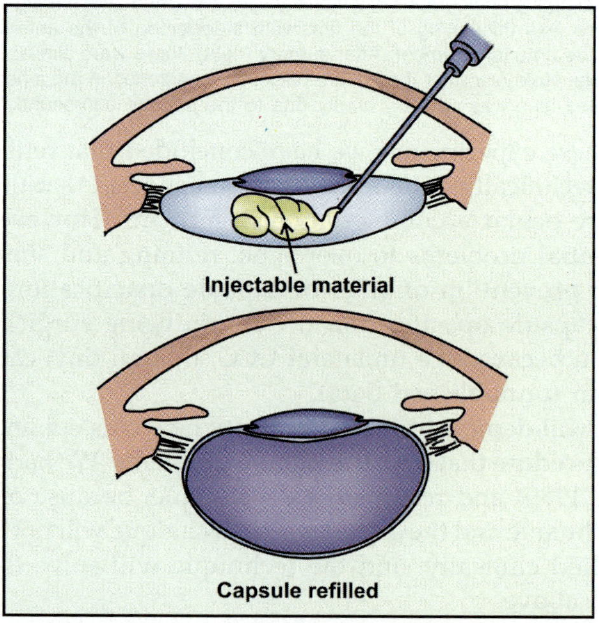

Fig. 22.5: Surgical lens refilling procedure using anterior capsule-supported IOL (Reprinted by permission of Graefe's Archives of Clinical and Experimental Ophthalmology)[9]

CCC edge is put in this groove, which chokes the IOL, preventing leakage of the injected material. Figure 22.5 illustrates the procedure. Figure 22.6 shows the most recent foldable version of the IOL.

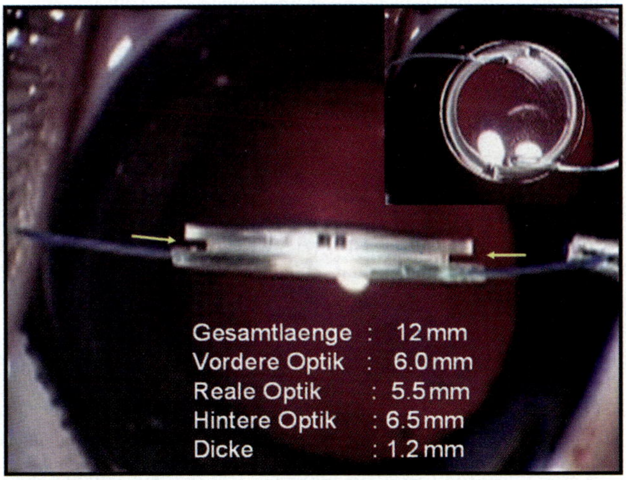

Fig. 22.6: Anterior capsule-supported foldable IOL and its dimensions

Surgical Procedure

As in conventional cataract surgery, CCC, around 4 mm in diameter, is created in the middle of the anterior capsule. After phacoemulsification aspiration, viscoelastics are injected into the capsular bag in the usual manner. The folded IOL is introduced entirely into the capsular bag. A Sinskey hook is introduced underneath the IOL, and the IOL is lifted by the hook, so that the optic edge groove of the lower half of the IOL is captured by the lower half of the CCC. The lower half of the groove is captured almost automatically while lifting the lower half of the IOL, because the IOL is firmly fixed in the middle by both haptics remaining in the capsular bag. Then, the viscoelastics are completely removed by aspiration, during which an I/A cannula is introduced underneath the upper half of the IOL, which is now outside of the capsular bag. Viscoelastics are injected into the anterior chamber onto the IOL. The upper half of the IOL is then captured by the CCC by pushing the IOL downward and posteriorly at the middle part of the IOL optic edge with a push-pull hook until the upper IOL clears the upper CCC edge to be captured. A small portion of the CCC edge at the optic groove is now hooked with the Sinskey hook and pulled slightly to introduce the injection cannula. The injectable material, actually a mix of two liquid silicones is then injected into the capsular bag. It polymerizes in 2 hr *in vitro*.

RESULTS AND DISCUSSION

We have refilled many pig cadaver eyes and rabbit eyes using this technique (Figs 22.7 to 22.10). After the IOL was correctly captured by

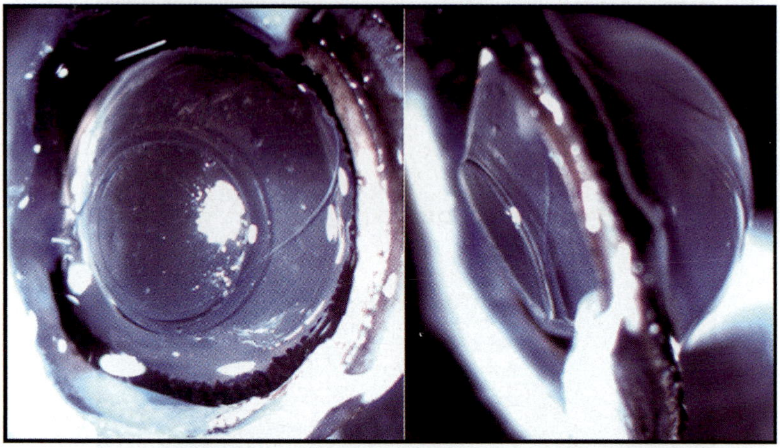

Fig. 22.7: A well-refilled pig cadaver capsule. The anterior capsule-supported IOL was firmly fixed, and there was no leakage of the material injected

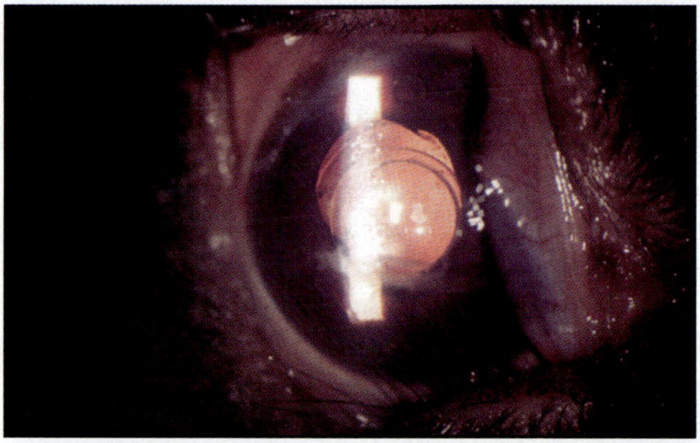

Fig. 22.8: A refilled rabbit crystalline lens. Three weeks after surgery. Note that the IOL was firmly and securely fixed. There was no leakage of the injected silicone compound. Posterior synechia

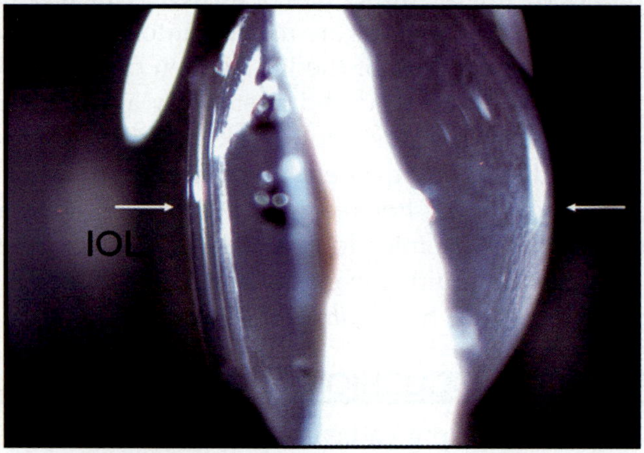

Fig. 22.9: An enucleated rabbit lens refilled

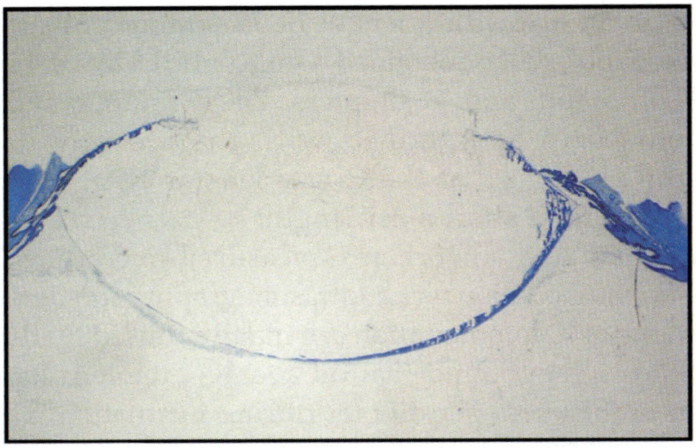

Fig. 22.10: Histopathological findings of an enucleated rabbit lens refilled. Three weeks after surgery

the CCC, there was no leakage of the injected silicone. Thus, the apropriate size for the CCC, not too small to capture but not too large to capture firmly the IOL, is crucial for surgical success. If the CCC is appropriately sized, the procedure is highly reproducible. We marked a 5 mm circle on the cornea using a Hoffer optic zone marker for 5 mm, according to the technique described by Wallace,[10] and used this mark as a guide for an appropriate CCC diameter around 4 mm.

Expected Mechanism of Accommodation

The expected mechanism of accommodation involves forward-movement of the IOL and thickening of the lens.

These expected mechanisms are based on two recent studies. Nawa and his coworkers[11] demonstrated the accommodation-amplitude obtained per 1 mm forward movement of the IOL. For this purpose, a ray-focusing equation for pseudophakic eyes was established using the ray-tracing method with dedicated computer soft ware. It was found that the amplitude depends on axial length and corneal power (Table 22.1). In eyes with an axial length of 21 mm and an IOL with 30 diopters, 1 mm forward movement yields 2.3 D of accommodation.

Table 22.1: The relationship between AL and dioptric power of an MA30BA IOL and amount of accommodation per 1.0 mm forward movement

	Axial Length (mm)						
Parameter	*21.0*	*22.0*	*23.0*	*24.0*	*25.0*	*26.0*	*27.0*
IOL power (IOL)	30.0	27.0	24.0	20.0	17.0	14.0	11.0
Accommodation per 1.0 mm forward IOL movement (D)	2.3	1.9	1.6	1.3	1.1	0.9	0.8

(Preprinted by permission of J Cataract Refract Surg 2003;29:2069-72)[11]

Accordingly, in an eye with a length of 23 mm and 24 diopters, 1.6 D of accommodation will be obtained, while only 0.8 D will be obtained with values of 27 mm and 11 diopters. These findings indicate that improvements may be obtained with the recently developed accommodating IOL such as the Crysta lens or 1CU, specifically in hyperopic eyes with a short axial length.

van der Heijde and coworkers[12] measured microfluctuations of steady-state accommodation using ultrasonography, and demonstrated that fluctuations in accommodation are mainly caused by fluctuations of lens thickness. They found that on average, the lens increases by about 56 μm in thickness per diopter during fluctuation. That means that 3 diopters could be obtained by about 0.17 mm change in thickness.

Enhancement of Accommodation-amplitude and PCO Prevention by Dual-optic

To prevent PCO and possibly to augument accommodation-amplitude being attained, we have drafted a dual-optic concept, as Figure 22.11 shows. First, a conventional foldable IOL with sharp edges and the enhanced haptic angulation is implanted into the capsular bag. It has a concave optic with a minus dioptric power, which may imperatively give a greater power to the anterior optic, achieving emmetropia. During accommodation, the anterior capsule moves forward, while the posterior capsule stays relatively unmoved, so that an anterior optic with a greater power may enhance the accommodation-amplitude attained. A large angulation of the haptic will press the sharp optic edge against the posterior capsule to create a strong compression on it for the prevention of PCO. The injected silicone mix will additionally press the IOL onto the posterior capsule. As an alternative technique,

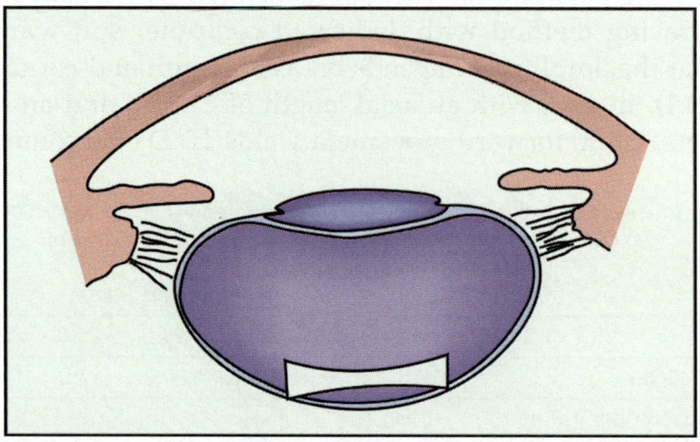

Fig. 22.11: Dual-optic refilling concept I. The concave posterior IOL with a minus power and sharp edges is pressed on the posterior capsule, so that LEC migration might be prevented

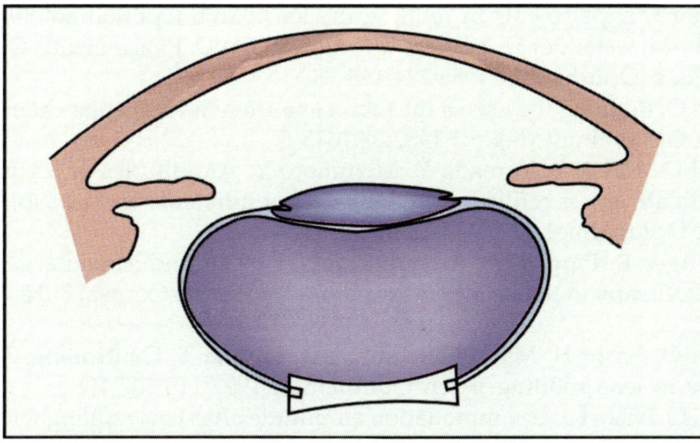

Fig. 22.12: Dual-optic refilling concept II. The concave posterior IOL optic is captured by the posterior CCC. The posterior visual axis is expected to remain PCO-free

the same CCC-capturing IOL can be implanted after a posterior CCC is performed (Fig. 22.12). Then, a CCC-capturing IOL is introduced into the capsular bag which contains the IOL being implanted previously and captured by the anterior CCC, as already described. To refill the bag, silicone mix is injected between two IOLs that are captured by the anterior and posterior CCCs.

SUMMARY

To summarize, the novel anterior capsule-supported IOL is technically quite feasible. Some accommodation might be obtained by forward movement and thickening of the lens. We will test this procedure in primate eyes. Anterior and posterior capsule opacification at least in the optical axis can be avoided. Postoperative emmetropia is supposed to be achieved more easily due to the predetermined optic. One of the advantages is that postoperative *in vivo* power change may be possible using an adjustable IOL.

In conclusion, restoration of accommodation by refilling the lens capsule is a goal of refractive cataract surgery. Technical feasibility has been repeatedly demonstrated by obtaining some useful accommodation in primates and will be further facilitated by modern technology. Capsular opacification is one of the essential problems to be overcome. The technique shown here may provide a breakthrough for possible clinical application to refilling of the lens capsule.

REFERENCES

1. Ludwig K. Physiological premises of current concepts regarding restoration of accommodation. In Guthoff, R; Ludwig, K, (Eds): Current Aspects of Human Accommodation II. Kaden, Heidelberg, 2003;pp39-48.

2. Kessler J. Experiments in refilling the lens. Arch Ophthalmol 1964;71:412-7.
3. Parel J-M, Gelender H, Treffers WF, Norton EWD. Phaco-ersatz. Graefes Arch Clin Exp Ophthalmol 1986;224:165-73.
4. Nishi O. Refilling the lens of the rabbit eye after endocapsular cataract surgery. Folia Ophthalmol (Japan) 1987;38:1615-8.
5. Nishi O, Nakai Y, Yamada Y, Mizumoto Y. Amplitudes of accommodation of primate lenses refilled with two types of inflatable endocapsular balloons. Arch Ophthalmol 1993;111:1677-84.
6. Haefliger E, Parel J-M. Accommodation of an endocapsular silicone lens (PhakoErsatz) in the aging rhesus monkey. J Refract Corneal Surg 1994;10:550-5.
7. Nishi O, Nishi K, Mano C, Ichihara M, Honda T. Controlling the capsular shape in lens refilling. Arch Ophthalmol 1997;115:507-10.
8. Nishi O, Nishi K. Accommodation amplitude after lens refilling with injectable silicone by sealing the capsule with a plug in primates. Arch Ophthalmol 1998;116:1358-61.
9. Nishi O, Sakka Y. Anterior capsule-supported intraocular lens. A new lens for small incision surgery and for sealing the capsular opening. Graefe's Arch Clin Exp Ophthalmol 1990;228:582-8.
10. Billotte C, Berdeaux G. Adverse clinical consequences of neodymium; YAG laser treatment of posterior capsule opacification. J Cataract Refract Surg 2004;30:2064-71.
11. Nawa Y, Ueda T, Nakatsuka M, et al. Accommodation obtained per 1.0 mm forward movement of a posterior chamber intraocular lens. J Cataract Refract Surg 2003;29:2069-72.
12. van der Heijde GL, Beers APA, Dubbelman M. Microfluctuations of steady-state accommodation measured with ultrasonograhy. Ophthalm Physiol Opt 1996;16:216-21.

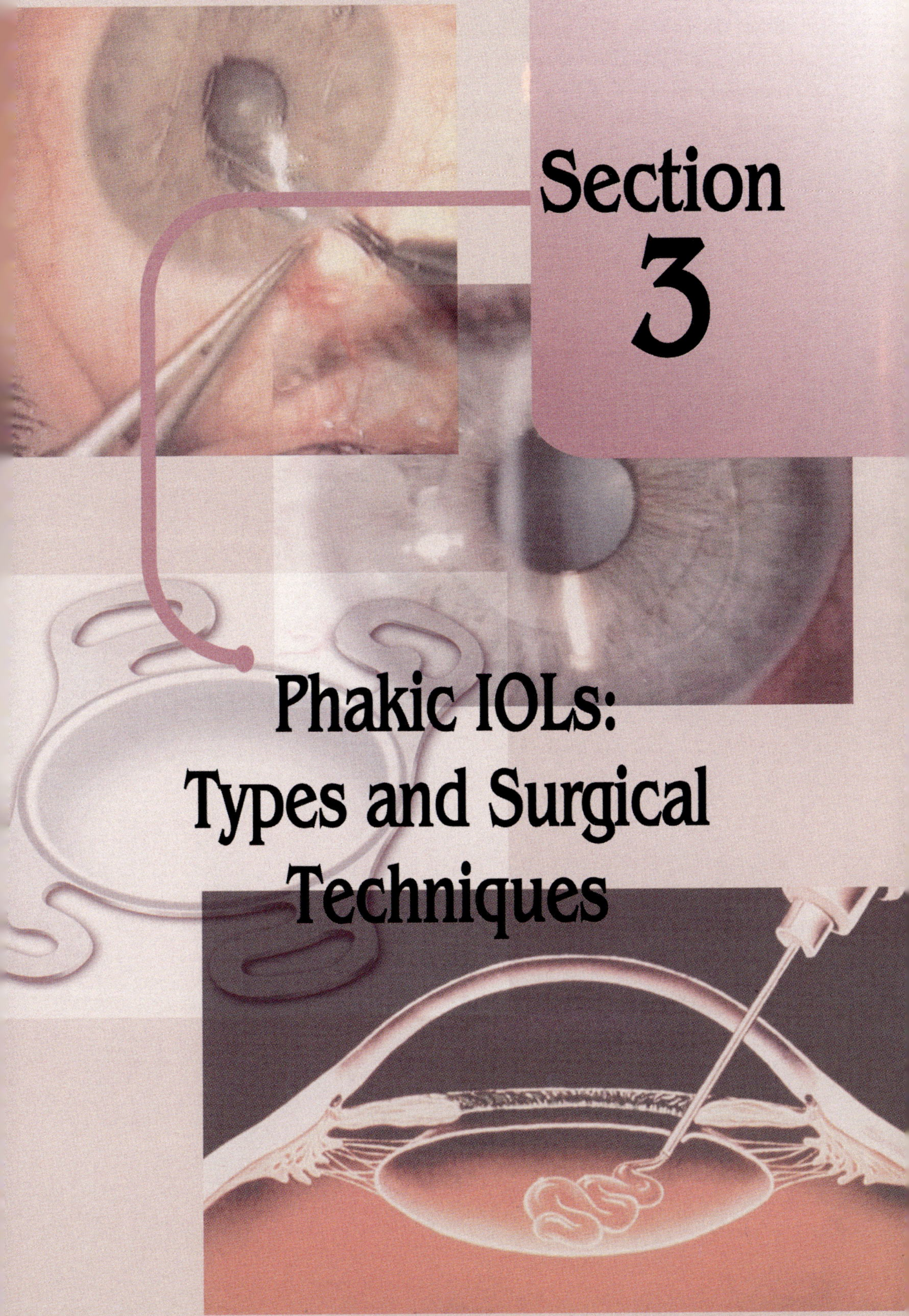

Section 3

Phakic IOLs: Types and Surgical Techniques

CHAPTER

23

Jairo Hoyos-Chacon, Melania Cigales,
Jairo E Hoyos (Spain)

Evaluation of Phakic Lenses

INTRODUCTION

The use of phakic lenses for the correction of high ametropia has recently gained popularity, owing to the poor efficacy of corneal techniques used to treat large refractive errors and the good visual quality achieved with intraocular lenses, along with the benefit of preserving the patient's accommodation ability. Since the middle of the last century, when Strampelli[1] implanted the first phakic intraocular lens, the materials and designs used have undergone extensive development. Phakic lenses may be implanted in the anterior chamber (between the cornea and iris) or the posterior chamber (between the iris and crystalline lens). The evolution of ophthalmologic microsurgery toward the small incision has been a determining factor for the widespread use of flexible phakic lenses, to the detriment of rigid lenses.

ANTERIOR CHAMBER PHAKIC LENSES

These lenses are implanted in the anterior chamber of the eye, that is, in the space between the iris and the cornea. Strampelli[1] implanted the first anterior chamber lens in the middle of the 20th century. In the years to follow, many researchers improved this initial design by evaluating different materials in an effort to increase biocompatibility and thus reduce the incidence of both chronic iridocyclitis and cataract. New models also emerged designed to enlarge the optical zone and smoothen the lens edges to minimize visual disturbances. The angulation of the haptics was gradually modified to increase the distance between the lens and endothelium and try to resolve the problem of corneal decompensation, and different designs were worked on to attempt to avoid secondary glaucoma, which occurred in most implant series.

During this development process, many lenses entered the market only to quickly be discontinued, while others survived due to the constant improvements made in successive generations. Today, we have at our disposition anterior chamber lenses supported by the iridocorneal angle, denoted *angle-supported lenses*, or fixed at the iris, known as *iris-fixated lenses*. Let us briefly review the anterior chamber phakic lenses available at present.

Vivarte/GBR Lens

These two lenses are practically the same, but were initially marketed by two different companies. Ciba Vision© (Duluth, GA, USA) sold the *Vivarte*, while the *GBR* was distributed by IOLtech© (La Rochelle, France), which currently markets both lenses under the same name.

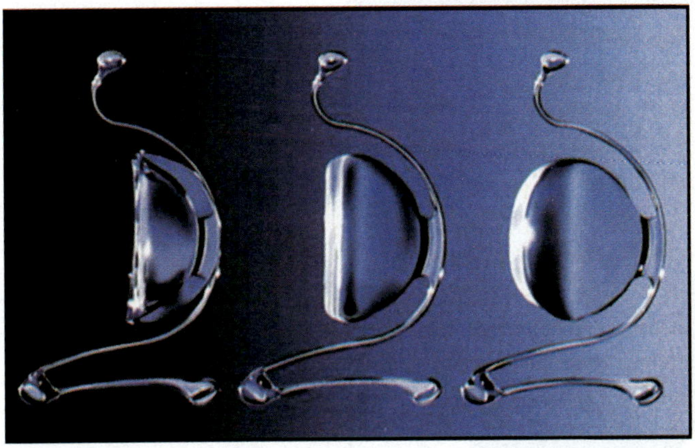

Fig. 23.1: Vivarte/GBR lens (IOLtech© — La Rochelle, France)

Designed by Baikoff, this is a one-piece angle-supported lens that has a foldable hydrophilic acrylic optic and haptics made of a rigid hydrophobic acrylic material (Fig. 23.1). The lens is implanted through a 3.2 mm clear corneal incision. It has soft acrylic angle support bearings, improving contact at the iridocorneal angle, to diminish local fibrosis, which can lead to iris retraction and consequently produce pupillary distortion. The lens has an optical zone of 5.5 mm and is available in three lengths (12.0, 12.5 and 13.0 mm). The manufacturing company recommends a minimum safety distance between the lens and endothelium of 1.55 mm and proposes a minimum anterior chamber depth depending on the lens power (Table 23.1).

Table 23.1: Minimum recommended anterior chamber depth (ACD) for the implantation of a Vivarte/GBR lens according to lens power

Lens power (D)	*ACD (included corneal thickness) (mm)*	*ACD (excluded corneal thickness) (mm)*
–7.0 to –13.0	3.2	2.7
–13.5 to –18.0	3.4	2.9
–18.5 to –22.0	3.6	3.1

There are two current models, one for myopia with powers in the range –7.00 to –22.00 D, and a multifocal lens to correct presbyopia.

The multifocal lens is marketed under two names, *Vivarte Presbyopic* and *Newlife*, but at present both are dependent on the company IOLtech© (La Rochelle, France). The multifocal model (Fig. 23.2) has three optic zones: the central and more peripheral zones for distance vision and the intermediate zone for near vision, and is available in powers of –3.00 to +3.00 D, with an addition for near vision of +2.5 D.

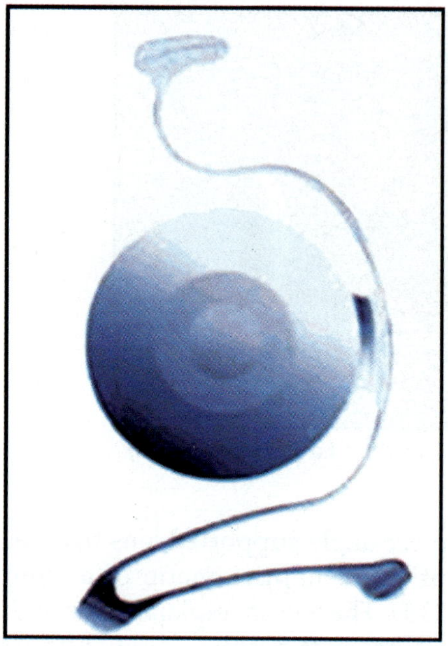

Fig. 23.2: Vivarte Presbyopic lens – Newlife lens (IOLtech© — La Rochelle, France)

Safety Flex Phakic 6 Lens

This lens was developed by several modifications made by Dr Alessio to Baikoff's ZB lens and is marketed by Ophthalmic Innovations International©© (Claremont, CA, USA).

The lens has an optical zone of 6.0 mm, a very flexible haptics that rest on the angle and it is supplied in lengths of 12.0 to 14.0 mm (Fig. 23.3). The distance of the lens to the anterior crystalline lens capsule has to be 1 mm, such that the manufacturers recommend a minimum anterior chamber depth of 3.2 mm. The powers available to correct myopia range from –2.00 to –25.00 D and to treat hyperopia from +2.00 to +10.00 D.

The lens surface is treated with heparin, which being an endogenous carbohydrate is not recognized by the immune system as foreign yet impairs bacterial adhesion to the lens surface, thus reducing the risk of endophthalmitis.

JMJ Lens

This lens was designed by J García-Sánchez, MT Iradier and J García-Feijoo, and is produced by the company AJL© (Vitoria, Spain).

The JMJ is a polymethylmethacrylate (PMMA) angle-supported lens for the correction of myopia that has a plano-concave optic and haptics in the shape of a Z with a curved step (Fig. 23.4). It has an overall optical

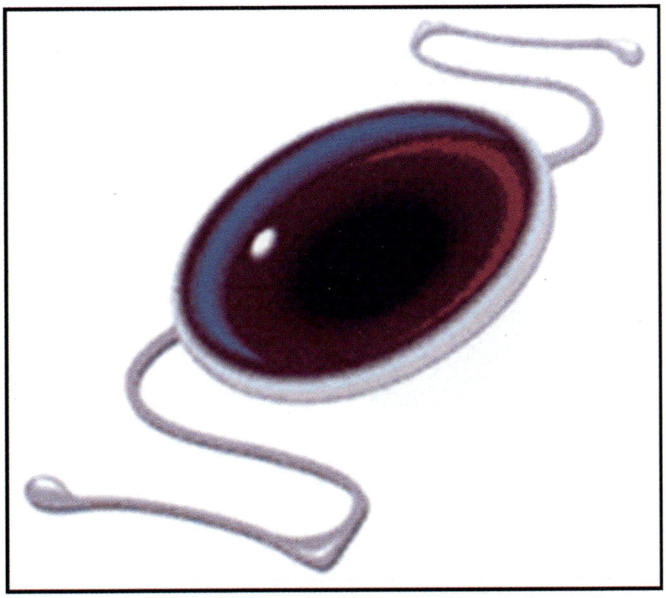

Fig. 23.3: Safety flex phakic 6 lens (Ophthalmic Innovations International© — Claremont, CA, USA)

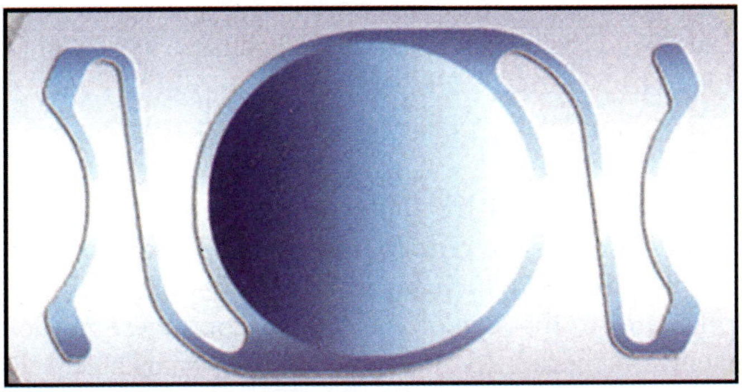

Fig. 23.4: JMJ lens (AJL© — Vitoria, Spain)

zone of 6.0 mm and effective zone of 5.5 mm, and can be obtained in 4 different lengths (12.0, 12.5, 13.0 and 13.5 mm). To calculate lens power a constant "A" of 115.5 is used and it is available in powers between –5.00 and –25.00 D in increments of 1.0 D.

LN-2000 Lens

This one-piece angle-supported lens was designed to correct myopia and is manufactured by Lenstec© (St. Petersburg, Fl, USA). The angulation of its haptics is 0° and its optic is meniscus-shaped with a diameter of 5.0 mm (Fig. 23.5). It is available in powers of –7.00 to

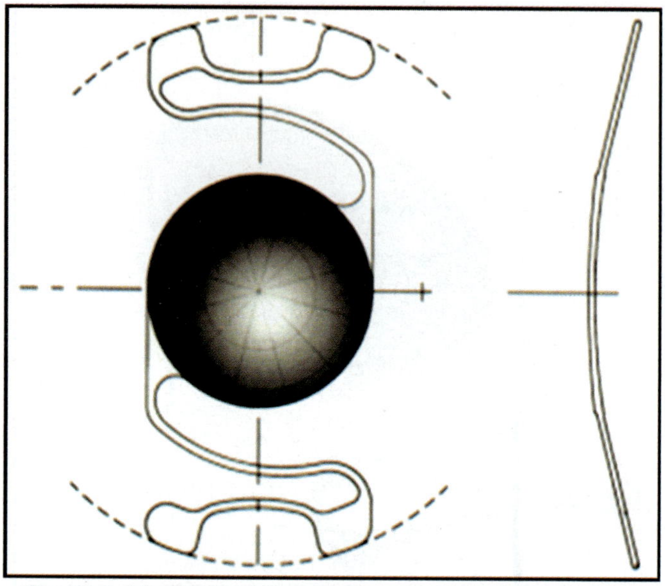

Fig. 23.5: LN-2000 lens (Lenstec© — St. Petersburg, Fl, USA)

–20.00 D and there are 4 different models depending on the length of the lens: LN-2010 (12.0 mm), LN-2020 (12.5 mm), LN-2030 (13.0 mm) and LN-2040 (13.5 mm).

ZSAL-4 Lens

This lens was developed by JJ Pérez-Santonja and JL Ali© from Kelman's multiflex anterior chamber implant. Its development started in the mid 1990s, during which several modifications to the angulation of the haptics and to the size of the optical zone were made until the fourth generation model *ZSAL-4* was created, marketed by Morcher GMBH© (Stuttgart, Germany).

This lens is a one-piece PMMA angle-supported implant with a plano-concave optic and haptics angulation of 19º (Fig. 23.6). Its Z-shaped haptics are 0.18 mm thick and very flexible, promoting the dispersion of compression forces on the angular structures as an attempt to reduce the incidence of pupillary distortion. The size of the optical zone is 5.5 mm total and effective 5.0 mm, and has a triple-surface edge to minimize glare.[2] The mean distance from the endothelium achieved is 1.54 mm. It comes in 2 diameters (12.5 and 13.0 mm) and powers in the range –6.00 to –22.50 D in steps of 0.50 D.

From the development of this lens emerged the *ZSAL-4/Plus* (Fig. 23.7), marketed by the same company. In this model, the optical

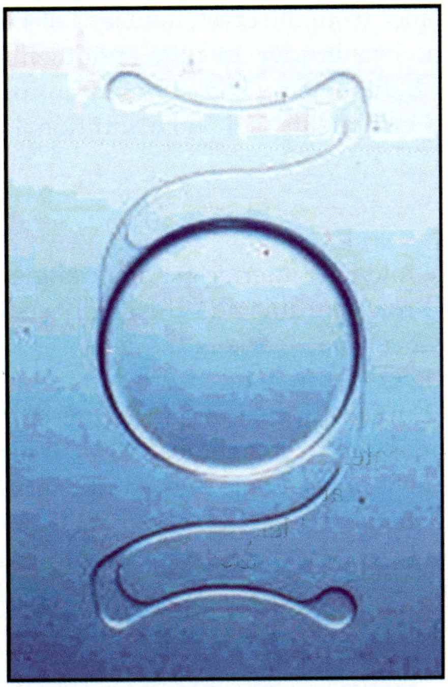

Fig. 23.6: ZSAL-4 lens (Morcher GMBH© — Stuttgart, Germany)

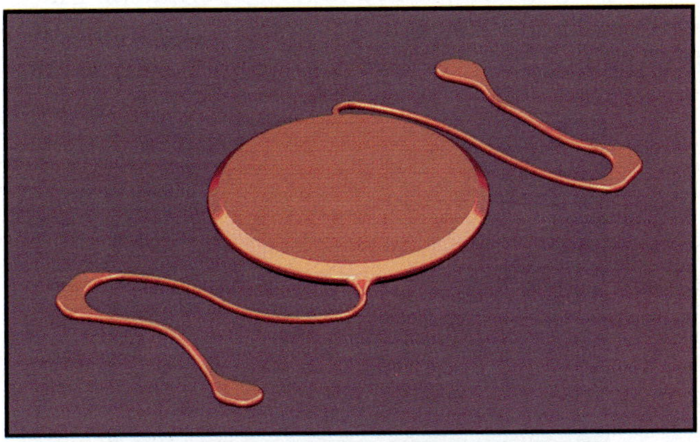

Fig. 23.7: ZSAL-4/plus lens (Morcher GMBH© — Stuttgart, Germany)

zone is larger (overall optic zone size 5.8 mm, effective 5.3 mm) in an attempt to reduce halos and night vision problems. In the periphery, the transition zone still has 3 surfaces to reduce halos and reflections. Its haptics are thin and long in the shape of a Z to enhance flexibility and their geometry is such that they reduce compression of the angle structures and therefore diminish the risk of pupillary ovalization[8]. Its total height is 1.2 mm, which avoids possible contact with the iris and allows a central distance from the crystalline lens of 1.0 mm. The mean distance between the lens border and the endothelium is 1.5 mm. It is manufactured in 2 diameters (12.5 and 13.0 mm), and powers of –6.00 to –22.50 D (in increments of 0.50 D; additional dioptric powers can be ordered).

ICARE Lens

This is the first fully foldable anterior chamber angle-supported lens. It was designed by Prof. Sourdille and the engineers of the company Corneal© (Paris, France) that markets the lens.

It is a one-piece lens that may be inserted through a clear corneal incision of 3.0 to 3.2 mm with the help of an injector. Comprised of hydrophilic acrylic material (water content 26%), it has 4 symmetrical footplates for placement at the angle and an optical zone of 5.75 mm (Fig. 23.8). It is available in 4 lengths from 12.0 to 13.5 mm in 0.5 mm increases. The mean distance from the optic center to the endothelium is 2.07 mm, from the lens border to the endothelium is 1.85 mm and from the posterior lens surface to the crystalline lens is 0.84 mm. It is supplied in powers from –5.00 to –20.00 D in –0.25 D increments. A new model for the correction of hyperopia is soon to be launched.

For this type of anterior chamber lens, unlike the case for the previous lenses, it is recommended that two peripheral iridotomies be conducted at 10:00 and 2:00 hours (personal communication by Dr. Alessandro Mularoni).

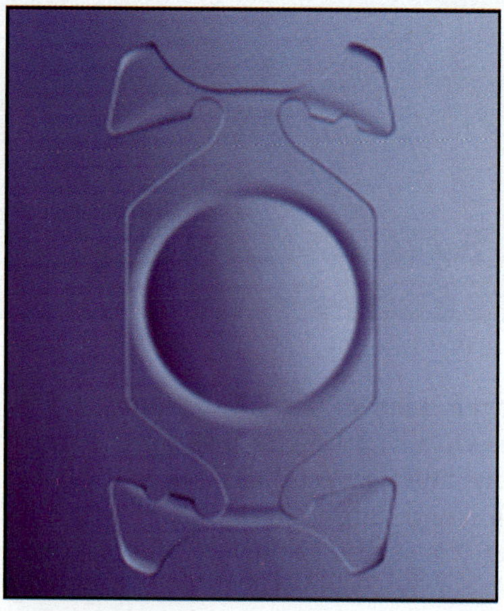

Fig. 23.8: ICARE lens (Corneal© — Paris, France)

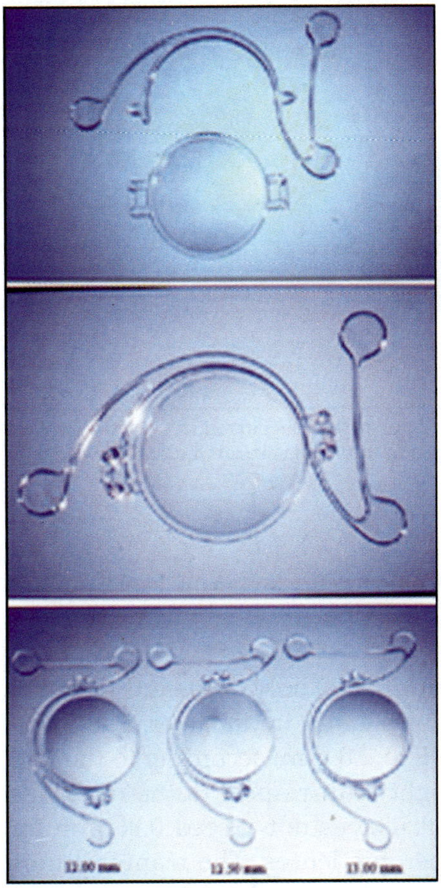

Fig. 23.9: Kelman Duet implant lens (Tekia© — Irvine, CA, USA)

Kelman Duet Lens

This lens, designed by CD Kelman and marketed by Tekia© (Irvine, CA, USA), is an anterior chamber, angle-supported two-piece model, whose two sections are separately introduced and fitted together once inside the anterior chamber (Fig. 23.9).

The Kelman Duet lens has a foldable silicon 5.5 mm optic and rigid PMMA haptics. It is available in lengths of 12.0, 12.5, 13.0 and 13.5 mm. For their implant, first, the haptics are inserted through an incision under 2.0 mm and, once rested on the angle, the lens optic is injected and connected to the haptics inside the anterior chamber (Fig. 23.10). The lens is presently available for the correction of myopia in powers of –8.00 to –20.00 D. In the future, the company intends to produce toric lenses, low power lenses for myopia and lenses for hyperopia.

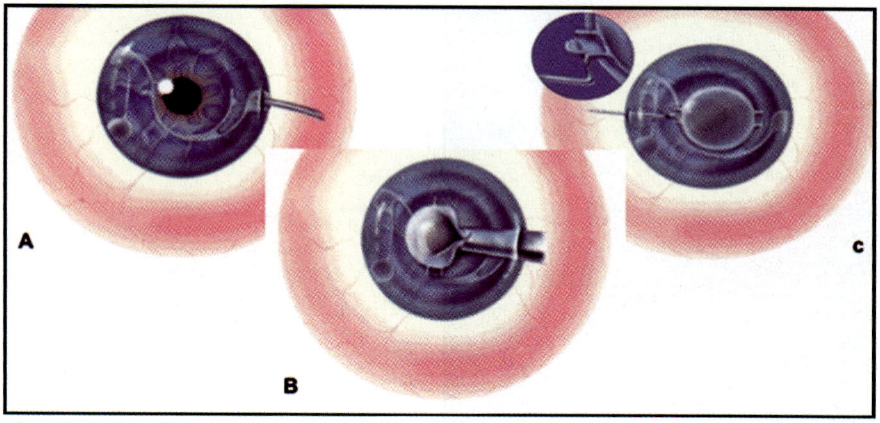

Fig. 23.10: Insertion technique for the Kelman Duet implant: (A) Introduction of the haptics. (B) Introduction of the optic. (C) Joining the optic to the haptics inside the anterior chamber

Artisan Lens

The *Artisan* lens is marketed by Ophtec© (Boca Raton, Fl, USA) but is also sold under the name of *Verysise*™ by Advanced Medical Optics, Incs (Santa Ana, Ca, USA).

It is a one-piece PMMA design supplied in only one length, 8.5 mm. Its concave-convex optic can be 5.0 or 6.0 mm in diameter. The optic-endothelium distance varies from 1.5 to 2.0 mm, according to the lens dioptric power. Maximum lens height with respect to the iris plane differs depending on its power, but it does not exceed 0.96 mm for myopic lenses and 1.0 mm for hyperopic lenses. The manufacturers recommend a minimum anterior chamber depth of 2.6 mm for its implantation. The lens design allows 4 outflow points for aqueous humor to pass from the posterior to the anterior chamber (Fig. 23.11), but it is still recommended that a surgical iridectomy or Yag laser iridotomy be undertaken.

The lens is introduced through a scleral-corneal tunnel 5.0 to 6.0 mm long. The haptics are secured at the mid-periphery of the iris, which is the avascular zone and also the "mute" zone of the pupil's dilatory muscle, such that pupillary excursions are not impeded [3]; they can be fixed across a horizontal, vertical or oblique axis. The lens powers available for the correction of myopia span from –5.00 to –20.00 D, and for hyperopia from +3.00 to +13.00 D, with the option of correcting astigmatism with toric lenses.

The latest generation of the Artisan family is *Artiflex*, a foldable lens that can be implanted through a 3.2 mm clear corneal incision. Its optic is made of silicon (soft and foldable) and PMMA haptics are rigid allowing them to extend their securing function to the iris stroma

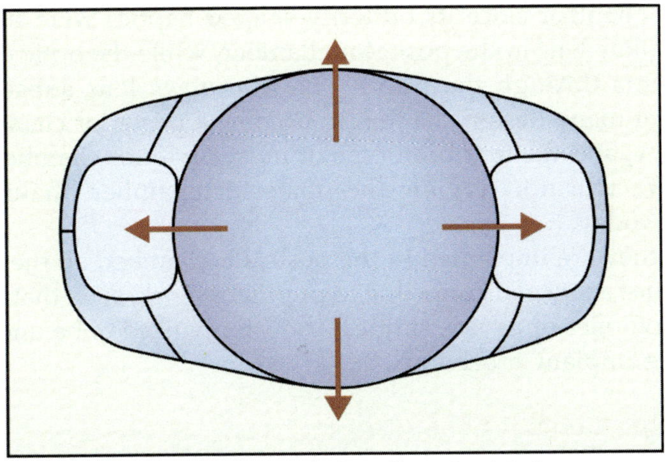

Fig. 23.11: The Artisan lens design allows 4 points for aqueous humor to pass from the posterior to the anterior chamber

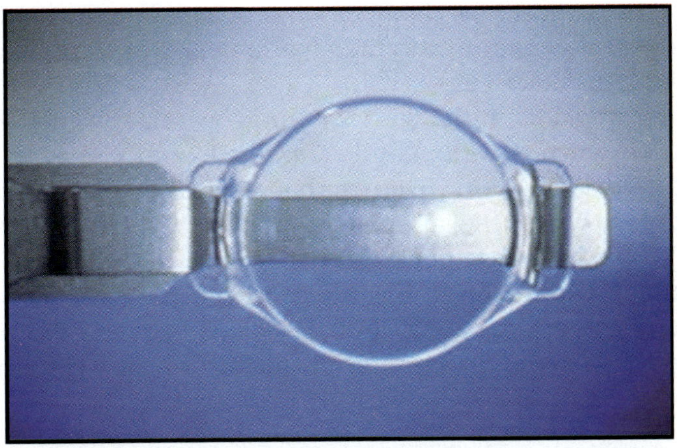

Fig. 23.12: Artiflex lens (Ophtec© — Boca Raton, Fl, USA) (Advanced Medical Optics, Incs — Santa Ana, Ca, USA)

(Fig. 23.12). This lens arose from the merging of the technologies of Ophtec© (Boca Raton, Fl, USA) and Advanced Medical Optics, Incs (Santa Ana, Ca, USA), since the silicon used for the optic was patented by Advanced Medical Optics, Incs. Its launching on the international market is forecast for the middle of 2005 after clinical trials.

POSTERIOR CHAMBER LENSES

These lenses are implanted in the posterior chamber of the eye, that is, between the iris and the crystalline lens. The first phakic posterior chamber lens was the *Mushroom* lens designed by Fyodorov and Zuev[4] in 1985. However, in practice this lens was not only implanted in the posterior chamber since its butterfly-shaped haptics were placed on the crystalline lens in the posterior chamber, while the optic extended beyond this through the pupil. The *Mushroom* lens subsequently underwent many design changes to become a posterior chamber lens exclusively, and the first prototype of most posterior chamber phakic lenses. We will now review the posterior chamber phakic lenses available today.

Since they are implanted in the posterior chamber, all these lenses can produce acute glaucoma due to pupillary block, such that two Yag laser iridotomies or a wide surgical iridectomy need to be undertaken before the implant procedure.

Implantable Contact Lens (ICL)

It was in 1993, when the company Staar© (Monrovia, CA, USA) acquired the marketing rights to one of the lenses developed by Fyodorov, that a posterior chamber lens appeared on the market. This lens made of a collagen polymer (collamer) was given the name "Implantable Contact Lens" (ICL).

The first implants in the western world were performed by Paolo Pesando, Vincenzo Assetto, Guido Caramello and Christian Skorpik using the model IC2020-M[5]. This lens had a biconcave 3.5 mm diameter optic and gave rise to the subsequent models: ICM(H)V1, ICM(H)V2, ICM(H)V3 and the last generation ICM(H)V4 (Fig. 23.13). In its development, the intention has always been to try to increase the diameter of the optical zone, and the space between the posterior surface of the lens and the anterior surface of the crystalline lens

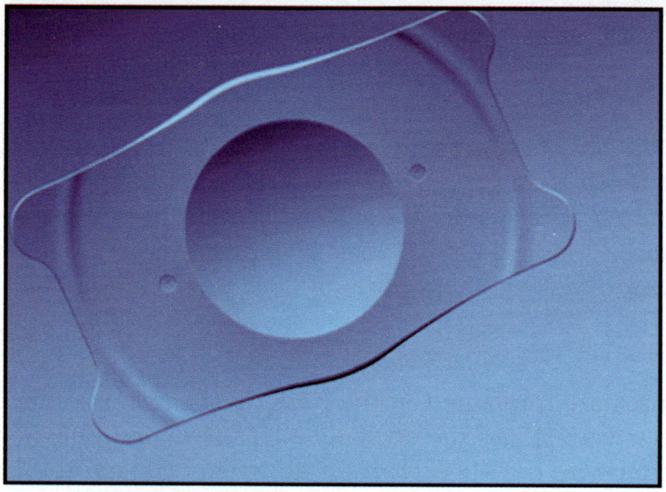

Fig. 23.13: Implantable contact lens (ICL) (Staar© — Monrovia, CA, USA)

(the vault). This new design was prompted by reports of the development of cataract[6,7] in eyes with a small vault, provoked by the inherent hydrophilic nature of the lens material.

The collagen polymer from which the lens is manufactured (63% polyhydroxymethylethylacrylate, 34% water, 0.2% porcine collagen, 3.4% benzophenone) confers the lens 37.5% hydrophilia and good permeability to gases and nutrients. It allows 99% light transmission and has a refraction index of 1.452.

The ICL is implanted in the posterior chamber and has 4 small plateforms at the end of the haptics so that it can rest on the sulcus. The posterior lens surface is concave and adopts the shape of a dome over the anterior crystalline capsule to create a space for the free movement of aqueous humor. This avoids contact with the crystalline lens inducing cataract formation.

The 5 lengths available: 11.5, 12.0, 12.5, 13.0 and 13.5 mm, mean the lens can be adapted to the different white-to-white measures (approximately the sulcus-to-sulcus distance). The optical zone varies from 4.5 to 5.5 mm depending on the lens power. The thickness of the optic is 100 to 600 microns and the thickness of the haptics is 60 to 80 microns. It has the advantage that it can be implanted using an injector through a self-sealing 3 mm corneal incision. The lens powers available for myopia run from –3.00 to –23.00 D and for hyperopia from +3.00 to +22.00 D (in 0.50 D increases).

There is currently also a toric lens, *Toric ICL,* that allows us to correct astigmatism associated with the spherical myopic defect. The lens has marks to help align the lens as it is implanted on the sulcus (Fig. 23.14). It can be purchased in the same length as the lens for spherical correction and is available for a myopia of –6.0 to –23.0 diopters with +1.0 to +6.0 diopters of cylinder in 0.5 diopter increments.

Phakic Refractive Lens (PRL)

Developed by the company Medenium Inc© (Irvine, CA, USA) since 1987 from one of Fyodorov's designs[8], the PRL was internationally launched by CIBA Vision© (Duluth, GA, USA), which then sold the patent to IOLtech© (La Rochelle, France), its current marketing company.

This is a one-piece lens made purely of silicon, a soft, elastic, hydrophobic material. Its refraction index is 1.46. The lens was designed to float in the posterior chamber but studies performed with the UBM indicate the lens is generally placed on the sulcus, zonula or ciliary body.[9] For the implant of the PRL, an anterior chamber depth equal to or greater than 3.0 mm is recommended (excluding corneal

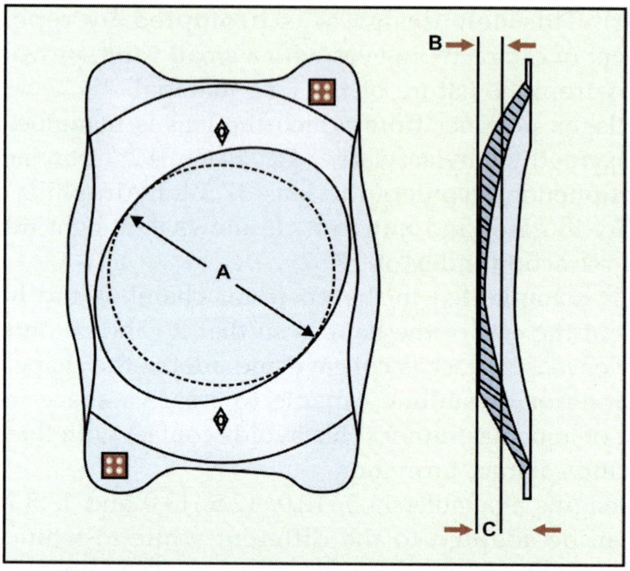

Fig. 23.14: Toric ICL (Staar© — Monrovia, CA, USA)

thickness), as well as two Yag laser iridotomies or a surgical iridectomy before lens implant.[10]

There are three different models available (Fig. 23.15): one to correct hyperopia (model PRL-200) and two for the treatment of myopia (models PRL-100 and PRL-101). Model PRL-200 is 10.6 mm long,

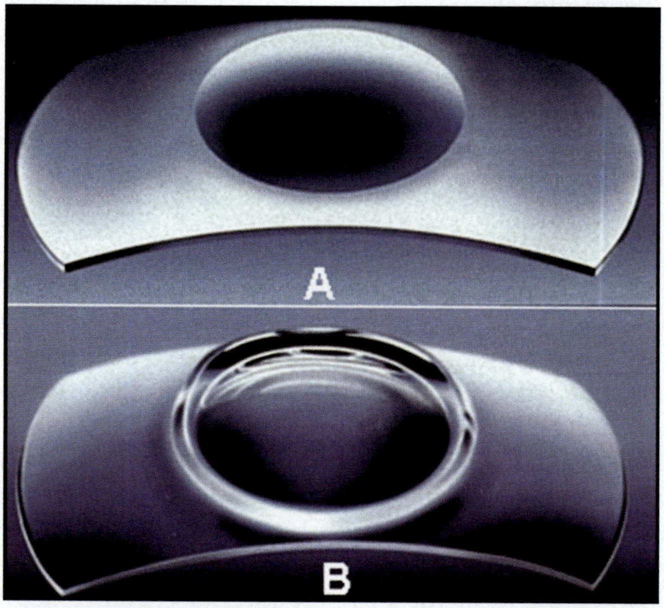

Fig. 23.15: Phakic refractive lens (PRL) (IOLtech© — La Rochelle, France). (A) PRL 200 for hyperopia. (B) PRL 100 for myopia

6.0 mm wide, has an optical zone of 4.5 mm and comes in powers of +3.00 to +15.00 D in 0.50 D increments, allowing a maximum correction of +11.00 D of hyperopia. The properties of the PRL-100 and PRL-101 models respectively for myopia are: length 10.8 mm and 11.3 mm, optical zone 4.5 to 5.0 mm for both depending on lens power, width 6.0 mm for both, dioptric power –3.00 to –20.00 D in 1.00 D (PRL-100) and 0.50 D (PRL-101) increments and maximum correction for both of –23.00 diopters of myopia. The main difference between the two models is the length of the lens and the choice of model is based on the white-to-white distance of the eye[9]. The manufacturers suggest the measurements provided in Table 23.2 to select the most suitable model.

Table 23.2: Selecting the best PRL model for myopia according to the white-to-white (W-W) distance

W-W distance	Model
W-W < 10.5 mm	No PRL
W-W from 10.5 to 11.3 mm	PRL-100
W-W > 11.3 mm	PRL-101

Although some injector models have been used to implant this lens, at present the company recommends their placement using forceps through a self-sealing corneal incision 3.5 to 4.0 mm long.

Precrystalline Lens

In 1995, Joaquín Barraquer in collaboration with Corneal WK© (Paris, France) developed a rigid posterior chamber lens fixed on the sulcus, which is now in its third generation.

The lens is composed of PMMA and has a rigid 6.0 mm optical zone with flexible haptics that rest on the sulcus. Its anterior surface is slightly convex and the posterior side is concave. Its overall diameter is 14.0 mm, with a lens body 9.0 mm long and 6.0 mm wide, and two plateforms in the optic that rest above the anterior crystalline lens capsule, which help the excursion of the iris and avoid pupillary capture of the lens. The body of the second generation lens is 8.0 mm long and pupillary capture has been observed during spontaneous pupil dilation.[11] Attempts to avoid this complication by lengthening the platforms by 0.5 mm to give a final length of 9 mm have led to the third generation lens (Fig. 23.16).

The main complication of the first generation of this lens was the adhesion of the lens to the crystalline through a vacuum effect. This gave rise to myopization as the anterior crystalline surface bellowed and to an increased incidence of cataract, since the space between the lens and the anterior surface of the crystalline lens was lost.[9] This problem was resolved in the second generation by creating drainage

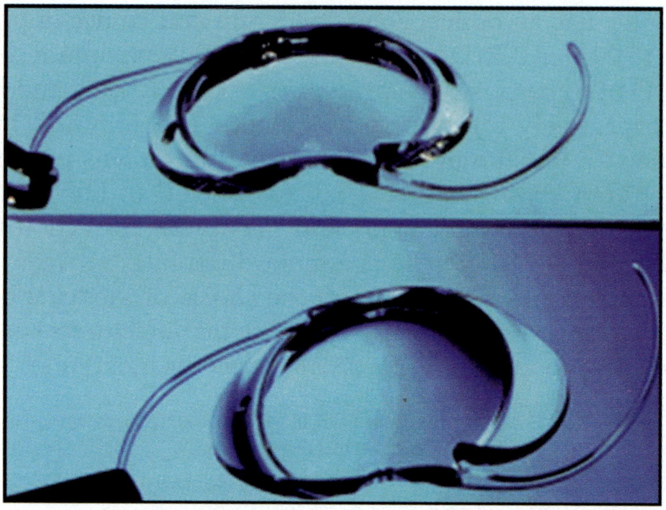

Fig. 23.16: Second and third generation models of the precrystalline lens (Corneal WK© — Paris, France)

ducts on the posterior lens surface such that the aqueous humor could freely circulate between the lens and the anterior surface of the crystalline lens.

Since this lens is rigid, its implant in the posterior chamber requires a wide incision. Two iridotomies using the Yag laser are recommended prior to surgery to avoid pupillary block and secondary glaucoma due to angular closure. This lens allows the correction of severe myopia from –10.00 to –30.00 D.

REFERENCES

1. Strampelli B. Lentilles camerulaires après années d'expériences. Acta Cong Ophthal Belgica (Brussels) 1958; 11:1692-8.
2. Rodríguez A, Cardoner A. Lente intraocular fáquica ZSAL-4 para la correcci©n de la alta miopía. In Menezo JL, Guell JL, (Eds): Correcci©n quirúrgica de la alta miopía. Barcelona: Espaxs 2001; pp 296-303.
3. Menezo JL, et al. Lente de sujeci©n iridiana tipo Artisán. In: Menezo JL, Guell JL, (Eds): Correcci©n quirúrgica de la alta miopía. Barcelona: Espaxs 2001; 19:305-23.
4. Fyodorov SN, Zuev VK, Azanabayev BM. Intraocular correction of high myopia with negative posterior chamber lens. Ophthalmosurgery 1991; 3: 57-8.
5. Merlin F, Caramello G. Lenti intraoculari per la correzione della miopia in occhi fachici: premessa e cenni storici. In Merlin F, Caramello G (Eds): Chirurgia refrattiva. Principi e tecniche. Italia: Fabiano Editore, 2000; pp 491-5.
6. Trindade F, Pereira F. Cataract formation after posterior chamber phakic intraocular lens implantation. J Cataract Refract Surg 1998; 24:1661-3.

7. Fink AM, Gore C, Rosen E. Cataract development after implantation of the Staar Collamer posterior chamber phakic lens. J Cataract Refract Surg 1999; 25:278-82.
8. Dementiev D, Hoffer KJ, Sborgia G, et al. Phakic Refractive Lens for correction of myopia and hyperopia. In Agarwal S, Agarwal A, Pallikaris IG, Neuhann TH, Knorz MC, Agarwal A, (Eds): Refractive Surgery, New Delhi: Jaypee Brothers, 2000; 440-61.
9. Hoyos J, Cigales M, Castanera F, et al. Ultrasound biomicroscopy evaluation of the PRL. New technologies in phakic refractive lenses. Ocular Surgery News. Europe/Asia-Pacific Edition. Marzo 2002; 11-3.
10. Hoyos JE, Dementiev DD, Cigales M, et al. Phakic refractive lens experience in Spain. J Cataract Refract Surg 2002; 28:1939-46.
11. Barraquer J, Ux© M. Correcci©n quirúrgica de la alta miopía. Indicaciones, técnica, complicaciones y resultados. Arch Soc Canar Oftal 2000; 11:109-15.

CHAPTER

24

Carlo Francesco Lovisolo (Italy)

Custom ICLs

INTRODUCTION

Since the celestial engineer provided the eye with two lenses, the surgical solutions to correct refractive errors may exploit two anatomical objectives (by modifying the optical behavior of the cornea or the crystalline lens) or a prosthetic one (by inserting a supplementary lens inside the eye). The lifelong stable, elliptical architecture of the cornea has been designed to deliver very high vergence (more than 70% of the total focusing power of the eye), while minimizing optical aberrations. Even with highly sophisticated optimized and/or customized laser treatments, corneal procedures are subject to physical limitations and challenging complications, mostly related to the issues of wound healing and biomechanics.[1] The optical quality of the outcomes may therefore be less than ideal when treating high ammetropias (myopia higher than 6-7 diopters, hyperopia higher than 3 diopters) and patients with large mesopic pupil sizes.[2,3] Newcomer keratoplasty techniques, using tissue engineered or synthetic lenticules as refractive onlay[4] or intrastromal inlay[5] have, so far, only shown the potential to overcome these drawbacks.

The crystalline lens gives one fourth of the power and is responsible of the autofocus mechanism of the eye's optical system. It grows and becomes sclerotic throughout life, causing changes of refraction and progressive loss of the accommodating power.[6,7] The benefits of its irreversible extraction (CLE)[8,9] and substitution with an artificial toric, aspheric, multifocal or accommodating implant is still controversial among eye-care providers. Accommodating IOLs have so far clinically failed to solve the main complication of lens removal, presbyopia. Multifocal optics inherently decrease contrast sensitivity and require neuroadaption. Beyond the unpleasant loss of accommodation in young people, long-term safety is a major concern for CLE, risk of influencing retinal detachment and macular pathology in eyes naturally prone to posterior segment pathology (i.e. high myopia).[8-11]

Instead, a supplementary intraocular lens (phakic IOL) implanted between the cornea and the lens has several theoretical advantages.[12] It allows the crystalline lens to retain its function without risking vitreoretinal side effects; since the quality of the implant surfaces is above the optical limits of the eye, its nodal points are nearer the pupil and the optic can be conveniently wide, may improve the natural properties of the eye's optical system to enhance the quality of the retinal image, allowing excellent vision even in all light conditions.[13-16] It is removable and exchangeable, permitting potential reversibility to the preoperative condition.[17,18] The result is highly predictable,[19-25] easily adjustable with complementary fine-tuning corneal surgeries[26-28] and immediately stable, because the refractive outcome depends less on healing processes. The major drawbacks of a phakic IOL surgery are essentially related to the intraoperative and early postoperative risks of an open-eye procedure and to the long term tolerability of the lens implant. There is enough evidence that the dangers of an intraocular procedure may be properly managed and minimized with proper care and proctoring of an accomplished surgical team and environment.[29]

THE CONCEPT OF CUSTOM PHAKIC IOL

There is no doubt that the same concepts behind the universal trend toward customization of corneal refractive surgery[50] must be immediately applied to phakic IOL procedures. Considering the wide variability of biological presentations, the variety of anatomical shapes and sizes and range of optical errors, the need for a custom-made lens implant would appear even more obvious than personalized corneal laser treatment.[30] Custom-designed lenses that perfectly fit the individual anatomy of each single eye are obviously safer than conventionally-sized ones, as late postoperative complications relate mainly to unstable implants and less than ideal distances from the internal structures.[30] Once inside the eye and over time, without a perfect fit, each site of haptic fixation has its own area of unique concern[30] and accurate preoperative assessment of the lens implant-to-tissue clearances becomes vital to avoid safety concerns.

Angle-fixated and iris-supported IOLs may induce acute and recurrent subchronic iritis, ischemic subatrophy of the iris, pupil distortion, progressive endothelial cell loss, secondary glaucoma, and breakage of the blood/aqueous barrier with persistent aqueous flare and cystoid macular edema.[31-39] When too long, posterior chamber phakic, like the Visian ICL™ (Staar, Monrovia, CA, USA), excessively vaulted between the iris' posterior pigmented layers and the anterior crystalline lens, may cause the iris diaphragm to bulge forward, with narrowing of the iridocorneal angle, chafing of the posterior iris surface, pigment dispersion and subsequent risk of angle closure and pigmentary glaucoma, ocular pain or tenderness due to nerve irritation by excessive pressure in the ciliary sulcus, cyclitis and macular edema[40-47] (Fig. 24.1). On the other hand, lack of vaulting because of short has caused iatrogenic anterior subcapsular cataract by preventing the nutritional turnover on the lens surface (Fig. 24.2) and implant decentration.[48,49] We should be aware that the vast majority of these iatrogenic damages to the delicate inner structures depend on human errors: the wrong selection of an unwelcome intraocular environment or the wrong choice of the overall length of the implant.[29]

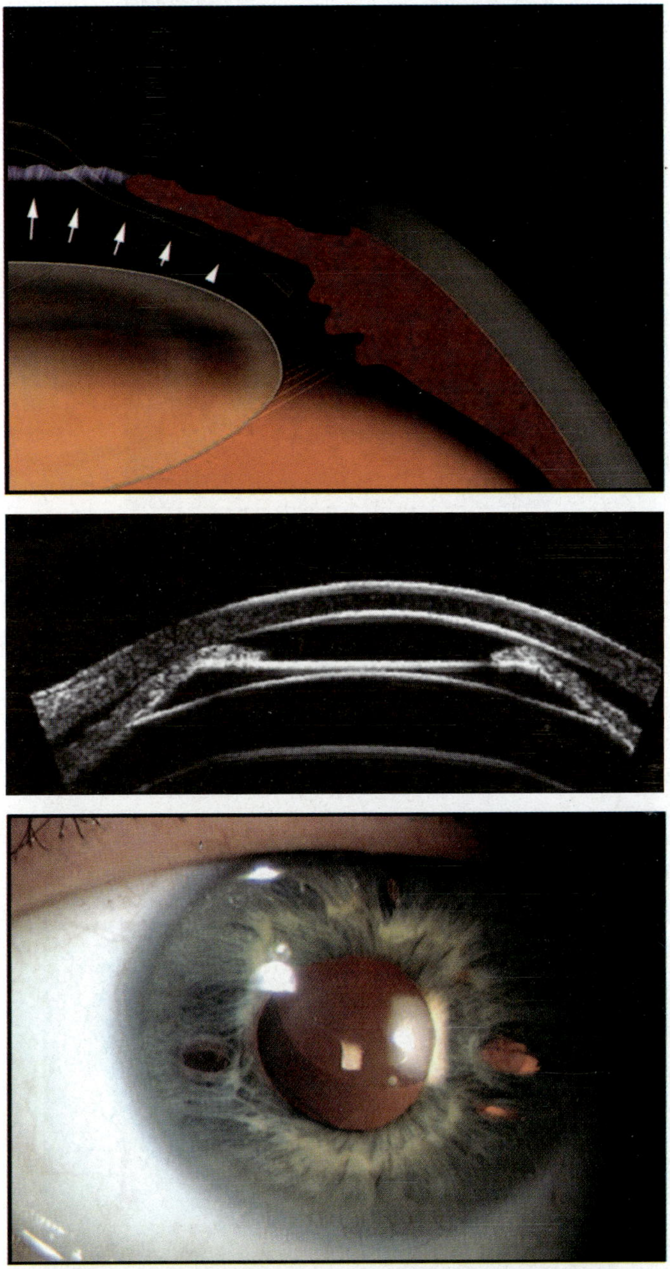

Fig. 24.1: Oversized ICLs may lead to angle closure glaucoma: (A) Artist's view of the bulging of the iris diaphragm induced by the lens implant; (B) VHF echography image of an ICL-induced papillary block; (C) Urgent lens explantation or multiple iridotomies are required

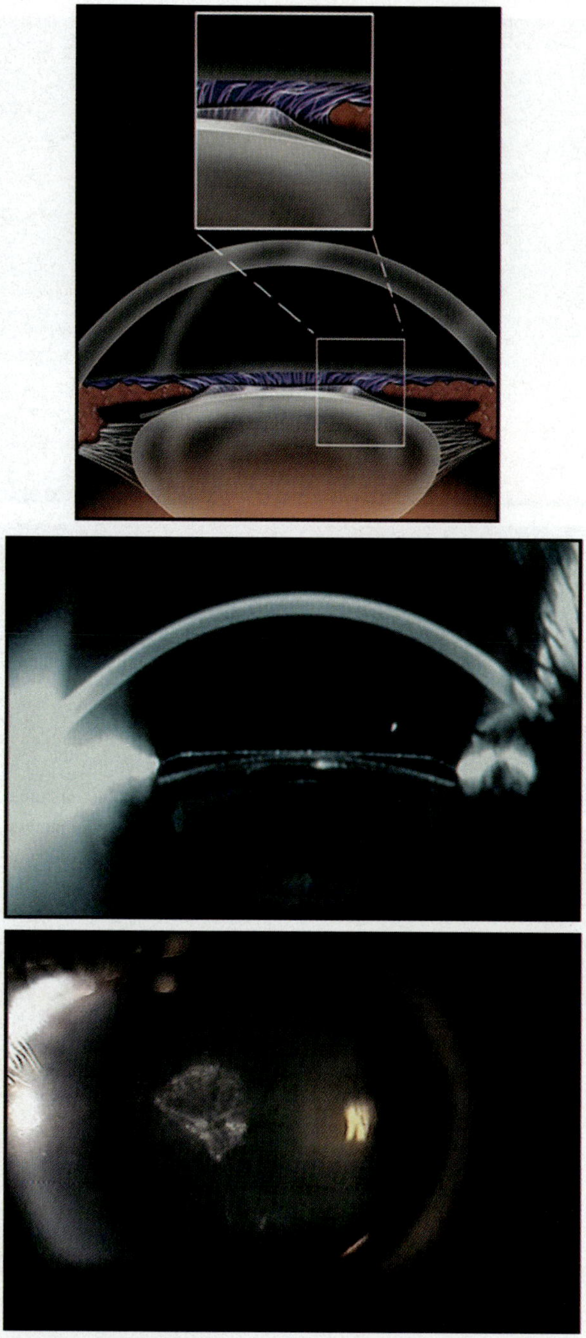

Fig. 24.2: (A) Artist's view; (B) Scheimpflug camera and (C) Slit lamp images of typical iatrogenic anterior subcapsular opacities of the crystalline lens caused by the lack of vaulting of an undersized ICL

CUSTOM SIZING THE OVERALL LENGTH

Since the prophetic words of Benedetto Strampelli[59] of the early 1950s (*"...the choice of the implant overall length appears particularly critical.... Unfortunately, proper measurements of the inner diameters are not achievable by any means...'* at the Società Oftalmologica Lombarda, December 1953) proper sizing has been considered for decades the 'mission impossible' to optimize safety of phakic IOL surgery. Anachronistically, after more than half a century and despite the lack of scientific proof behind it, the vast majority of surgeons worldwide still behave like him, selecting the overall diameter of the ICL according to the 'golden rule of thumb', by empirically adding 0.5 to 1.0 mm to the horizontal corneal diameter (white-to-white distance, *W-to-W*) obtained externally. Whether measured at the slit lamp by comparison with a ruler or gauge, or under the operating microscope using the surgical caliper, white-to-white is an unreliable landmark, as the points where white begins and gray starts at the limbus are open to each surgeon's personal interpretation. More standardized strategies, based on the analysis of digital photographs from videokeratography or laser partial coherence interferometry images have slightly improved the precision achieving acceptable reproducibility tolerances. Nevertheless, numerous findings from *in vivo* ultrasound[60] and MRI[61] studies, anatomic observations on cadaver eyes[62] have definitely showed that, regardless of the accuracy of the measurement of *W-to-W*, there is no proportional anatomical correspondence between external measurements and internal dimensions of the anterior segment compartment.[12,30,60] Internal anatomy cannot be predicted by external measurements. As a consequence, *W-to-W* distance alone is totally adequate for sizing ICL[63] (Fig. 24.3). Instead, the exact internal linear sulcus-to-sulcus *(S-to-S)* distance, the iris-to-crystalline lens relationship (distance between the iris and the ciliary processes, width of the irido-corneal angle and of the iris-crystalline angle) measured point-by-point at different levels, should be used. Accurate imaging of these hidden anatomical sites can be obtained with high-resolution ultrasound devices that use very high frequency (VHF) waves in the 35-to-50 MHz range, like the Artemis 2 (Ultralink, St. Petersburg, FL, USA)[64] and the Vu-Max (Sonomed, New York, NY, USA). Optical devices like slit scanning systems with or without rotating Scheimpflug camera (like the Precisio, Ligi, Taranto, Italy, the Pentacam, Oculus, Germany and the Galilei, Ziemer, Germany) (Fig. 24.4), or infrared light optical coherence tomography systems (OCT Visante®, Zeiss-Meditec, Jena, Germany) permit high-resolution cross-sectional anterior segment imaging with excellent reproducibility of measurements by using the interference profile of

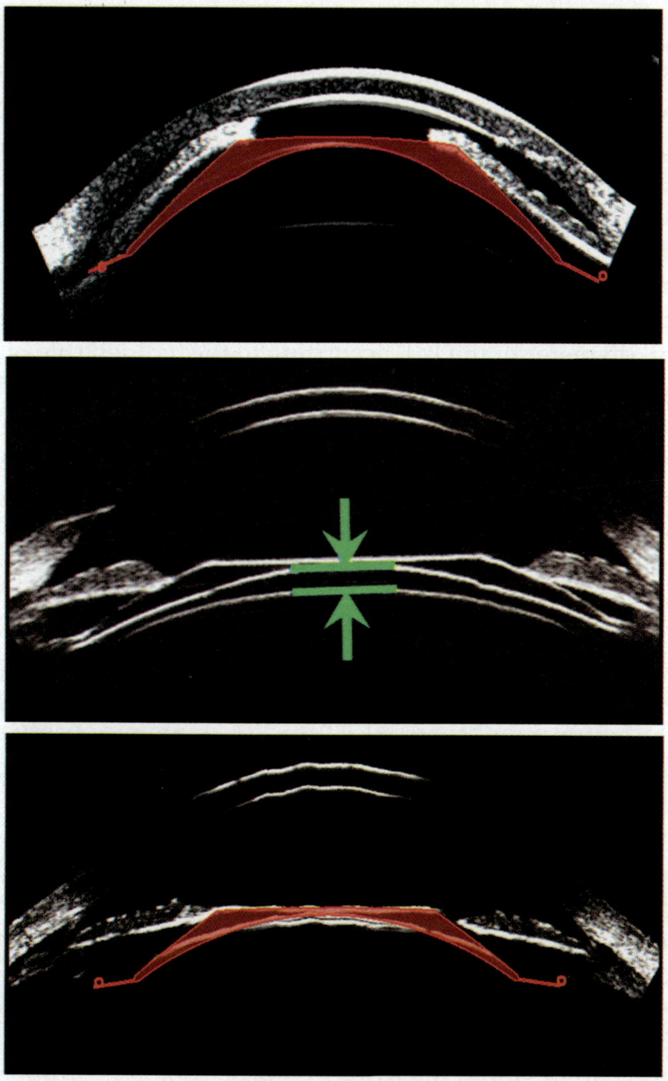

Fig. 24.3: In a series of 200 patients where the W-to-W distance was accurately measured with the Orbscan and the 'golden rule' (W-to-W + 0.5 mm = overall length) meticulously applied, we achieved the desired outcome (vault height between 200 and 700 microns) in 59% of cases (A); in 24% of cases we got significant overvault, superior than 700 microns (B); and in 17% an insufficient vault, inferior than 100 micron (C)

the reflections from the cornea, the iris and the crystalline lens.[65] These methods are not interesting for sizing the ICL, since the retroirideal space cannot be perfectly visualized by optical devices and the statistical correlation between angle and sulcus diameters is as poor as between external white-to-white and internal dimensions.[30]

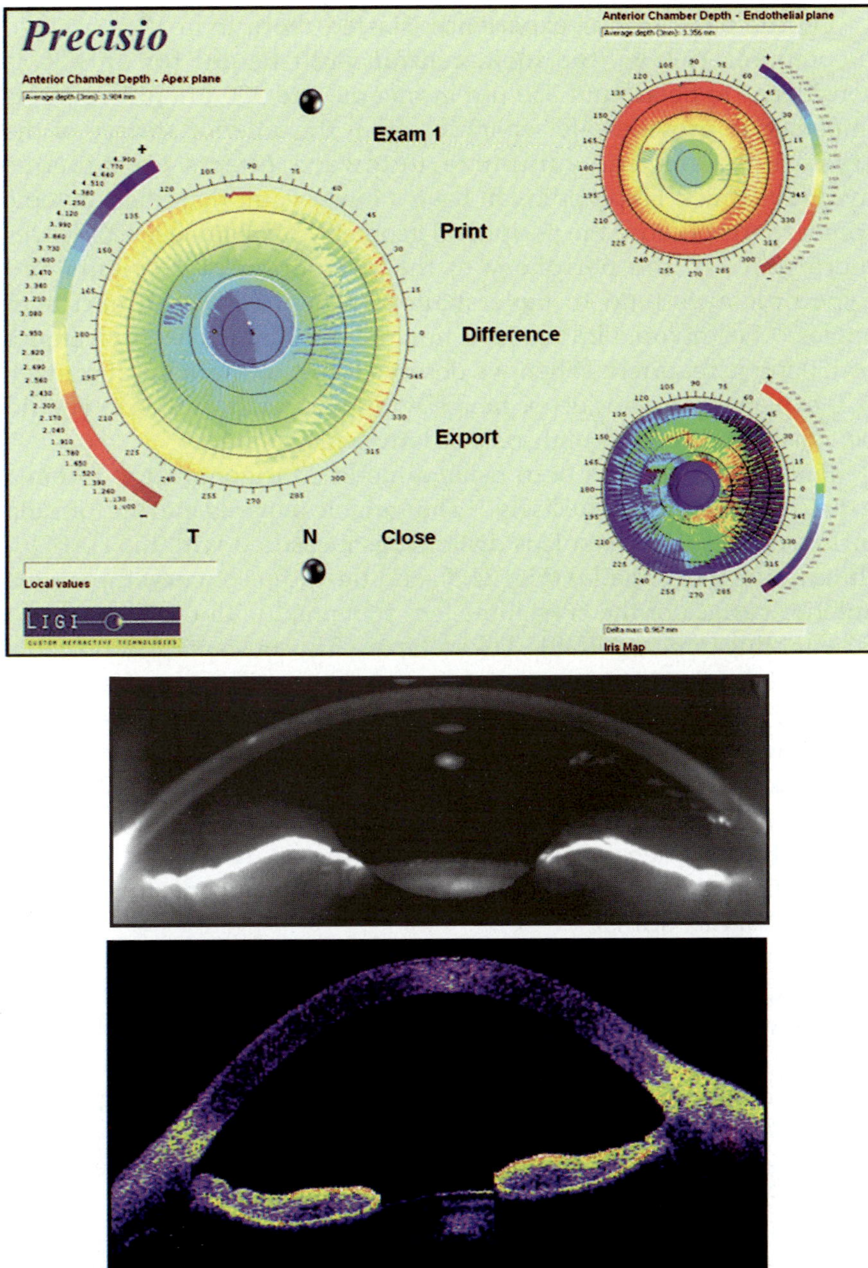

Fig. 24.4: Bidimensional maps (A) and cross-sectional scan (B) of the anterior chamber provided by the Precisio rotating Scheimpflug camera (LIGI, Taranto, Italy); author's left eye OCT Visante image

On the basis of our experience, started more than 13 years ago (September 1993)[12], the ideal central vault height for an ICL is considered to be around 350 μm in myopic and 250 μm in hyperopic implants, to provide safe separation from the anterior surface of the crystalline lens and minimize untoward effects on aqueous hydrodynamics. Hyperopic can have a lower vault than their myopic counterparts because the peripheral geometry of positive lenses leaves more space in the periphery to the circulation of nutrients and hyperopic eyes tend to have shallower chambers with narrower angles.[66] For myopic implants, a minimum mid-peripheral clearance of 150 μm is required. When we observe lower or mechanical contact, ICL explantation and/or exchange with a larger overall size should be considered for the high risk of iatrogenic cataract.

Since 1997, we have been using a modified trigonometric formula to predict vault height precisely.[12] The variables entered into the formula included the sulcus-to-sulcus distance, as measured with the I^{3}ABD™ (Innovative Inc, Canada) (Fig. 24.5), and the radius of curvature of the anterior surface of the crystalline lens (obtained with the EAS 1000™ Scheimpflug camera, NIDEK, Tokyo, Japan). The constants in the formula included the elasticity (elongation factor) of the collamer and the base-curve of the ICL. Since then, we have improved the formula and now are using a proprietary software to simulate the expected clearances between corneal endothelium, iris and crystalline lens.[76] The last *LOVISOLO ICL SIZER®* software (Fig. 24.6) takes into consideration:

- The three-dimensional map of the biometric data of the patient's anterior segment as obtained from VHF ultrasonography (Artemis 2 or VuMax scans)
- The specific features of the chosen lens implant (overall length, vault, central and peripheral optic thickness, flexibility); a corrective factor, considering the variation of ICL dimension from the labelled size (as measured *in vitro* at 20°C) when going into the aqueous environment. Intraocularly, for instance, a 125V4 ICL enlarges from 12.5 to 13.2 mm
- Its behavior under compression, as predicted by finite element analysis (Fig. 24.7)
- The age and the life expectancy of the patient. As the human lens gradually grows, doubling its thickness and displacing anteriorly by 0.4 mm during the lifetime of a 90-year old,[74] due to the life-long mitotic activity of the sub-capsular epithelial cells at the lens equator, the anterior chamber depth drops by 0.75 mm over a 50-year span.[4,74,75] An average reduction of the anterior chamber depth of 0.015 mm per year is calculated to predict the anatomic relationships even after 50 years

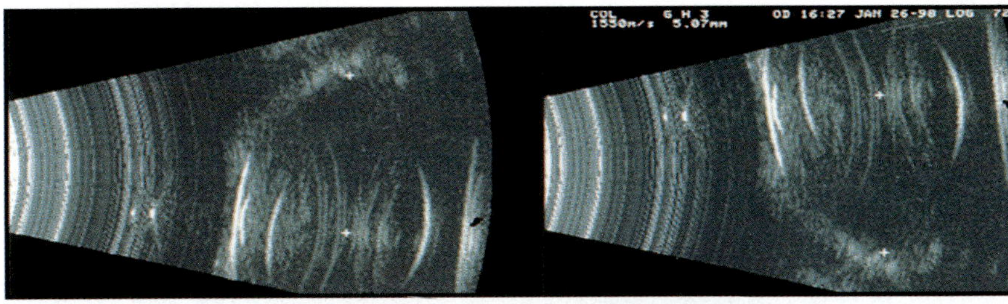

Fig. 24.5: The first generation of the Lovisolo ICL Sizer® software. As the ultrasound cone width was limited to 8 mm, two scan images were pasted together to measure the sulcus diameter (from left and right ciliary recesses to the geometrical center of the crystalline lens) and the anterior curvature of the crystalline lens was measured (A, B) then the trigonometric Fumagalli sag formula was applied (C)

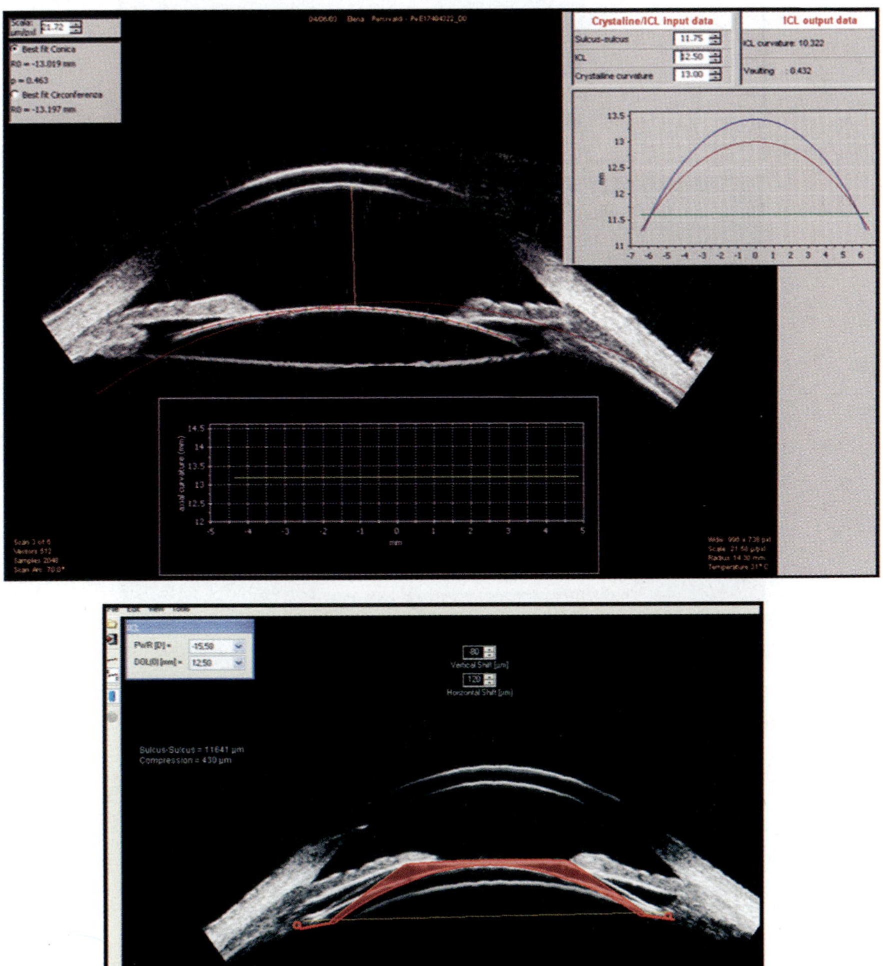

Fig. 24.6: Snapshots of the second (A) and last (B) generation of the Lovisolo ICL Sizer®. In (B) a predicted versus obtained vault is shown

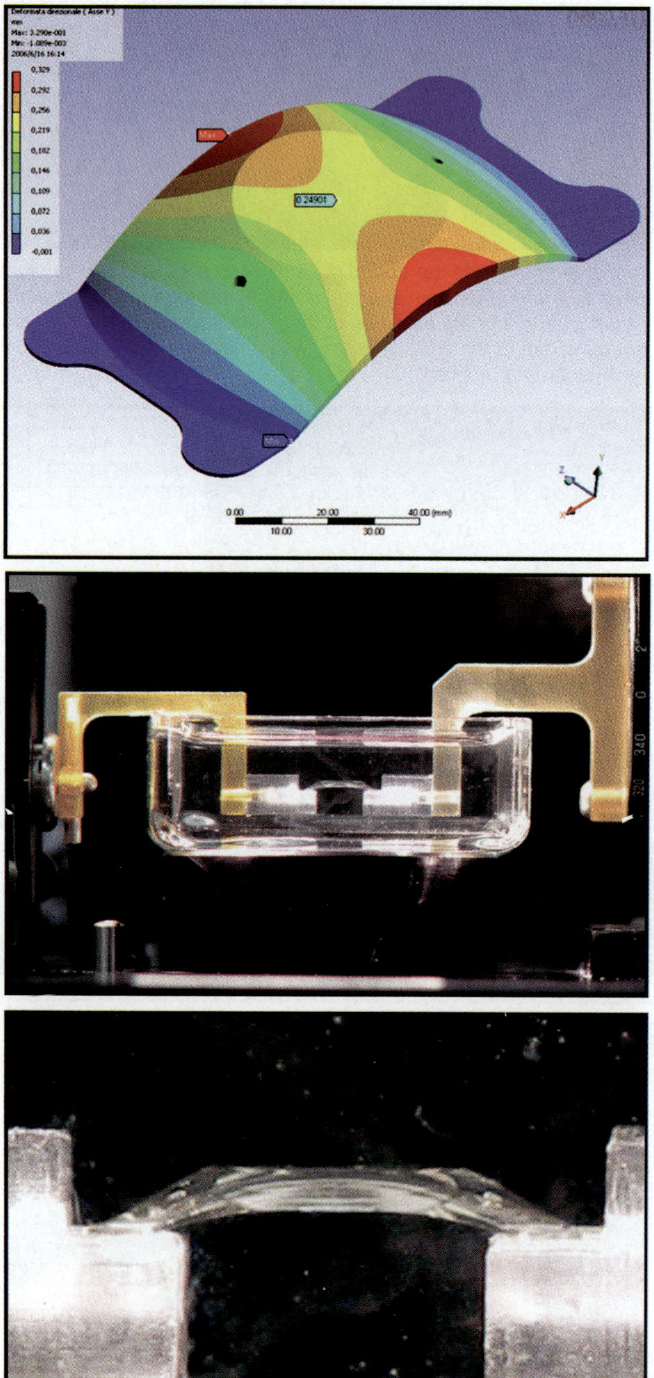

Fig. 24.7: Ansys™ finite element analysis (A) and mechanical compression data (B) were compared to get the intraocular behavior of every lens

- New anatomical safety parameters are introduced (Table 24.1); a warning signal if more than one parameter shows a difference higher than 20% from normal value.

Table 24.1: Normal values of anatomic parameters for ICL implantation

- Crystalline lens rise over the iris plan (cycloplegia): 0.4 mm
- Iris configuration (sclero-iris angle): 28.1°
- Ciliary body position (sclero-ciliary angle): 53.1°
- Iridocorneal angle: 31.3°
- Crystalline lens anterior curvature:

R = 12.08 mm (cycloplegia)
R = 10.3 mm (non-accommodating miosis)

In our most recent personal series on 394 eyes implanted with the ICL V4, after a maximum follow-up of almost 9 years (since April 1998) and a mean follow-up of 39 months, we have not yet observed any cases of iatrogenic cataract, pigmentary dispersion or angle closure glaucoma. The mean central vault height was 386 μm, with a standard deviation of ±113 μm. The minimum vault obtained was 189 μm. In the 95% confidence interval, an expected vs. achieved vault height in the ±150 μm range was obtained in the 95% confidence interval. In comparison with the group control of 237 eyes, where the ICL was implanted on the basis of the W-to-W, the mean central vault height was 406 μm (not statistically significant), but the standard deviation was highly significant (±667 μm). The minimum vault achieved was 0 μm and the incidence of size-related complications (angle closure glaucoma, cataract and clinically significant pigmentary dispersion) was around 8%. The reference point of the 95% confidence interval as referred to the expected vs. achieved vault height was reached for the range of ±730 μm.[77] For further comparison, the reader should know that similar values could be easily obtained from multivariate regression analysis by sizing the ICL on the basis of anterior chamber depth, corneal pachymetry, opening of the iridocorneal angle, angle-to-angle distance, axial length, but also shoe, hat, or glove size.

While recognizing that researchers are still far from fully understand the detailed mechanisms of ICL-induced cataract formation, we attribute these results to the meticulous selection of the anatomic features of each single eye and to the precise sizing of the implanted lenses, allowing an ideal prediction of lens vaulting.

With the extraordinary confidence the system provides to our practice, we now consider as relative contraindications and evaluate on a case-by-case analysis many of the conditions that have been considered exclusion criteria (Table 24.2). Pediatric age, for instance, is not an absolute preclusion to surgery any more. An original excess of caution made it wise to avoid implanting phakic in children, but special cases of unilateral ammetropia or high anisometropia with contact lens intolerance and functional strabismus are worth reassessing, to prevent amblyopia.[12,67-69]

Table 24.2: Generally accepted inclusion criteria (Safety guidelines) for phakic IOL surgery

- Age > 21 years
- Stable ametropia, not amenable to excimer laser surgery
- Intolerance of contact lenses or spectacles
- Central ACD ≥2.8 mm
- Irido corneal angle aperture ≥30°
- Endothelial cell count >2,000 cells/mm^2
- Overall length based on external white-to-white distance
- No previous ocular surgery
- No ocular pathology (glaucoma, uveitis, cataract, etc)
- No systemic diseases (diabetes, autoimmune disorders, etc)

Old absolute contraindications have now proved too conservative, like in the case of stable ectatic corneal disorders (keratoconus, pellucid marginal degeneration, iatrogenic ectasia) and sequelae from trauma, infection or unsatisfactory previous corneal surgeries (like PKP, LKP, RK, ALK, epikeratoplasty, LTK, PRK, LASIK)[12,70,71] that may be dealt with successful outcomes (Fig. 24.8).

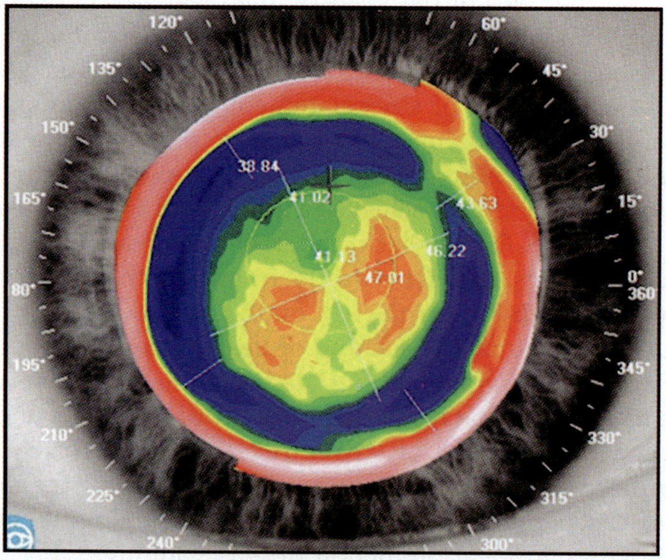

Fig. 24.8: A toric ICL was implanted three months after a couple of intrastromal corneal ring segments (INTACS) were inserted in an advanced stage case of pellucid marginal degeneration. Preoperatively, the BSCVA was 20/80 with –13.00 –12.00 x 115°; after INTACS implantation BSCVA was 20/30 with –11.25 –6.75 x 98°; 6 months after ICL surgery UCVA was 20/20

Eyes with anterior chamber depth (ACD, endothelium to anterior crystalline central distance) less than 2.8 mm can also be implanted with an excellent safety ratio. Although still a preclusive medicolegal reference point, a single measurement of the central ACD, usually obtained by conventional A-scan ultrasound biometry, cannot help in preventing angle closure glaucoma after ICL surgery if no information is provided on the opening of the iridocorneal angle, the shape of the anterior segment, the crystalline lens rise over the pupil plane. No complication was encountered in a series 61 eyes, where the ACD was lower than 2.8 mm, but the other parameters were considered safe.

Eyes with endothelial cell count lower than 2000 cells/mm^2 (post-keratoplasty ammetropias for instance are excellent candidates) may safely undergo ICL surgery as the iris-barrier between the ICL and the cornea protects against corneal decompensation. Our long-term (based on more than 10 years of maximum follow-up) cell losses are completely similar to physiological decay (0.6% per year). Moreover, in the retrospective analysis of our last 6 years series, we observed that no intraoperative endothelial cell sacrifice is required any more. The mean postoperative cell loss was 0.4%, with as much as 46% of eyes whose count and morphometric indices improved. Apart from some unavoidable endotelioscopy bias, these apparently paradoxical findings are probably due to the postoperative centrifugal migration of peripheral endothelial cells and to the cell enhanced metabolism after stopping contact lens wear.

Using VHF echotomography (Artemis 2) and scanning slit optical tomography (Orbscan II)[72,73] we realize that there is no precise correlation between central and peripheral depths of the anterior chamber (*Sizing Phakic*, presented by Lovisolo CF at the ASCRS meeting, San Francisco, April 2003). A certain number of eyes show a progressive narrowing from center to periphery, with the nasal regions about 20% shallower than the temporal counterparts. However, some are strangely shallower in the center and each single eye seems to have its own anterior chamber shape and volume, with no general rule (Fig. 24.9). In a sample of 288 eyes scanned with VHF Echography, the largest cross-sectional internal sulcus diameters was found horizontally in 27%, obliquely in 15%, vertically in 58% of cases. The largest external diameter (white-to-white) was found to be horizontal in 100% of cases. W-to-W was found larger than S-to-S in 59%, the opposite was found in 41% of eyes examined (Fig. 24.10).

As regarding efficacy and functional performance, the same concerns about the quality of vision in kerato-refractive surgery apply equally to phakic. To prevent the symptoms of the 'GASH-tetrad

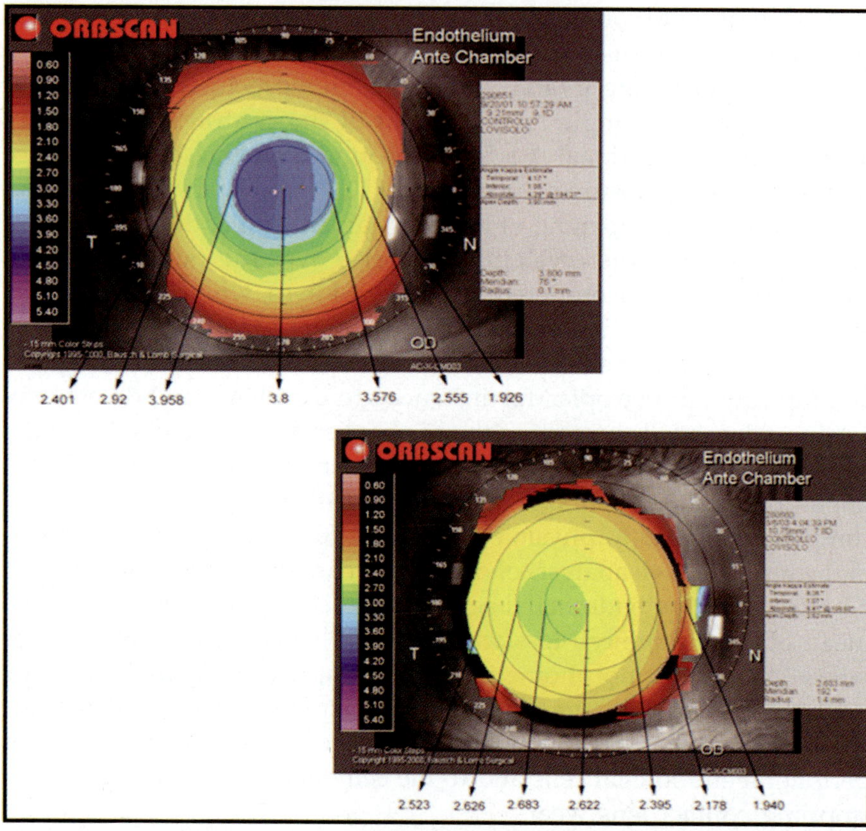

Fig. 24.9: As can be seen from the two Orbscan maps (A, B), similar peripheral narrowing of the anterior chamber (depths equal to about 1.9 mm at 3 mm of eccentricity) corresponds to completely different shapes and volumes of the anterior segment (central depth of 3.8 mm in A, 2.6 mm in B)

syndrome' (glare, arcs, starbursts, halos), the customized optic would have:

1. The necessary spherocylinder power. Like in secondary IOL implantation in aphakic eyes, or piggy-back pseudophakic implantation, the power of an ICL positioned intraocularly is equivalent to the power of the lens measured at a given distance from the corneal vertex. It is not necessary to determine the axial length, the crystalline lens thickness and the vitreous chamber length, as they remain completely unchanged. This calculation depends very much on precise refractive measurements, but also on the ability to predict the intraocular position of the nodal points of the lens (*ELP* or *Effective Lens Position,* the distance between the secondary principal plane of the cornea and the principal plane of the IOL) to avoid over or undercorrection.

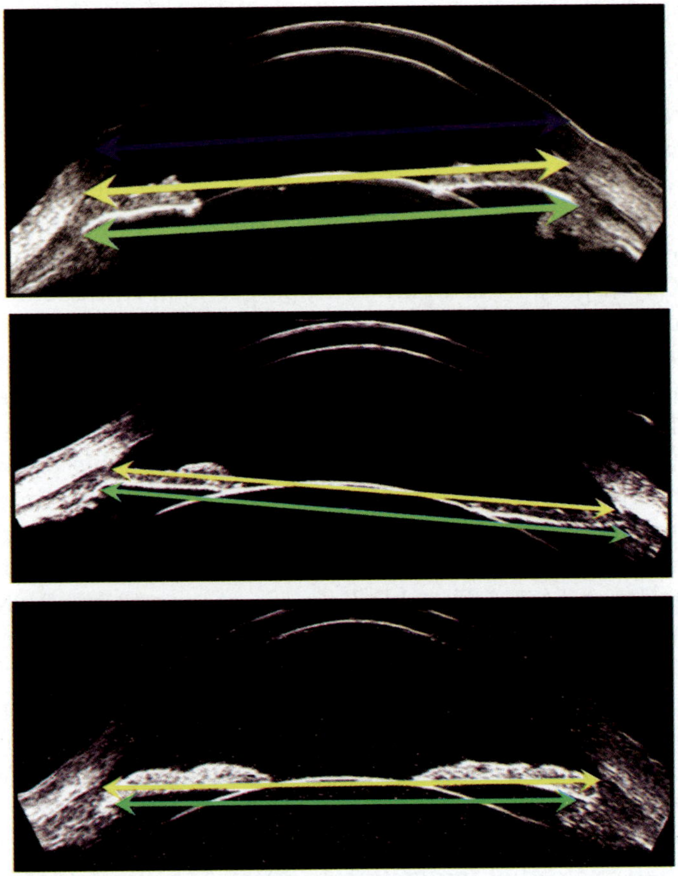

Fig. 24.10: Artemis 2 (Ultralink) images of external, white-to-white (*W-to-W*) and internal measurements, angle-to-angle (*A-to-A*) and sulcus-to-sulcus (*S-to-S*) distances, relevant for sizing ICLs. Without a statistical correlation or a rule, some eyes show almost identical A-to-A and S-to-S distances (A); in the majority of cases A-to-A is larger than S-to-S (B), in the minority the opposite is true (C)

Currently available refined toric lens implantation[51] requires an astigmatically neutral surgical incision and robust fixation site to provide rotational stability over time. For that reason the 6 to 7 mm opening of the eye needed for implanting the Artisan PMMA lens seems too challenging for the average surgeon, while the minimal size (2.5 mm) achievable with the ICL seems ideal. The rotational stability of the toric ICL is even more important, as the cylinder correction decreases with increasing deviation of the lens implant from the target axis by following a non-linear relationship. As shown in a study where the positions of a group of sized with VHF echography were documented by superimposable slit-lamp photographs (Carlo Lovisolo, unpublished data), the mean lens deviation from the original meridian over time (three years) is less than 5°, i.e. compatible with a maximum of 10% loss of astigmatic correction. Once again, as small implants may rotate, accurate sizing is mandatory.

2. An effective diameter at least as large as the mesopic entrance pupil diameter. Infrared pupillometry has shown that scotopic pupil diameter in young myopic patients — the average candidates to ICL surgery — is significantly larger than in the emmetropic group. Our observations on more than 3,000 Caucasians myopic eyes, ranging from 21 to 39 years of age, showed a mean scotopic pupil diameter of 6.87 ±0.72 mm, the range of minimum-maximum value going from 5.6 to 8.9 mm. For that reason, due to the limited diameter of the optical zone, all currently available phakic have been reported to induce different degrees of night time visual disturbances (mainly halos and glare when driving vehicles).[52-53] The successful trend of combining different surgical approaches (Bioptics and/or Adjustable Refractive Surgery) has highlighted not only the concept of fine-tuning residual refractive errors after implantation but also the need for a wide functional optical zone. For a –17.00 correction in a patient with a 6.0 mm mesopic pupillary diameter, for instance, postoperative quality of vision is unquestionably better if we select a wide-optic implant (a –12.00 ICL has a 5.5 mm diameter and corrects approximately –10.00), and combine it with a –7.00, 6.0 mm optical zone excimer laser ablation, instead of implanting a –20.00, 4.65 mm optic ICL, fully correcting the –17.00 dt ammetropia. As a trend, taking advantage of new designs and higher index materials, it is easy to foresee that the average effective optical zone of future lenses will soon be made larger.

3. A proper geometric shape factor (asphericity) to respect physiology.[3,54] Conventional high-power (more than –12.0 and +7.0 D of correction) spherical phakic with an average optic size of about 5.0 mm inevitably induce moderate amounts of spherical aberration and coma, thus reducing contrast sensitivity and increasing glare and halos for the average mesopic pupil.[55] An aspheric phakic lens can be designed on the basis of theoretical assumptions (to limit spherical aberration without reducing the depth of focus[56]), or wavefront analysis from aberrometers (to correct not only on-axis aberrations like spherical aberration, but also higher-order aberrations like trefoil and coma). The weak point of aspheric lenses is the need for perfect alignment with the

cornea and crystalline lens (centration and tilt). When measured as a modulation transfer function, the optical performance of an aspheric IOL is not degraded if the IOL is decentered less than 0.4 mm and tilted less than 7°. Larger discrepancies between lens optical center and visual pathway could cause significant symptoms. Our observations with infrared photography and VHF echography on a group of patients implanted with different phakic showed that pupil decentration is 0.32 mm and tilt is 5° on average (Carlo Lovisolo, unpublished data). However, in patients with largely positive angle kappa[57], even an accurate sizing could cause a significant misalignment with the line of sight. Once this becomes more accurate and standardized, we can foresee a demand even for haptic customization, with asymmetrical loops and wings to match individual pupil decentration. Otherwise iris-fixated lenses that can be nicely centered over the pupil will be preferred to sulcus-supported lenses.

4. Quality of the surfaces higher than the eye's optical limits, possibly designed on the basis of wavefront detection. Custom ICL could be therefore indicated in piggybacking pseudophakic eyes with significant residual ammetropia[58], as well as in pediatric patients with aniridia, albinism, anisometropic amblyopia or in eyes with naturally occurring or iatrogenic, stable corneal disorders (keratoconus, marginal pellucid degeneration, post-RK hyperopic shift, post-LASIK iatrogenic keratectasia, post-trauma or post-keratoplasty astigmatism...), which cause significant higher-order aberrations and may theoretically be tackled by making the compensating corrections intraocularly instead of on the corneal surface (Fig. 24.11).

CONCLUSION

We can roughly estimate that around 100,000 phakic have been implanted to date throughout the world. Many surgeons worldwide actually share my opinion that, so far, the Visian-ICL is the winner of every competitive analysis of the products available on the market. Its collamer material offers the best biocompatibility; the surgeon's learning curve and experience in sorting out intraoperative difficulties is not as steep as for other models; its foldability allows minimally invasive, smooth insertions as well as safe removals under topical anesthesia and through anastigmatic small incision, with absolute patient comfort and the fastest rehabilitation among anterior segment procedures; it produces excellent results in terms of precision, predictability (the percentage of eyes obtaining ±1.00 D from the

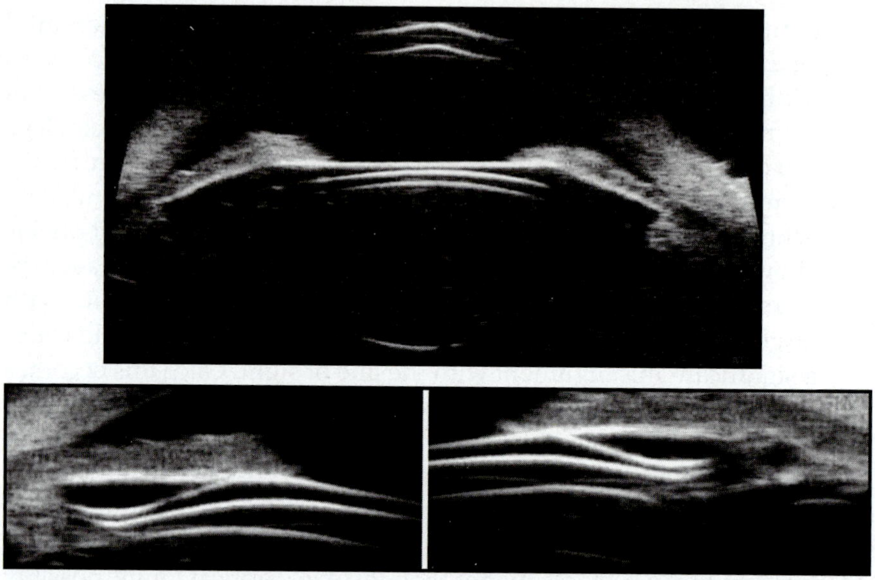

Fig. 24.11: VuMax (Sonomed) VHF echography images of a perfectly sized toric Visian ICL with a central vaulting of 355 microns (A) and retroirideal details of haptic positioning in the ciliary sulcus (B, C)

desired refraction is 100%), and stability of the refractive outcome; a toric optic may correct high degree of astigmatism with unbelievable outcomes in 'desperate' cases; the iris-barrier protects against the most feared complication of phakic IOLs, progressive endothelial cell loss; the incidence of catastrophic events like endophthalmitis and retinal detachment (only anecdotal reports) is acceptably low; provided that a perfect lens sizing guarantees a smooth, uniform distribution of minimal pressures at the fixating points without losing intraocular stability, the long-term risk/benefit ratio is more than acceptable, as late complications, iatrogenic cataract in particular, are mainly due to human errors in sizing, so they can be expected to become less frequent as surgeons gain experience. The absence of synechiae and chronic inflammatory phenomena encapsulating the haptics will facilitate future implant exchange or the 'bilensectomy' procedure when the time comes for cataract surgery in these subjects. The reported nighttime visual symptoms (halos, arcs and glare) are disabling only in a minority of cases and are destined to become minor issues with the latest and future generations of wide-optic customized lenses. Since the implant is generally inserted into pristine, young patients' eyes, the ethical endeavor to ensure a life long enduring harmonious relationship with the internal structures is mandatory. Only a Custom ICL, perfectly designed on the individual anatomic and optical features of each single eye may accomplish all these goals. At last, after almost a decade of sterile debate, I sincerely hope that times are mature to:

- Abandon empirical technique, like the 'junk' White-to-White' based state of the art sizing method
- Perform the most crucial choice (size the overall length of the ICL) on the basis of anatomically correlated measurements, obtained with the newest high resolution biometry devices (VHF Echography) (Fig. 24.11) and calculated by an accomplished software
- Ask the firm marketing the ICL to provide at least the intermediate sizes (0.25 mm steps) and a wider range (from 11 to 14 mm) of lens diameters
- Closely monitor the ICL implant-to-tissue clearances yearly, with the same High-Res instruments and decide for prompt removal/ exchange if vault height values are outside the safety limits.

REFERENCES

1. Moller-Pederson T, Vogel M, Li HF, Petroll WM, et al. Quantification of stromal thinning, epithelial thickness, and corneal haze after photorefractive keratectomy using in vivo confocal microscopy. Ophthalmology 1997; 104:360-8.
2. Artal P, Marcos S, Inglesias I, et al. Optical modulation transfer function of the human eye for the different pupil diameters: an analytical expression. J Opt Soc Am A 1994;11(1):246-9.
3. Marcos S. Aberrations and visual performance following standard laser vision correction. J Refract Surg 2001;17:596-601.
4. Jackson WB. Bioengineered tissue onlay holds promise for refractive correction. EuroTimes 2006;11(11):38.
5. Ismail MM. Correction of hyperopia by intracorneal lenses: two-year follow-up. J Cataract Refract Surg 2006;32:1657-60.
6. Glasser A, Campbell MC. Presbyopia and the optical changes in the human crystalline lens with age. Vision Res 1998;38:209-29.
7. Yamamoto S, Adachi-Usami E. Senile changes of crystalline lens: effects on the delayed latency of pattern visually evoked potentials in phakic and pseudophakic eyes. Acta Ophthalmol 1991;69(2):205-9.
8. Goldberg MF. Clear lens extraction for axial myopia: an appraisal. Ophthalmology 1987; 94:571-81.
9. Gris O, Guell JL, Manero F, et al. Clear lens extraction for severe myopia. J Cataract Refract Surg 1996;22:686-9.
10. Barraquer C, Cavelier C, Mejia LF. Incidence of retinal detachment following clear lens extraction in myopia patients. Retrospective analysis. Arch Ophthalmol 1994;112:336-9.
11. Colin J, Robinet A, Cochener B. Retinal detachment after clear lens extraction for high myopia: seven-year follow-up. Ophthalmology 1999;106(12): 2281-4.
12. Lovisolo CF, Pesando PM. The implantable contact lens (ICL™) and other phakic IOLs. Fabiano Ed S. Stefano Belbo (CN) Italy; 2000; 84.
13. Heijde GL Van der. Some optical aspects of implantation of an IOL in a myopic eye. Eur J Implant Ref Surg 1989;1:245-8.

14. Holladay JT. Refractive power calculations for intraocular lenses in the phakic eye. Am J Ophthalmol 1993;19:700-12.
15. Holladay J. Power calculation and optics of phakic IOLs. In Lovisolo CF, Pesando PM (Eds): The implantable contact lens (ICL) and other phakic IOLs, S. Stefano Belbo, Italy Fabiano Ed 2000; pp 295-302.
16. Sarver EJ, Sanders DR, Vukich JA. Image quality in myopic eyes corrected with laser in situ keratomileusis and phakic intraocular lens. J Refract Surg 2003;19(4):397-404.
17. Ibrahim O, Waring GO. Successful exchange of dislocated phakic intraocular lens. J Refract Surg 1995;11(4):282-3.
18. Trindade F, Pereira F. Exchange of a posterior chamber phakic intraocular lens in a highly myopic eye. J Cataract Refract Surg 2000;26(5):773-6.
19. Alexander L, John M, Cobb L, et al. US clinical investigation of the Artisan myopia lens for the correction of high myopia in phakic eyes. Report of the results of phases 1 and 2, and interim phase 3. Optometry 2000;71(10): 630-42.
20. Arne JL, Lesueur LC. Phakic posterior chamber lenses for high myopia: functional and anatomical outcomes. J Cataract Refract Surg 2000;26(3): 369-74.
21. Dick HB, Aliò J, Bianchetti M, et al. Toric phakic intraocular lens: European multicenter study. Ophthalmology 2003;110(1):150-62.
22. Perez-Santonja JJ, Aliò JL, Jimenez-Alfaro I, et al. Surgical correction of severe myopia with an angle-supported phakic intraocular lens. J Cataract Refract Surg 2000;26(9):1288-302.
23. Pesando PM, Ghiringhello MP, Tagliavacche P. Posterior chamber collamer phakic intraocular lens for myopia and hyperopia. J Refract Surg 1999;15(4):415-23.
24. Uusitalo RJ, Aine E, Sen NH, et al. Implantable contact lens for high myopia. J Cataract Refract Surg 2002; 28(1):29-36.
25. Zaldivar R, Davidorff JM, Oscherow S. Posterior chamber phakic intraocular lens for myopia of –8 to –19 diopters. J Refract Surg 1998;14:294-305.
26. Arne JL, Lesueur LC, Hulin HH. Photorefractive keratectomy or laser in situ keratomileusis for residual refractive error after phakic intraocular lens implantation. J Cataract Refract Surg 2003;29(6):1167-73.
27. Guell JL, Vázquez M, Gris O. Adjustable refractive surgery: 6 mm Artisan lens plus laser in situ keratomileusis for the correction of high myopia. Ophthalmology 2001;108(5):945-52.
28. Zaldivar R, Oscherow S, Piezzi V. Bioptics in phakic and pseudophakic intraocular lens with the Nidek EC-5000 excimer laser. J Refract Surg 2002;18(3 Suppl) 336-9.
29. Lovisolo CF. Ten years of ICLs. Paper presented at the winter ESCRS meeting Barcelona Jan 2004.
30. Lovisolo CF, Reinstein DZ. Phakic intraocular lenses. Surv Ophthalmol 2005;50:549-87.
31. Aliò JL, de la Hoz F, Pérez-Santonja JJ. Phakic anterior chamber lenses for the correction of myopia: a seven years cumulative analysis of complications in 263 cases. Ophthalmology 1999;106:448-56.
32. Benitez del Castillo JM, Iradier MT, Hernandez JL, et al. Corneal endothelial permeability after implantation of angle-fitted anterior chamber lenses in myopic phakic eyes. Preliminary results. Doc Ophthalmol-96 1995;91(3): 201-6.

33. Gelender IL. Corneal endothelium cell loss, cystoid macular edema and iris-supported intraocular lenses. Ophthalmology 1984;91:841-6.
34. Pérez-Santonja JJ, Iradier MT, Benitez del Castillo JM, et al. Chronic subclinical inflammation in phakic eyes with intraocular lenses to correct myopia. J Cataract Refract Surg 1996;22:183-7.
35. Pérez-Santonja JJ, Hernandez JL, Benitez del Castillo M, et al. Fluorophotometry in myopic phakic eyes with anterior chamber intraocular lenses to correct severe myopia. Am J Ophthalmol 1994;118:316-21.
36. Pérez-Santonja JJ, Iradier MT, Sanz-Iglesias L, et al. Endothelial changes in phakic eyes with anterior chamber intraocular lenses to correct high myopia. J Cataract Refract Surg 1996;22:1017-22.
37. Perez-Santonja JJ, Ruiz-Moreno JM, de la Hoz F, et al. Endophthalmitis after phakic intraocular lens implantation to correct high myopia. J Cataract Refract Surg 1999; 25(9):1295-8.
38. Perez-Santonja JJ, Bueno JL, Meza J, et al. Ischemic optic neuropathy after intraocular lens implantation to correct high myopia in a phakic patient. J Cataract Refract Surg 1993;19(5):651-4.
39. Werner L, Apple DJ, Izak AM, et al. Phakic anterior chamber intraocular lenses. Int Ophthalmol Clin 2001; 41(3):133-52.
40. Abela-Formanek C, Kruger AJ, Dejaco-Ruhswurm I, et al. Gonioscopic changes after implantation of a posterior chamber lens in phakic myopic eyes. J Cataract Refract Surg 2001;27(12):1919-25.
41. Brandt JD, Mockovak ME, Chayet A. Pigmentary dispersion syndrome induced by a posterior chamber phakic refractive lens. Am J Ophthalmol 2001;131(2):260-3.
42. Bylsma SS, Zalta AH, Foley E, et al. Phakic posterior chamber intraocular lens pupillary block. J Cataract Refract Surg 2002;28(12):2222-8.
43. Keuch RJ, Bleckmann H. Pupil diameter changes and reaction after posterior chamber phakic intraocular lens implantation. J Cataract Refract Surg 2002;28(12):2170-2.
44. Kodjikian L, Gain P, Donate D, et al. Malignant glaucoma induced by a phakic posterior chamber intraocular lens for myopia. J Cataract Refract Surg 2002;28(12):2217-21.
45. Sanchez-Galeana CA, Zadok D, Montes M, et al. Refractory intraocular pressure increase after phakic posterior chamber intraocular lens implantation. Am J Ophthalmol 2002;134(1):121-3.
46. Visessook N, Peng Q, Apple DJ, et al. Pathological examination of an explanted phakic posterior chamber intraocular lens. J Cataract Refract Surg 1999;25(2):216-22.
47. Werner L, Apple DJ, Pandey SK, et al. Phakic posterior chamber intraocular lenses. Int Ophthalmol Clin 2001;41(3):153-74.
48. El-Sheikh HF, Tabbara KF. Cataract following posterior chamber phakic intraocular lens. J Refract Surg 2003;19(1):72-3.
49. Sanchez-Galeana CA, Smith RJ, Sanders DR, et al. Lens opacities after posterior chamber phakic intraocular lens implantation. Ophthalmology 2003;110(4):781-5.
50. Waheed S, Krueger RR. Update on customized excimer ablations: recent developments reported in 2002. Curr Opin Ophthalmol. 2003;14:198-202.
51. Aliò JL, Galal A, Mulet ME. Surgical correction of high degrees of astigmatism with a phakic toric-iris claw intraocular lens. Int Ophthalmol Clin 2003;43(3):171-81.

52. Maroccos R, Vaz F, Marinho A, et al. Glare and halos after "phakic IOL" surgery for the correction of high myopia. Ophthalmologe 2001;98(11): 1055-9.
53. Tester R, Pace NL, Samore M, et al. Dysphotopsia in phakic and pseudophakic patients: incidence and relation to intraocular lens type (2). J Cataract Refract Surg 2000;26(6):810-6.
54. Packer M, Fine IH, Hoffman RS, Piers PA. Prospective randomized trial of an anterior surface modified prolate intraocular lens. J Refract Surg 2002;18(6):692-6.
55. Brunette I, Bueno JM, Harissi-Dagher M, et al. Optical quality of the eye with the Artisan phakic lens for the correction of high myopia. Optom Vis Sci 2003;80(2):167-74.
56. Holladay JT, Piers PA, Koranyi G, van der Mooren M, Norrby S. A new intraocular lens design to reduce spherical aberration of pseudophakic eyes. J Refract Surg 2002;18:683-91.
57. Von Noorden G, Maumenee AE. Atlas of Strabismus (2nd ed). The CV Mosby Company St. Louis 1973; pp 32-3.
58. Chiou AG, Bovet J, de Courten C. Pseudophakic ametropia managed with a phakic posterior chamber intraocular lens. J Cataract Refract Surg 2001;27(9):1516-8.
59. Strampelli B. Sopportabilità di lenti acriliche in camera anteriore nella afachiae nei vizi di refrazione. Ann Ottalmol Clinic Oculist 1954;80:75-82.
60. Artola A, Jimenez-Alfaro I, Ruiz-Moreno, Lovisolo CF, Reinstein DZ. Proper patient assessment: selection and preparation. In Aliò JL, Perez-Santonja JJ (Eds): Refractive Surgery with Phakic IOLs. Fundamentals and practice. Highlights of Ophthalmology International. El Dorado, Panama 2004; pp 37-53.
61. Fea AM, Annetta F, Cirillo S, et al. Magnetic resonance imaging and Orbscan assessment of the anterior chamber. J Cataract Refract Surg 2005 Sep;31(9):1713-8.
62. Werner L, Apple DJ, Pandey SK, et al. Phakic posterior chamber intraocular lenses. Int Ophthalmol Clin 2001;41(3):153-74.
63. Pop M, Payette Y. Predicting sulcus size using ocular measurements. J Cataract Refract Surg 2001;27:1033-8.
64. Reinstein DZ, Silverman RH, Raevsky T, et al. A new arc-scanning very high-frequency ultrasound system for 3D pachymetric mapping of corneal epithelium, lamellar flap and residual stromal layer in laser in situ keratomileusis. J Refract Surg 2000;16:414-30.
65. Bechmann M, Ullrich S, Thiel MJ, et al. Imaging of posterior chamber phakic intraocular lens by optical coherence tomography. J Cataract Refract Surg 2002;28(2):360-3.
66. Rabsilber TM, Becker KA, Frisch IB, Auffarth GU. Anterior chamber depth in relation to refractive status measured with the Orbscan II Topography System. J Catar Refract Surg 2003;29(11):2115-21.
67. Ben Ezra D, Cohen E, Karshai I. Phakic posterior chamber intraocular lens for the correction of anisometropia and treatment of amblyopia. Am J Ophthalmol 2000;130(3):292-6.
68. Chipont EM, Garcia-Hermosa P, Aliò J. Reversal of myopic anisometropic amblyopia with phakic intraocular lens implantation. J Refract Surg 2001;17(4):460-2.

69. Lesueur LC, Arne JL. Phakic intraocular lens to correct high myopic amblyopia in children. J Refract Surg 2002;18:519-23.
70. Colin J, Velou S. Implantation of Intacs and a refractive intraocular lens to correct keratoconus. J Cataract Refract Surg 2003;29(4):832-4.
71. Fink AM, Gore C, Rosen ES. Overcorrected radial keratotomy treated with posterior chamber phakic intraocular lens and laser thermal keratoplasty. J Refract Surg 1999;15(6):683-6.
72. Rabsilber TM, Becker KA, Frisch IB, et al. Anterior chamber depth in relation to refractive status measured with the Orbscan II Topography System. J Catar Refract Surg 2003;29(11):2115-21.
73. Vetrugno M, Cardascia N, Cardia L. Anterior chamber depth measured by two methods in myopic and hyperopic phakic IOL implant. Br J Ophthalmol 2000;84(10):1113-6.
74. Okabe I, Taniguchi T. Age related changes of the anterior chamber width. J Glaucoma 1992;1:100.
75. Fontana ST, Brubaker RF. Volume and depth of the anterior chamber in the normal aging human eye. Arch Ophthalmol 1973; 98:1803.
76. Lovisolo CF. Posterior chamber phakic IOLs. ISRS/AAO 2003 Refractive Surgery comes of age. American Academy of Ophthalmology 33-41.
77. Lovisolo CF. ICL sizing based on VHF Ecography is safer than 'White-to-White' rule of thumb. Free paper presented at the AAO annual meeting, Las Vegas 2006.

CHAPTER

25

Dimitrii D Dementiev (Italy)

Phakic Refractive Lens (PRL™) for Myopia and Hyperopia Correction

INTRODUCTION

The last years more and more refractive surgeons are looking to use not only the corneal refractive procedures (RK, KM, LASIK, PRK, LASEK) for myopia and hyperopia correction, but also the phakic implants. It was just approved that the quality of vision after the refractive implants is much better that after corneal procedures, especially in high refractive error eyes .The evidence of reversibility, stability (no regression was noticed) and high predictability of the final refractive effect of the implants make this kind of surgery to become more popular among the refractive surgeons all over the globe.

In this chapter we want to describe our experience with Phakic Refractive Lenses (PRL Medennium-Carl Zeiss/Meditec) implantation and to show the evolution of the phakic refractive lenses we have worked with, to compare the different models of the lenses we used in the past and we use today, to analyze the follow-up and complications we had, to present the instrumentation we developed for this surgery.

HISTORY OF PRLs BACKGROUND AND DEVELOPMENT

Pupil-fixated Lens (Mushroom) (Fig. 25.1)

In 1986, in Moscow Research Eye Institute Drs V Zuev and S Fyodorov proposed a new phakic silicone IOL, named the *mushroom* lens, which was implanted from 1986 until 1990 in Russia. The lens was fixated in the pupil. The main idea was to avoid contact between the lens and the endothelium. We implanted more than 120 lenses with good refractive results. A new era of phakic correction using a lens in the posterior chamber was started. The diameter of the optic zone of this lens was 3.2 mm and the total length of the PRL was 8.0 mm. The haptic was placed in the PC and the optic part remained in the AC; the lens being fixated by the pupil (Fig. 25.2).

Despite of the good refractive results many complications were manifested. The complications such as iridocyclitis (the material was toxic), night glare, night vision acuity loss, pupillary block, endothelial cell loss, cataracts in several cases, and inflammation reaction in long term follow-up were the serious reason to stop the study of this implant design.

Posterior Chamber Phakic Lens Made in Russia (Fig. 25.3)

Based on the work with the *Mushroom* lens the concept of a purely posterior chamber PRL was proposed at MERI in Russia and was made

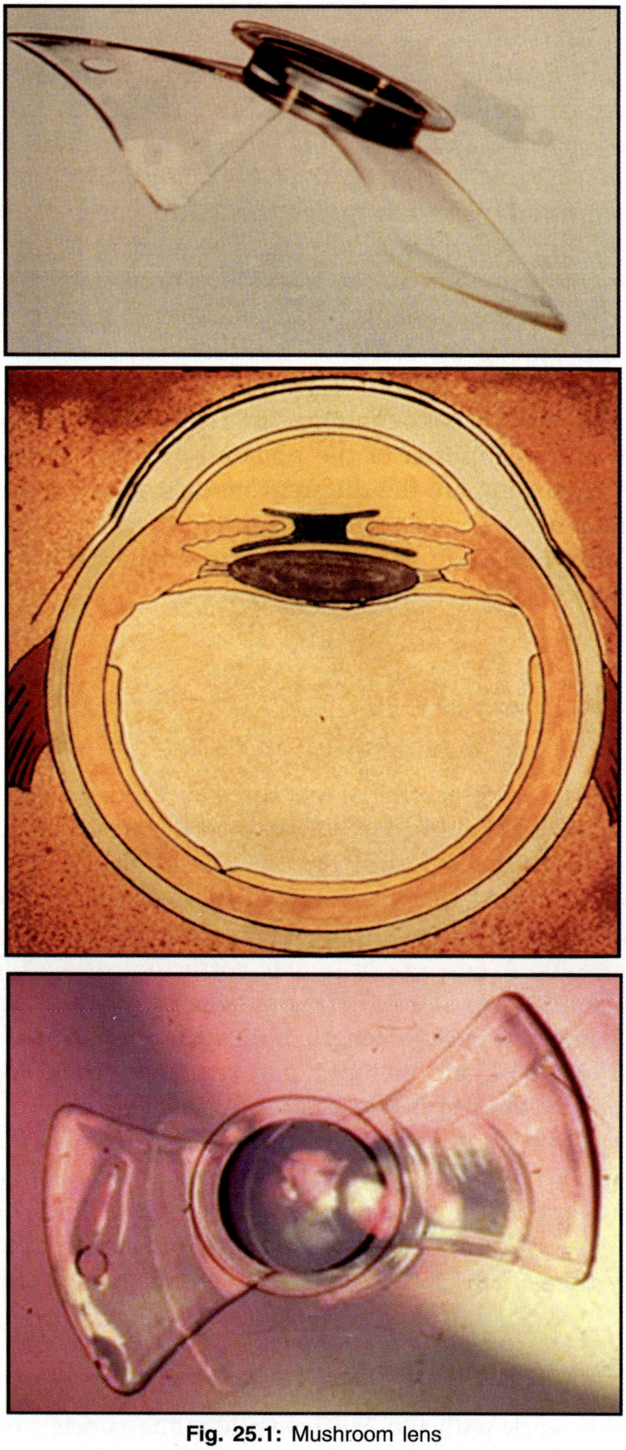

Fig. 25.1: Mushroom lens

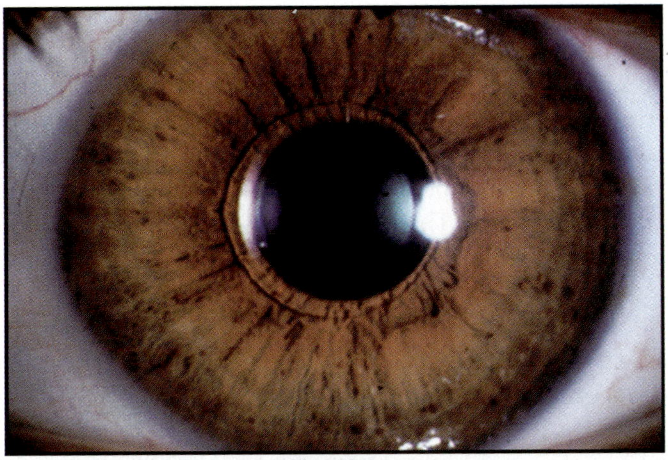

Fig. 25.2

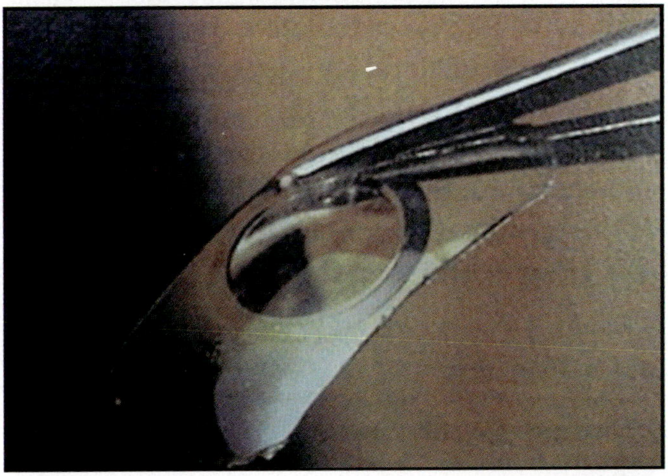

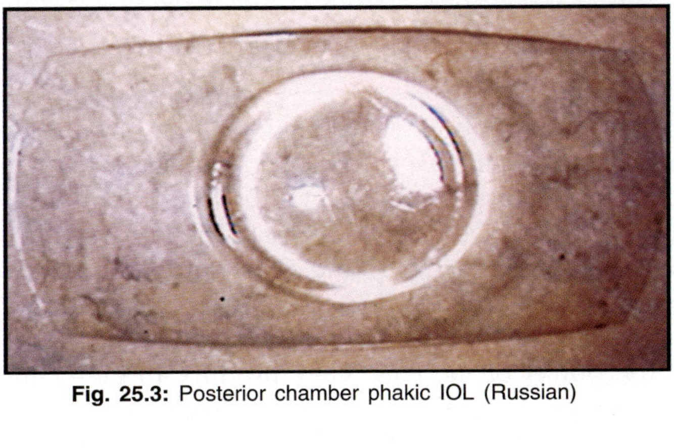

Fig. 25.3: Posterior chamber phakic IOL (Russian)

from a completely new silicone material, which was not toxic but biocompatible and had a higher refractive index than previous silicon.

Its configuration, parameters and the mechanism of fixation of this PRLs were completely different from the previous *Mushroom* model. It was intended for implantation entirely in the posterior chamber with fixation on the zonular fibers. The OZ diameter was 4.5 mm and the total length was 10.6 mm. The lens was created for surgical high myopia correction starting from –10.0 D. This lens was the first prototype of all other posterior chamber PRLs available on the market today.

The problems with endothelium cells loss, cataract formation, severe glare were resolved. But a new complication like an implant decentration occurred in many cases (Fig. 25.4).

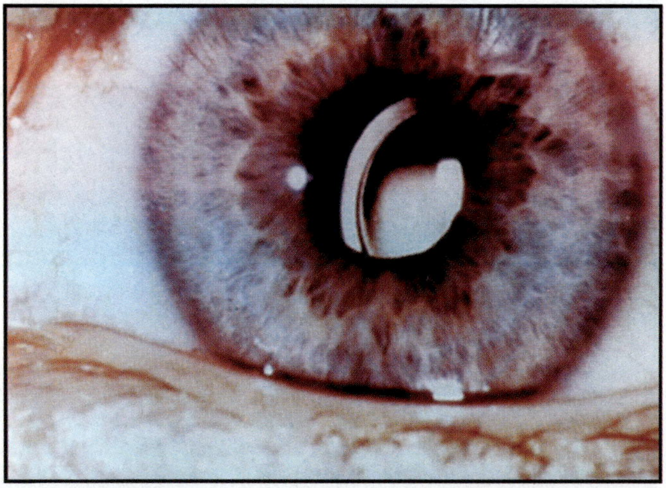

Fig. 25.4: Decentration of the PC phakic IOL

Posterior Chamber Phakic Lens (PRL™) by IVI- Medennium (Fig. 25.5)

International Vision, Inc

This company was set up in Cincinnati, Ohio to produce the PC PRL that we have been using for the past 6 years. The idea of PRL design was moved from Russia to USA, modified and improved according to the complications we had in the past. The size and the curvature of the implant were changed, and FDA study started. The phakic refractive lens (PRL) is made from silicone with a 1.46 refractive index. The diameter of the optic zone is from 4.5-5.5 mm depending upon the dioptric power of the lens. They produce PRLs for myopia and hyperopia (range from+3.5 to+13.5 and from –5.0 to –20.0), which permits a maximum correction of 27.0 D of myopia and 11.0 D of

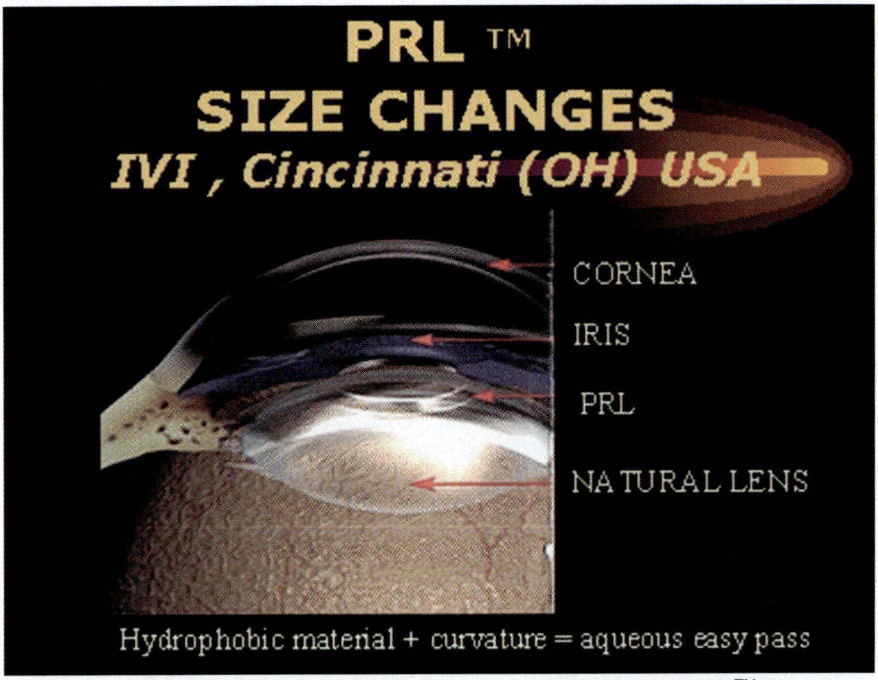

Fig. 25.5: The last modifications of phakic refractive lens PRL™

hyperopia. The material is soft, elastic, and hydrophobic. It is easy to perform the implantation through a 3.0-3.5 mm clear cornea incision. The lens does not contact the anterior capsule of the crystalline lens. Beeing done from hydrophobic material and having the curvature that repeats the curvature of the crystalline lens the edges of the PRL are lying on the zonulars and all the body floats in the posterior chamber keeping the space between the implant and anterior capsule of the lens. This floating phenomena let the aqueous easy to pass under the PRL keeping the lens metabolism unchanged (Fig. 25.6). No synechiae have been noted in long term follow-up. It is easy to remove if it should become necessary. After changing the size parameters of the PRL, decentration has not been observed. Other possible complications are cataract formation and pigmentary glaucoma..

PRL Medennium/IOL Tech/Carl Zeiss (Fig. 25.7)

Today the PRL has received the CEE mark and available on the markets of Europe and south America. In the USA it is under the phase III FDA study. Manufactured by IVI/Medennium Inc. Irvine, CA, USA and distributed by IOL Tech /Carl Zeiss (Laroshele, France).

When implanted PRL functions as an optical element to correct refractive error and avoids contact with the natural lens of the eye.

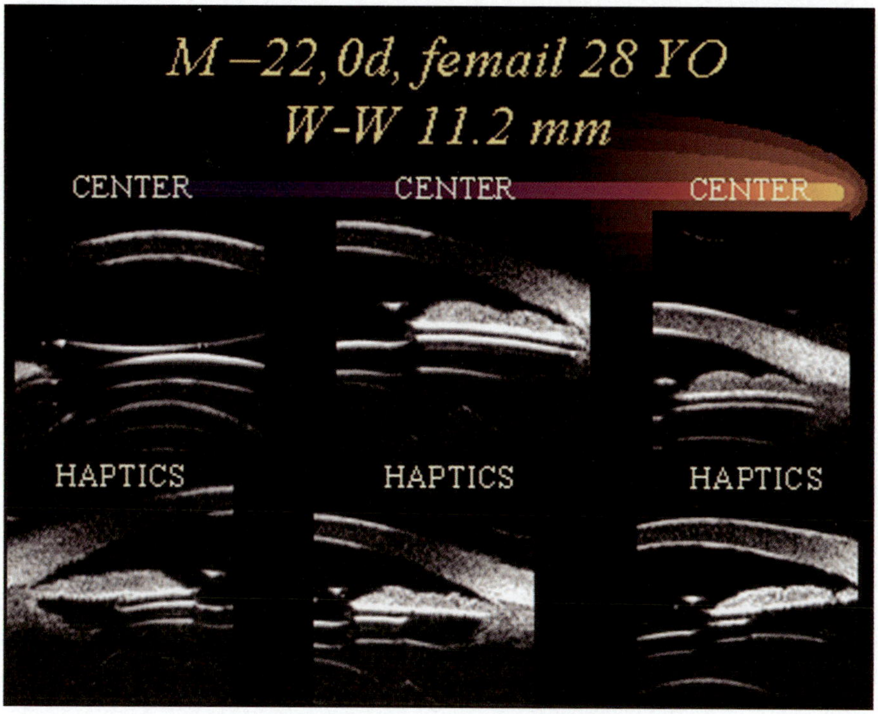

Fig. 25.6: UBM picture shows floating of PRL in PC. No contact with the anterior capsule, contact with the iris

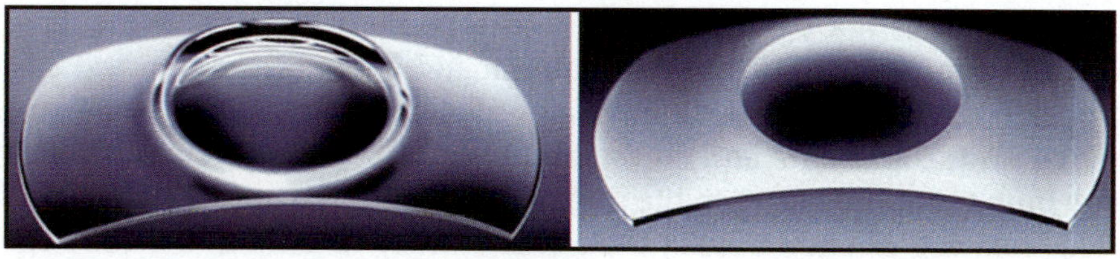

Fig. 25.7

PRL does not have the contact with the anterior capsule of the crystalline lens. PRL myopic and hyperopic implants are available. PRL is done from high refractive index (1.46) highly purified, optically clear silicone elastomer that has undergone biocompatibility testing in Russia and USA. The specific gravity of the PRL is 0.99. PRL has spherical, thin, flexible and elastic haptic for ease of insertion and conformance to the natural shape and dynamic changes of the eye. The PRL is not fixed in the ciliary sulcus, but floats in the posterior chamber touching the natural lens zonulars with its edge. The implant's width is 6.0mm. Myopic implant (MI) is 11.3 mm length (one size fits all) and hyperopic implant (HI) is 10.6 mm length (one size fits all).

The optic diameter of MI is varying from 5.0 mm to 4.5 mm.
HI has 4.5 mm diameter in all the implants.
The Power of MI is from –3.0 D to –20.0 D
The power of HI is from +3.0 D to +15.0 D
With 0.5 D increment both MI & HI.

MYOPIC PRL HYPEROPIC PRL

MODEL	*OPTIC DIA*	*LENGTH*	*WIDTH*	*POWER D*	*INCREMENTS*
Myopic	4.5-5.0 mm	11.3 mm	6.0 mm	–3.0 – 20.0	0.5 D
Hyperopic	4.5 mm	10.6 mm	6.0 mm	+3.0 + 15.0	0.5 D

PATIENT SELECTION

Myopic Range

From –3.00 D to –30.00 D.

Hyperopic Range

From +3.00 to +16.00 D.

A +16.0 D hyperope is the maximum we have corrected.

Because the anterior chamber of the hyperopic patients is usually shallow, it is safer to limit the hyperopic correction for PRL implantation to a maximum of +11.00 D unless there is a deep AC.

Unilateral High Myopia with Amblyopia in Children

So far we have performed seven implantations for correction of unilateral high myopia in children with amblyopia. In cases of progressive myopia, scleral reinforcement surgery is recommended.

Combined Astigmatism

In cases with astigmatism greater than 1.0 D we performed PRL implantation with additional AK surgery.

Keratoconus Correction and Correction of the Refractive Error of the Previous Surgery

PRL implantations can be performed for keratoconus correction with a high myopia component and for overcorrection of a previous refractive procedure such as RK, PRK, or LASIK. It is an exchange of a previous model of PRL.

Poor Candidates

1. Clouded or non-transparent cornea
2. Cataract

3. Lens subluxation
4. Glaucoma or ocular hypertension
5. Shallow anterior chamber (less then 2.5 mm)
6. Vitreo-retinal problems that would preclude good vision or require posterior segment intervention
7. Previous ocular surgery: vitreo-retinal surgery, glaucoma filtration, etc.
8. Age limited to age 60.

PREOPERATIVE PREPARATION

PRL Power Calculation

It is important to obtain a precise refraction of the eye (with accurate vertex distance measurement) as well as an accurate axial length and corneal power readings to use the various methods.

Vertex Chart

The spherical equivalent of the most accurate refraction of the eye is used to interpolate the power of the posterior chamber PRL. These powers are based on a simple vertex correction from 12 mm to the corneal plane. This does not seem to make sense optically, but so far has resulted in excellent accuracy in our experience.

Iridectomy

Surgical

Usually we recommend performing a surgical iridectomy at the time of PRL implantation. We feel it should be a basal iridectomy made at 12:00 and we prefer to perform it after the PRL is inserted. It is of the utmost importance to make sure that it is a complete iridectomy by checking to be sure the pigment layer has been cut through. This must be done carefully so as not to damage the crystalline lens.

Laser

Those surgeons who prefer not to make it surgically must do it by YAG-laser. It is recommended that two YAG iridectomies always be performed at around two weeks before the surgery and that they be made at 10:00 and 2:00. To avoid light and additional images passing through the iridectomies, it is very important not to make them too large and to make them as peripheral as possible. We had one patient with severe complaints of night glare. The iridectomy was found to be too large and located nearer to the pupil. We decided to suture it and after it became smaller, the patient complained much less. We have

Table 25.1: PRL power

Based on 12 mm Vertex Formula: PRL=Rx/(1-0.012*Rx)

EACH PRL CAUSES WHAT RX?				EACH Rx NEEDS WHAT PRL?			
MYOPIA		HYPEROPIA		MYOPIA		HYPEROPIA	
PRL	RX	PRL	RX	RX	PRL	RX	PRL
-3.0	-3.11	**3.0**	2.90	**-3.0**	-2.90	**3.0**	3.11
-3.5	-3.65	**3.5**	3.36	**-3.5**	-3.36	**3.5**	3.65
-4.0	-4.20	**4.0**	3.82	**-4.0**	-3.82	**4.0**	4.20
-4.5	-4.76	**4.5**	4.27	**-4.5**	-4.27	**4.5**	4.76
-5.0	-5.32	**5.0**	4.72	**-5.0**	-4.72	**5.0**	5.32
-5.5	-5.89	**5.5**	5.16	**-5.5**	-5.16	**5.5**	5.89
-6.0	-6.50	**6.0**	5.60	**-6.0**	-5.60	**6.0**	6.47
-6.5	-7.00	**6.5**	6.00	**-6.5**	-6.03	**6.5**	7.05
-7.0	-7.64	**7.0**	6.50	**-7.0**	-6.46	**7.0**	7.64
-7.5	-8.24	**7.5**	6.88	**-7.5**	-6.88	**7.5**	8.24
-8.0	-8.85	**8.0**	7.30	**-8.0**	-7.30	**8.0**	8.85
-8.5	-9.50	**8.5**	7.71	**-8.5**	-7.71	**8.5**	9.47
-9.0	-10.09	**9.0**	8.12	**-9.0**	-8.12	**9.0**	10.09
-9.5	-10.72	**9.5**	8.50	**-9.5**	-8.53	**9.5**	10.72
-10.0	-11.36	**10.0**	8.93	**-10.0**	-8.93	**10.0**	11.36
-10.5	-12.00	**10.5**	9.33	**-10.5**	-9.33	**10.5**	12.01
-11.0	-12.67	**11.0**	9.72	**-11.0**	-9.72	**11.0**	12.67
-11.5	-13.34	**11.5**	10.11	**-11.5**	-10.11	**11.5**	13.34
-12.0	-14.00	**12.0**	10.50	**-12.0**	-10.49	**12.0**	14.02
-12.5	-14.71	**12.5**	10.87	**-12.5**	-10.87	**12.5**	14.71
-13.0	-15.40	**13.0**	11.25	**-13.0**	-11.25	**13.0**	15.40
-13.5	-16.11	**13.5**	11.62	**-13.5**	-11.62		
-14.0	-16.83	**14.0**	12.00	**-14.0**	-11.99		
-14.5	-17.50	**14.5**	12.35	**-14.5**	-12.35		
-15.0	-18.29	**15.0**	12.71	**-15.0**	-12.71		
-15.5	-19.00	**15.5**	13.07	**-15.5**	-13.07		
-16.0	-19.80	**16.0**	13.42	**-16.0**	-13.42		
-16.5	-20.50			**-16.5**	-13.77		
-17.0	-21.36			**-17.0**	-14.12		
-17.5	-22.15			**-17.5**	-14.46		
-18.0	-23.00			**-18.0**	-14.80		
-18.5	-23.78			**-18.5**	-15.14		
-19.0	-24.61			**-19.0**	-15.47		

Contd...

Contd...

-19.5	-25.50	**-19.5**	-15.80
-20.0	-26.32	**-20.0**	-16.13
		-20.5	-16.45
		-21.0	-16.77
		-21.5	-17.09
		-22.0	-17.41
		-22.5	-17.72
		-23.0	-18.03
		-23.5	-18.33
		-24.0	-18.63
		-24.5	-18.93
		-25.0	-19.23
		-25.5	-19.53
		-26.0	-19.82
C 2001 Hoffer-Dementiev		**-26.5**	-20.11

CLINICAL RULES

1. Cycloplegic Rx must be less minus than manifest Rx in myopes.
2. Cycloplegic Rx must be more plus than manifest Rx in hyperopes.
3. If cycloplegic Rx is different, see if patient can accept full cycloplegic correction.
4. Best to attempt correction of cycloplegic Rx in hyperopes and manifest Rx in myopes.
5. Hyperopic patients 18-35 can accommodate a small undercorrection (up to +1.00).
6. Myopic patients 18-35 should not be overcorrected but left emmetropic or small myopia.
7. All patients 36-50 must obtain emmetropia or slight overcorrection (up to -1.00)
8. If cylinder is not to be corrected, using the SE plans for PO mixed astigmatism.
9. If correcting cylinder prior to PRL, use the SE of the resultant healed refraction.
10. If correcting cylinder after the PRL:
    a. If your astigmatic surgical correction will not change the average K, use the SE
    b. If your astigmatic surgical correction will change the average K (flatten), use the sphere only.

concluded that the iridectomy's size and placement is very important.

INSTRUMENTATION (FIG. 25.8)

A. **INCISION**

Incision trapezoid diamond Dementiev blade for clear cornea incision 3.0-3.2-3.5 mm (Rumex Int, USA).

B. **PARACENTESIS**

Dementiev diamond paracentesis 1.0 mm blade (Rumex Int).

C. **IMPLANT LOADING**

PRL titanium loading block (DK, UK) (Fig. 25.9).

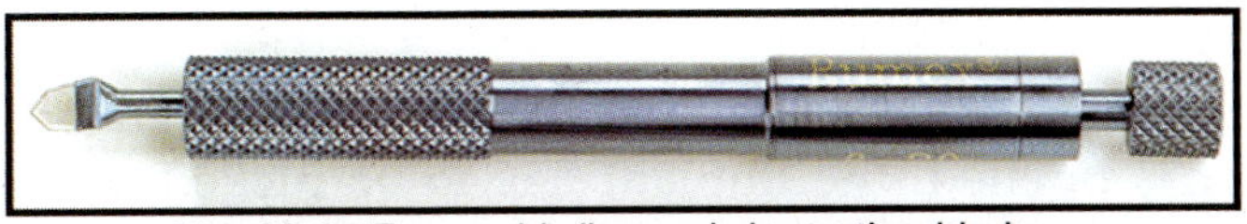

Fig. 25.8: Trapezoid diamond dementiev blade

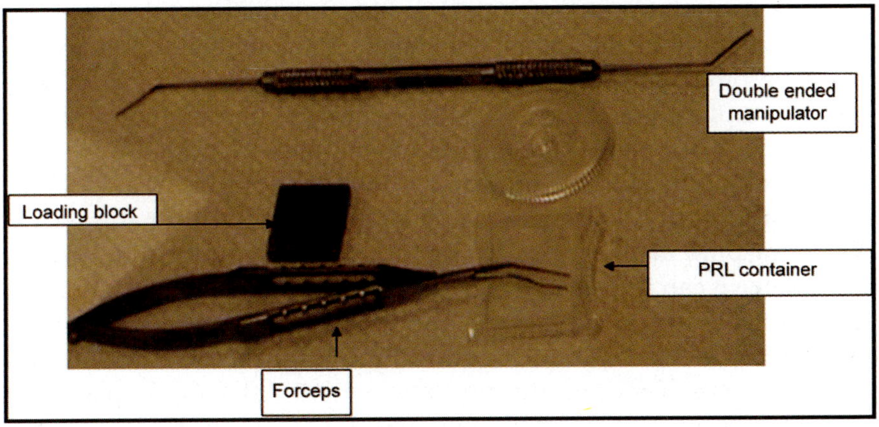

Fig. 25.9

D. **INSERTION**
Titanium Dementiev forceps for PRL implantation (DK, UK). Titanium diamond dust covered Dementiev PRL forceps (Rumex Int, USA) (Figs 25.10A and B).

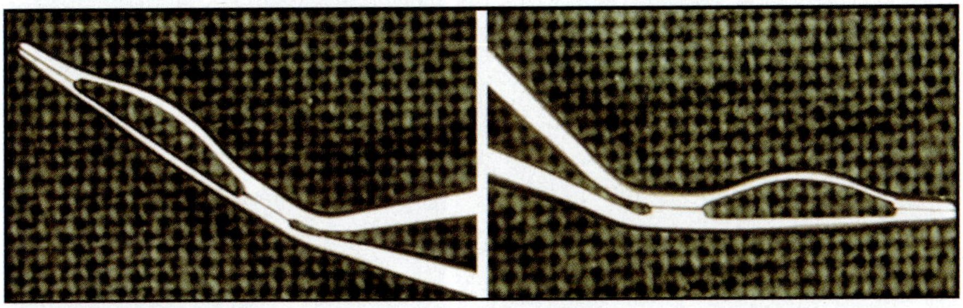

Figs 25.10A and B: Titanium diamond dust covered Dementiev PRL forceps

E. **MANIPULATION**
Dementiev PRL titanium double ended haptic spatula (DK,UK). Dementiev PRL titanium diamond dust covered manipulator (Rumex Int, USA).

F. **IRIDECTOMY**
PRL set for manual iridectomy (iris scissors + iris forceps) (Rumex Int, USA).

G. **OTHER** Standard blepharostat and eye fixation forceps (Rumex Int, USA).

Handling the Implant

The PRL implant is supplied in a plastic sterile container. After the container is opened, the implant has to be picked up using PRL Dementiev forceps. It is important to be careful to be sure that the lens does not come into contact with the skin, conjunctiva, lids, lashes or epithelium of the cornea because some microelements can be attracted to and become deposited on the lens surface. It is necessary to be sure that the implant is grasped with the forceps in the correct position. The anterior surface of the lens should be up and posterior surface should be down. This can be seen by observing the fact that the PRL has a similar convexity (curvature) paralleling that of the natural lens. While grasping the lens with the forceps, do not squeeze too hard it's optics since it can be easy damaged. Implant is put on the PRL loading block, after that is grasped by the forceps in length.The edge of the implant has to correspond to the end of the forceps. We do not fold the lens; it is self-folding during its insertion. After the implant has been grasped in the correct manner and orientated in the forceps, we irrigate it profusely using BSS from a syringe. It is important to inspect it carefully and with fine forceps gently remove any foreign particulate matter or fibers that may have become attached to its surface. The lens is now ready for insertion (Fig. 25.11).

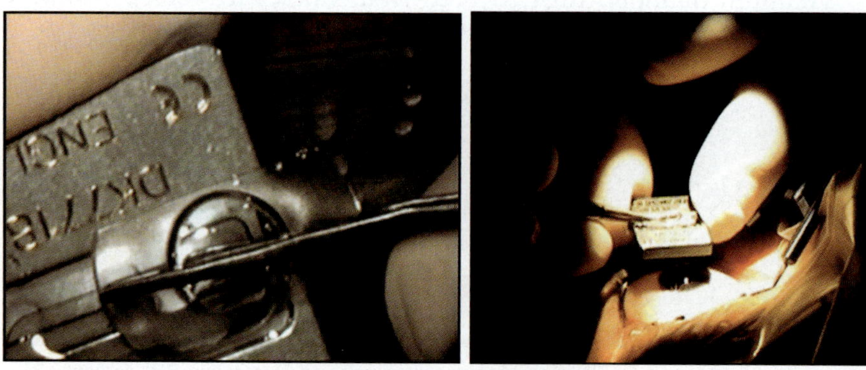

Fig. 25.11: Handling the PRL

SURGICAL STEPS

Do not start the surgery if the pupil is not wider than 5.0 mm.

Incision

Usually, the incision is placed at the temporal cornea. Our experience recommends performing a clear corneal, self-sealing incision of 3.0-3.2 mm in width. The incision can be made with either a diamond or stainless steel blade.

Any method of fixation may be used to ensure that there is no possibility of the blade contacting the anterior lens capsule since the pupil is widely dilated. The incision architecture should be one the surgeon is familiar with for self-sealing cataract surgery. Non-suture closure is the intended aim.

Viscoelastic Insertion

Next the anterior chamber should be filled with viscoelastic to achieve a chamber of not less than 3.0 mm in depth. It is also helpful to place some viscoelastic under the iris to make more room to facilitate lens insertion in the posterior chamber.

Paracentesis (Figs 25.12A to C)

This incision is needed to perform the iridectomy and to create an additional entry point for the lens manipulator that will be needed in the next step to position the PRL in the posterior chamber.

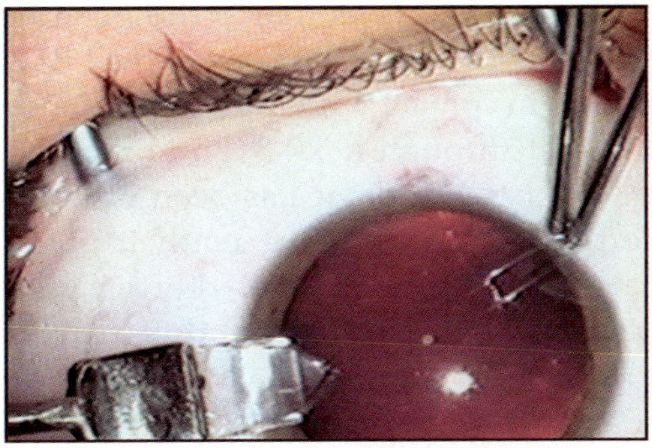

3.0 mm clear cornea incision

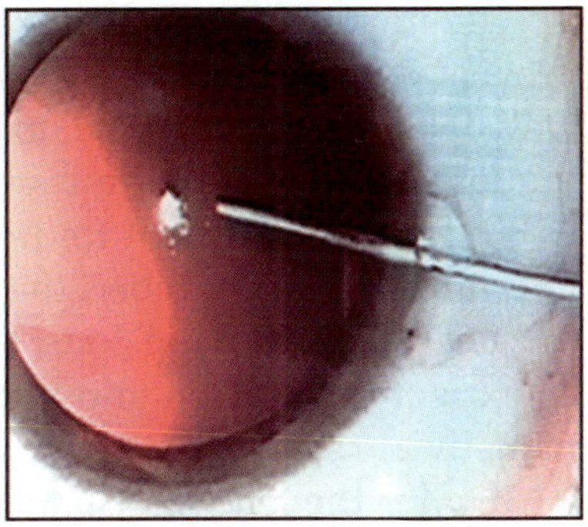

Visco insertion

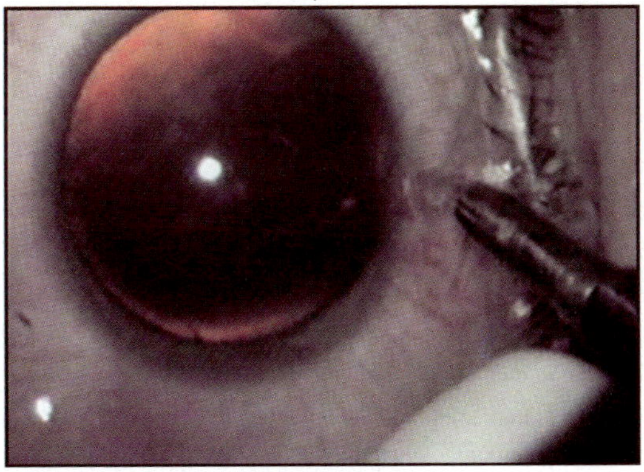

Paracentesis

Fig. 25.12

We make it no larger than 0.5 mm and it should be placed at the 12:00 position. It can be made with a stainless steel or diamond knife. The position of the knife has to be perpendicular to the cornea surface and the cut has to be made at the limbus so that the iridectomy will be more basal. This will avoid:

1. Light passing through the iridectomy and the upper lid will cover it (less halos),
2. The possibility of the iridectomy being blocked by the edge of the PRL (pupillary block).

Lens Insertion

This is the most important and delicate step of the procedure.

The surgeon has to be extremely careful:

1. Not to damage the implant (very soft, thin and rather expensive),
2. Not to damage the anterior capsule with the forceps,
3. Not to touch the endothelium with the implant or the forceps.

The implant is grasped by the special forceps that is designed to prevent damage to the PRL (protection of the optical zone of the PRL). Only the haptic area of the implant is in contact with the forceps. Since the lens is very thin, we can insert it through a 3.0-3.2 mm incision without any additional folding. After the implant has been inserted into the anterior chamber, the forceps must be opened gently to allow for the release of the lens. Care must be taken that there are no unexpected sudden movements of the eye during this crucial maneuver.

If, after the lens is inserted, it is discovered that it is upside down it, is necessary to correct this (Figs 25.13A to D).

Retro-iris Placement and Centration

Next, we must manipulate the peripheral edges of the implant under the iris. Using the spatula-PRL manipulator (entered through the paracentesis at 12:00), we move the two lateral edges of the lens under the pupil margin and under the iris. In this step, it is very important to pay maximum attention so as not to put pressure on the crystalline lens capsule. It is important to avoid anterior capsule and cortical damage. It is very important not to push too hard to get it under, but rather try to fold it with the spatula and then release it under the iris to avoid damage to the zonular fibers. When all four "feet" are under the iris satisfactorily, the PRL optic zone is then gently centered using the same manipulator.

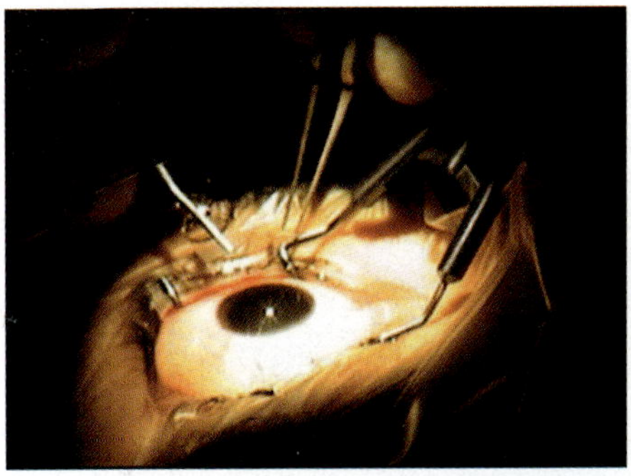

PRL is loaded in the forceps

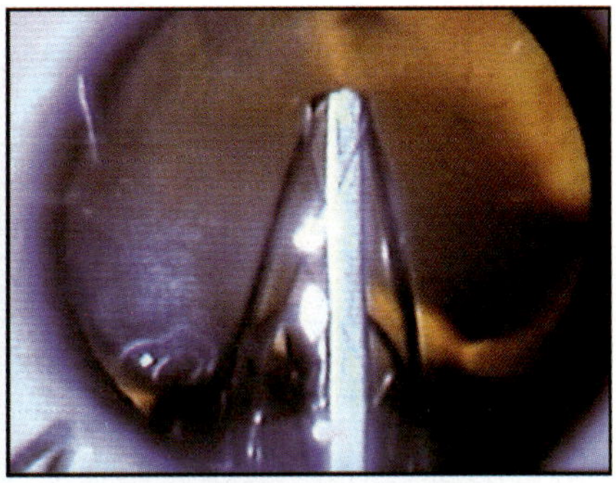

PRL insertion (self folded)

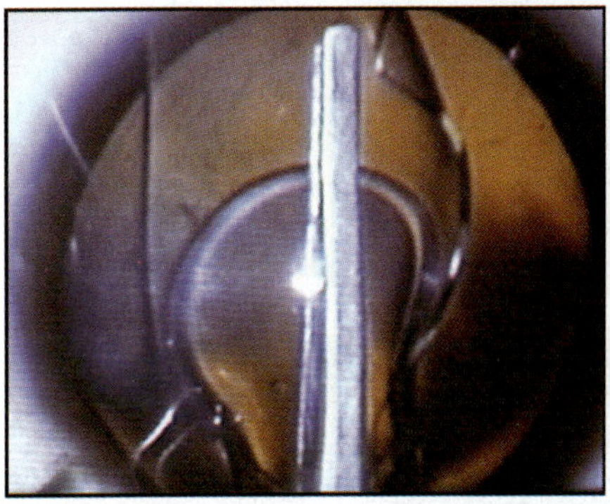

PRL opening in the AC

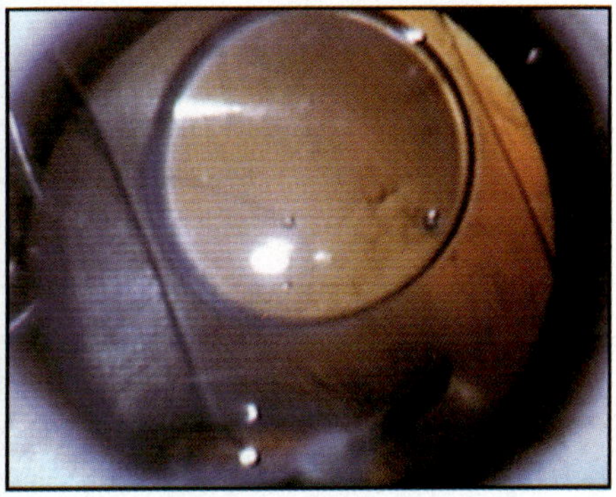

Under iris placement

Fig. 25.13

Iridectomy

I prefer to perform the iridectomy at 12:00 through the paracentesis site. The iridectomy has to be as peripheral as possible. This decreases the risk of the PRL blocking it. During this step, bleeding is possible. If this should happen, I prefer to reinject viscoelastic in the area of bleeding to act as a tamponade. After an appropriate waiting period (and clotting has occurred), the viscoelastic must again be removed (Fig. 25.14).

Viscoelastic Removal

We now must try to remove all the viscoelastic by irrigation. It is extremely important to remove as much as possible and not to leave any in the anterior or posterior chamber. If this is not accomplished it may create (Fig. 25.15).

1. Postoperative IOP increase,
2. Viscoelastic crystallization between the anterior capsule and the posterior surface of the implant.

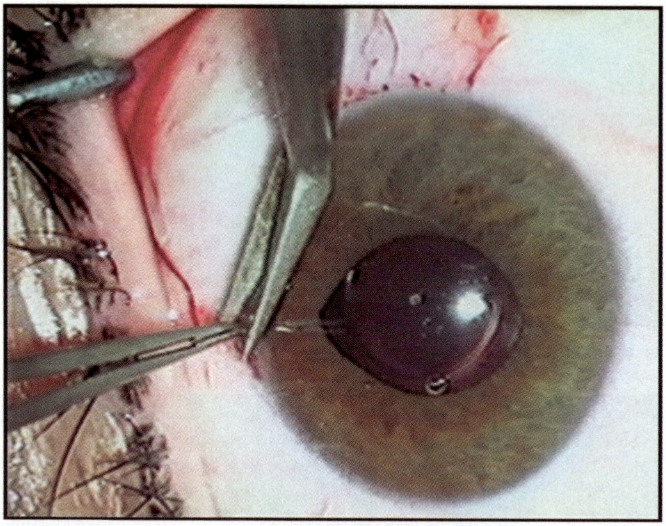

Fig. 25.14: Surgical PI

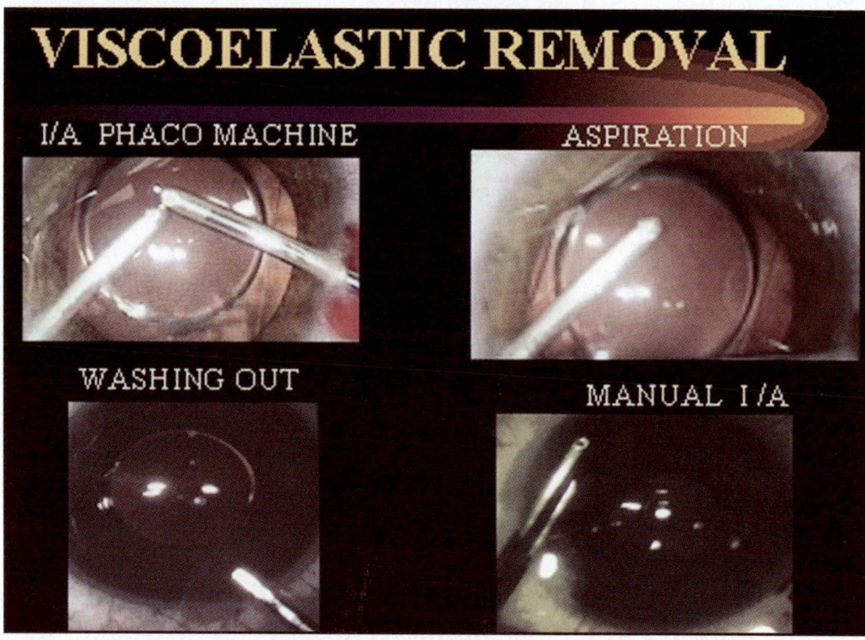

Fig. 25.15: Viscoelastic removal

If it is not possible to remove all the viscoelastic by irrigation, irrigation-aspiration may be used, but be thoughtful of damaging the endothelial cells.

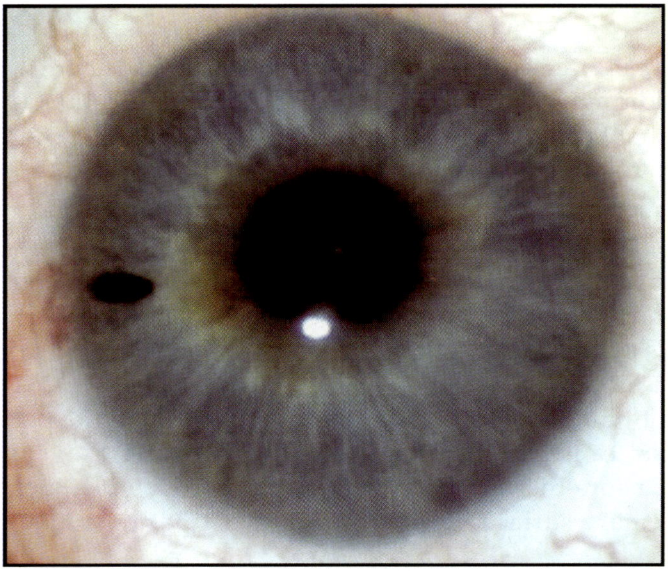

Fig. 25.16: No stitches are needed

Pupil Constriction

It is important to constrict the pupil as much as possible before the iridectomy is performed. We recommend injecting acetylcholine solution into the AC to accomplish this.

Incision Closure

Is not necessary unless security of wound closure is in doubt (Fig. 25.16).

Patch

Placing a patch on the eye is not obligatory.

OPERATIVE COMPLICATIONS

Implant Damage

Damage to the implant can occur during its insertion into the AC if the special forceps are not used. It can also happen during its release and manipulation under the iris. Both the surgeon and the technician must be very careful when the lens is taken from the package and inserted into the forceps. Do not forget that the implant is very thin and rather expensive and can be damaged easily.

Hemorrhage

Bleeding can occur during the manual surgical iridectomy. It should not be common. If it happens, is recommended injecting some viscoelastic through the paracentesis and wait several minutes for the bleeding to stop, then remove it.

Iris Damage

It is possible to damage the posterior pigment surface of the iris with the implant, so we recommend injecting viscoelastic under the iris to avoid this complication. The surgeon has to be very careful during the manual iridectomy:

1. Do not pull and tear the iris strenuously through the paracentesis; this can cause iris damage and actual bleeding,
2. But, be sure that the iridectomy is completely open including the pigmentary surface of the iris, to prevent postoperative pupillary block.

Lens Damage

The worst complication that the surgeon can have during the actual procedure is the immediate creation of lens damage and a cataract. One must always be ready to convert the surgery (in case of lens damage) to phacoemulsification with IOL implantation.

The lens can be damaged in the following steps of the surgery:

1. Corneal incisions: due to sudden knife insertion or eyeball movement.
2. Paracentesis: due to insufficient viscoelastic in the AC, too quick blade movement, or eyeball movement.
3. Implant insertion: due to contact between the forceps and the anterior capsule of the lens.
4. Implant manipulation: due to pushing the implant on the lens.
5. Viscoelastic removal: due to inadvertent movement of irrigation or aspiration needle, and excessively forceful BSS irrigation.

Endothelial Damage

Inadequate viscoelastic protection may allow endothelial cell damage during the implant insertion. It is necessary to be sure to avoid contact of the forceps with the endothelium. The implant lens is soft, but it is made of silicone and studies have shown that silicone contact can be damaging to endothelial cells. My experience has shown, however that even if the edge of the lens touches the endothelium damage has not been noticed. This may be due to the high endothelial cell density in this age range.

Zonular Fiber Damage

Pushing the implant too strenuously under the iris may cause the edge of the implant to damage the zonular fibers. We have to remember that there are a large number of zonular fibers that stretch across the anterior periphery of the lens capsule. This could lead to implant dislocation and optic zone decentration in the future. That is why we try to fold and then release the implant allowing it to go under the iris never pushing it there with force.

UNUSUAL SITUATIONS AND POSTOPERATIVE COMPLICATIONS

IOP Increase on First or Second Day PO

The patient feels pain in the eye, complains of vision loss, or headache in the temple.

Slit lamp examination: The chamber may be shallow, pupil does not react to light or is sluggish, residual viscoelastic is noted in the AC or PC, the gap between the PRL and the anterior capsule is larger.

Be sure to check the patency of the iridectomy (visual and red reflex).

What to do?

a. Treat the iridectomy: If it is small or closed by making it larger or making an additional one (possible YAG).
b. Residual viscoelastic in the chamber: Diamox up to 1.0 g a day and keep the pupil dilated to help reabsorb the viscoelastic. Use betablocker drops until the pressure is normalized.

Traumatic Catract (Lens Damage During Surgery)

What to do?

Be ready to convert the procedure to phaco with IOL implantation, keep an IOL ready in the OR with all IOL power calculations done in advance.

CONCLUSIONS

PRL implantation is:

1. Safe
2. Predictable
3. Reversible
4. Inexpensive for the doctor or the patient.
5. Able to achieve immediate and stable refractive effect.
6. Able to increase BUCVA and BCVA.

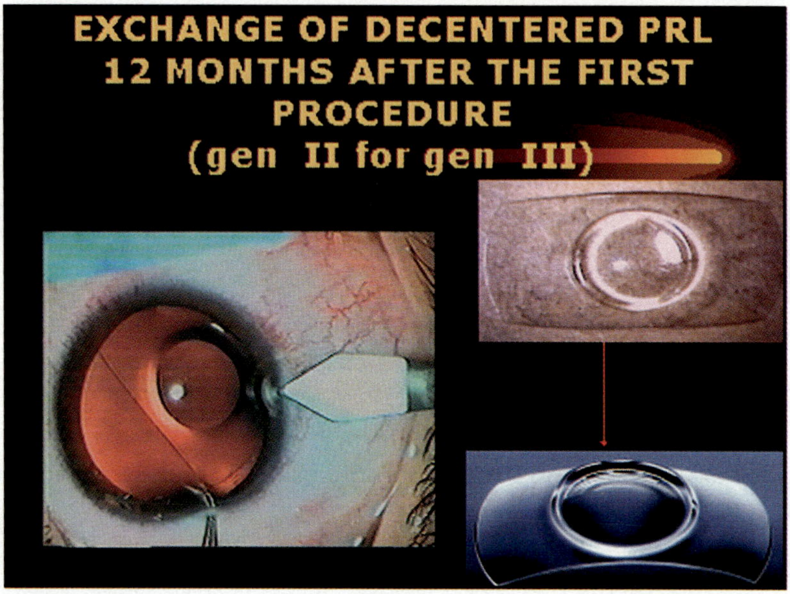

Fig. 25.17

The technique is relatively safe and easy to perform for any skilled cataract surgeon. The complications we have seen are not serious and have been treatable. The two main problems we need to look for in longer follow-up are subcapsular opacity (till now we have only one) and pigment dispersion that may lead to glaucoma. Our study shows that there is not pigment dispersion in negative-powered silicon PRLs but some slow dispersion in the positive-powered PRLs. The UBM ultrasound study showed us that the implant does not touch the anterior capsule, but we need to know more about contact between the PRL and the capsule and iris.

The goal of any refractive procedure is emmetropia, and the predictability of the PRL implantation is very promising in providing stable long-term emmetropia.

The most important point concerning PRL implantation is it reversibility. There are no refractive procedures which can be reversed. With the promising results, and more modern materials, surgical and diagnostic equipment, it will be one of the most exciting areas of ocular surgery.

PEDIATRIC USAGE

In cases of high unilateral myopia in children, PRL implantation (Fig. 25.18) can be used instead of amblyopia treatment with aniseikonic spectacles or forcing a contact lens.

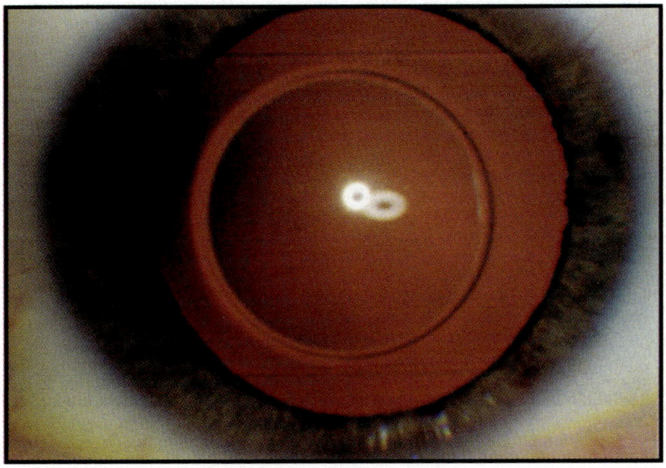

Fig. 25.18: Myopic PRL

The youngest patient in which we have implanted a myopic PRL was -14.00 D at the age of seven. Twenty months PO, 20/40 vision without correction was obtained in this amblyopic eye which was 20/100 best corrected preoperative. There are not many reasonable alternatives today to help these young patients. Spectacle correction is practically impossible and it is not easy to make them wear contact lenses. These eyes are destined to become strabismic with deep amblyopia for life. With PRL implantation, we can not only correct myopia but treat amblyopia and prevent strabismus. We prefer and recommend performing scleral reinforcing surgery one to two months prior to implantation for the purpose of slowing the growth of the eyeball. Even if the refractive error changes when the child grows to adulthood, the PRL implant can be easy exchanged and the procedure can be repeated.

We are planing to start correcting hyperopia in the near future (Fig. 25.19), but up to now, we do not have any clinical experience in hyperopic correction with PRL implantation in children. The surgical technique is the same that we use for our adult patients. The only difference is that general anesthesia is recommended, and manual iridectomy at the time of surgery is preferable.

FUTURE APPLICATIONS

Piggyback Over IOLs

When two IOLs are necessary, it is certainly conceivable that the second lens could be a posterior chamber PRL that could be easily inserted in the capsular bag or in the ciliary sulcus. In such special eyes that require piggyback lenses the calculations of IOL power are often not

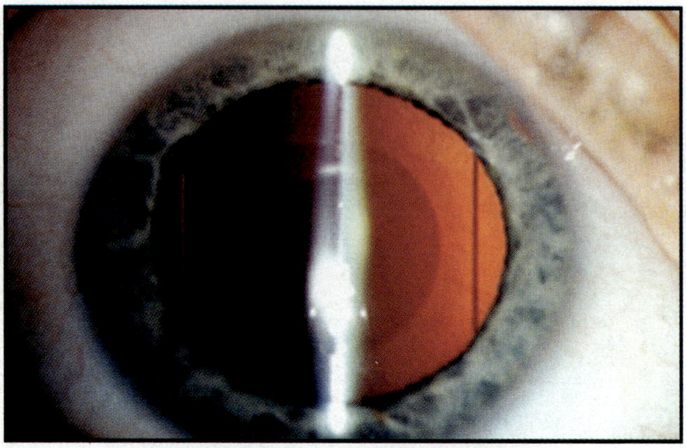

Fig. 25.19: Hyperopic PRL

as accurate and it may be necessary to exchange the more anterior lens. A PRL is much easier to remove and replace than an IOL is.

Pseudophakic Ametropia Correction

Every patient who is unhappy with the refractive results of their cataract/IOL surgery could be offered a rather simple procedure of posterior chamber PRL implantation over the top of the IOL. This would open a whole new market for the anterior segment surgeon and replace the dangers inherent in removing and replacing a well-placed IOL in the bag. Patients could be almost assured of obtaining the refractive result they desire.

Those patients that wish to try monovision could have the non dominant eye implanted with an additional appropriate plus power PRL over the emmetropic IOL. If they could not tolerate the monovision, the PRL could be easily and atraumatically slipped out.

Multifocal Correction

The posterior chamber PRL could open two fronts in the use of multifocal IOLs.

1. Any and all patients could try the concept by having an emmetropic IOL implanted with a multifocal PRL placed on top of it during their cataract removal. After the patient has had sufficient time to become accustomed to it, they could decide whether they wish to keep it or have it easily slipped out.
2. All patients who have missed the chance for getting a multifocal IOL could now have a multifocal PRL placed on top of their IOL to try it out. Again, if they did not like it, it could be easily removed. Perhaps any over or under-correction in the original IOL could also be taken into account in the PRL distance power.

PRL IMPLANTATION FOR THE CORRECTION OF HIGH AMETROPIA

Informed Consent

All visual errors can be corrected by refractive-surgery. The most advantageous application of surgery, apart from the simple esthetic-practical aspects of being able to abandon the use of spectacles and contact lenses, are the ocular and environmental conditions that prevent the optimal use of visual capacity. This understanding is critical for the high dioptric values of the visual error that tie the patient tightly to the vision-aid, in the marked differences in refraction between one eye and an other, limit binocular vision and the visual field, particularly where there is intolerance to comfortable contact lenses wearing and in some types of activity where the traditional optical aids are unquestionably contraindicated.

According to the specialist who has been treating you, you may benefit from the implantation *of a so-called Phakic Refractive Lens*, a soft, flexible implant inserted surgically inside the eye, between iris and the crystalline.

This technique, when performed correctly, has the following **advantages:**

1. The operation is rapid. It lasts 10-15 minutes. It is performed in Day-Hospital on outpatient basis, under topical anesthesia, more specifically with the sole instillation of anesthetic eye-drops and peri-ocular infiltration of anesthetic. The PRL is implanted through a small self-sealing incision measuring about 3.0 mm that normally does not require sutures. The lens is inserted with a special forceps, if it is necessary the PRL can be removed through the same incision, restoring the clinical situation and the refraction as before.
2. It is reversible technique: contrary to what happens with the corneal refractive surgery (incisional or laser), the natural structures of the eye are not modified in a unidirectional manner.
3. Visual rehabilitation is rapid. The patient can normally appreciate the visual result the next day of the surgery and the result is stable in time. We did not see the cases of vision fluctuation, it is no regression of the obtained result in follow-up.
4. The predictability of the results is high.

The Risks and Possible Problems

1. Some patients, with particularly large pupils under low light conditions complain of haloes with night vision, similar to those reported by contact lens wearers, but the brain usually adapts to this problem during the first 2-6 months after the surgery.

2. In order to avoid pupilary block and intaocular pressure increase after the PRL implantation,the periphery iridectomy will be performed (small hole in the iris) or during the surgery or by YAG laser 1-week before the procedure.
3. As we are dealing with a surgical operation that requires the eye-globe to be opened, and even through very small incisions, the risk of infection persists. In order to avoid this potentially complication preoperative and postoperative prophlaxis is necessary. (drops installation, oral medications or I/M injections in some cases).The slight inflammation is possible in immediate postoperative period.
4. The implantation of PRL runs the risk of developing opacities in the crystalline lens (cataract) in time. It should be remembered that in subjects with serious errors, especially myopic,the risk of developing a natural cataract is much higher and more precocious than in the 'normal' population. Moreover, the surgical replacement of the cataractous lens is now considered to be a routine technique, it is well-known, safe and simple, and in the vast majority of cases produces excellent results, with simultaneous correction of the myopia and the removal of the cataract.
5. There is also possible that the PRL may provoke intraocular pressure increase. In the more serious cases, the patient may feel severe pain along the trigeminal nerve irradiating from the eye to the forehead, accompanied by nausea and vomiting. This situation should be treated immediately with the oral medicamentations and drops.

Issued by Dr Dimitrii Dementiev.

The undersigned, expressing his/her full, free, unconditioned will,

First name and family name of patient.......................

Date and place of birth...

Place of residence..

Consent of the surgery of the PRL implantation. He/she declares that the information provided regarding the implications of the operation has been full and thorough. He/she declares that he/she has carefully evaluated the possible benefits and potential risks inherent to this type of surgery.

Signature of patient...

Date...

BIBLIOGRAPHY

1. A Chatitterjee, S Shah. Predictability of spherical PRK based on initial refraction. Journal of Refractive Surgery Apr 1998, 14(2) (supl).
2. A Hatsis. Silicon Posterior Chamber Intraocular Lens (P-PCIOL), American Blind Eye Study." ASCRS annual meet April 1998, San Diego, USA.
3. A Marinho, et al. Phakic IOLs: The state of the art. ASCRS annual meeting 1998, April, San Diego, USA.
4. A Marinho, M C Neves, M C Pinto, Fernando Vaz. Posterior chamber silicon phakic intraocular lens. Refrac Surg, May/June 1997, 13(3).
5. A Tereschenko. Complications of minus silicon posterior chamber phakic Lenses. ASCRS annual meet 1997, Boston, USA.
6. A.Hatsis. Phakic Posterior IOLs for the correction of high hyperopia and high myopia. ASCRS 1997, Boston,USA.
7. Asseto, Benedetti, Pesando. Collamer intraocular contact lens to correct high myopia. J Cataract Refract Surg1996;22.
8. Baikoff G, Colin J. Intraocular lenses in phakic patients. Ophthalmol Clin North Am, 1992;5.
9. Baikoff G, Joly P. Comparison of minus power anterior chamber intraocular lenses and myopic epikeratoplasty in phakic eyes. Refract Corneal Surgery 1990;6:252-60.
10. D Brown. Use of the Staar Surgical Implantable Contact Lens for High Myopia. Ascrs annual meeting 1997, April, Boston USA.
11. D Dementiev, G Rozakis, A Hatsis, K Hoffer, G Sborgia, P Marucchi. The 5 Years Experience in the Phakic Refractive Posterior Chamber IOL. Implantation for the correction of High Ametropia. Binkhorst Symposium during XXVIII International Congress of Ophthalmology, 1998 June, Amsterdam, Holland.
12. D Dementiev. Comparison of three generations of Posterior Chamber Phakic Lenses for the Correction of high myopia and hypropia. ASCRS 1997; Boston,USA.
13. D Dementiev. Silicone Phakic Posterior Chamber Intraocular Lens (P-PCIOL) and the management of pediatric Anisometropia. ASCRS annual meeting Apr1998, San Diego, USA.
14. D J Apple Complications of Phakic IOLs. AAO annual meet 1998 New Orleans.
15. E K Vorotnikova, V V Kurenkov,G S Polunin. Retreatment of regression after photorefractive keratectomy for myopia. Journal of Refractive Surgery, Apr1998, 14(2) (Sup).
16. E Tumanian, VK Zuev, TV Koslova. Hydrodynamics before and after implantation of Negative IOL in highly myopic phakic eye. Ophthalmosurgery,1997;4:50-6.
17. F Lavery. Laser in situ Keratomilesusis for Myopia. Journal of Refractive Surgery, Apr 1998, 14(2) (Sup).
18. Fechner PU. Intraocular lenses for the correction of myopia in phakic eyes: short long success and long term caution. Refract Corneal surgery 1990; 6:242-44.
19. Fechner PU. Phakic IOLs is promising for high myopia by Schonfeld AR. Ocular Surgery News 1993,4:12.
20. Fyodorov, Zuev, Aznabaev. Intraocular correction of high myopia with negative posterior chamber lens. Ophthalmosurgery 1991;3:57-8.

21. Fyodorov,Zuev, Tumanian,Suheil. Clinical and functional follow-up of minus IOL implantation in high grade myopia. Ophtalmosurgery 1993;2: 12-7.
22. G Avalos. Comparison Between LASIK and Phakic Posterior Chamber Intraocular Lenses in High Myopia and High Hyperopia. ASCRS annual meet April 1998, San Diego, USA.
23. G Avalos. Silicone Posterior Chamber Intraocular Lens(P-PCIOL) in the management of LASIK complications. ASCRS annual meet April 1998, San Diego, USA.
24. G Baikoff, et al. Angle Fixated Anterior Chamber Lens for Myopia of –7.0 to –19.0 Diopters. Journal of Refractive Surgery May/June 1998, 14(3).
25. G Baikoff. 5 years follow-up on anterior chamber phakic IOLs Chiron's ZB5-XXVIII International Congress of Ophthalmology, Amsterdam, June 1998.
26. G Baikoff. Anterior Chamber Phakic IOLs. AAO annual meeting 1998,New Orleans,USA.
27. G Baikoff. Contrast sensitivity in patients with PRK in one eye and refractive implant in the fellow eye, Last evaluation of the Phakic Myopic Baikoff lens. ASCRS annual meeting April 1997, Boston, USA.
28. G Rozakis, D Dementiev, G Avalos, A Hatsis. Complicaqtiopns of Silicon Phakic Posterior Chamber Intraocular Lens (P-PCIOL) for the Correction of High Ametropia. ASCRS annual meet Apr1998, San Diego, USA.
29. G Rozakis,D Dementiev, A Hatsis, G Avalos. Complications of Silicon Phakic Posterior Chamber Lenses for the Correction of high ammetropia. ASCRS 1998, San Diego, USA.
30. Gelender H. Corneal Endothelial Cell Loss, Cystoid Macular Edema, and irissuported intraocular lenses. Ophthalmology 1984;91: 841-6.
31. Grabby, Deitz, Fyodorov. Staar implantable contact lens(ICL). In Martin RG, Dills JP, Sanders DR (Eds.). Foldable Intraocular Lenses. Slack, INC, Thorafare, NJ 1993,pp 251-5.
32. Holladay JT. Refractive power calculation for intraocular lenses in the phakic eye. Amer J Ophthalmol 1993; 116(24):63-6.
33. I Pallicaris. Barraquer lecture. AAO annual meeting 1997, San Francisco,USA.
34. Izak M. Worst Myopia Iris Claw IOL implantation. ASCRS annual meeting, April 1997, Boston, USA.
35. J L Guell. Cataract formation after phakic IOL Implantation. World Refractive Surgery Symposium,Orlando 1998 in Eurotimes pg.15 from Oct.98.
36. J M Davidorf, R Zaldivar, S Oscherow. Posterior Chamber Phakic Intraocular Lenses for Hyperopia of +4 to +11 Diopters and Posterior Chamber Phakic Intraocular lenses for Myopia of –8.0 to –19.0 Diopters J. Refract Surg May/June 1998, 14(3).
37. JGF Worst. Iris Anatomy and its Surgical Implications. XXVIII International Congress of Ophtalmology, June 1998,Amsterdam, Holland.
38. JGF Worst. Recent improvements in phakic refrative correction with Iris Claw Lens. ASCRS annual meeting 1998, San Diego USA.
39. JJ Saragoussi, M Puech, M Assouline, G Reard, Y Pouliquen. Ultrasound Biomicroscopy of Baikoff Anterior Chamber Phakic Intraocular Lenses. Journal of Refractive Surgery, March-April 1997, 13(2).
40. K J Hoffer. Predicting silicon phakic posterior chamber IOL power in the management of high hyperopia" ASCRS ann. meet Apr1998 San Diego, USA.
41. Kanski J. Clinical Ophthalmology. Butterworth Ltd., 1989, 360.

42. Landesz M., Worst JGF, Siertsema JV, Van Rij G. Correction of High Myopia with the Worst Myopia Claw Intraocular Lens. XXVIII International Congress of Ophtalmology, June 1998, Amsterdam, Holland.
43. Luger M H A. The Staar Collamer phakic posterior chamber IOL to correct myopia and hyperopia. XXVIIIth ICO, Amsterdam 1998.
44. M Alberti. PRK and Lasik Versus Intraocular Contact Lenses for High Myopia Correction Ascrs annual meeting Boston,USA.
45. M Hodkin, M.M.Lemos, M.B. McDonald, J.Holladay, S.H.Shhidi. Near vision sensitivity after photorefractive keratectomy. J.of Cataract Refractive Surgery, March 1997, 23(2).
46. P Brauweiler, M Busin, T Wehler. High incidence of cataract formation after implantation of a silicon Posterior Chamber Lens in Phakic, highly myopic eyes. AAO annual meeting 1998 New Orleans, USA.
47. Phakic high myopia correction, J.Worst ASCRS meet 1997 Boston.
48. R Zaldivar, J Davidorf, S Osheraw. Intarocular Contact Lens" in Lasik 2000 of L Buratto. M.Ferrari.Fabiano Editore, Belbo(CN), 1998.pp 359-75.
49. Saragoussi JJ, et al. Damage to the Corneal Endothelium by Minus Power Anterior Chamber Intraocular Lenses. Refract Corneal Surg 1991;7.
50 Sosnier Z. Evaluation of the effect of Synder-Thompson scleroplasty based on the behavior of the axial dimension of the eye ball. Klin Oczna 1989 Jan;91:19-20.
51. Strampelli B. Supportalita di lenti acriliche in camera anteriore nella afachia e nai vizi di r refrazione. Ann Ottalmol Clin Oculist 1954;80:70-82.
52. T Werblin "Barraquer lecture" AAO annual meeting 1998, New Orleans, USA.
53. Tarutta E, Saksanova E.Peripheral segments of the fundus oculi in highly myopic patients after scleroplasty. Vestn Opht1991 Jul-Aug;107 (4):19-23.
54. Tratta E, Shamlokova E.An analysis of the late results of scleroplasty in progressive myopia. Ophthal Zh1989; (4):204-7.
55. Tumanian E. Surgical correction of high myopia by the method of implantation of negative phakic IOL. In Russian, Diss Kand Medic 1989; 15864.
56. U Kariger. Refractive Baikoff Anterior Chamber Lenses Implantation. ASCRS 1997.
57. Woo GC., Wilson MA. Current methods of treating and preventing myopia. Optometry and vision science. 1990;67 (9):719-27.
58. Y Wang, K Zhao, H Wang. 14(2) (Sup). Histopatoplgy of corneal wound healing after PRK in rabbit eyes. Jornal of Refractive Surgery, Apr.1998 Vol 14, N.2 (supl.)
59. Zaikova M, Molokova N.Scleroplasty results in progressive myopia with use of allogenic. Vestn Opht 1990 May-June;106(3):16-9.

CHAPTER

26

Juan C Rocco (Argentina)

Anterior Chamber Phakic IOL with Angle Fixation

ADVANTAGES

The validity of the concept of a myopic implant has been proven by 30 years of experience with the Kelman's multiflex implant (Fig. 26.1).

Nowadays we have near of 20 years of use of the first Baikoff model and a lot of happy ex-high myopic patients.

With these techniques we have a lot of advantages like: excellent visual results; fast visual recovery; preservation of accommodation; easy operation technique to anterior chamber surgeon; reversibility; the possibility to combine with excimer laser surgery in very high myopic patients; the option to correct astigmatism with the phakic IOL and the predictability of visual result.

Since the standard deviation of the residual postoperative refraction is in near one diopter, in almost all the patients, which appears to be the best of all the refractive surgical techniques and also is a very reproducible surgery (Fig. 26.2).

In the past there was concern about the long-term potential damage to anterior chamber structures, meanly the endothelial loss, but with the new lens design are safer and this problem is almost disappear. In these last years we can see a lot of very good result and with a precise technique is a very useful options for patients with high myopia (Fig. 26.3).

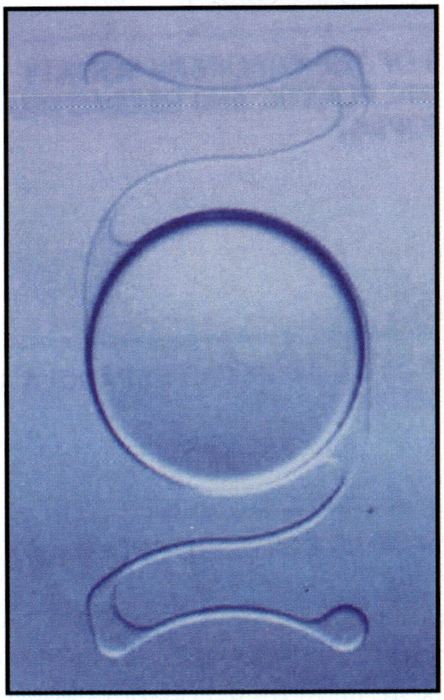

Fig. 26.1

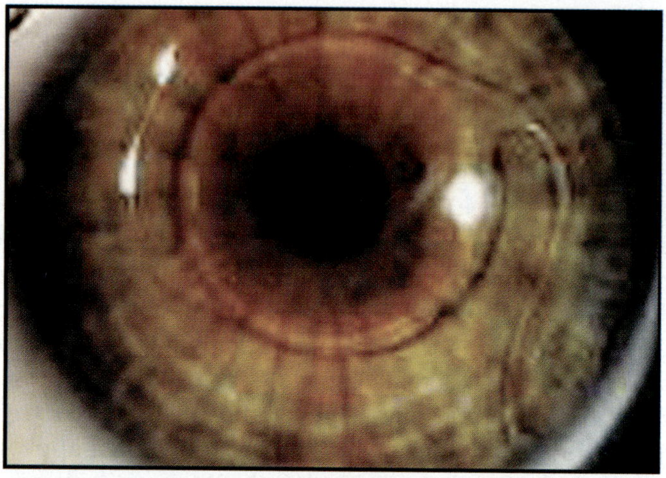

Fig. 26.2

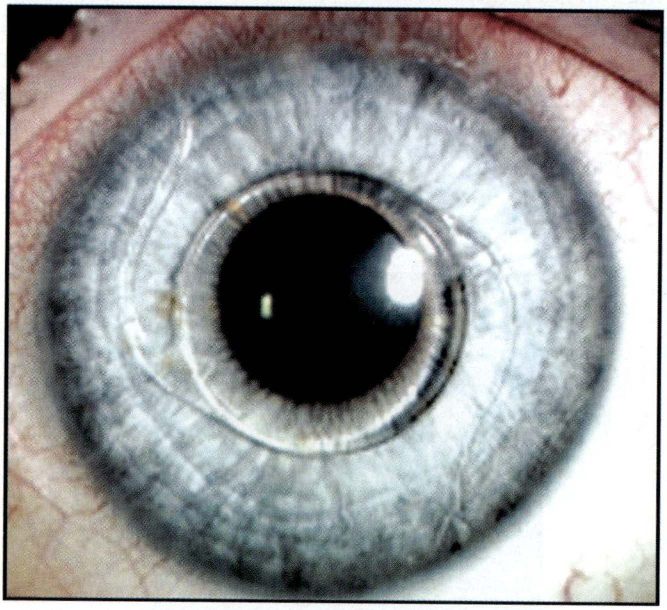

Fig. 26.3

HISTORY

The use of anterior chamber lens to correct myopia was developed first time in 1950s by Strampelli et al and Barraquer and Choyce et al, also Fechner and colleagues with the "Worst-Fechner iris claw"(Fig. 26.4). and Praeger and Baikoff, all of them collaborated to develop this option for high myopic patients.

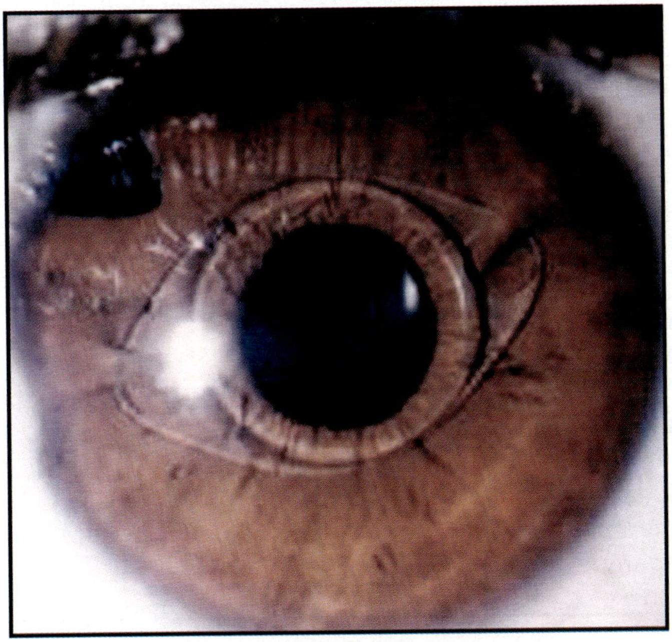

Fig. 26.4

After that Joly in 1987 modified the Kelman Multiflex four-point fixations lens that was used to cataract surgery and now it is used in anterior chamber to correct high myopia.

The first generation of this kind of lens to correct myopia was designed by Dr George Baikoff and the Company Domilens in France, and was called Baikoff ZB Lens.

This was a Z shaped haptic derived from the Kelman's Multiflex type, which allows a certain suppleness of the lens that can adapt to the different dimensions of the anterior chamber. The footplates were too large to avoid the iris wrapping. This model was designed with 25 degree vaulting to project in front and very near of pupil and have to maintain a distance about 2 mm back from the central cornea and about 1 mm in front of the pupil. Its optic was 4.50 mm and the thickness of the edges is 0.7 mm.

There was a lot of complications with this model, mainly a high rate of endothelial loss because an excessive contact between the optic edge and the peripheral endothelium.

Dr Baikoff realized of this problem and modificated the angle of the lens and was born the new model ZB5M, to reduce the contact between the lens and the peripheral epithelium and gained 0.6 mm of space between the cornea and the lens, in comparation with the ZB lens.

The first model has to be explanted in several patients for high rate of endothelial loss, but the last model was safer and predicable because the loss of endothelial cells occurs only mainly during the operation, but the first model the endothelial loss appeared during and after the surgery.

TYPES OF PHAKIC LENS

Morcher GMBH 93 A (Fig. 26.5)

- Plano concave
- PMMA
- UV rays block
- Length: 12.50 mm to 13.00 mm
- Posterior angle 19º
- Optic size: 5.50 mm
- Diopters range: –6.00 diopters to – 22.00 diopters
- Company: Morcher GMBH.

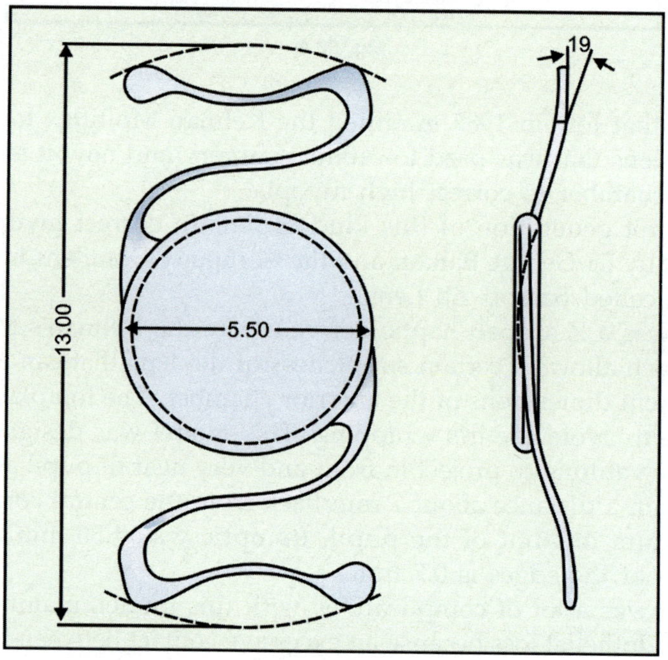

Fig. 26.5

Baikoff Model ZB5MF(Fig. 26.6)

- Biconcave
- PMMA
- UV rays block

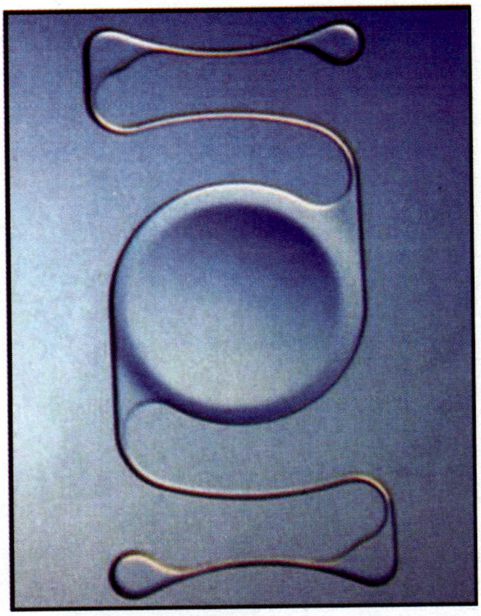

Fig. 26.6

- Length: 12.50 mm, 13.00 mm, 13.50 mm
- Posterior angle 20º
- Optic size: 5 mm
- Diopters range: – 7.00 diopters to – 20.00 diopters
- Company: Domilens.

Phakic 6 Model 130 (Fig. 26.7)

- Biconcave
- PMMA
- UV Block
- Length: From 12.00 mm to 14.00 mm
- Posterior angle 14º
- Optic size: 6 mm
- Diopters range: –2.00 diopters to – 25.00 diopters
- Company: Ophthalmic Innovations International Inc.

Nuvita Baikoff MA 20 (Fig. 26.8)

- Biconcave
- PMMA
- UV block
- Length: From 12.50 mm to 13.50 mm
- Optic size: 4.50 diopter
- Diopter range: From – 7.00 diopters to – 20.00 diopters
- Company: Bausch & Lomb.

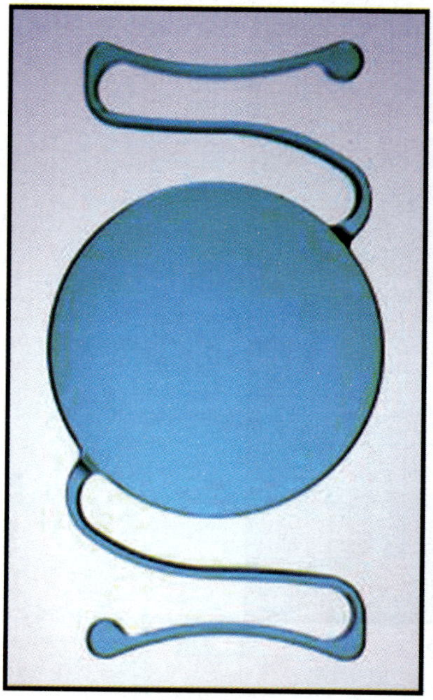

Fig. 26.7

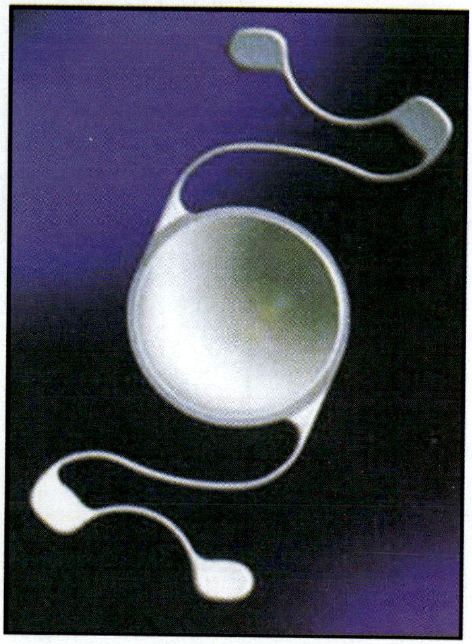

Fig. 26.8

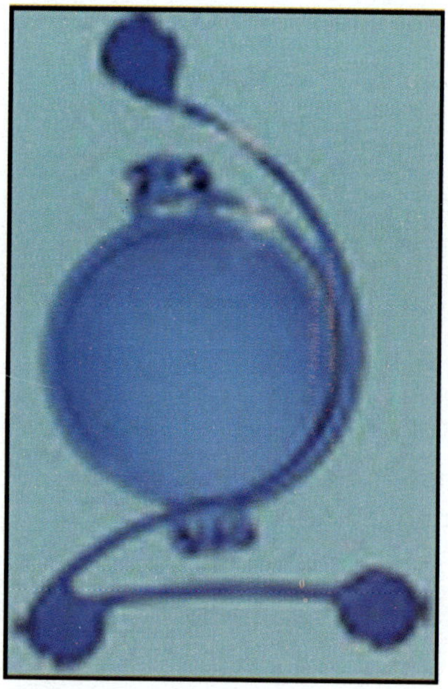

Fig. 26.9

Kelmnan Duet (Fig. 26.9)

- Two pieces
- Haptic PMMA
- Optic foldable

- Length: 12.00 mm – 13.00 mm – 13.50 mm
- Optic size: 5.50 mm
- Diopter range: From – 8.00 diopters to –20.00 diopters
- Company: Tekia, Inc.

INCLUSION CRITERIA

The selection process must be very strict and the patients must have real expectative before surgery.

The patient will be refraction stable atleast 8 months; older than 21 years old, has a myopia between – 4.00 diopters to – 22.00 diopters; has problem with using contact lens; can not wear spectacles (for a physic appearance or work restriction); endothelial cell density greater than 2.500 cell/mm; anterior chamber depther than 3.4 mm; without any eye disease like: glaucoma, uveitis, retinal detachment, conjunctivitis, autoimmune disease; any retinal problem must be treated before the surgery (retinal photocoagulation).

Before surgery we need know exact manifest and cycloplegic refraction, visual acuity, slit lamp examination, direct and indirect ophthalmoscopy,occular pressure, pupil diameter.

SURGICAL TECHNIQUE

The patient has to firm informed consent.

The decision to use phakic lens to correct myopia should be rigorously studied. The power of the implant can be determined using a mathematical calculation, using the formula of Van der Heijde and coauthors, that takes into account the keratometry, the depth of the anterior chamber and the amount of refraction.

Same manufacturer advice the use of theoretical tables to determine the exact diopters of each phakic lens.

A much simpler and useful way to do it is take the refraction of the patient's eyeglasses in spherical equivalent very precise, is recommended use autorefractometry and skiascopy using cycloplegic drops. If a patient has –10.00 diopters of myopia, we have to use a –10.00 diopters phakic lens, for a-15.00 diopters of myopia we have to use a phakic lens of –14.00 and for a myopia of –22.00 diopters we use a –20.00 diopters phakic lens.

In any case is preferable to leave the patient slightly under corrected by 1 or 2 diopters that are better than over correction.

Each phakic lens company use different approach to calculate the lens.

To choose the phakic lens's length was selected by measuring the horizontal white-to-white distance and we add 1.00 mm to this distance, in general 60% of the lens is of 12.50 mm; 30% of 13.00 mm and 10% of 12.00 mm.

One day before surgery the patient received 500 mg of acetazolamide orally and ciprofloxazine (drops) four times a day.

Who wear contact lenses, this will be remove ten days before surgery. Is recommended gave sedation via oral for a quiet surgery.

One hour before surgery, we constrict pupil with 2% pilocarpine for a easy and non-complication introduction of lens.

Clean the whole eye zone and lashes with betadine 2%. Before the introduction xilocaine intracamerular, we use topic proparacaine five drops.

Collocation speculum and drape de lid's border.

Paracenthesis in anterior chamber and introduction of 2 cc. Xilocaine 10% and filled with viscoelastic material.

A 6 mm corneoscleral incision was made in the steeped meridian if the patient has astigmatism.

Introduction a special silicone glide in the anterior chamber and re-fill with viscoelastic substance, then with a forceps the phakic IOL is inserted in anterior chamber in front of the iris, with very carefully to touch any structure of anterior chamber like iris, lens, endothelium or angle iridocorneal.

We use the silicone glide to push the lens very slowly into the eye until the upper portion of the lens and with the help of forceps, is introduced behind the limbus in contact with the angle iridous-corneal.

After that introduce a air bubble in anterior chamber with the object to put back the Phakic lens and ensure a good position and it is rotate with Sinskey hook to get a good centration with the pupil.

A small peripheral iridotomy is performed with mini scissors (Vannas) to prevent any rise of intraocular pressure in the post-operative period (Fig. 26.10).

It is very important to carefully remove all the viscoelastic material of the anterior chamber, because if remain, same of this substance can produce endothelium edema and increase intraocular pressure.

A single nylon 10.0 was used to close the incision and the eyes were not occluded after surgery.

We prescribe drops of ciprofloxacine and prednisolone 1% four times a day, during 15 days and are examined in 1,3,6 and 15 days.

The suture is removed when the astigmatism is controlled.

COMPLICATIONS

Pupil ovalization: Pupil ovalization is discrete and non-progressive, occurred along the axis of the lens. In general has no symptoms, only the appearance (Fig. 26.11).

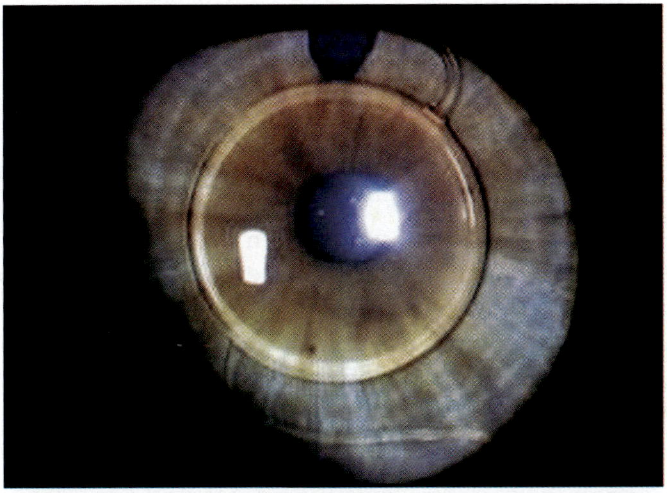

Fig. 26.10

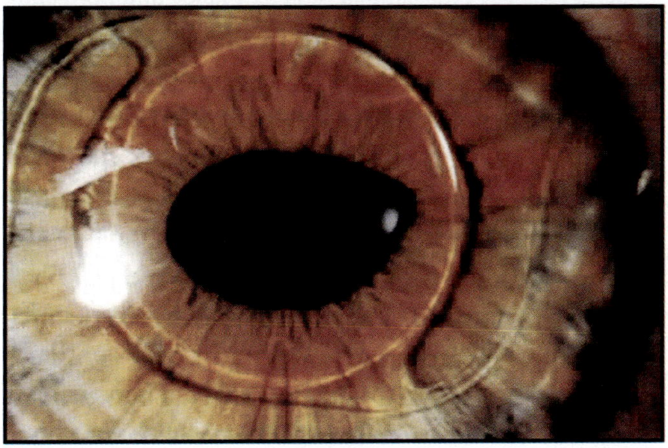

Fig. 26.11

Halos and glare: These may appear in any time,this phenomenon is because the small diameter of the optic zone; more common in lights eye color and it is relation with pupil diameter in dim light.

Giant papillary conjunctivitis: It is related with nylon suture, but if you use only one suture and hide the knot, is very strange that appear.

Postoperative uveitis: Only appear in 2% of the cases, one can see cells in anterior chamber, but disappear with use of corticosteroid eye drops.

Elevated intraocular pressure: In 22% of the operated eyes; is transitory and is related with the use of corticosteroid eye drops and material viscoleastic that isn't removed after the surgery.

Lense rotation: Lens rotation is rare (only 4%) if one made a good measurement of white to white to choose a good phakic lens, it appear when the lens is too small. If the rotation is evident and persist, the lens will be replace for a bigger one.

CONCLUSION

The essential problem with this technique remains the long-term effect on the endothelium, although with the new models this damage is very low and is not a real problem now like in the past. The results in all authors is very satisfactory and was determined that endothelial damage mainly is produced during the surgery and improving the technique and using correct instruments and viscoelastic material, this is an efficiency, precise, predictable, reproducible, stable and safety option to correct myopia.

BIBLIOGRAPHY

1. Alió JL, de la Hoz F, Perez-Santoja JJ, et al. Phakic anterior chamber lenses for the correction of myopia; A 7 years cumulative analysis of complication in 263 cases. Ophthalmology 1999; 106:458-66.
2. American Academy of Ophthalmology. Keratophakia and keratomileusis: safety and effectiveness. (Ophthalmic Procedures Assessment). Ophthalmology 1992; 99:1332-41.
3. Arenas-Archilla E, Sánchez-Thorin JC, Naranjo-Uribe JP, Hernandez-Lozano A. Myopic keratomileusis in situ: a preliminary report. J Cataract Refract Surg 1991; 17:424-35.
4. Ayala-Espinosa MJ, Claramonte Meseguer P, Artola Roig A, et al. Queratectomía fotorrefractiva en ojos implantados con lente intraocular de cámara anterior en ojos fáquicos. Arch Soc Esp Oftalmol 1998; 73:515-20.
5. Baikoff G, Arne JL, Bokobza Y, et al. Angle-fixated anterior chamber phakic intraocular lens for myopia of –7 to –19 diopters. J Refract Surg 1998; 14:282-93.
6. Baikoff G, Joly P. Comparison of minus power anterior chamber intraocular lenses and myopic epikeratoplasty in phakic eyes. Refract Corneal Surg 1990; 6:252-60.
7. Baikoff G. The refractive IOL in a phakic eye. Ophthalmic Pract 1991; 9:58-61,80.
8. Barraquer J. Anterior chamber plastic lenses. Results and conclusions from 5 years´experience. Trans Ophthalmol Soc UK 1959; 79: 393-424.
9. Barraquer J. Anterior chamber plastic lenses. Results of and conclusions from five years'experience. Trans Ophthalmol Soc U K 1959; 79:393-424.
10. Barraquer JI. Keratomileusis for myopia and aphakia. Ophthalmology 1981; 88: 701-8.
11. Bas AM, Nano HD Jr. In situ myopic keratomileusis, results in 30 eyes at 15 months. Refract Corneal Surg 1991;7:223-31.
12. Choyce DP. Polysulfone corneal inlays to correct refractive errors. Cataract 1985; 2(6): 6-11.
13. Choyce DP. The present status of intracamerular and intracorneal implants. Can J Ophthalmol 1968; 3: 295-321.

14. Collin J, Mimouni F, Robinet A, et al. The surgical treatment of high myopia: comparison epikeratoplasty, keratomileusis and minus power anterior chamber lenses. Refract Corneal Surg 1990; 6:245-51.
15. Fechner PU, Van der Heijde GL, Worst JGF. Intraokulare linse zur Myopiekorrektion des phaken Auges. Klin Monatsbl Augenheilkd 1988; 193:29-34.
16. Fechner PU, van der Heijde GL, Worst JGF. Intraukulare Linse zur Myopiekorrektion des phaken Auges. Klin Monatsbl Augenheilkd 1988; 193:29-34.
17. Fechner PU, van der Heijde GL, WorstJGF. The correction of myopia by lens implantation into phakic eyes. Am J Ophthalmol 1989; 107:659-63.
18. Fukala V. Operative Behandlung der Höchstgradien Myopice durch Aphakie. Albrecht von Graefes Arch Klin Exp. Ophthalmol 1980; 36:230-44.
19. Fyodorov SN Zuev VK, Tumanyan ER (Intraocular correction of high myopia with negative posterior chamber lens), (Russian). Ophthalmosurgery 1991;3:57-8.
20. Güell JL, Vazquez M, Gris O, et al. Combined surgery to correct high myopia: iris claw phakic intraocular lens and laser in situ keratomileusis. J Refract Surg 1999; 15:529-37.
21. Hanna KD, Chastang JC, Pouliquen Y. A rotating slit delivery system for excimer laser refractive keratoplasty. Am J Ophthalmol 1987; 103:474.
22. Joly P, Baikoff G, Bonnet P. Mise en place d'un implant négatif de chambre antérieure chez des sujets phakes. Bull Soc Ophalmol Fr 1989; 89:727-33.
23. Kelman CD. Anterior chamber lens design concepts. In Rosen ES, Haining WM, Arnott E, (Eds): Intraocular Lens Implantation. St Louis: Mosby, 1984:239-45.
24. Kim WJ, Lee JH. Long-term results of myopic epikeratoplasty. J Cataract Refract Surg 1993; 19:352-5.
25. Krumeich JH, Swinger CA. Non-freeze epikeratophakia for the correction of myopia. Am J Ophthalmol 1987; 103 (3): 397-403.
26. Lindstrom RL, Lane SS. Polysulfone intracorneal lenses. In Sanders DR, Hofman RF, Salz JJ, (Eds): Refractive Corneal Surgery. Thorofare, NJ: Slack Inc, 1986: 551-63.
27. Mardelli PG, Piebenga LW, Matta CS, et al. Corneal endothelial status 12 to 55 months after excimer laser photorefractice keratectomy. Ophthalmology 1995, 102:544-8.
28. Maxwell WA. Myopic keratomileusis: initial results and myopic keratomileusis combined with other procedures. J Catraract Refract Surg 1987; 13: 518-24.
29. Mc Carey BE, Waring Go, Street DA. Refractive keratoplasty in monkeys using intracorneal lenses of various refractive indexes. Arch Ophthalmol 1987; 195: 123-6.
30. Mimouni F, Colin Koffi V, Bonnet P. Damage to the corneal endothelium from anterior chamber intraocular lenses in phakic myopic eyes. Refract Corneal Surg 1991; 7:277-81.
31. Nordan LT, Fallor MK. Myopic keratomileusis: 74 consecutive non-amblyopic cases with one year of follow-up. J Refract Surg 1986;2:124-8.
32. Pérez- Santoja JJ, Bueno JL, Zato MA. Surgical correction of high myopia in phakic eyes with Worst- Fechner myopia intraocular lenses. J Refract Surg 1997; 13:268-84.

33. Praeger DL. Innovations and creativity in contemporary ophthalmology-preliminary experience with the phakic intraocular lens. Ann Ophthalmol 1988; 20: 456-62.
34. Romanet JP, Albinet P, Mouillon M. Utilisation du collagéne humain (type IV) en chirurgie conrnéenne refractive. Etude expérimentale. Ophthalmologie 1988; 2:285-9.
35. Saragoussi J-J, Cotinat J, Renard G, et al. Damage to the corneal endothelium by minus power anterior chamber intraocular lenses. Refract Corneal Surg 1991; 7:282-5.
36. Sher NA, Barak M, Daya S, et al. Excimer laser photo refractive keratectomy in high myopia: a multicenter study. Arch Ophthalmol 1992;110:935-43.
37. Stark WH, Worthen DM, Holladay JT. The FDA report on intraocular lenses. Ophthalmology 1983;90:311-7.
38. Strampelli B. Lentilles camerulaines après 6 années d´expériences. Acta Conc Ophthal Belgica (Brussels) 1958;11:1692-8.
39. Strampelli B. Sopportabilitá di lenti acriliche in camera anteriore nella afachia e nei vizi di refrazione. Ann Ottamol Clin Oculist 1954; 80:75-82.
40. Thompson KP, Hnna K, Waring GO. Emerging technologies for refractive surgery: laser adjustable synthetic epikeratoplasty. Refract Corneal Surg 1989; 5(1): 46-8.
41. Trokel SL, Srinivasan R, Braren B. Excimer laser surgery of the cornea. Am J Ophthalmol 1983; 96:710-5.
42. Verzella F. Microsurgery of lens in high myopia for optic purposes. Cataract 1984; 1(2): 8-12.
43. Warning GO III, Lynn MJ, Nizam A, et al. Results of the prospective evaluation of radial keratomy (PERK) study five years after surgery. Ophthalmology 1991; 98:1164-76.
44. Werblin JP, Klyce SD. Epikeratophakia: the surgical correction of myopia. Lathing of corneal tissue. Curr Eye Res 1981; 1 (10): 397-592.
45. Werblin TP, Peiffer RL, Fryczkowski A. Myopic hydrogel keratophakia-preliminary report. Cornea 1984-85; 3 (3): 197-204.

CHAPTER

27

Johan A de Lange (South Africa)

Artisan, Toric Artisan and Artiflex Phakic Intraocular Lenses

GENERAL DISCUSSION

What is a Phakic IOL?

It is an IOL which is inserted into the eye without removing the normal crystalline lens of the eye.

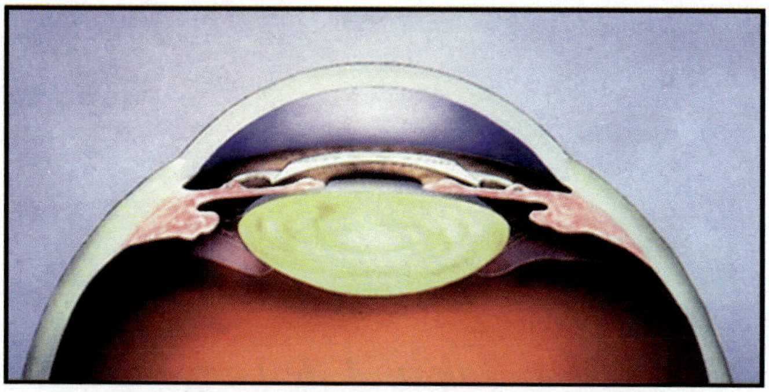

Fig. 27.1: Schematic drawing of Artisan PIOL attached to iris in a phakic eye

The main indication for use of a phakic IOL is the treatment of refractive abnormalities such as myopia and hyperopia, with or without astigmatism.

DIFFERENT TYPES OF PHAKIC IOLs (PIOLs)

1. Anterior chamber PIOLs
   - 1.1. Angle supported anterior chamber PIOLs.
   - 1.2. Iris fixated PIOLs.
2. Posterior chamber PIOLs.

Anterior Chamber PIOLs

Angle supported PIOLs are placed in the anterior chamber and have 3 or 4 haptics resting anterior of the iris in the anterior chamber angle. The optic of this IOL is also in the anterior chamber. Typical examples are the Vivarte and Baikof PIOLs.

Iris fixated PIOLs are placed in the anterior chamber but they are attached to the iris and do not reach the angle of the anterior chamber. They have their haptics as well as the optic in the anterior chamber. The Artisan PIOL is an excellent example of this PIOL. In the USA and elsewhere the Artisan PIOL is also marketed under license by AMO as the Verisyze PIOL.

Posterior Chamber PIOLs

Posterior chamber PIOLs are inserted into the posterior chamber. It means that their haptics as well as optics are behind the iris in the area between the iris and the normal crystalline lens of the eye. The STAAR ICL is the best known example.

This chapter will concern itself with the Artisan group of **Iris fixated PIOLs.**

HISTORY

In February 1986 a group of Dutch ophthalmologists, gathering in a French ski resort discussed the possibilities of designing a phakic IOL. It seemed appropriate as most of them had a problem with radial keratotomy, which was at that moment the treatment for the correction of myopic refractive errors.

The concept of the iris claw lens seemed a good basis for such a design. They formulated the main conditions for the design as follows:

- Smooth claws to avoid damage to the delicate iris
- Ample space for natural aqueous humor flow
- Sufficient space between PIOL and cornea
- Sufficient space between PIOL and natural lens
- Overall diameter limited to 8.5 mm.

Three types of Artisan Iris fixated PIOLs are available:

1. Artisan spheric
2. Artisan toric
3. Artiflex foldable.

Originally only the spheric Artisan PIOLs were designed. Myopic as well as hyperopic lenses were developed. These PIOLs had a number of excellent qualities:

- Between the enclavation site and the peripheral cornea an iris bridge is formed
- This iris bridge protects the endothelium from touching the PMMA, because the lens does not reach the periphery where the AC is shallow
- It has safe clearance from the crystalline lens
- Unrestricted pupil dilatation and constriction is possible
- Unique possibility to position the lens in the optical centre of the eye
- Excellent centration. Once fixated the lens will not decenter
- Lens axis direction can be varied, allowing for astigmatism correction
- Maximal surgical visibility, accessability and controllability
- Optimal postoperative visibility of lens and lens fixation
- The Artisan PIOL is cosmetically invisible
- It is easy to reposition, reversible and exchangeable

- There is no interference with the vascular iris physiology (no leakage of iris vessels was demonstrated on fluorescein angiography)
- High predictability of postoperative results
- One size fits all.

We will discuss these Iris fixated PIOLs of the Artisan group in sequence.

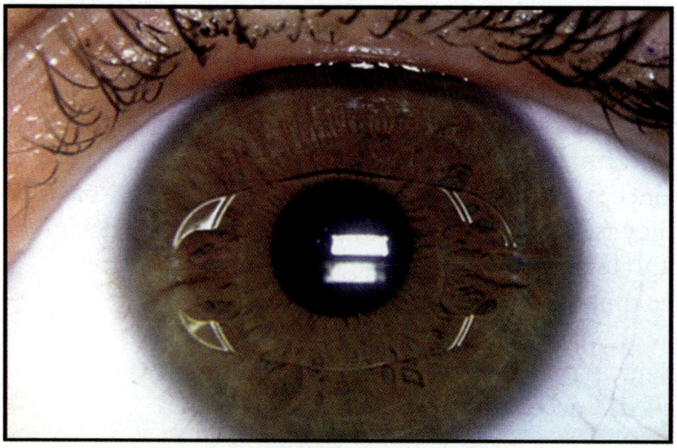

Fig. 27.2: Artisan spheric phakic intraocular lens

QUALITIES OF THE ARTISAN SPHERIC PIOL

The Artisan spheric PIOL is a PMMA (perspex CQ-UV) PIOL.

Myopic as well as hyperopic Artisan IOLs are available.

The myopic Artisan is available in 0.5 D increments from -23.5 to -1.0 D. The optic diameter is 5 mm or 6 mm; the overall diameter 8.5 mm; the height is 0.96 mm.

The hyperopic Artisan is available from +1.0 to +12 Dioptres in 0.5 D increments. Optic diameter is 5 mm, overall diameter 8.5 mm, total height is 1.0 mm.

The thickness of the lens can vary depending on the dioptric power of the lens.

Indications for the Artisan Spheric PIOL

Myopic or Hyperopic refractive errors. Patients with stabilized axial myopia or hyperopia who will not achieve satisfactory visual correction with glasses, contact lenses or refractive excimer laser.

Requirements for the Artisan Spheric PIOL

1. ACD more than 3.2 mm.
2. Normal corneal endothelium and corneal clarity.

3. Corneal astigmatism of –1.75 D or less.
4. Flat normal iris.

Contraindications

1. Corneal endothelial dystrophy.
2. Endothelial cell count < 2000 per square mm.
3. ACD less than 3.2 mm.
4. Bulging iris.
5. Small ACD, i.e. deep enough centrally but white to white less than 10.5 mm.
6. Cataract.
7. Recurrent or chronic uveitis.
8. Angle closure glaucoma.
9. Wide angle glaucoma.
10. Small refractive errors. In this case Lasik may be better.
11. Astigmatism of more than –1.75 D (better to use **toric** Artisan PIOL)
12. Insufficient iris to support PIOL, abnormal iris or pupil.
13. Spherical equivalent outside the available dioptres of the Artisan PIOLs
14. Previous retinal detachment.
15. Patient younger than 18.

Surgery for the Artisan PIOL

Anesthesia

This surgery can be performed under topical, peribulbar or general anesthesia.

It is the surgeon's choice but will naturally be influenced by patient expectations and preferences. In the USA and Europe topical anesthesia is popular.

However, patients receiving Artisan PIOLs are often young people who may not tolerate topical anesthesia very well. For them general anesthesia may be a very good alternative.

Incision

More than one incision type is possible.

My preferred incision is a superior scleral tunnel under a limbal based conjunctival flap.

The incision width is 0.5 mm larger than the diameter of the lens optic, e.g. 5.5 or 6.0 mm (Fig. 27.3).

Two limbal clear corneal parasyntheses are made at the 3 and 6 o' clock positions. These are used to introduce the enclavation forceps to enclavate the iris.

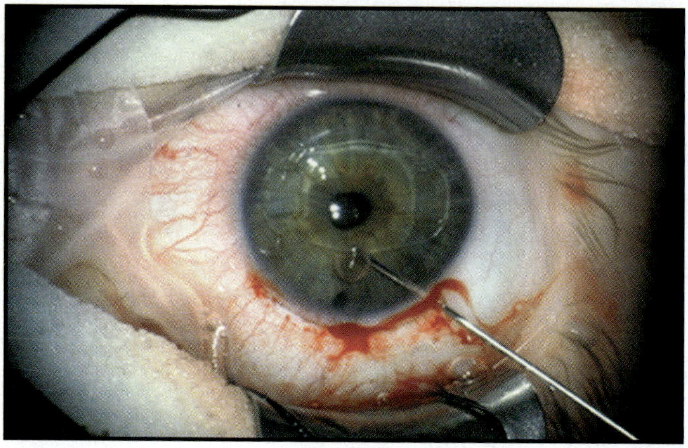

Fig. 27.3

Some surgeons prefer to make vertical limbal parasyntheses at the 2 and 10 o' clock positions. Through these they introduce a special enclavation needle to do the enclavation.

After making the incisions, acetylcholine is injected into the anterior chamber to create instant miosis.

This is followed by an OVD (Ophthalmic viscosurgical device previously known as a visco-elastic) into the anterior chamber to fill the AC. It should be a cohesive OVD to prevent adhesion to the intra-ocular structures. It is mandatory that this OVD should be easily removable after the PIOL has been inserted.

Then the PIOL is removed from its container and introduced into the AC (Fig. 27.4).

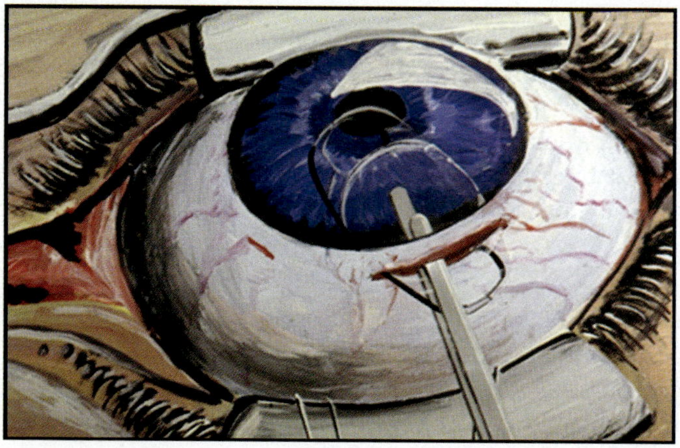

Fig. 27.4

In the anterior chamber it should be rotated to a horizontal position and must be well centered over the pupil (Fig. 27.5).

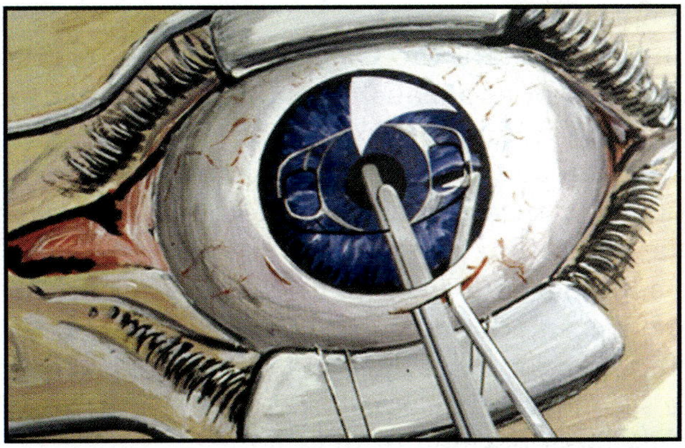

Fig. 27.5

At this stage the PIOL is held with a special holding forceps and the first pair of haptic claws are attached to the iris by enclavating iris between the two curved haptic claw tips.

This procedure is repeated for the second pair of haptic claws.

Now the PIOL is securely attached to the iris and the peripheral iridotomy can be done at the 12 o'clock position.

Then it is time to remove the OVD which should be done very thoroughly.

This is followed by wound closure, with sutures if necessary, as well as closure of the conjunctiva.

Follow-up

This is done after 1 day, 1 week, one month, 3, 6, 12 months.

Complications

Preoperative complications

1. Anesthetic complications
   - Some patients cannot tolerate topical anesthesia and must receive peribulbar or general anesthesia
   - For young patients the peribulbar injections may also be a problem and they may prefer general anesthetic.
2. Calculating the power of the PIOL. This is done by the manufacturer Ophthec. It is based on refractive information provided by the surgeon.

Intraoperative complications

1. Wound complications
   - The incision should be the correct size (0.5 mm larger than the lens optic) and as small as possible to avoid unnecessary post-operative astigmatism
   - Leaking of the wound can occur and will require a suture.

2. OVD complications
   - During enclavation the OVD may escape from the AC and should be kept at adequate volume to facilitate surgery
   - Inadequate volume of OVD in the AC will not protect the endothelium and may lead to endothelial damage
   - Enough OVD is necessary to elevate the PIOL to make it possible for the surgeon to grasp it
   - If an adhesive OVD is used, it will be very difficult to remove it from the anterior chamber
   - Insufficient removal of the OVD may cause postoperative wide angle secondary glaucoma.
3. Complications of position of the PIOL
   - In some cases it may be difficult to place the PIOL directly over the centre of the pupil. Any decentration should be avoided but if it does happen it is better to err towards the nasal side because most eyes have a slight nasal displacement of the visual axis
   - Sometimes the first attempt to enclavate the PIOL results in a wrong position of the PIOL. If this happens it should be rectified immediately. It is very easy to disenclavate the PIOL by just pushing the iris bach through the claws of the PIOL.
4. Complications of the peripheral iridotomy/iridectomy

   It may happen that the iridotomy/iridectomy is not patent and this may lead to postoperative acute pupillary block glaucoma.

   If a peripheral iridectomy is performed it may be too large and give rise to various postoperative symptoms like awareness of the PI, glare, etc.
5. Postoperative complications
   - Postoperative mild uveitis will occasionally be present
   - In case of a non-patent peripheral iridotomy, acute pupillary block glaucoma may develop within hours after the surgery
   - Corneal edema is rare but in case of excessive manipulation it is possible
   - Traumatic cataract may be caused by lens touch during careless surgery
   - Hemorrhage (hyphema) is very rare but not impossible
   - Infection, e.g. endophthalmitis is also rare but the usual precautions must be taken
   - Decentration of the PIOL will impact negatively on visual acuity and will also lead to various optical disturbances such as halo, glare, monocular diplopia, etc.
   - A frequently encountered complication is the presence of unwanted postoperative astigmatism. This is usually the result of too tight sutures in the superior scleral tunnel. This creates

with-the-rule astigmatism. As time goes by this astigmatism reduces to acceptable levels but most patients find it very disturbing. That is one of the very good reasons why the **Artiflex** foldable PIOL has been developed.

Results of the Spheric Artisan PIOL

Predictability excellent. If the preoperative refractive measurements are correct, the predictability is excellent and >95% of eyes are within 1 D of emmetropia.

Efficacy excellent. UCVA as well as BSCVA are significantly better than preoperative. Improvement in BSCVA is very common and also occurs in eyes that were previously regarded as amblyopic. This happens more often in the myopia group and the improvement in best corrected vision is probably caused by the magnification effect of the PIOL.

Safety. In most reports no eyes lost any line of BSCVA. Serious complications are rare. Please refer to complications.

ARTISAN TORIC PHAKIC INTRAOCULAR LENS

ARTISAN® Toric 5/8.5

ARTISAN® toric phakic IOLs are available with a 0° or a 90° cylinder.

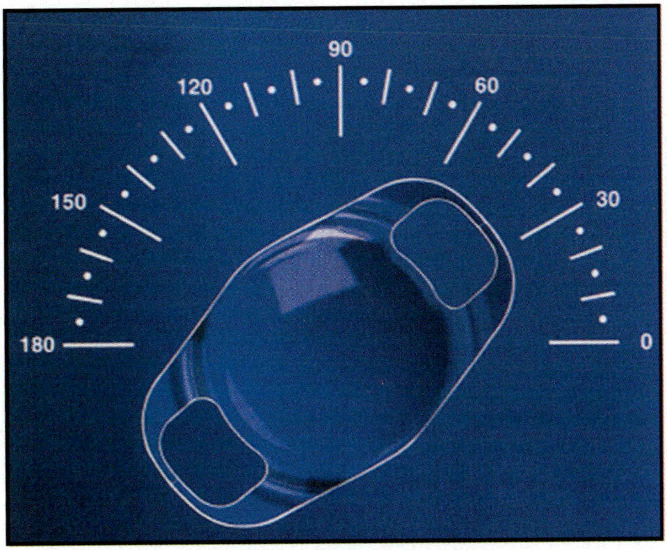

Fig. 27.6: ARTISAN® PTIOL

Qualities of the Artisan Toric PIOL

This is also a PMMA PIOL.

The optic diameter is 5.0 mm.

The length of the IOL including the haptics is 8.5 mm.

The thickness of the lens varies between 0.96 and 1.2 mm depending on the dioptric power of the lens.

It is available in 0.5 dioptre spheric increments from –2.5 to –21.0 dioptres as well as from +2.00 to + 7.5D combined with the required cylinder. The cylinder is available from –2.0 Dioptre to –7.5D at whatever axis necessary.

The toric Artisan is custom made and delivery is 8-10 weeks after order approval.

A unique feature of this PIOL is the variation of the cylinder position relative to the shape of the PIOL. The cylinder can be ordered in such a way that the surgeon can only implant the PIOL in a horizontal position to ensure the correct cylinder axis. But this may vary and the surgeon should be aware of the possible variation in cylinder position.

The lens is also fixated to the iris in two spots using an iris enclavating technique.

Material:	Perspex CQ-UV
Optic diameter:	5 mm
Overall diameter:	8.5 mm
Total height:	0.96 mm
Weight (–10D):	± 9 mg
Sterilization:	EO

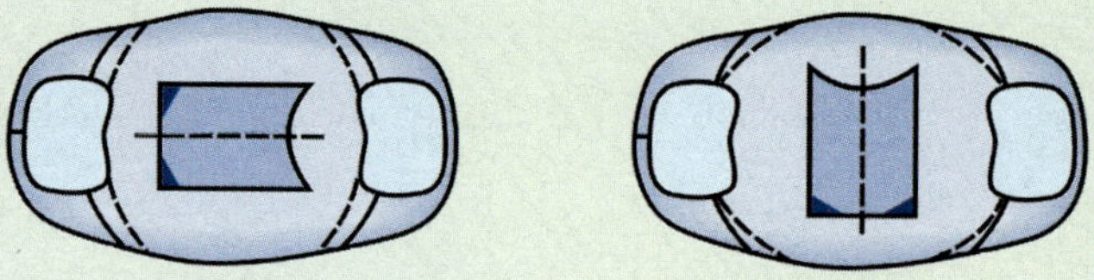

PTIOL-0° PTIOL-90°

Figs 27.7A and B

Indications for the Artisan Toric PIOL

1. Myopic or hyperopic astigmatism with sphere of –20.0 to –2.0 as well as +2.00 to +6.00 combined with.
2. Astigmatism of –2.0 to –7.5D dioptres.
3. Phakic eyes.
4. ACD more than 3.2 mm.
5. Normal corneal endothelium.
6. Normal iris.

7. Stable keratoconus with good BSCVA.
8. Correction after Lasik overcorrection.
9. Correction after PKP.

Contraindications for Toric Artisan (same as for Artisan PIOL)

1. ACD less than 3.2 mm.
2. Bulging iris.
3. Small ACD, i.e. deep enough but because of short white-to-white and high K-readings the peripheral haptic of the PIOL will be too close to the endothelium.
4. Cataract.
5. Recurrent or chronic uveitis.
6. Angle closure glaucoma.
7. Wide angle glaucoma.
8. Small refractive errors. In this case Lasik may be better.
9. Astigmatism of less than -1.75 D (Here we use Artiflex PIOL).
10. Patient younger than 18.
11. Spherical or astigmatic error outside the available dioptres of the Artisan PIOLs.
12. Endothelial cell count < 2000 per square mm.
13. Corneal endothelial dystrophy .
14. Insufficient iris to support PIOL.

Surgery for Toric Artisan PIOL

The surgery is essentially the same as for spheric Artisan PIOL.

A few important adjustments must be made for the fact that this is a toric PIOL.

Preoperative Marking of the Enclavation Sites

The surgeon must be aware of the axis of the cylinder relative to the shape of the PIOL. This means that every PIOL may potentially be implanted in a different axis.

A simple way of marking the enclavation sites of the PIOL is to make small YAG laser burns on the iris at the correct spots preoperative

An alternative for marking the correct cylinder axis is to use a surgical marker to mark the limbus.

Anesthesia

As for spheric Artisan this surgery can be performed under topical, peribulbar or general anesthesia.

Incision

A superior 5.5 mm scleral tunnel under a limbal based conjunctival flap.

The incision width is 0.5 mm larger than the diameter of the lens optic.

Two limbal clear corneal parasyntheses are made at the correct positions, keeping in mind the marked enclavation sites and the surgeon's technique.

After making the incisions, acethylcholine is injected into the anterior chamber to create instant miosis.

This is followed by an OVD into the anterior chamber to fill the AC.

It should be a cohesive OVD to prevent adhesion to the intraocular structures.

This OVD should be easily removable after the PIOL has been inserted

Then the PIOL is introduced into the AC. In the anterior chamber it should be rotated to the correct position and must be well centered over the pupil.

At this stage the toric Artisan is held with a special holding forceps and the first pair of haptic claws are attached to the iris at exactly the correct spot as marked preoperation with the YAG laser. This procedure is repeated for the second pair of haptic claws, once again making sure that it is enclavated at exactly the correct position.

Now the peripheral iridotomy can be done superiorly but not always precisely at 12 o'clock.

Then the OVD is removed completely.

The incision as well as conjunctiva is closed.

Follow-up

Visits are scheduled for 1day, 1 week, one month, 3, 6, 12 months.

Complications

Preoperative complications

1. Anesthetic complications
   - Some patients, particularly young people, cannot tolerate topical anesthesia and must receive peribulbar or general anesthesia
   - Young patients may prefer general anesthesia to peribulbar injections.
2. Calculating the power of the toric PIOL
   This is done by the manufacturer Ophthec. It is based on refractive information provided by the surgeon.

Intraoperative Complications

1. Wound complications
   - Some scleral tunnels may leak without the use of sutures.
2. OVD complications
   - During enclavation the OVD may escape from the AC and should be kept at adequate volume to facilitate surgery
   - Inadequate volume of OVD in the AC will not protect the endothelium and may lead to endothelial damage
   - Insufficient OVD is necessary to elevate the PIOL to make it possible for the surgeon to grasp it
   - Insufficient removal of the OVD may cause postoperative wide angle secondary glaucoma.
3. Complications of position of the toric Artisan PIOL
   - Any decentration should be avoided and more so because this is a toric lens
   - Misalignment of the cylinder axis: If the PIOL is not positioned in the correct axis, a postoperative refractive error will be the result
   - Sometimes the first attempt to enclave the PIOL results in a wrong position of the PIOL. If this happens it should be rectified immediately. It is very easy to disenclavate the lens by just pushing the iris bach through the claws of the lens.
4. Complications of the peripheral iridotomy/iridectomy
   - A peripheral iridotomy is better than an iridectomy
   - However it may happen that the iridotomy is not patent and this may lead to postoperation acute pupil block glaucoma
   - A peripheral iridectomy may be too large and give rise to various postoperative symptoms like awareness of the PI, glare, etc. PPP PI.

Postoperative Complications

These are very similar to those of the Artisan spheric PIOL

- Postoperation mild uveïtis will occasionally be present
- In case of a non-patent peripheral iridotomy acute pupillary block glaucoma may develop within hours after the surgery
- Corneal edema should not occur but in case of excessive manipulation it is possible
- If the crystalline lens is touched during surgery it may cause early postoperative traumatic cataract
- Hemorrhage (hyphema) is very rare
- Infection, e.g. endophthalmitis is also rare
- Decentration of the PIOL will impact negatively on visual acuity and will also lead to various optical disturbances such as halo, glare, monocular diplopia, etc.

- A frequently encountered complication is the presence of unwanted postoperative astigmatism. This is usually the result of too tight sutures in the superior scleral tunnel which creates with-the-rule astigmatism. As time goes by this astigmatism reduces to acceptable levels but most patients find it very disturbing. That is one of the very good reasons why the Artiflex foldable PIOL was developed.

Results of the Toric Artisan PIOL

Predictability excellent. If the preoperative refractive measurements are correct, the predictability is excellent and >90% of eyes are within 1 D of emmetropia.

Efficacy is excellent. UCVA as well as BSCVA are significantly better than preoperation. As with the other PIOLs some patients gain as many as 3 or more lines of best corrected vision.

Safety. In most reports no eyes lost any line of BSCVA. Complications can happen as discussed. However, the complication rate is low and very few serious complications occur.

ARTIFLEX FOLDABLE IRIS CLIP PIOL

Qualities of the Artiflex Spheric PIOL

It is also an Iris fixated PIOL.

It has a foldable optic made of polysiloxane.

The optic diameter is 6 mm.

The length of the IOL including the haptics is 8.5 mm.

The Artiflex PIOL has PMMA haptic claws into which iris must be enclavated in a similar fashion as with the Artisan PIOL.

A special spatula is provided with the Artiflex PIOL to fold the PIOL before introducing it into the AC.

The Artiflex IOL is only a myopic spheric PIOL and is available in 1 dioptre increments from –14.5 to –2.00 dioptres.

Indications for use of the Artiflex PIOL

These indications are basically the same as for the Artisan spheric PIOL.

The Artiflex PIOL will probably soon replace the Artisan PIOL for myopia.

Indications

1. Refractive errors between –2 to –15.0 (Lens is –2.0 to –14.5).
2. Phakic eyes
3. Anterior chamber depth more than 3.2 mm.

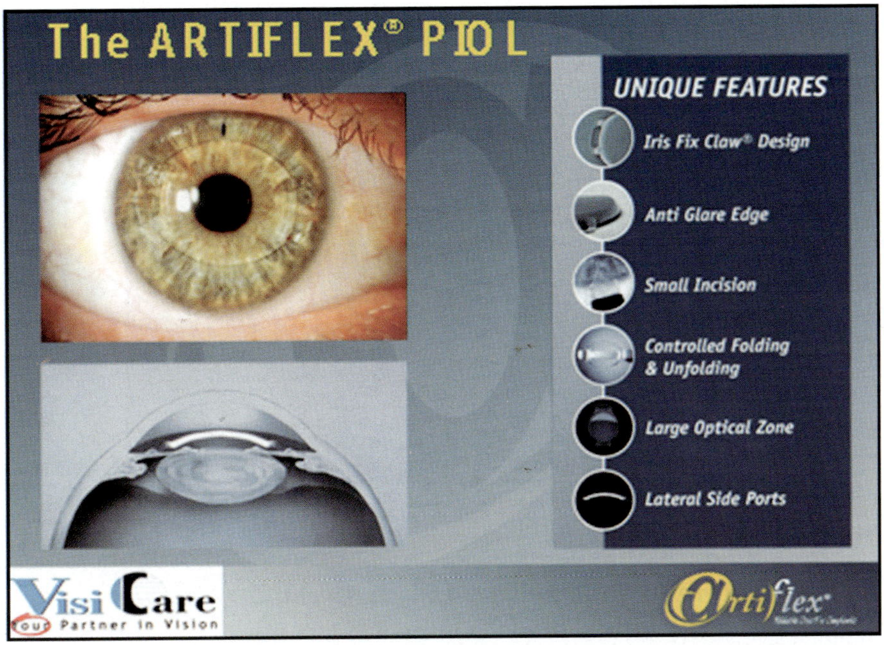

Fig. 27.8A

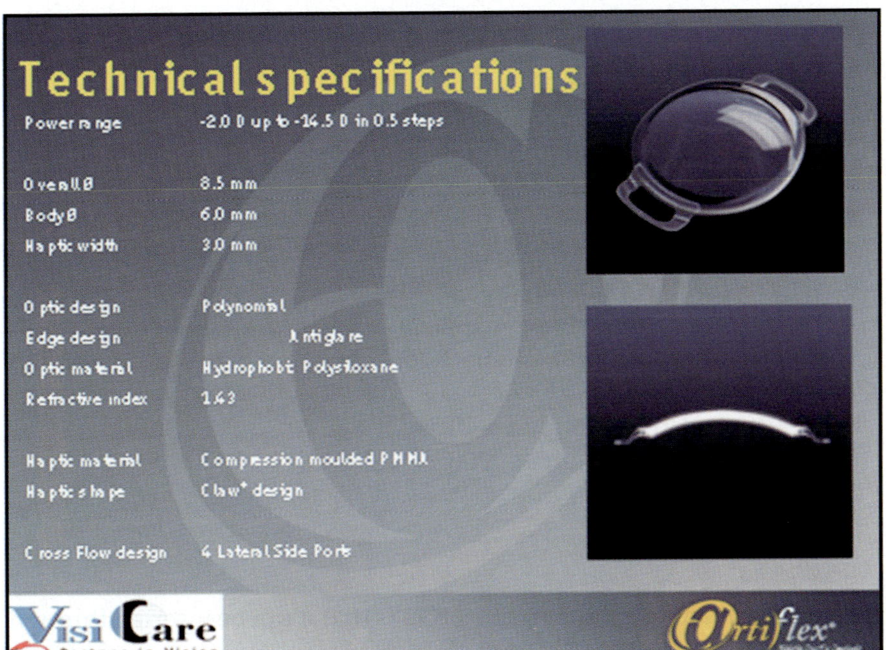

Fig. 27.8B

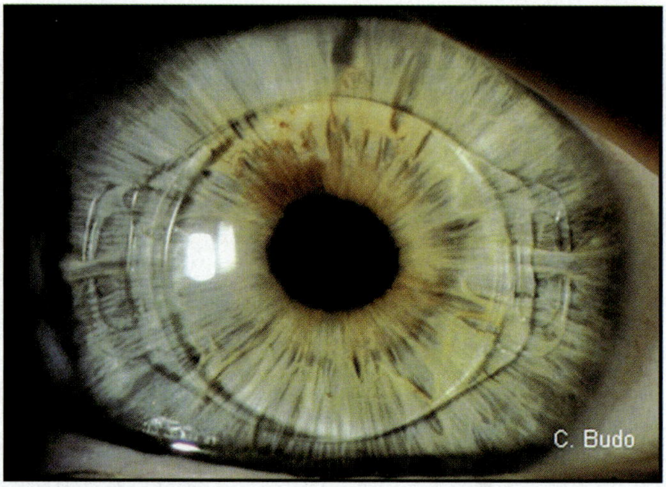

Fig. 27.9

4. Normal corneal endothelium and clarity ECC >2000.
5. Corneal astigmatism of -1.75 D or less.
6. Normal pupil and flat iris.

Contraindications

1. ACD less than 3.2 mm.
2. Bulging iris.
3. Small ACD, i.e. deep enough but white to white too short to provide ample space in the AC.
4. Cataract.
5. Recurrent or chronic uveitis.
6. Angle closure glaucoma.
7. Small refractive errors. In this case Lasik may be better.
8. Astigmatism of more than -1.75 D (Here we use toric Artisan PIOL).
9. Insufficient iris to support PIOL.
10. Endothelial cell count < 2000 cells/mm^3.

Surgery

Anesthesia

The main advantage of the Artiflex IOL is that it can be inserted through a clear corneal incision.

Therefore, the operation can quite comfortably be done under topical anesthetic combined with intracameral lignocaine.

This surgery can also be performed under peribulbar or general anesthesia.

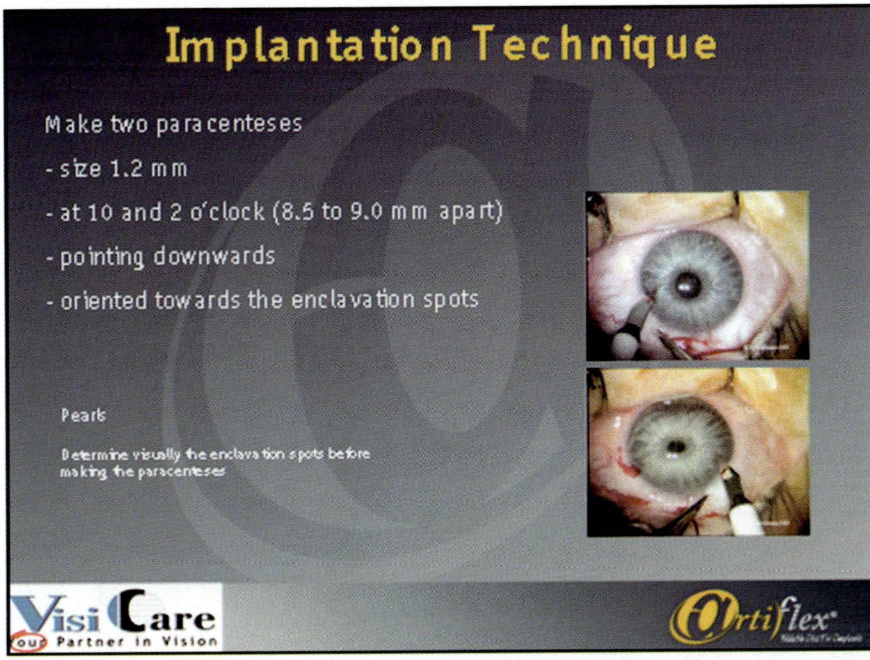

Fig. 27.10

As with the Artisan lens it is the surgeon's choice but will naturally be influenced by patient expectations and preferences. In the USA and Europe topical anesthesia is popular.

Incision

More than one incision type is possible.

An excellent option is a superior clear corneal incision. It can be made with a diamond knife and the aim is to make the incision 3.2 mm wide and 1.5 to 2 mm in length.

This is followed by two limbal clear corneal paracenteses at the 3 and 6 o'clock positions. These are used to introduce the enclavation forceps to enclavate the iris.

Some surgeons prefer to make vertical limbal paracenteses at the 2 and 10 o'clock positions.Through these they introduce a special enclavation needle to do the enclavation.

After making the incisions acethylcholine (miochol or equivalent) is injected into the anterior chamber to create instant miosis.

This is followed by an OVD into the anterior chamber to fill the AC. It should be a cohesive OVD to prevent adhesion to the intraocular structures. It is mandatory that this OVD should be easily removable after the Artiflex lens has been inserted.

Then the Artiflex PIOL is removed from its container and loaded onto the insertion spatula. This little procedure is very easy but needs to be executed correctly.

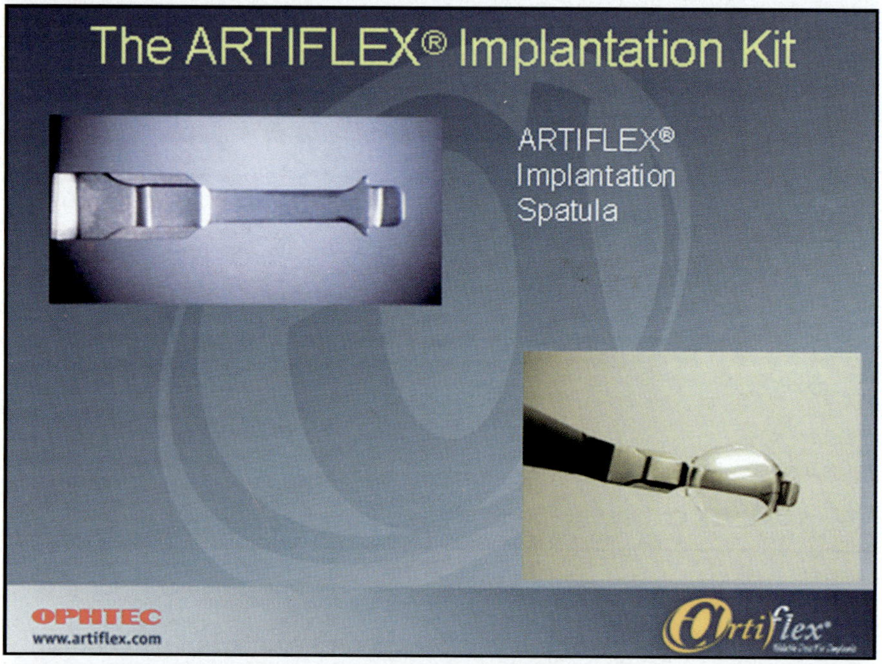

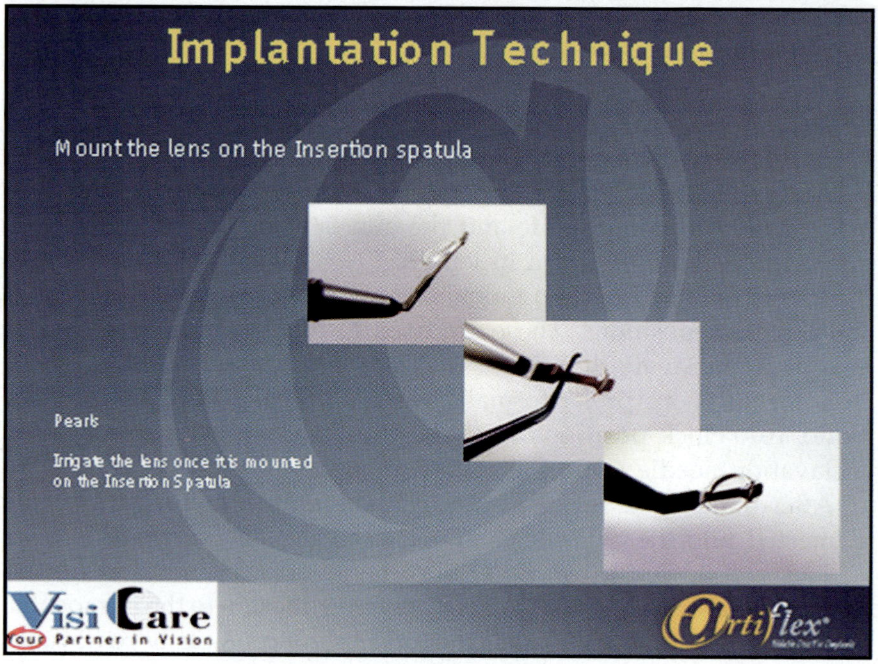

Figs 27.11A and B

The Artiflex PIOL is gently introduced into the AC with the help of the injector.

When the optic of the Artiflex PIOL is well into the AC, the injector can be retracted. This maneuver will leave the Artiflex lens in the AC. In some cases the following haptics could still be outside the eye and can gently be moved forward into the AC.

It may well be asked: why would the following haptics not enter the AC with the PIOL? The problem is that the injector's tip may reach the inferior AC angle before the haptics are altogether in the AC superiorly. It is then safer to retract the injector rather than damage the inferior AC angle. If the following haptics are still outside the AC it can be moved inwards without a problem.

Once in the anterior chamber the Artiflex PIOL should be rotated to a horizontal position. Care should be taken to make sure it is well centered over the pupil.

At this stage the PIOL is held with a special holding forceps. These holding forceps are different from those used for the Artisan PIOL. It is important to note that only the haptics are held and the optic should never be touched with these forceps.

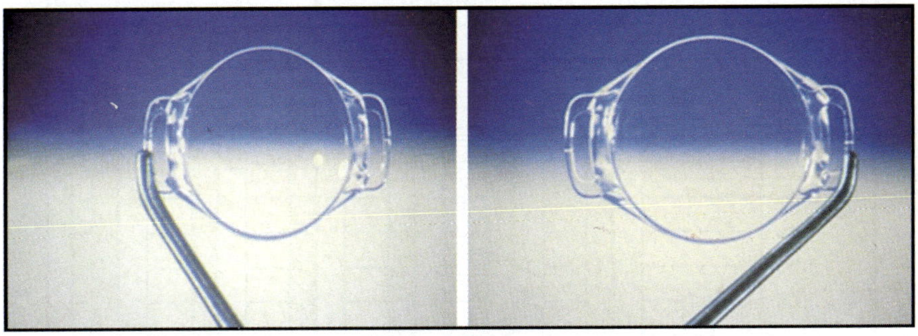

Figs 27.12A and B

As with the Artisan PIOL the first pair of haptic claws are attached to the iris by enclavating iris between the two curved haptic claw tips. The enclavation can be done using special forceps or a special enclavation needle.

This procedure is repeated for the second pair of haptic claws.

Now the PIOL is securely attached to the iris and the peripheral iridotomy can be made at the 12 o'clock position.Then the OVD is removed very thoroughly and the AC is filled with BSS. If required the incision edges may be hydrated.

No suturing is necessary.

Follow-up

One day, 1 week, 1 month, 3, 6, 12 months.

Results

Fast visual recovery: Because the clear corneal incision induces very little astigmatism the visual recovery is very quick. Many patients wil have 1.0 unaided vision the day after surgery.

Efficacy: Excellent visual acuity results.

The efficacy index (UCVA postoperative/BCVA preoperative) was measured as 1.01 in one series. Due to the high quality of the Artiflex lens and the stability and predictability of the lens the visual acuity is excellent. Final UCVA after 3 months is often 20/20 or better and BSCVA is often better than preoperative. As with other lenses of the Artisan group a high percentage of patients will experience upto 3 or more lines of improvement of BSCVA, probably due to magnification of retinal images.

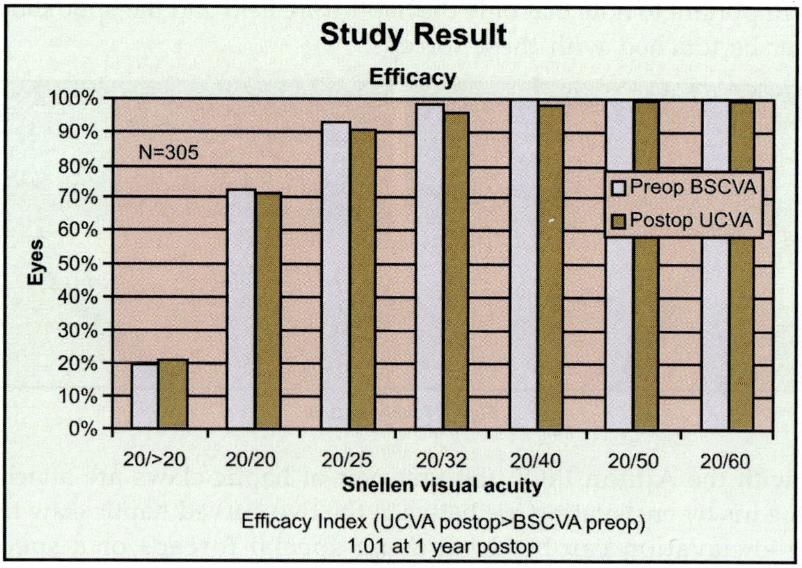

Fig. 27.13

High predictability: The preoperative calculations are extremely accurate and it provides exceptionally good predictability.

Safety: The surgery is fast, smooth and atraumatic. Very few significant complications are reported. The safety index was 1.10 at 1 year post-operation.

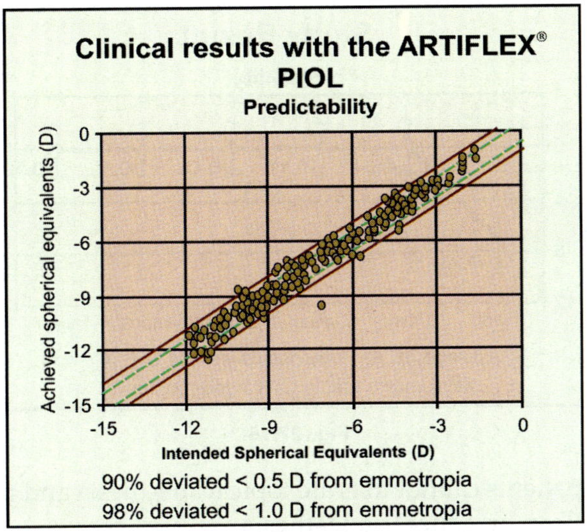

Fig. 27.14

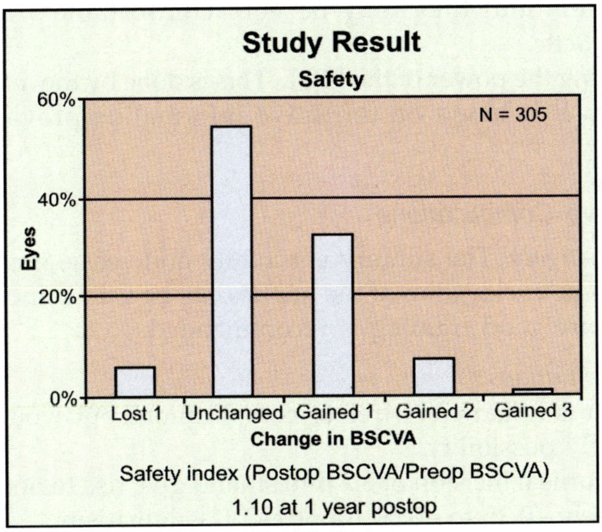

Fig. 27.15

Stable results: The enclavation technique is remarkably stable and the lens position will not change during any normal physical activity (boxing is not advocated). Therefore, the result is maintained over many years.

Complications

Preoperative

1. Anesthetic complications

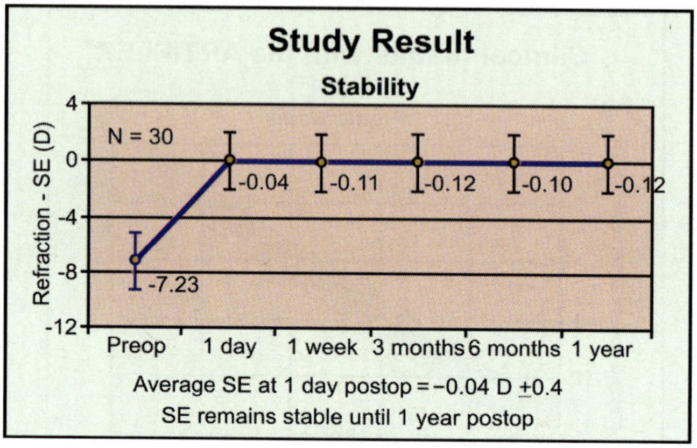

Fig. 27.16

- Some patients cannot tolerate topical anesthesia and must receive peribulbar or general anesthesia
- For young patients the peribulbar injections may also be a problem and they may be very comfortable with general anesthetic.

2. Calculating the power of the PIOL. This is done by the manufacturer Ophthec. It is based on refractive information provided by the surgeon.

Intraoperative Complications

Demanding surgery: The surgery is actually quite easy, except for one maneuver. The enclavation of the haptics can be very difficult, and for this procedure good training is recommended.

Wound complications

The incision is remarkably free of complications but wound leakage is an unlikely possibility.

A clear corneal incision of 3.2 mm should give rise to not more than approximately –0.25 to –0.50 dioptres of astigmatism.

OVD complications

During enclavation the OVD may escape from the AC and should be kept at adequate volume.

Insufficient volume of OVD will lead to endothelial touch and damage. It will also make it very difficult to pick the PIOL up with the holding forceps when manipulating the lens.

A cohesive OVD should be used to facilitate removal of the OVD from the AC.

Removal of the OVD at completion of the operation is very important to avoid postoperative acute secondary wide angle glaucoma.

Complications of position of the PIOL

It is extremely important to place the PIOL over the centre of the pupil. Any decentration should be avoided but if it does happen it is better to err towards the nasal side because most eyes have a slight nasal displacement of the visual axis.

Sometimes the first attempt to enclavate the PIOL results in a wrong position of the PIOL. If this happens it should be rectified immediately. It is very easy to disenclavate the PIOL by just pushing the iris bach through the claws of the PIOL.

Complications of the peripheral iridotomy/iridectomy

A peripheral iridotomy is preferred to an iridectomy. However it may happen that the iridotomy is not patent and this may lead to post-op acute pupillary block glaucoma.

A peripheral iridectomy may be too large and give rise to various postoperative symptoms like awareness of the PI, glare, etc.

Postoperative complications

Postoperative mild uveïetis will occasionally be present.

In case of a non-patent peripheral iridotomy acute pupillary block glaucoma may develop within hours after the surgery.

Corneal edema might occur after excessive manipulation during surgery.

Lens touch during surgery may cause a traumatic cataract.

Hyphema is very rare.

Infection, e.g. endophthalmitis is also rare.

Decentration of the PIOL may cause reduction of visual acuity as well as various optical disturbances such as halo, glare, monocular diplopia, etc.

Late complications

- At 1 year the following complications were reported
- Pigment deposits: 5.6%
- Haloes: 5.2%
- Glare: 3.6%
- Non pigment deposits: 3.6%
- Synechiae 0.3%
- Explantation 0.3%
- Lens exchange 0.3%.

EFFECTS OF ARTISAN AND ARTIFLEX PHAKIC IOLs ON THE EYE

Effects on the Endothelium

A main concern for any IOL in the anterior chamber would always be its effect on the endothelium. A number of good studies have been done to evaluate this. The concensus of opinion is that the initial surgery will cause a loss of endothelial cells of 0% to 4%.

After this initial loss of endothelial cells the endothelial cell count will not show any significant deterioration for as long as 10 years post-operation.

A recent multicentre study done on the Artiflex PIOL has shown 0% endothelial cell loss after the first year postoperation.

The present belief is that the PIOL may not anywhere be closer to the endothelium than 1.0 mm. That is why an AC depth of 3.2 mm preoperation is so important. If the AC is shallower, the peripheral edges of the PIOL will be too close to the endothelium.

Effects on the Iris

The claw-haptic of the PIOL does cause some iris depigmentation at the site of enclavation, but if enough iris is enclavated, this will not lead to any problems. Iris necrosis and PIOL dislocation is extremely unlikely.

If the initial enclavation is not well done and only a very thin piece of iris is enclavated, it may well lead to erosion of the iris by the claw-haptics, which in turn will cause disinsersion of one or both haptics and therefore dislocation of the PIOL into the AC.

The peripheral iridotomy or iridectomy will cause some pigment dispersion into the AC and this pigment will be most visible on the PIOL as well as the crystalline lens and the endothelium.

No reports of secondary pigmentary glaucoma due to the small amount of pigment dispersion have come to our attention.

Effects on the Crystalline Lens

The main concern for the patient's crystalline lens is of course the formation of cataract.

The most dangerous time is during surgery. If the crystalline lens is inadvertently touched it may lead to instantaneous traumatic segmentary cataract.

In case of good successful surgery the chances of development of cataract at a later stage is not more than that of the normal population.

The fact that the PIOL is in the AC, has very little effect on the crystalline lens.

Effects on the Intraocular Pressure

The main concern is postoperative pupillary block glaucoma in the presence of a non-patent peripheral iridotomy. Obviously prevention is better than cure. Make sure the PI is open during surgery.

The Artisan and Artiflex PIOLs have no proven long term direct effects on the IOP.

These PIOLs should not be used in the presence of angle closure glaucoma.

Effects on the Anterior Chamber Angle

These PIOLs do not touch the anterior chamber angle and will have no effect on the angle.

A REVIEW OF THE BENEFITS OF THE ARTISAN OR ARTIFLEX PIOLs COMPARED TO OTHER PIOLs

- **Longest clinical history.** It has the longest clinical history of all the PIOLs. The first Artisan PIOL was implanted on November 2, 1986
- **One size fits all**. Other PIOLs need sizing for a proper fit. This applies to the anterior chamber as well as posterior chamber PIOLs
- **Extremely versatile**. The Artisan lenses are designed for aphakia, myopia, hyperopia as well as astigmatism
- **Reversibility of fixation**. Easy to reposition or exchange
- **Safe distance from crystalline lens**. Virtually no PIOL related lenticular opacifications occur
- **Safe distance from endothelial cells**. The initial cell loss is surgery related
- **High predictability**. 98% of patients obtain a refractive result within 1 Dioptre of emmetropia
- **Excellent centration**. Once fixated the lens will not decenter

ARTISAN® lens manufacturing information

PMMA lens are manufactured by using compression molding technology. During the compression molding process the molecular structure of PMMA (A) is enhanced by redistributing the molecules into longer chains (B). This results in a much stronger material.
Compression molding technology gives a high tensile strength, combined with superb flexiblity of the lens haptics. The risk of fracture is minimal.
The tumbling process gives a special surface treatment to the PMMA lenses. Ultra smoothness of the haptics is the result.

A

B

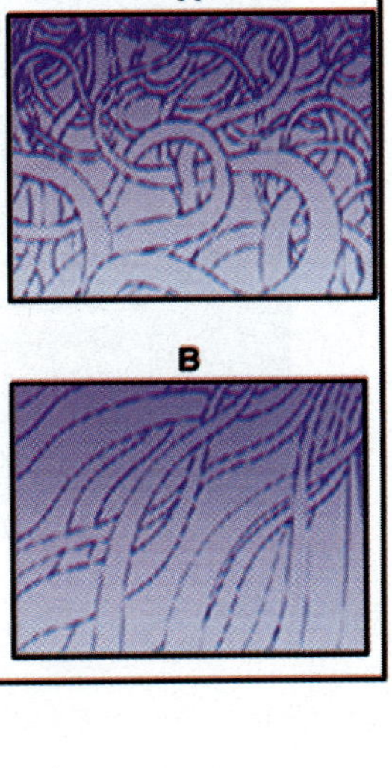

Figs 27.17A and B

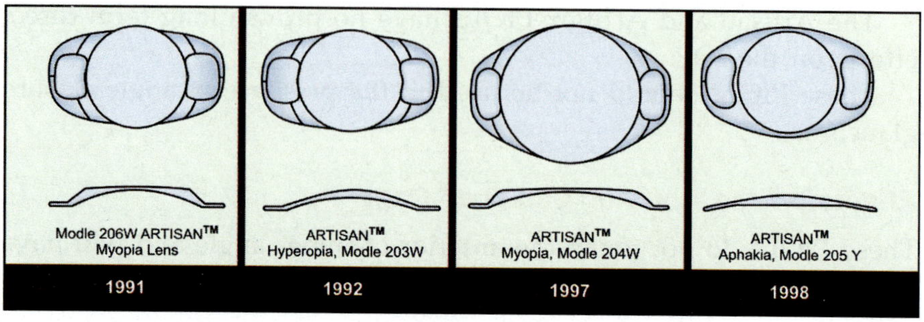

Fig. 27.18

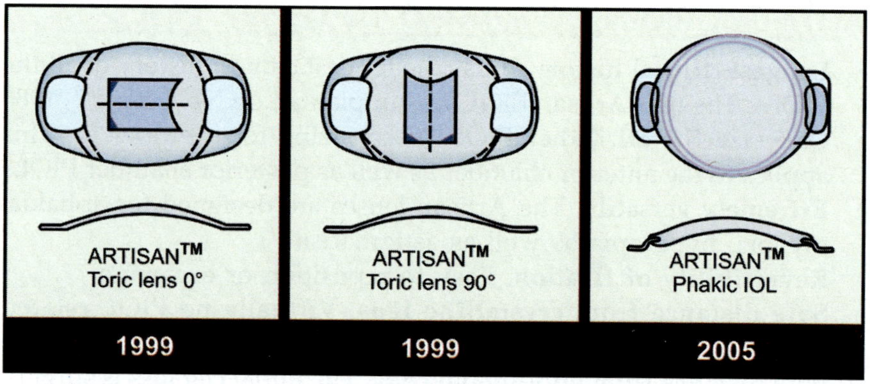

Fig. 27.19

Comparison Chart

	ARTISAN®	ARTIFLEX®
Power Range (S)	+12.0 D up to -23.5 D	-2.0D up to -14.5 D
Power Range (C)	2.0D up to 7.5D	none
Body Ø	5.0mm / 6.0mm	6.0mm
Overall Ø	7.5mm / 8.5mm	8.5mm
Optic Material	PMMA	Hydrophobic Polysiloxane
Refractive Index	1.49	1.43
Optic Design	Spherical	[illegible]
Optic configuration	Convex-concave	Convex-concave
Anti Glare Edge Design	no	yes
Haptic shape	Claw	Claw
Cross Flow Design	4 Lateral Side Ports	4 Lateral Side Ports
Recommended Incision width	5.2mm / 6.2mm	3.2mm
Passport system	none	Insertion Spatula™
Instruments	ARTISAN® Kit	ARTIFLEX® Kit
Viscoelastics	ArtiVisc™ / ArtiVisc Plus™	ArtiVisc™ / ArtiVisc Plus™

Fig. 27.20

- **Normal pupil**. The lens does not affect dilatation or constriction of the pupil.

SUMMARY

The Artisan group of iris fixated PIOLs is an excellent option when considering refractive surgery. It is very effective, safe, predictable and stable and can be often used when other modalities may be inadequate.

BIBLIOGRAPHY

1. Antonio Leccisotti. Angle supported phakic intraocular lenses in hyperopia. JCRS Aug 2005.
2. E Yusbasioglu, et al. Fixed dilated pupil after phakic IOL implantation. J Cat Refr Surg Jan 2006.
3. Georges Baikoff. Anterior segment OCT and phakic intraocular lenses. JCRS Nov 2006.
4. I Jimenez-Alfaro, et al. Safety of posterior chamber phakic Intraocular Lenses for the correction of high myopia. Anterior segment changes after posterior chamber phakic intraocular lens implantation. Ophthalmology Jan 2001.
5. J L Guell, et al. Adjustable refractive surgery : 6 mm Artisan lens plus laser in situ keratomileusis for the correction of high myopia. Ophthalmology May 2001.
6. M Bartels, et al. Toric phakic intraocular lens for the correction of hyperopia and astigmatism. JCRS Feb 2006.
7. M Kolhaas, S Druschel. Intraocular pressure after phakic posterior chamber intraocular lens implantation: 5 year follow-up. JCRS Nov 2005.
8. Mana Tehrani, H Burkhard Dick. Changes in higher order aberrations after implantation of a foldable iris claw lens in myopic phakic eyes. JCRS Feb 2006.
9. MC Bartels, et al. Toric phakic intraocular Lens for correction of hyperopia and astigmatism. JCRS Feb 2006.
10. Mihai Pop, et al. Ultrasound biomicroscopy of the Artisan phakic intraocular lens in hyperopic eyes. JCRS Oct 2002.

CHAPTER

28

Emanuel Rosen, Mark Wevill
Christa Gore, Elizabeth Kowaleski (UK)

Phakic IOLs

INTRODUCTION

Phakic IOLs are utilized to correct significant ametropia and are an accepted facet of the refractive surgeon's armamentarium. However, the role of pseudophakia to correct aphakia is only a relatively recent event in the history of ophthalmic surgery. Less than three decades ago lens implantation for aphakia was still a hostile concept; "a time bomb waiting to explode!" In spite of almost universal hostility, pseudophakia not only survived but also blossomed to become the unquestioned answer for cataract affected patients. The impetus of lens implantation could not simply be erased like a mistake in spelling. Unlike so many ideas that perished in their infancy, phakic lens implantation has also survived earlier negative exaggerations which attempted to condemn but ultimately served to market the proposition. Prescient leaders of refractive surgery, rather than associating themselves with the chilly disapprobation of the majority, generated their own frisson of excitement for what phakic lens implantation might achieve for many disadvantaged ametropic patients. They were not to be deterred or so easily distracted from their intended purpose by the bleak insufficiency of a one dimensional approach to refraction, whilst others were excited by the commercial opportunity born. Phakic implantation was not an idea condemned to perish in its infancy.

Technological advances and pseudophakic experience have each played their part to complement the pioneering efforts of George Baikoff in France and Svyatoslov Fyoderov in the then Soviet Union, amongst others. Their contributions were fundamental and have finally lead to universal acceptance of the role of phakic implantation which now complements pseudophakic surgery.

In an age where corneal refractive surgery has exploded on the back of increasingly sophisticated laser surgical technologies, so there has been a much slower but parallel development of phakic implantation. Phakic implant surgery is additive surgery and therefore potentially reversible, a safety aspect appealing to surgeons and patients alike. The optical quality of phakic IOL vision would seem to be superior to oblate corneal vision, so much so that the parameters for corneal laser surgery have receded whilst those for phakic implantation have advanced.

Phakic IOLS may be located in the anterior chamber – angle supported. Arguably this is the simplest of the surgical procedures but requires a substantial incision and therefore the skills to control the prospect of induced astigmatism; anathema to the refractive surgeon. Similarly, the iris supported 'lobster claw' artisan type phakic implant also requires not only a sizeable incision, but additional skills to fixate the IOL by subtle surgical manoeuvres. Prevention of induced astigmatism represents a further surgical challenge. A toric version adds to its potential value aiding the neutralisation of pre-existing astigmatism. Further, a foldable version is imminent. Finally the posterior chamber, which always seemed to be the most unlikely location for phakic implants, has proved to have important advantages for their use. Small, self sealing incisions avoid induced astigmatism, the IOL is invisible to the naked eye and arguably the optical quality is superior because of its proximity to the crystalline lens.

Each type of phakic implant has its advocates and surgeons being creatures of habit adopt one of the versions for their own particular reasons and then the added experience of continued usage invariably persuades them to become advocates for that particular process. This outcome confirms that all the systems are effective, the pros and cons offering the opportunity for continued animated debates amongst refractive surgeons as well as providing an opportunity for novice enlightenment.

REFRACTIVE SURGERY

Refractive surgery is a process wherein one intervention may not suffice to obtain the optimum visual result. When a fair proportion of ametropic eyes have intrinsic astigmatism, this has to be dealt with primarily by surgical means at the time of phakic IOL implantation either by one form of astigmatic surgery or another or use of a toric implant. It follows that many eyes will have a residual error that requires refractive fine tuning. The advent and successful application of corneal laser surgery has by and large provided a satisfactory means of enhancement. Accordingly a major principle of refractive surgery of which phakic IOL implantation is an additive example is that patients are properly informed of the potential need to carry on with staged procedures until the desired outcome is achieved.

ROLE OF PHAKIC IOLs

Phakic IOLs really apply as a solution when corneal laser surgery (CLS) is not safely indicated. This means eyes out of range for CLS for whatever reason – high ametropia or thin cornea etc. Phakic IOLs are an additive solution for a refractive error problem and there are a number of options for surgeons to contemplate namely (a) the location of the IOL — anterior chamber, iris support or posterior chamber; (b) Thereafter, the surgeon is faced with the further choice of rigid or flexible implant plus various manufacturers options rematerials and design.

INDICATIONS

Correction of ametropia too extreme for application of corneal laser surgery preferably, it is a technique which is applied in eyes retaining useful accommodation. Phakic IOLs are an additive solution for the problem of ametropia which means that a degree of reversibility is possible. The case for application in presbyopic eyes is controversial as refractive lens exchange may be the better solution.

CONTRAINDICATIONS

The main contraindication to insertion of a phakic IOL is a shallow anterior chamber depth. A shallow anterior chamber is a contra-indication because of the ultimate proximity of the IOL to the corneal endothelium or in the case of a posterior chamber IOL its proximity to the anterior surface of the crystalline lens and the compromise it may make on aqueous drainage.

RETINAL EFFECTS OF PHAKIC IOLs

Does the insertion of a phakic IOL into myopic eyes in particular (with their extra vulnerability to retinal detachment) increase the risk of retinal breaks and therefore retinal break or detachment compared with un-operated eyes and compared with similar eyes undergoing refractive lens exchange? As a prospective trial to answer these questions is ethically impossible an indirect answer has to be gleaned largely from retrospective studies and epidemiological studies.

Martinez-Castillo V,and colleagues in a study 'Rhegmatogenous retinal detachment (RRD) in phakic eyes after posterior chamber phakic intraocular lens implantation for severe myopia.'Ophthalmology 2005 Apr;112(4):580-5 suggested that the incidence of RRD after PC PIOL implantation was 2.07% over time. In their study the mean patient age was 32.9 years (range, 23-46years). A primary RRD developed in 16 eyes of 15 patients despite prophylactic laser photocoagulation which was performed in 3 eyes of 3 patients (18.75%). The mean preoperative spherical equivalent (SE) was -17.3±2.47 D (-13.75 to -22D.) RRD occurred from 1 to 70 months after PC PIOL implantation (mean: 29.12 months).Each of 11 RRDs (68.75%) had 1 causative break. Fourteen breaks (60.86%) were horseshoe tears (traction tears) and 9 (39.14%) were atrophic holes. Scleral buckling was performed in 10 eyes (62.5%).

Pars plana vitrectomy alone was performed in 5 cases (31.25%) with posterior breaks the initial reattachment rate was 90.9% but the final retinal reattachment was 100%. The mean postoperative BSCVA was 20/28 (0.72±0.25). and mean follow-up after retinal detachment surgery was 35.25±17.29 months (12 - 67 months).

Ruiz-Moreno reporting on RRD in myopic eyes after phakic IOL implantation in JRS 22 2006 247-252 studied 522 eyes retrospective study. There was a RRD of 2.9% with a mean postoperative time of 24 months (range 1-92 months). 0.57% occurred at 3 months, 1.64% by 12 months, 2.73% by 36 months and 4.06% at 92-145 months.

They concluded that the risk of retinal detachment in eyes implanted with phakic lenses for the correction of high myopia was higher in eyes with axial length >30.24 mm.

STAAR COLLAMER ICL

THE Staar Collamer Implantable Contact Lens (Fig. 28.1) is a derivative of the professor Fyderov posterior chamber phakic IOL which he used from the late 1980's until in 1993. Thereafter the Staar company acquired the patents and modified the material and design. The lens used today is the 4th version of the IOL. The modifications have largely solved some initial problems such as ICL induced anterior sub-capsular lens opacities.

Indications

The correction of ametropia both myopia and hyperopia beyond the reach of CLS.

Contraindications

The ICL requires an anterior chamber depth (corneal endothelium to anterior lens surface) of atleast 3 mm.

Technique (Figs 28.1 to 28.7)

Either prior YAG iridotomies 90 degrees apart (10.30 and 1.30) with horizontal location of the ICL or surgical iridactomy at 12 o'clock iris periphery.

ICL loaded in delivery cartridge filled with mixture of BSS and Healon for lubrication.

Paracentesis at 90 degrees.

Anterior chamber deepened with Healon. Temporal incision 2.4 mm in clear cornea.

ICL injected into anterior chamber and relocated into posterior chamber by gentle manipulation of ICL foot paltes over dilated pupil margin. Thereafter, Healon expressed by injection of Miochol into anterior chamber through paracentesis incision.

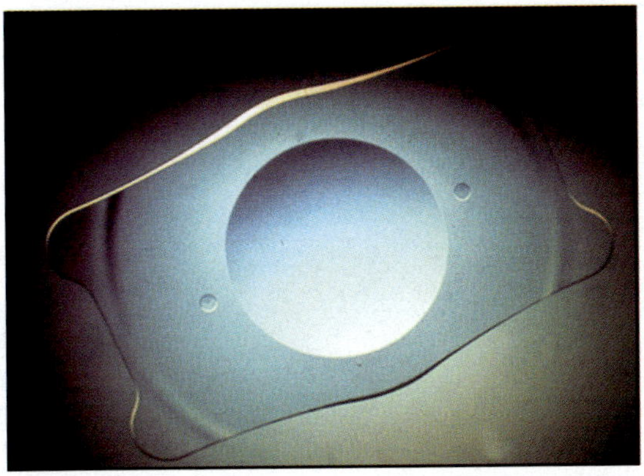

Fig. 28.1: Staar Collamer ICL Collagen-HEMA Polymer = COLLAMER™
62,9% p-HEMA, 33,4% water, 0,2% porcine-collagen, 3,4%UV-absorber, refractive index @35°C = 1.452, hydrophilic and foldable

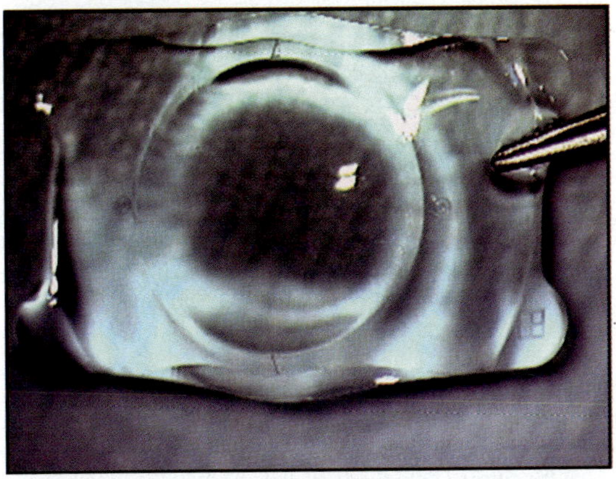

Fig. 28.2

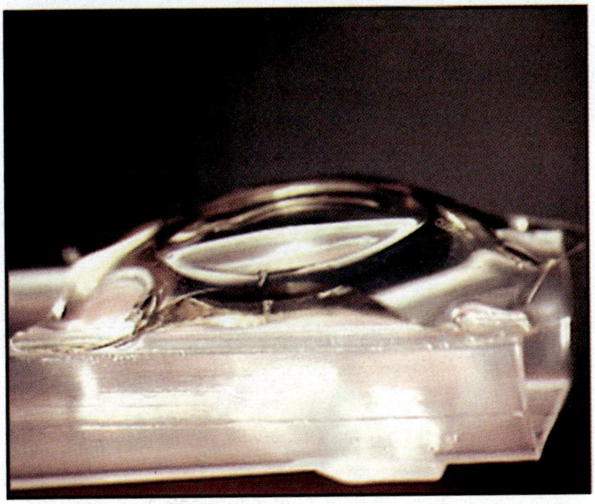

Figs 28.2 and 28.3: ICL preparatory to cartridge loading

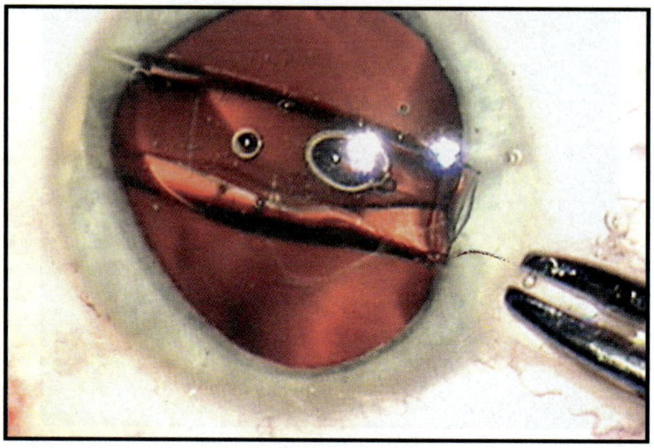

Fig. 28.4: ICL rolled and injected into Healon filled AC

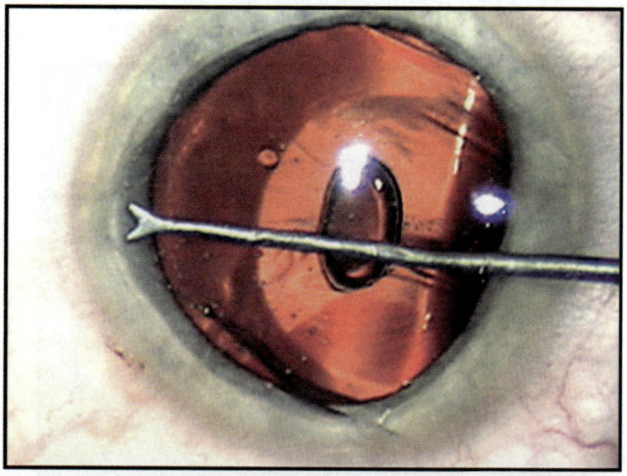

Fig. 28.5: Relocation of ICL footplates into PC

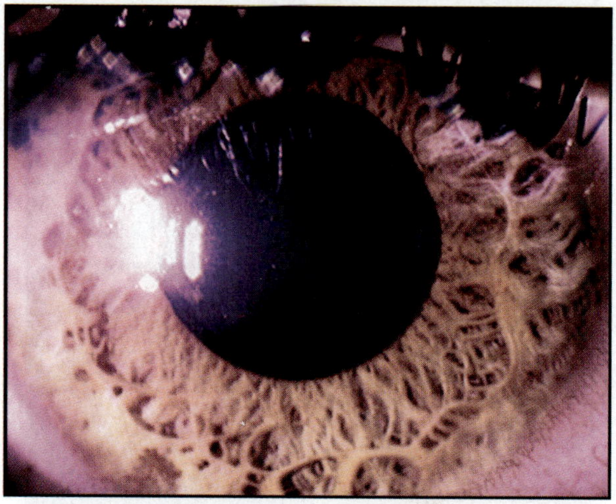

Fig. 28.6: ICL *in situ* week 1

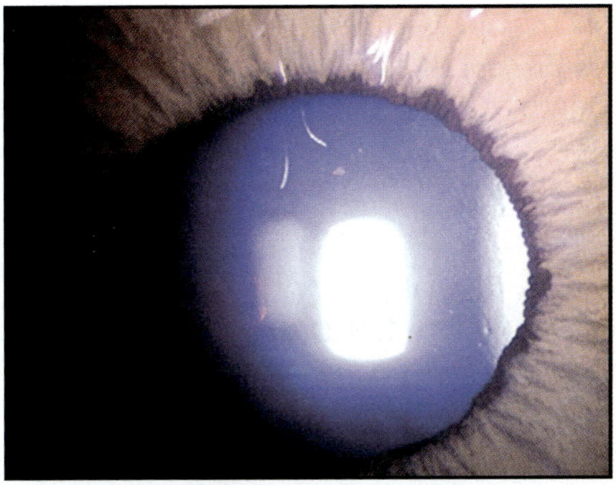

Fig. 28.7: ICL *in situ* day 1

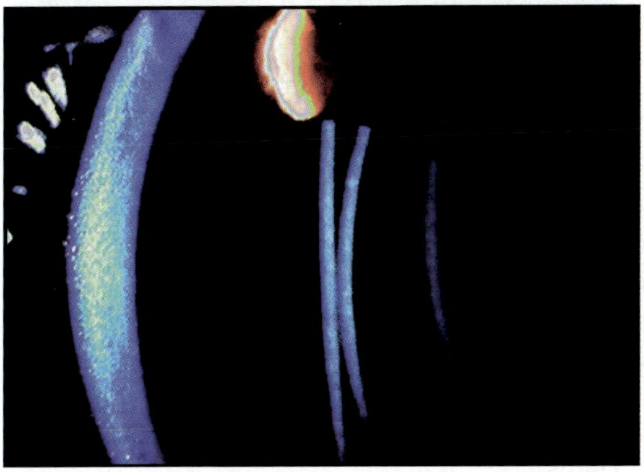

Fig. 28.8: S/L profile of myopic ICL in PC

EXPERIENCE AT ROSEN EYE ASSOCIATES CLINIC MANCHESTER UK

Demography

Number of myopic eyes preop: 291

age	average	36 years (from 17 to 68)
sex	female	63.6% or 185 eyes
	male	33.7% or 98 eyes
eye	left	48.5% or 141 eyes
	right	51.5% or 150 eyes

pre SR equiv: mean –10.29 D ± 3.82 D (from –25.50 to –2.25)
pre SR sph: mean –9.69 D ± 3.73 D (from –24.50 to –2.25)
pre SR cyl: mean –1.20 D ± 1.15 D (from –5.50 to plano)

Hyperopic Eyes

number of eyes pre op: 64

age	average	35 years (from 21 to 66)
sex	female	35.9% or 23 eyes
	male	62.5% or 40 eyes
eye	left	50.0% or 32 eyes
	right	50.0% or 32 eyes

pre SR equiv: mean 5.08 D ± 1.56 D (from 1.25 to 8.25)
pre SR sph: mean 4.51 D ± 1.54 D (from 0.75 to 7.75)
pre SR cyl: mean 1.14 D ± 0.87 D (from 0.00 to 3.50)

Outcomes

291 myopic eyes and 64 hyperopic eyes treated with atleast 3 months follow-up
19 eyes with complications (7%)
1 uveitis
4 exchanges due to incorrect lens diameter (1xV3, 3xV4)
12 cataract surgery 3.4% (Anterior sub-capsular lens opacities in 37% of ICL V2, 14% of ICL V3 and 2% of ICL V4)
1 exchange due to incorrect power
2 explanted due to insuperable glare (same case)
1 glare needing PI suture
No retinal detachments
Hyperopic eyes pupil block (early cases)
3 eyes
Brown irides
Prior YAG iridotomies
1 further YAG resolved the block
1 surgical PI resolved the block
1 block persisted despite YAG iridotomy and surgical iridectomy and progressed to malignant glaucoma requiring resolution by lensectomy and secondary lens implant with 20/20 uncorrected acuity outcome.

Figures 28.6 to 28.8 show ICL *in situ*.

Figures 28.9 to 28.13 Illustrate lens opacities with earlier versions of ICL (V3 and V2).

Figure 28.14: Illustrates rare pigment dispersion on ICL.

Figure 28.15: Illustrates unique example of inspissated Healon which failed to be removed at the end of the surgical procedure.

CONCLUSION

Phakic IOLs are an important element in the armamentarium of the refractive surgeon. The experience in this chapter relates to the posterior chamber Collamer ICL of Staar Company of California and

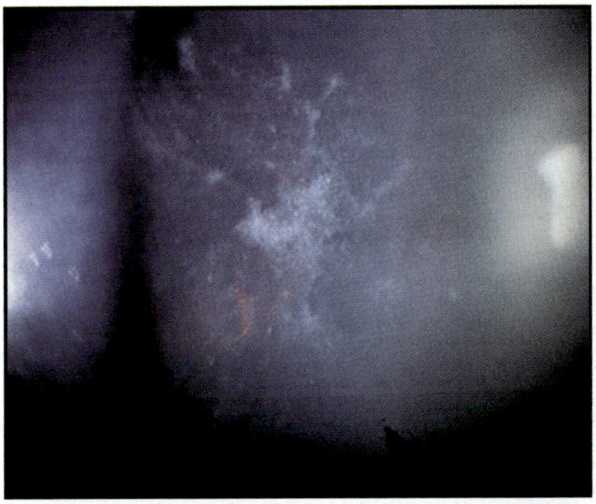

Fig. 28.9: Anterior subcapsular opacities in presence of posterior chamber ICL V2

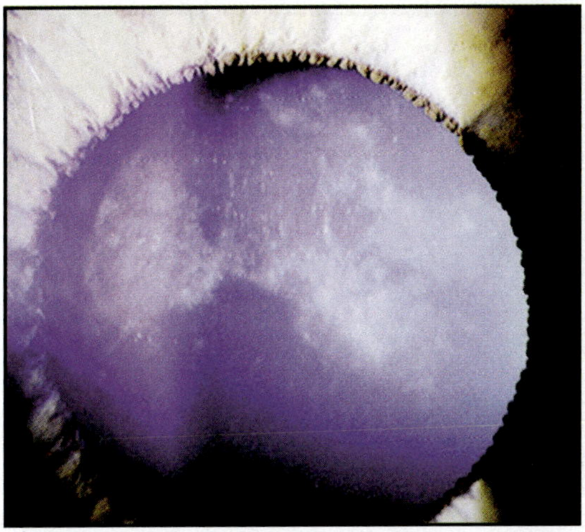

Fig. 28.10: Month 12 anterior subcapsular lens opacities changing over time

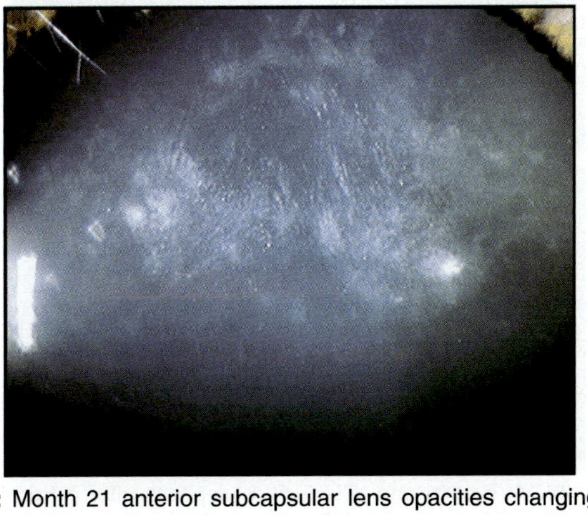

Fig. 28.11: Month 21 anterior subcapsular lens opacities changing over time

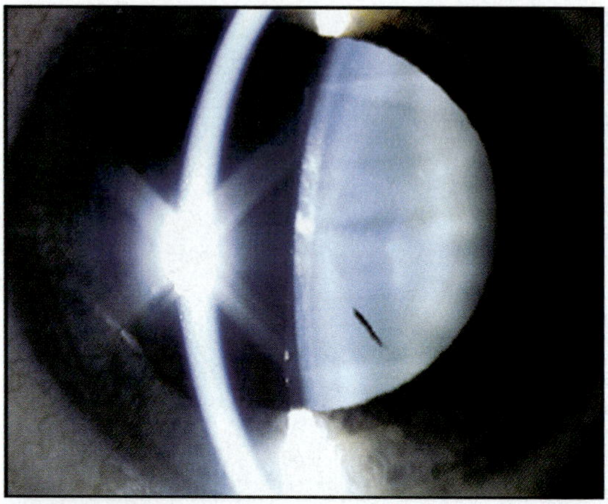

Fig. 28.12: Anterior subcapsular lens opacities caused by early version of ICL

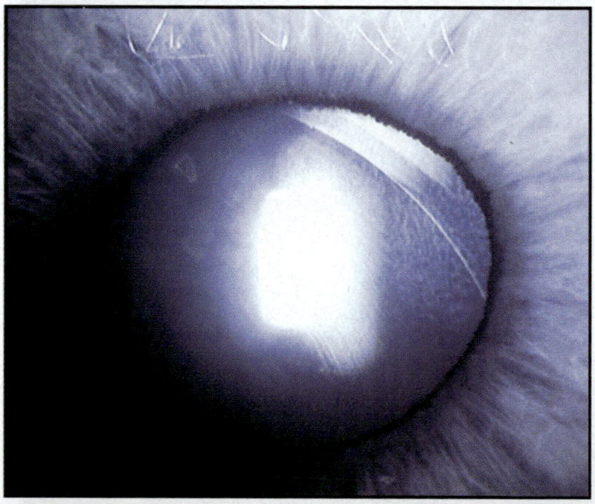

Fig. 28.13: ICL too short and subluxated required uneventful exchanges

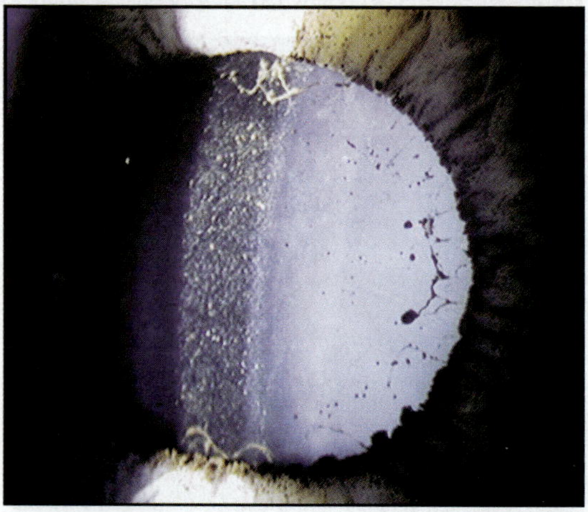

Fig. 28.14: Biofilm and ICL surface deposits after a transient uveitis vision remains 6/6 with no night vision problems

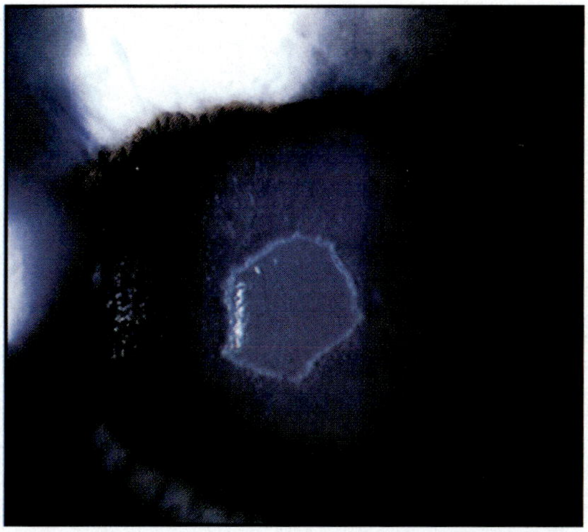

Fig. 28.15: Plaque of inspissated Healon between ICL and anterior lens capsule 2 weeks post surgery. Plaque disappeared by month1

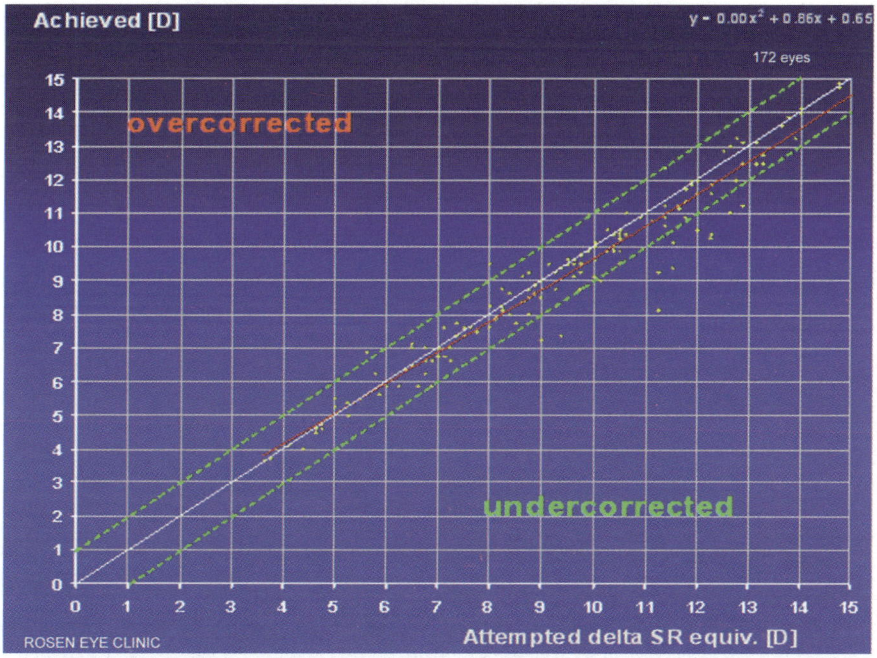

Fig. 28.16: Attempted v achieved. Correction: ICL myopic eyes 6 months postop

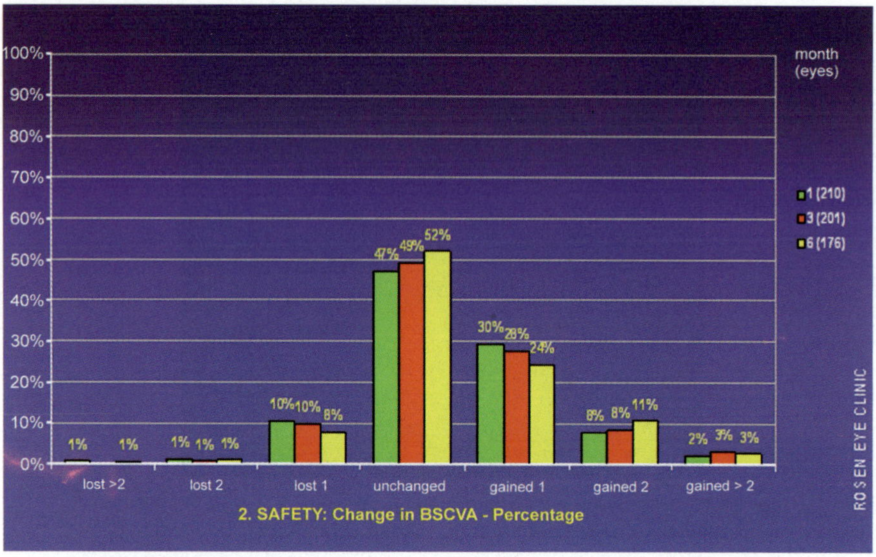

Fig. 28.17: BCVA gained/lost-ICL myopic eyes 1,3 and 6 months postop

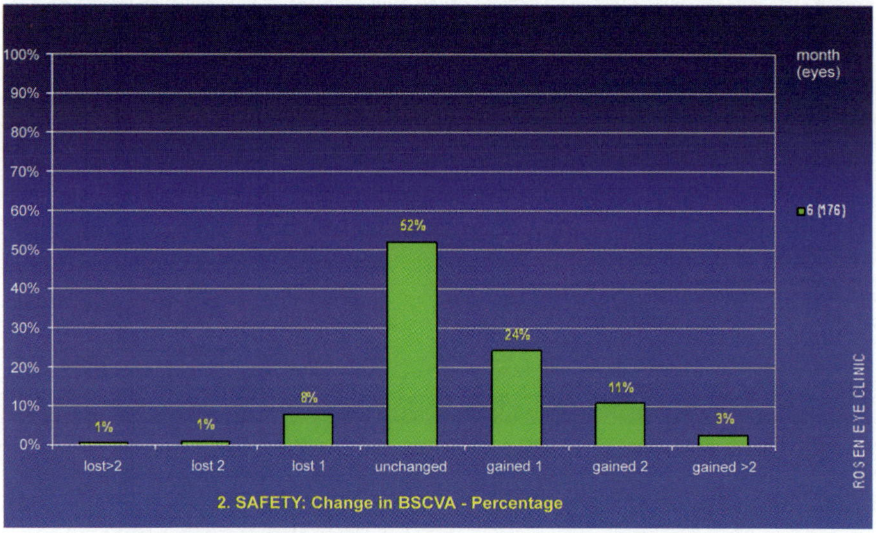

Fig. 28.18: BCVA gained/lost-ICL myopic eyes 6 months postop

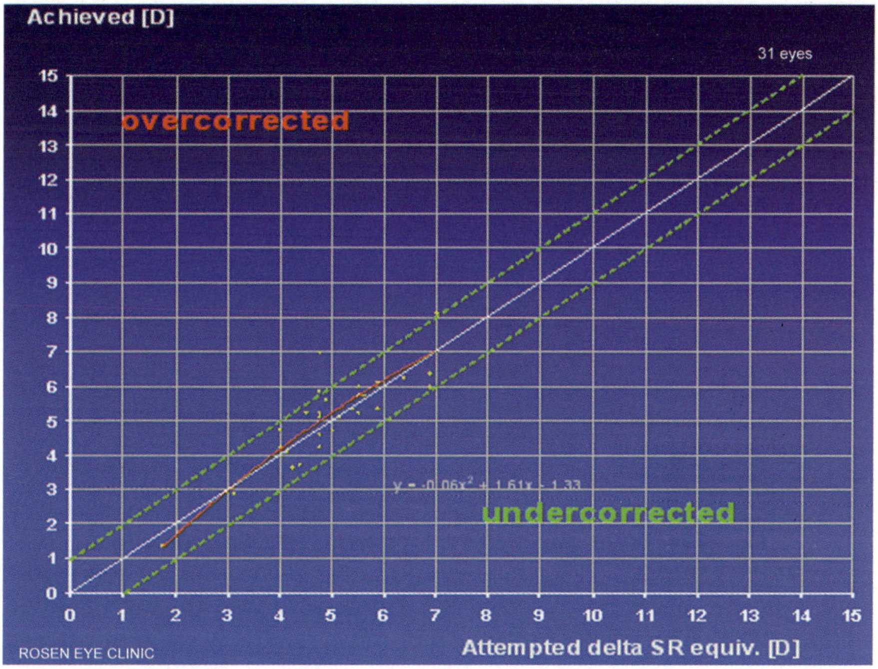

Fig. 28.19: Attempted v achieved. Correction: ICL hyperopic eyes 6 months postop

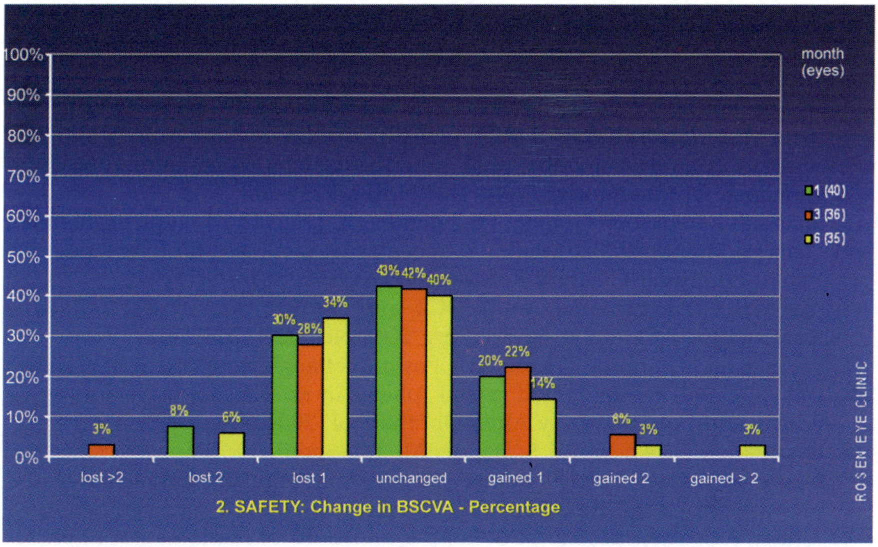

Fig. 28.20: BCVA gained/lost-ICL hyperopic eyes 1,3 and 6 months postop

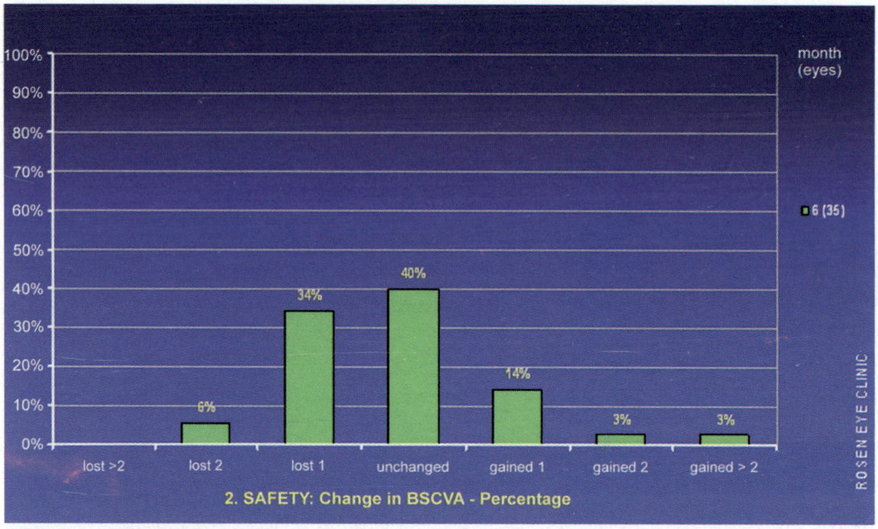

Fig. 28.21: BCVA gained/lost-ICL hyperopic eyes 6 months postop

Switzerland. This is because the ICL offers insertion through a small astigmatically neutral clear corneal incision, a relatively straightforward surgical process with the added benefit of the availability of a toric version for myopic astigmatic eyes. Version 4 of the lens seems to have solved the problem of anterior sub-capsular lens opacities which plagued the earlier versions. Patient acceptance is enthusiastic there being excellent function and no cosmetic issue. Other surgeons will have other preferences based on their own experience. The refractive surgeon has an enviable choice of options.

BIBLIOGRAPHY

1. Alio JL, Abdelrahman AM, Javaloy J, Iradier MT, Ortuno V. Angle-supported anterior chamber phakic intraocular lens explantation causes and outcome. Ophthalmology 2006 Dec;113(12):2213-20.
2. Baikoff G, Bourgeon G, Jodai HJ, Fontaine A, Lellis FV, Trinquet L.Pigment dispersion and Artisan phakic intraocular lenses: crystalline lens rise as a safety criterion.J Cataract Refract Surg 2005 Apr;31(4):674-80.
3. Baikoff G.Anterior segment OCT and phakic intraocular lenses: a perspective. J Cataract Refract Surg 2006 Nov;32(11):1827-35.
4. Baumeister M, Buhren J, Kohnen T.Position of angle-supported, iris-fixated, and ciliary sulcus-implanted myopic phakic intraocular lenses evaluated by Scheimpflug photography.Am J Ophthalmol. 2004 Nov;138(5):723-31.
5. Brazitikos PD, Androudi S, Balidis M, Tsinopoulos L, Papadopoulos NT, Stangos AN, Georgiadis N. Retinal complications of phakic intraocular lenses. Semin Ophthalmol 2003 Sep;18(3):97-102.
6. Cheng AC, Yuen KS, Lam DS. Long-term results of implantation of phakic posterior chamber IOLs.J Cataract Refract Surg 2006 Jan;32(1):4.

7. Coppens JE, van den Berg TJ, Budo CJ. Biometry of phakic intraocular lens using Scheimpflug photography.J Cataract Refract Surg 2005 Oct;31(10):1904-14.
8. Fink A, Rosen ES, Gore C, Cataract formation after Staar Collamer Implantable Contact Lens UK Clinical Experience Jl Cataract & Refractive surgery Feb 1999.
9. Fink A, Rosen ES, Gore C. Staar Collamer Implantable Contact Lens UK Clinical Experience Jl Cataract & Refractive surgery April 1998.
10. Goldsmith JA, Li Y, Chalita MR, Westphal V, Patil CA, Rollins AM, Izatt JA, Huang D.Anterior chamber width measurement by high-speed optical coherence tomography.Ophthalmology 2005 Feb;112(2):238-44.

CHAPTER

29

Frank Jozef Goes (Belgium)

Phakic IOLs: Personal Experience with the Verisyse-Artisan, Veriflex-Artiflex Lens

INTRODUCTION

Visual correction with spectacles or contact lenses is often unsatisfactory or impractical and corneal refractive surgery is not always an option for high myopia or hyperopia. Although LASIK surgery is the most commonly performed refractive procedure,[1-2] concerns of postoperative ectasia limit the procedure in patients who have high myopia and whose corneas do not have adequate thickness or adequate steepness to undergo excimer ablation. Additional potential complications of **LASIK** include microkeratome-related problems, irregular astigmatism, unstable refractions, and the need for enhancements.[3] Although, photorefractive keratectomy –**PRK** can be performed in patients with corneas too thin for LASIK, complications from PRK performed on eyes with high myopia include corneal scarring, an increased risk of ectasia, regression and loss of best spectacle-corrected visual acuity.[4] Furthermore, all refractive surgical interventions, with the exception of the intrastromal corneal ring and phakic IOLs are **irreversible.**

In patients who are not ideal candidates for excimer laser refractive surgery, insertion of **PHAKIC IOLs** offer the possibility of achieving best visual potential without the aid of spectacles or contact lenses, **maintains accommodation, is reversible and is predictable**.

PHAKIC IOLs — HISTORY

Research on Phakic IOLs began in 1986 and includes 3 major designs: (1) posterior chamber lenses (ICL, Fyodorov); (2) anterior chamber angle-supported lenses (Nuvita, Baikoff); and (3) iris-stroma-supported lenses (Artisan-Verisyse Worst).

The first use of **a posterior chamber phakic IOL** to correct myopia was performed by Fyodorov in 1986.[5] In 1990 a second generation unfoldable lens replaced the first generation lens. This lens incorporated collagen into silicone to make the lens hydrophilic.[6] Since 1990, there have been several other posterior chamber lenses employed to correct high myopia including the Collamer Staar IOL. This posterior chamber IOL has undergone many modifications.[7] The Visian ICL (Visian ICL 4, STAAR Surgical Co, Monrovia, CA), was approved by the FDA, December 23, 2005. It is made from a new generation of biocompatible IOL material termed Collamer. Collamer is comprised of a proprietary, hydrophilic porcine collagen (<0.1%)/hydroxyethyl methacrylate copolymer into which an ultraviolet-absorbing chromophore has been incorporated into the polymer chains The implantable collamer lens (ICL) is designed to vault anteriorly to the crystalline lens to have minimal contact with the natural lens.

The first **anterior chamber phakic IOLs** in the 1950s had significant complications including poor fit, increased weight, poor lens quality, and poor surgical technique. Early lenses had **angle fixation** in contrast to the present anterior chamber phakic IOL, the Verisyse lens (AMO), which is fixated to the **iris** in the midperiphery.Angle supported IOLs have as major drawback iris retraction, pupillary ovalization, halo's and glare and endothelial cell loss[8] and they are difficult to reposition and to remove. In contrast, the iris fixated lens or "**iris claw**" anterior chamber phakic Verisyse lens, which is marketed outside the United States as the Artisan lens (Ophtec BV, Groningen, The Netherlands) minimizes the problems of angle fixation, is stable and reversible.

The Artisan lens was introduced in 1991 after a 5-year trial. It had a concave-convex configuration, which decreased the risk of endothelial damage. The lens has a track record of safety with over 15 years of experience.

Verisyse and Veriflex are the AMO market brand of Artisan and Artiflex.Artisan and Artiflex are sold worldwide except in the US.AMO has the right to sell only Verisyse, no Ophtec products are in the US market. In many other markets AMO and Ophtec distributors are competitors.

The Verisyse lenses available in the United States are nonfoldable with a 5.0 mm or 6.0 mm optic with a split haptic at each end to allow for enclavation (or insertion) of a small amount of iris tissue to fixate the lens in the anterior chamber. The enclavation site is typically 1.5 to 2.0 mm from the corneal endothelium at the angle so as to allow adequate distance from the epithelium while allowing the pupil to widely dilate. The Verisyse phakic lens is positioned in the anterior chamber and held in place by fixation to the midperipheral iris stroma, creating a bridge over the optical axis. The enclavation site is typically 1.5 to 2.0 mm from the corneal endothelium at the angle. This location provides ample distance from the epithelium while enabling the pupil to widely dilate.

The vault of the lens does not change with the lens power. The range is 0.35 to 0.93 mm and occupies approximately 30% of the anterior chamber. The 5.0 mm optic is available in powers from – 1.00 to – 23.5 D in 0.50 increments and the 6.00 mm optic is available from – 1.00 to – 15.50 D also in 0.50 increments. The 6.0 mm optic is thicker than the 5.0 mm optic and is limited in power to provide enough distance between the optic and the corneal endothelium. The overall length of both lenses is 8.5 mm.The lens material is Perspex CQ-UV.

Development Artisan-Verisyse:Artiflex-Veriflex

The Artisan / Artiflex Lens design is developed by Prof. Jan GF Worst MD, winner of the prestigious Binkhorst Award for innovation in ophthalmology in 1976. The current lens is the result of over 20 years of clinical experience with a unique fixation concept.

In 1978, the first Artisan Lens, originally called 'Iris Claw" was introduced. This model was developed for the correction of aphakia following cataract surgery. The lens has been implanted in approximately 300,000 aphakic eyes worldwide. Nowadays Artisan aphakia Lenses are increasingly used as the back-up lens of choice by many cataract surgeons.

In 1986, the first Artisan Phakic lens for the correction of myopia was implanted in November 2 by Paul U Fechner, Germany. It had a biconcave design.

In 1991, following a 5 year feasibility study, modifications were incorporated into the phakic lens design, resulting in a convex-concave Artisan Myopia lens. The new design decreases the potential for complications, improves the optical performance and makes the surgical implantation easier.

In 1992, the first Artisan Hyperopia Lens was implanted. In 1996 a redesigned Artisan Aphakia Lens was developed.

In 1999, an Artisan Toric Lens was developed and introduced to the market in 2001.

In 2003 a flexible Artisan lens, the Artiflex Lens, was developed. The lens obtained FDA approval in 2004 and was since 2005 introduced to the market as the Artiflex Myopia lens.

The Verisyse phakic IOL is the first lens of its kind to receive FDA approval, with a new option for treating myopic patients .The Verisyse lens is suitable for the reduction or elimination of myopia in adults from –5.0 to –20.0 dioptres and in patients aged 21 and over.

The lens design was introduced in Europe more than 17 years ago. More than 150,000 been safely implanted worldwide.

Artisan lenses are available from –1 to –23.5 in 0.5 D step for **myopia** and from +1 to +12 D for **hyperopia.**The **toric myopic** lens is available till 7.5 D of astigmatism. The **foldable version Artiflex** is available from –2 to –14.5 D (Figs 29.1 to 29.3).

Specifications-Verisyse-Veriflex

The ARTISAN Intraocular Lenses are substantially different from all pupil-supported lenses of the past. ARTISAN Intraocular Lenses are peripheral "**iris bridge**" supported lenses, and not "iris/pupil supported" lenses ARTISAN Phakic Intraocular Lens haptics (fixation

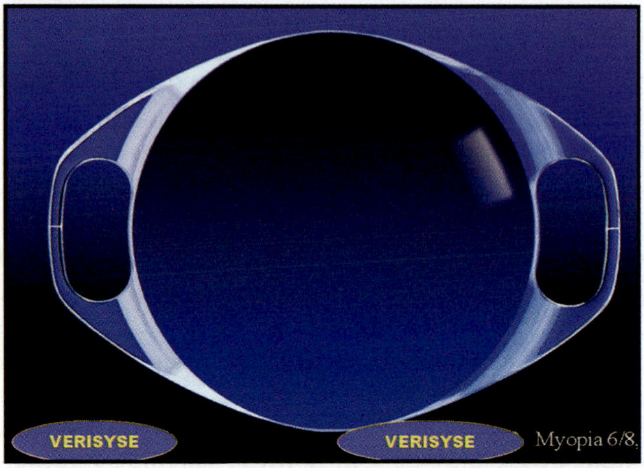

Fig. 29.1: Verisyse IOL: Optic-haptic and enclavation slits

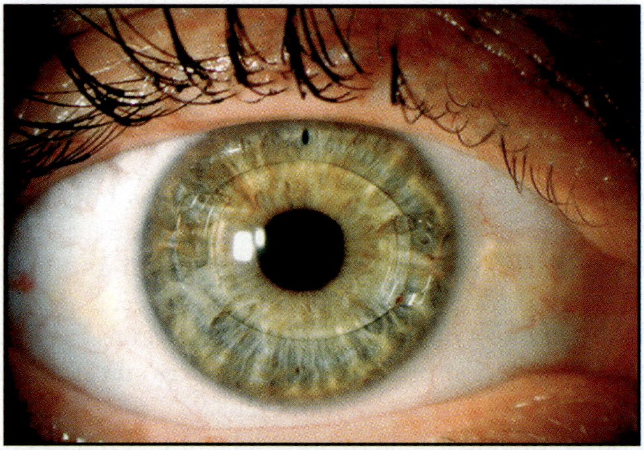

Fig. 29.2: Verisyse IOL in the eye: Notice the peripheral iridotomy

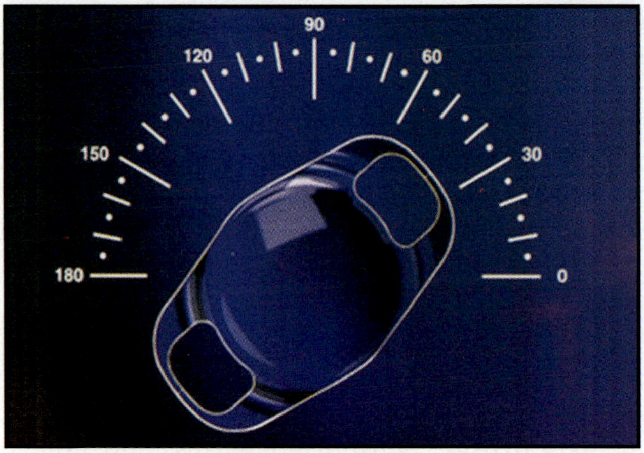

Fig. 29.3: Toric IOL

arms) attach to the midperipheral virtually immobile iris stroma, thus allowing the pupil unrestricted ability to dilate and constrict.

The two diametrically opposed haptics ensure stable **fixation to the iris**, preventing pseudo-phakodonesis and the risk of post-operative decentration. The fixation concept permits the ARTISAN Phakic Intraocular Lenses to be centred on the pupil. The system is extremely **versatile,** as ARTISAN Phakic Intraocular Lenses may be fixated horizontally, vertically or obliquely. Since its inception 25 years ago, the fixation principle of the ARTISAN Lens has remained unchanged.

The vaulting of ARTISAN Phakic Intraocular Lenses provides optimum clearance between the PIOL and the crystalline lens, and between the PIOL and the cornea. At the same time ARTISAN Phakic Intraocular Lenses show a low cross-sectional profile within the eye. The distance from the rim of the optic and the corneal endothelium is approximately 1.0 to 2.0 mm, depending on the AC depth and dioptric power. A free flow of aqueous is ensured by the vaulted lens design. The lens has four side-ports, thereby minimizing the potential risk of pupillary block. Nevertheless, it is important to perform an iridectomy or iridotomy; an iridectomy is preferred.

The **ARTIFLEX PIOL** design is the latest step in development of the iris fixation concept. The ARTIFLEX Myopia is a three-piece lens consisting of a flexible optical part made of ultraviolet absorbing Polysiloxane and rigid haptics made of Perspex CQ–UV polymethylmethacrylate (PMMA).Because the design of the ARTIFLEX PIOL was based on the ARTISAN concept, it includes all the advantages of the ARTISAN PIOL, such as: reversibility, one-size fits all, excellent centration, iris bridge to protect the endothelium and safe clearance from vital tissue.

The **ARTIFLEX** Myopia Intraocular Lens is designed with a flexible 6 mm body. The flexibility of the body allows for a small incision of 3.2 mm. Due to the **small incision**, the frequency of surgically induced astigmatism can be reduced, faster visual recovery can be achieved and there is no need for suturing. This allows an extremely rapid postoperative recovery and a reduction of risk of glare and halos because of the special edge design.

Technical details of the different **Verisyse Artisan lenses** go below:

ARTISAN Myopia 5/8.5
Material: Perspex CQ-UV
Optic diameter: 5 mm
Overall diameter: 8.5 mm
Powers available: –1.0 D to –23 .5 D (0.5 D increments)

ARTISAN Myopia 6/8.5
Material: Perspex CQ-UV
Optic diameter: 6 mm
Overall diameter: 8.5 mm
Powers available: –1.0 D to –15 .5 D (0.5 D increments)

ARTISAN Hyperopia 5/8.5
Material: Perspex CQ-UV
Optic diameter: 5 mm
Overall diameter: 8.5 mm
Powers available: +1.0 D to +12.0 D (0.5 D increments)

ARTISAN Toric 5/8.5
ARTISAN Toric Phakic IOLs are available with a 0° or a 90° cylinder.
Material: Perspex CQ-UV
Optic diameter: 5 mm
Overall diameter: 8.5 mm
The specifications of the **VERIFLEX-ARTIFLEX** are as follows: Dioptre Range: –2.0 to –14.5 D in 0.5 dioptre increments; Overall size: 8.5 mm; Optic size: 6.0 mm; Haptic width: 3.0 mm; Optic material: Polysiloxane; Refraction index: 1.43; Optic shape: Round, convex-concave; Edge shape: Anti-glare design; haptic material: Perspex CQ-UV (PMMA); Haptic shape: Iris claw design; Overall shape: Open port design.

The Veriflex

The Veriflex PIOL is suitable for patients who are 21 to 60 years old and have stable refraction, have good general health, seek independence from contact lenses or spectacles, are not good candidates for kerato-refractive surgery and like the idea of removable implants that offers high-quality vision.

The Artisan toric lens has a convex concave toric optic with a spherical anterior surface and a spherocylindrical posterior surface. This single-piece lens is composed of PMMA and is manufactured using a compression molding technology. The toric IOL is iris-claw fixated, and it has a 5 mm optical zone. The intraocular lens is available in dioptric powers of –3.00 D to –20.50 D; 2.00 D to 12.00 D; and in cylindrical powers of 2.00 D to 7.50 D (Figs 29.4 to 29.6).

Analysis of Phakic IOL Position

Pinault et al[9] evaluated the anatomic relationships of the implantable contact lens (ICL) (17 eyes) and the phakic refractive lens (PRL) posterior chamber phakic intraocular lenses (14 eyes) (PCP IOL) using

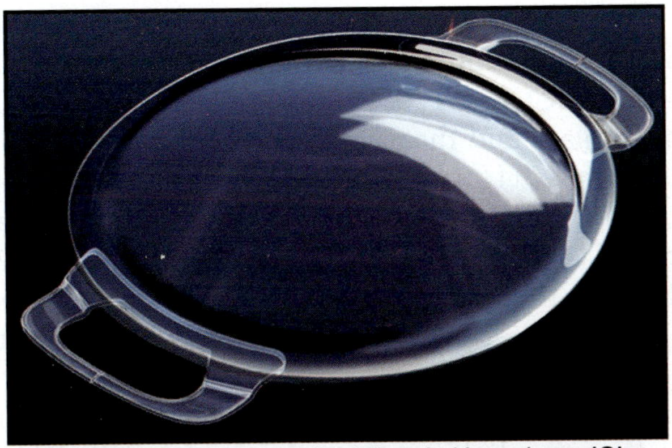

Fig. 29.4: Notice the vault of the phakic verisyse IOL

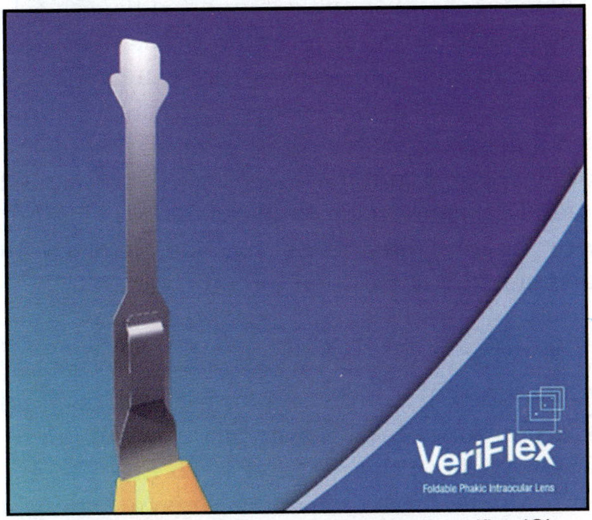

Fig. 29.5: Insertion spatula of the foldable veriflex IOL

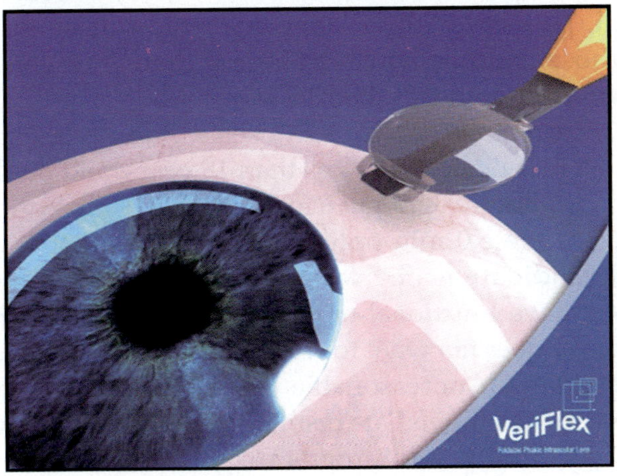

Fig. 29.6: Insertion of the veriflex IOL

ultrasound biomicroscopy (UBM).The mean distance between the PCP IOL and the central endothelium was 2398+/–203 micron and 2640+/230 micron in the ICL and PRL groups, respectively. The central vault between the implant and the crystalline lens was greater in eyes with ICL (ICL, 402+/–194 micron; PRL, 256+/–187 micron $p<0.05$). However, the incidence of lens contact on the peripheral level was higher in the ICL group (41%) than in the PRL group (29%).

According to these authors PCP IOL implantation is a safe procedure for the correction of high myopia with regard to refractive results.

Baumeister et al[10] examined the postoperative positional stability of different myopic phakic intraocular lenses (IOLs).46 eyes which received an anterior chamber angle-supported Bausch & Lomb NuVita lens –20 eyes which received an anterior chamber iris-fixated lens (Ophtec Artisan; 20 eyes) and 16 eyes with a sulcus-implanted phakic IOL(Staar ICL; 16 eyes).The angle-supported anterior chamber phakic IOLs showed a generally stable position regarding distance to cornea and natural lens, but rotation was observed in four IOLs. The iris-fixated phakic IOL showed the highest overall stability. In general intraocular lenses implanted in phakic eyes followed for 12 months demonstrated stable IOL position overall.

PATIENT SELECTION FOR PHAKIC IOLs IN MYOPIA

The Verisyse phakic IOL is **indicated** for use in patients who have had a stable refraction for at least a year, are a minimum of 18 years of age and have myopia in the range of – 4.5 to – 22.0 D.

Contraindications to insertion of the Verisyse lens include, cataract, patients with retinal detachment or family history of retinal detachment, patients with an abnormal pupil or abnormal cornea, patients whose endothelial count is less than 2000 cells/mm^2, low anterior chamber depth(less than 3.2 mm), elevated IOP, abnormal iris, chronic or recurrent uveitis/iritis, rubeosis irides, preexisting macular degeneration, retinopathy, age less than 18 years, and pupil size under mesopic conditions greater than 6 mm for the 5.0 mm optic and greater than 7 mm for the 6.0 mm optic.

A **good candidate** is one who is dissatisfied with the quality of vision, might have functional or cosmetic limitations with spectacles, and is unable or does not want to wear contact lenses. A poor candidate has inappropriate or unreasonable expectations and expects perfect vision and demands immediate results. Target postoperative refraction is – 0.50 D. A formula and program can be obtained from AMO to calculate IOL power.[30] Anisekonia may be an issue in patients who have surgery in one eye with dioptric powers above a – 7.0D and patients should consider bilateral procedures.

Besides that excellent candidates for the VERIFLEX lens are patients with preoperative astigmatism of less than 2.0 D.

IOL Power Calculation

This is based upon the van der Heyde formula.[11] The IOL power is dependent on the preoperative spectacle refraction, corneal power and postoperative position, but not on the axial length.

Correction of strongly myopic eyes is, at least optically, a simple matter. Precise measurement of preoperative spectacle refraction and corneal power will provide the power for an IOL for any location. In contrast with implants in phakic eyes, the negative power of an IOL needed for a myopic eye will decrease for more posterior positions in the anterior chamber (Figs 29.7 to 29.9).

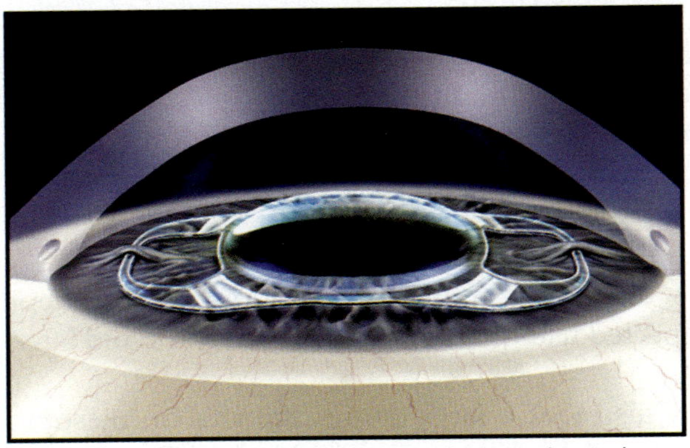

Fig. 29.7: The veriflex in place nicely enclavated

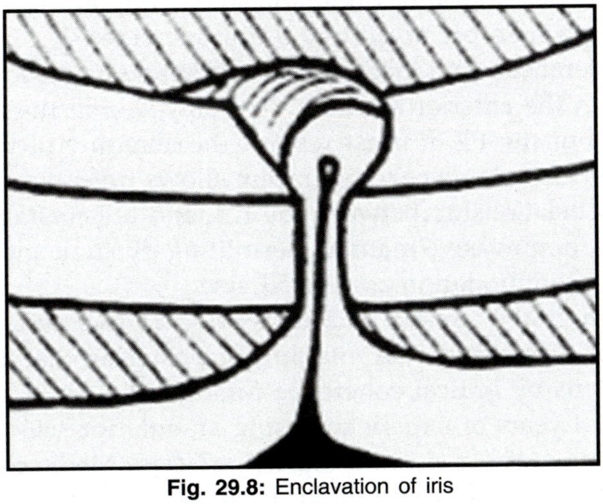

Fig. 29.8: Enclavation of iris

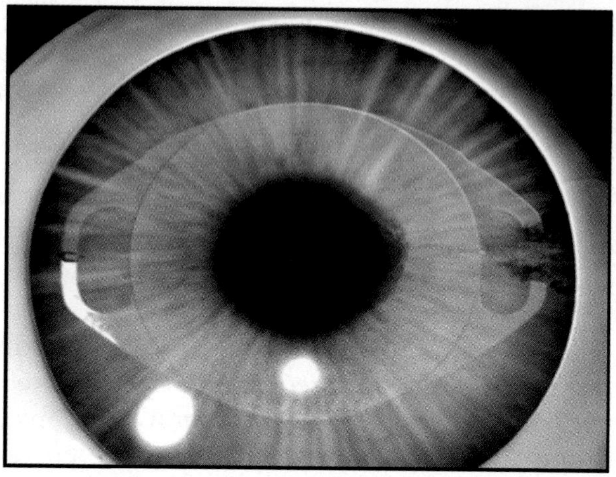

Fig. 29.9: Iris tissue enclavated:Left too little right too much

Preoperative Assessment

The standard surgical workup and measurement has to be performed, including refraction (without soft cl for 1 week and without GP cl for 3 weeks) precise keratometry, accurate biometry (IOL master or Immersion ultrasound) endothelial cell count and precise topography. The target is emmetropia for young people, and can be modified according to the age.

We know also that a minimum anterior chamber depth (3.2 mm) has to be respected using this surgery in order to avoid later endothelial damage.

We know also that a large pupil diameter in mesopic conditions will enhance the risk of later glare and halo's. That is the reason why we prefer to use the 6 mm optic and avoid implanting the lens in patients with a mesopic pupil of 7.0 mm or wider.

Perfect tolerance is expected when one implants a phakic intraocular lens (PIOL) in the anterior segment. Not only should the material be compatible, but the PIOL must respect the anatomy of the anterior chamber. Optical coherence tomography allows precise assessment of the anatomic relationship between the ICL and the crystalline lens in a noncontact, noninvasive manner, permitting dynamic monitoring of changes in accommodation and pupil size.

Bechmann et al[12] already in 2002 used OCT to assess the phakic IOL position discussing also imaging of posterior chamber phakic intraocular lens by optical coherence tomography.

Based on 3 years of experience using an anterior segment optical coherence tomographer (Visante OCT, Carl Zeiss Meditec), Baikoff et al[13, 14] have defined safety criteria for PIOLs. He proposes an objective measurement of the iris dome, the **crystalline lens rise** (CLR), which is the distance between the anterior pole of the crystalline lens and a line joining the 2 opposite iridocorneal angles. In a series with the Artisan IOL (Ophtec), pigment dispersion syndrome appeared in 70% of cases in which the CLR was greater than 600 micron. The higher the crystalline lens rise, the greater the risk for developing pigment dispersion in the area of the pupil. This complication occurred more frequently in hyperopic eyes than in myopic eyes. Results indicate there is little or no risk for pigment dispersion if the rise is less than 600 micron. Crystalline lens rise should be considered a new safety criterion for Artisan phakic IOL implantation and should also be applied to other types of phakic IOLs.

COMPLICATIONS

Maroccos et al[15] noticed that all currently available phakic IOLs, in particular the ICL and the NuVita lead to a decreased visual performance during night time causing **glare and halo's**; Therefore, this phenomenon must be explained to the patient prior to surgery. An increase in the size of the optic (which took place for the 6 mm version of Verisyse Veriflex lens) should lead to an improvement with reduction of postoperative glare and halos.

Alio et al[16] discussed the potential risk of nuclear **cataract** development after phakic AC IOL implantation angle supported intraocular lenses. Phakic IOL explantation, phacoemulsification, and PC IOL implantation successfully resolved this complication. In their analysis the benefits in terms of BSCVA and spherical equivalent obtained after phakic AC IOL implantation were preserved after cataract surgery.

Allemann et al[8] reported good efficacy for myopic angle-supported intraocular lenses correction of high myopia by the phakic IOL NuVita angle supported IOL used during the two years of follow-up. Long-term complications for this angle-supported such as **iris retraction** and **endothelial cell loss** remained a concern.

Menezo et al[17] in a retrospective study in 1998 of 111 phakic eyes (73 patients) implanted with the Worst iris-claw lens.1, 2, 3, and 4 years postoperatively concluded that **endothelial damage** occurred primarily during the surgical procedure.

Trindade and Pereira[18] reported **cataract** formation after posterior chamber phakic intraocular lens implantation and described a case of cataract formation 6 months after uneventful implantation of a Staar PCP IOL to correct high myopia. In their study the most common reason for explantation of phakic posterior chamber IOLs was cataract.

Other causes for explantation included, in decreasing order, IOL decentration/dislocation, inappropriate dioptric power, corneal edema, and pupil ovalization.

Of all respondents who reported lens opacities after phakic IOL implantation, 71.2% observed anterior subcapsular (AS) opacities and 12.3% observed **nuclear opacities** occurring in 1 to 20% of cases.[1]

Moshirfar et al[19] reported a **TASS** syndrome after Verisyse IOL.Toxic anterior segment syndrome has been reported after implantation of IOLs previously, but this new case of TASS should alert surgeons to the possibility of the syndrome after phakic IOL placement.

Tahzib et al[20] described **severe cell deposits** 1 week after implantation of a foldable Artiflex phakic intraocular lens (PIOL) for the correction of high myopia. A successful exchange with a PMMA Artisan PIOL was done. This highlights the importance of intensive steroid therapy first days after Artiflex implantation.

Dick et al[21] analysed **changes in pupil size** after implantation of an iris-fixated toric phakic intraocular lens for correction of myopia and hyperopia with astigmatism. Twenty-two myopic eyes and 9 hyperopic eyes were included in the study. The scotopic pupil size was measured with a handheld infrared pupillometer (Colvard, Oasis Medical) before and 6 months after implantation of the TPIOL.The scotopic pupil diameter decreased by a mean of 1.1 mm in myopic eyes and 1.0 mm in hyperopic eyes after implantation of the iris-supported TPIOL.The slightly smaller pupil diameter in the axis of enclavation suggests that this fixation method restricts pupil size under scotopic conditions.

Sekundo et al[22] studied the Influence of incision parameters on astigmatism during implantation of phakic-6-mm-iris-claw intraocular lenses. The superior corneal incision had a mean SIA of 1.2 D cyl. The sclerocorneal tunnel induced 0.75 D cyl, while the two-incisional techniques delivered nearly astigmatismus neutral results. A proper selection of an appropriate incision site and type allowed to correct the preexisting astigmatism or to keep a spherical refraction after an implantation of a 6-mm-rigid phakic iris-claw IOL. Of course the use of the **foldable** version will exclude this complication.

Tehrani et al[23] studied postoperative astigmatism and **rotational stability** after Artisan toric phakic intraocular lens implantation. The difference between the mean intended cylinder axis and achieved cylinder axis was 3.9 degrees (median 3 degrees; range to 13 degrees).During the 6-month follow-up, no significant rotation was observed after implantation of Artisan toric phakic IOLs to correct high ametropia.

Ardjomand et al[24] described a **pupillary** block after phakic anterior chamber intraocular lens implantation. Very severe and disturbing pupillary block glaucoma may occur after phakic IOL implantation without iridotomy, and we advocate that routine iridotomy be performed during phakic IOL and we use the **YAG** laser to perform it beforehand.

Morales et al[25] studied outcomes of simultaneous phakic implantable contact lens removal with cataract extraction and pseudophakic intraocular lens implantation.

We know that **lens opacities and cataract** formation are a potential complication of ICL surgery. This retrospective noncomparative interventional case series evaluated 14 eyes of 12 patients with ICL implantations who developed a cataract and had simultaneously ICL removal and cataract extraction with IOL implantation. The removal of the ICL and the cataract with IOL implantation was found to be safe, with predictable refractive results.

LITERATURE RESULTS VERISYSE ARTISAN-VERIFLEX-ARTIFLEX-TORIC PHAKIC IOL

Early Years

Worst JG et alin 1990[26] proposed refractive surgery for high myopia using The Worst-Fechner biconcave iris claw lens. The found that iris claw lens, fixed to the midperiphery of the iris, has proved its safety in aphakic eyes.

Fechner et al reported in 1990[27] one hundred and twenty-seven eyes of 70 patients using the worst biconcave phakic iris claw lens. A refractive outcome of +/–1.00 D was achieved in 51 eyes (75%). Seventeen eyes (13.4%) had a decrease in endothelial cell density and projection to 8-year follow-up resulted in a decrease in 27% of eyes. Four eyes needed a penetrating keratoplasty and 13.4% of implanted eyes suffered significant progressive reduction of endothelial cell density. This lens style is no longer in clinical use.

Landesz et al 1995[28] analysed outcomes of correction of high myopia with the Worst myopia claw intraocular lens. They studied 35 eyes in 18 patients with a preoperative myopia ranging from –6.00 to –28.00 dioptres (D). The follow-up ranged from 6 months (n = 15) to 12 months (n = 20). Implanting a Worst myopia claw IOL in high myopic eyes resulted in a stable, reasonably accurate refractive outcome.

In the study of Perez-Santonja et al[29] of surgical correction of high myopia in phakic eyes with Worst-Fechner myopia intraocular lenses the mean endothelial cell loss was 7.2% at 3 months, 10.6% at 6 months, 13% at 12 month and 17.6% at 24 months after surgery. Their results for the Worst-Fechner myopia lens confirmed earlier findings on the effectiveness of the refractive results. However, the study showed a continual decrease in endothelial cell density.

Modern Times

Myopia

Budo et al[30] assessed the Artisan intraocular lens to correct myopia in phakic eyes in a European Multicenter study sponsored by Ophtec BV, Groningen, The Netherlands in 2000.

In this prospective multicenter clinical study, the Artisan lens was implanted in 518 eyes between September 1991 and October 1999. The power of the lenses ranged from –5.0 to –20.0 dioptres (D). Follow-up ranged from 6 months (n = 454) to 3 years (n = 249). The preoperative mean best spectacle-corrected visual acuity (BSCVA) was 0.67 +/- 0.26 (SD).

A UCVA of 20/40 or better was observed in 76.8% of eyes regardless of the postoperative goal. A BSCVA of 20/40 or better was observed in 93.9% of eyes and remained stable throughout the follow-up. Of the eyes with extremely high myopia (> –15.0D) 63.3% gained 2 or more lines of BSCVA: of those with moderate myopia (-5.0 to –10.0 D), 23.5% gained 2 or more lines. The mean endothelial cell density change was 4.8% at 6 months, 2.4% at 1 year, 1.7% at 2 years and 0.7% at 3 years. Secondary surgical interventions included repositioning of the lens because of poor initial placement and lens exchange because of preoperative power calculation errors. Glare and halo effects during night driving were noted and were related to large pupils in young patients.

The degree of endothelial cell loss was confirmed in a subgroup of 129 eyes with a follow-up of 3 years. Postoperatively, the mean cell density change was 4.8% (2739 +/–431 cells/mm^2) at 6 months, 2.4% (2672 +/– 386 cells/mm^2) at 1 year, 1.7% (2626 +/– 424 cells/mm^2) at 2 years, and 0.7% (2607 +/– 442 cells/mm^2) at 3 years.

The Artisan model 206 with a 5.0 mm optic was used exclusively during this study. In 1997, a new model with a 6.0 mm optic was introduced to address potential glare/halos in patients with larger pupils. This model is more forgiving when the lens is somewhat decentered.

No rotation of the IOL, pupil ovalization, uveitis, or persistent corneal dystrophy was reported.

Maloney et al in 2002[31] in the USA evaluated the safety and efficiency of the Artisan iris-supported phakic intraocular lens for the correction of high myopia. Their short-term results suggested that the

Artisan lens was an accurate and safe method for the correction of high myopia. They highlighted that surgical skill is important in avoiding lens opacities.

The Verisyse US STUDY group[32,33] published results in 2004.This clinical study involved 440 subjects(myopia –5 to –20.0) in 22 centers.The mean refractive power was –12,6 D:over 86% of patients were within +/–1D. Minimal endothelial cell loss was reported after surgery. Contrast sensitivity was unchanged or improved after implantation. Adverse effects were uncommon.

Moshirfar et al[34] reported 2 cases in which an Artisan phakic intraocular lens (IOL) (Ophtec) was used to successfully treat high myopia after penetrating keratoplasty (PKP).

Lifshitz et al in 2004[35] reviewed thirty-one eyes (22 patients) with myopia from –5.25 to –19.00 dioptres. At 3 months BSCVA for 20 eyes (64.5%) had improved one or more lines in visual acuity. Mean endothelial cell loss at 3 months was 3.96%. According to them the Artisan lens is a safe, predictable, and efficacious method to correct high myopia. Postoperative gain in BSCVA was achieved for the majority of eyes.

Benedetti et al[36] reported a 2 year follow-up of myopia –7 to –24 corrected with Artisan. At 4 months, 83.8% in group 1,(myopia –6.75 to –15.50 D) and 68% in group 2,(myopia –16.0 to –23.0 D) of eyes achieved UCVA of > or =20/40. The BSCVA remained the same or improved in 100% of eyes. Mean endothelial cell loss was 2.8% at 4 months, 3.9% at 12 months, and 5.4% at 24 months. Their results confirmed that these lenses are safe and effective for the correction of high myopia, with a stable refractive outcome but with a higher than normal rate of endothelial cell loss during 2-year follow-up (Fig. 29.10).

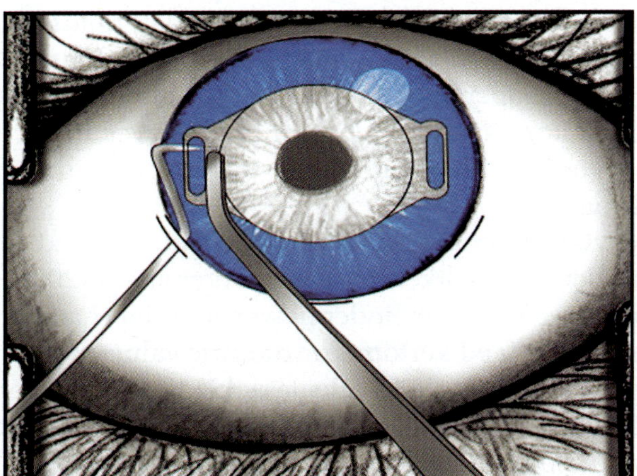

Fig. 29.10: Technique of two hand enclavation of phakic iris-fixated IOL

Hyperopia

Saxena et al[37] reviewed Artisan results in hyperopia. Twenty-six eyes of 13 self-selected patients with refractive error ranging from +3.00 to +11.00 dioptres (D) were followed for a mean of 22.4 months (range, 3-36 months). No patient lost 2 or more lines after the procedure. There was a significant negative correlation between anterior chamber depth and endothelial cell loss. Implantation of the Artisan Hyperopic lens leads to accurate and stable refractive results with no significant loss of vision. According to the authors more attention should be paid to convex irides and shallow anterior chambers during the preoperative screening to avoid unnecessary complications.

Pop and Payette[38] **compared outcomes of phakic IOL and Lensectomy**.They matched nineteen eyes (12 patients, 20 to 41 years old) with an Artisan phakic IOL (Model 203: 1.00-D increment) for hyperopia from +2.75 to +9.25 D to 19 eyes (15 patients, 26 to 46 yr) with hyperopia from +2.75 to +7.50 D, who had refractive lens exchange.

The coefficient of correlation showed statistically better accuracy (intended vs. achieved refraction; $P = .035$) for the Artisan phakic IOL ($R = 0.83$) than for refractive lens exchange/ pseudophakic IOL ($R = 0.50$). The Artisan phakic IOL in carefully selected patients provided a better overall outcome for young patients with high hyperopia whose accommodation was preserved, as compared to refractive lens exchange.

Results Toric

Dick et al[39] evaluated the change in **contrast sensitivity** after implantation (18 eyes) of the Verisyse toric phakic intraocular lens (IOL) (AMO) for the correction of myopia with astigmatism. The mean contrast sensitivity increased considerably at all spatial frequencies compared with preoperative levels. They concluded that Implantation of the Verisyse toric iris-claw lens in phakic eyes to correct high or moderate myopia with astigmatism has the potential to improve contrast vision.

Rudy Nuyts[40] described the technique and analysed results of the toric Artisan lens in postkeratoplasty astigmatism (2006) in 16 eyes. Refractive error, refractive cylinder power, anterior chamber depth, and topographically derived kertometric dioptric values were inserted into the van Der Heyde formula to calculate the dioptric power of the lens for two meridians. The axis of the cylinder identified by the subjective refraction was used to determine the axis of surgical enclavation. Before surgery the horizontal and vertical axis for lens enclavation should be marked. A two-plane 5.3 mm corneoscleral incision should be centred at 12 o'clock. Two stab incisions should be performed at 2 and 10 o'clock and directed toward the enclavation sites. After an intracameral injection of acetylcholine and under an ophthalmic viscoelastic device, the lens should be introduced by forceps. After gentle rotation, the lens should fixate with a disposable enclavation needle in the marked axis. The wound suture should consist of three to four interrupted 10/0 nylon sutures, and a topical antibiotic can be used four times daily for 3 weeks, and three times daily for 1 week after the procedure.

In his series there was no loss of BCVA and a gain of at least two line of vision in fifty percent of eyes. In 16 eyes spherical equivalent was reduced from –4.90+/–5 D before surgery to 0.96+/–0.86 at the final follow up. The mean +/– standard deviation of the preoperative cylinder of –6.66+/–1.93 was reduced to –1.42+/–0.78D after surgery. The percent reduction in refractive astigmatism was 78%+/–11.5.Their study showed that use of Artisan Toric IOL, with a power range of 7.50 D of cylinder and –20.50 D of myopia to 12.00 D of hyperopia, provides a wide field for correction. enhancements) is better than in most reported LASIK series. The reduction of refractive astigmatism after LASIK varies from 48 to 88%.

Still, the authors advised a cautious use of Artisan Toric lens implantation, because they found a progressive endothelial cell loss in these corneas with a compromised endothelium.

Results Artiflex

Coullet et al in 2006[41] compared, a randomized paired eye study, refractive performance of Verisyse-Artisan phakic intraocular lens and its foldable version, Veriflex-Artiflex, for the correction of moderately high myopia. In a series of thirty-one patients with myopia from –6 to –14 dioptres (D), one eye was implanted with an Artisan, Verisyse phakic intraocular lens (PIOL) and the other with an Artiflex Veriflex PIOLs.

One year after surgery, the percentage of eyes with UCVA of >20/40 was 51.6% (16/31 patients) for Artisan-treated eyes and 77.4% (24/31 patients) for Artiflex treated eyes (P = .033). One month after surgery, this same percentage was 42.9% (13/31 patients) and 77.4% (24/31 patients), respectively (P = .004). The safety index at one year was 1.13 +/–0.24 for Artisan-treated eyes and 1.12 +/–0.21 for Artiflex-treated eyes (not statistically significant P = 0.742). At one year after surgery, the changes of two lines or more of BSCVA and the endothelial cell loss were similar for both groups.

Their conclusion was that, the Veriflex-Artiflex foldable lens provided a faster visual recovery and a better UCVA than the Artisan non foldable lens.

The Artiflex International study group[42] discussed results for myopia in 2005; 23 surgeons reviewed 1000 implantations with 350 eyes analyzed at 1 year follow-up. The average implantation power was -7.9 (+/–2.6). The incision size varied between 3 and 4 mm: average 3.2 (+/– 0.1 mm); 90% of eyes deviated <0.5 from emmetropia and 98% deviated <1.0 D from emmetropia. The average SE at 1 day postoperative was 0.04 D (+/– 0.4) and remained stable until at least 1 year postoperatively. The Efficacy index (UCVA post / BSCVA preop) was 1.01 at 1 year. No significant cell loss was observed at 1 year. Complications, included glare 3.6%, halos 5.2%, pigment deposits 5.6%, non pigment deposits 3.6%, specula 0.3%, explantation 0.3%, and lensectomy 0.3%.

The clinical results were excellent, yielding a high predictability, safety and efficacy and stable results.

Hoa

Buhren et al[43] examined thirteen eyes of seven patients preoperatively and 1 month after implantation of an Artisan lens. After implantation of the Artisan lens HOA in myopic eyes increased slightly. Particularly, induction of Z 3,-3 and Z 4,0 contribute to the increase of HOA. The induction of trefoil (Z 3,-3) was a result of the incision, whereas the increase of spherical aberration was due to the implant.

Tehrani and Dick[44] evaluated the HOA in a prospective nonrandomized comparative self-controlled trial included 41 eyes that had implantation of a foldable iris-claw pIOL between July 2003 and November 2004. All patient data for HOAs (Zernike coefficient) were measured and calculated using the same pupil size preoperatively and postoperatively, and the root-mean-square (RMS) wavefront error was calculated. Over a 12-month follow-up, 3rd-order and 4th-order HOAs did not increase after foldable

Iris-claw PIOL implantation in myopic eyes.

Chandhrasi and Knorz[45] compared HOA in -Laser *in situ* keratomileusis- the Verisyse IOL, and the Array IOL. Higher order aberrations increased at large pupil sizes, but no increase occurred at small pupil sizes with LASIK or the Verisyse IOL. Contrast sensitivity in photopic conditions was normal with LASIK and the Verisyse IOL, but slightly reduced with the Array IOL due to the multifocal optic.

Results Bioptics

Although the Verisyse Artisan eyes comes into a very high myopia range (till –23.5 D for the 5 mm and –14.5 D for the 6 mm optic) the range may be insufficient for treatment of the very high myopes. For these eyes an excellent option is the combination of a Phakic IOL and Excimer laser (preferentially Lasik) treatment-**BIOPTICS.**

Zaldivar et al[46] was the first to describe bioptics, **combination of posterior chamber phakic intraocular lens and laser in situ keratomileusis** for severe myopia first in 1991. The mean preoperative spherical equivalent refraction was –23.00 +/– 3.60 D (range, –18.75 to –35.00 D). The mean postoperative spherical equivalent refraction at last examination after the LASIK portion of the two-part phakic IOL-LASIK procedure was –0.20 +/– 0.90 D (range, +1.75 to –5.13 D).

Eighty-five percent (57 eyes) were within +/– 1.00 D and 67% (45 eyes) were within +/– 0.50 D of emmetropia at last examination. A gain of 2 or more lines of spectacle-corrected visual acuity was seen in 51 eyes (76%) and no eyes lost 2 or more lines of spectacle-corrected visual acuity at last examination. They demonstrated that combined posterior chamber phakic IOL implantation with the STAAR Collamer plate lens and LASIK (bioptics) is an effective and reasonably predictable method for correcting myopia from –18 to –35 D.

Guell et al started in 1999[47] a prospective study of 6 patients (8 eyes) with high myopia who had Artisan phakic IOL implantation followed by LASIK.

After the second procedure (LASIK), uncorrected visual acuity ranged from 0.4 to 0.63 (mean, 0.5 +/– 0.07) at 1 month and from 0.6 to 0.7 (mean, 0.62 +/– 0.04) at 12 months. Spectacle-corrected visual acuity improved 2 or more lines in 62.5% (5 eyes) from preoperative values. All eyes were within +/–1.00 D of emmetropia.There were no major complications.

Guell et al reported in 2001[48] on twenty-six eyes of 18 patients with a preoperative spherical equivalent between –16.00 and –23.00 D. The second surgery was performed once refraction and topography were stable, between 3 and 5 months later. 80.70% of the eyes were within 0.50 D of emmetropia and 100% within 1.0 D. Twenty-six percent of the eyes gained 3 or more lines from their preoperative BCVA, and 42% gained 2 or more lines. No serious complications were observed. The combination of a 6 mm optic, 15 D Artisan lens, and LASIK appears to be a safe and highly predictable method for the correction of myopia greater than –15.00 D. In 2000 it was the best approach with the technology currently available.

Arne et al[49] performed Excimer laser treatment after Verisyse IOL implantation and reviewed bioptics outcomes **in** thirty-two eyes of 28 patients with extreme myopia or myopia combined with astigmatism were treated by implantation of a phakic posterior chamber IOL. The mean preoperative spherical equivalent (SE) refraction was –18.7 dioptres (D). After excimer laser treatment, the uncorrected visual acuity improved in all eyes but a loss of 1 line of the corrected vision after IOL implantation occurred in 22.2% of PRK-treated eyes and in 13.6% of LASIK-treated eyes. Bioptic treatment of extreme myopia and myopia associated with astigmatism appears to be safer and more predictable than other methods of treatment.

Munoz et al[50] used BIOPTICS to treat 39 eyes with a mean preoperative spherical equivalent (SE) of 7.39 diopters (D) +/–1.30 (SD) and a cylinder between 0 and –4.25 D. The Artisan iris-fixated phakic IOL (Ophtec) for hyperopia was implanted, and LASIK was performed 6 to 8 months later. At 1 year, 37 eyes (94.9%) were within +/–1.00 D of emmetropia and 31 eyes (79.5%) were within +/–0.50 D. Nine eyes (23.1%) lost 1 line of BCVA; 7 eyes (17.9%) gained at least 1 line. The combination of Artisan phakic IOL implantation and LASIK safely, predictably, and effectively reduced high hyperopia. A loss of 1 line of BCVA should be expected in about one third of eyes implanted with this IOL. Halos and glare at night remain a potential problem.

Personal Results

Surgery

In our center, The Goes Antwerp Eye Centre, all surgery was done on an outpatient basis under topical anesthesia; mostly simultaneously in the same setting. Only 5% of patients preferred both eyes at different sessions.

Preoperatively a **YAG LASER** iridotomy was performed at least one week beforehand. We preferred to do this before surgery in order to avoid an eventual bleeding peroperatevly; also the iridotomy can be performed more peripherally with the laser than with scissors.

Surgery was without complications in all cases. Since we know that most eventual complications arise from traumatic surgery extreme was paid to elegant and delicate surgery. A stepwise approach according to guidelines described in brochures was followed. Care was being taken that the visco-elastic material was completely washed out at the end of surgery in order to avoid postoperative intraocular pressure rise. However, this happened in two cases. Under extensive local medication the condition improved rapidly. In the Veriflex Artiflex group local anti-inflammatory (cortisone-antibiotic) medication was instilled more frequently (5 times daily) first 5 days, since we experienced more reaction the first days. A shield was prescribed at night during the first week.

Routine medication after surgery includes a topical antibiotic (Ciloxan® or Tobradex® combination antibiotic-cortisone 4ys.X day during at least 3 weeks-Diclofenac X3 one week and levobunolol X1 one week-Acetazolamide 1 co 2 d and a shield at night for one week.

Outcomes

We have experience and follow up of more then 12 months after implanting **114 Spherical Verisyse IOL's for myopia-8 toric Verisyse IOL's for myopia combined with astigmatism -and a fup of at least 6 months of 32 Veriflex IOL's for myopia** (Fig. 29.11).

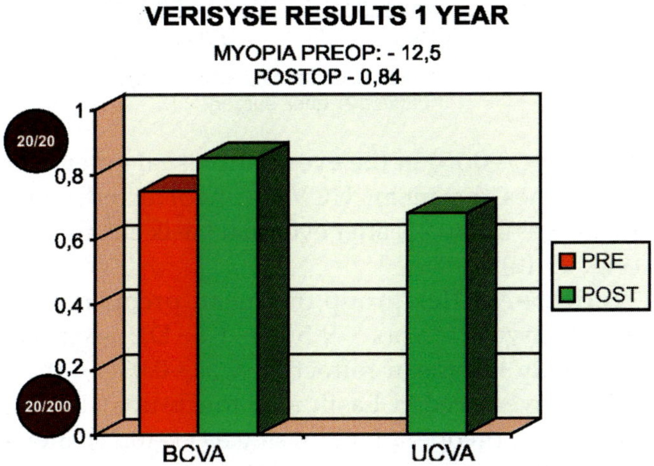

Fig. 29.11: Personal results of verisyse IOL: BCVA climbed from 0.75 (20/27)to 0.85(20/24) after surgery

In the spherical **Verisyse-Artisan group** the mean preoperative spherical equivalent of myopia was –12.5(+/–4.1 D); extremes –6 to –23): postoperatively the mean refraction wás –0.84(+/–1.47)D.

In this group 16/114 eyes needed **Lasik touchup**;some of these eyes were high myopes beforehand (2—23 D eyes). Mostly Lasik enhancement was done to get rid of the astigmatism. The mean refraction prelasik was –2.9 D: afterwards it was 0.13 D.Lasik was performed three months after surgery and after stitches removal. The lasiksurgery, using the microkeratome, was always uneventful as in normal phakic eyes; no touch was observed at any moment between the cornea and the phakic IOL.

Looking at the BSCVA (best spectacle corrected visual acuity) of the Verisyse Series the value was preoperatively 0.75((+/–0.21) and

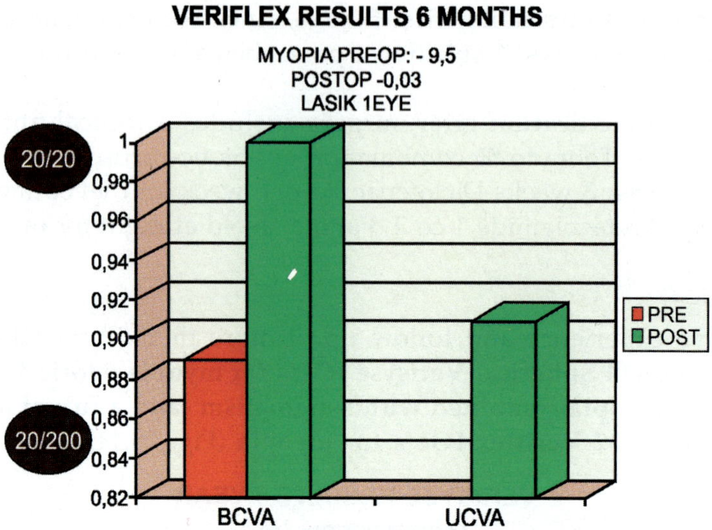

Fig. 29.12: Personal results of veriflex foldable IOL: BCVA climbed from 0.89(20/23) to 1.02(20/19) after surgery

after surgery 0.85(+/–0.15) in the eyes with visual potential of at least 20/40.In this series the mean UCVA (uncorrected visual acuity) postoperatively was 0.64(0.21):after eventual Lasik enhancement UCVA was 0.68 (Fig. 29.12).

In the **Veriflex-Artiflex** group,the mean preoperative spherical equivalent of myopia was –9.5(+/–1.5 D); extremes –6 to –12:postoperatively the mean refraction was –0.03(+/–0.23)D.In this group only1/32 eyes needed Lasik as a touch-up. 0.03 (0.23)

The Mean Bscva preoperatively was 0.89+/–(0.21):after surgery it was 1.02(+/–0.12)

The mean UCVA after implantation was extremely good: 0.91(+/ – 0.21); already at **DAY ONE** after surgery it was 0.88(+/–0,15) (Fig. 29.13).

In the **toric Verisyse group** the data were also excellent; the astigmatism decreased from 4 D preoperatively to 0.9 D after surgery; the myopia decreased from –13.5 to –0.42 D and the BSCVA improved from 0.65 before surgery to 0.88 after surgery. The obtained UCVA after surgery of 0.68 for this group with high astigmatism and important myopia was extremely good.

LITERATURE COMPARISON VERISYSE – OTHER IOLs

Zaldivar et al 1998[51] analysed outcomes of posterior chamber phakic intraocular (Staar Collamer plate lens) lens for myopia of –8 to –19

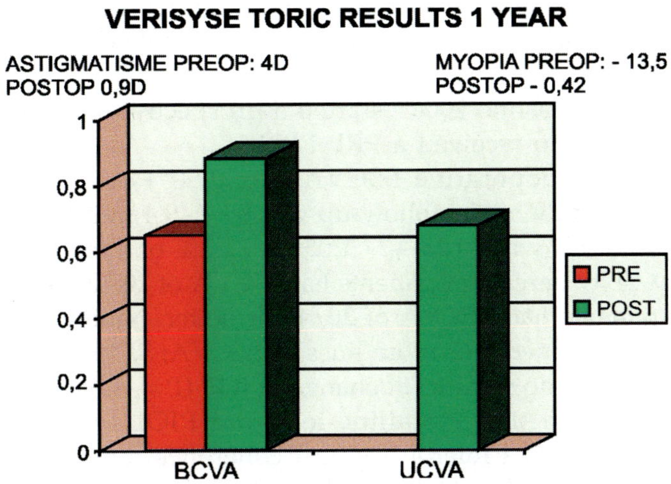

Fig. 29.13: Personal results of toric myopic phakic IOL: BCVA improved from 0.65(20/31) before to 0.88 (20/23) after surgery

dioptres. A gain of two or more lines of spectacle-corrected visual acuity was seen in 36% (45 eyes).

Uusitalo and Laatikainen[52] in 2002 reported results of Implantable contact lens (ICL) (Staar Collamer) as a posterior chamber phakic intraocular lens (IOL) to correct high myopia. The mean follow-up was 13.6 months (range 6 to 24 months). In eyes in which the preoperative myopia was less than -18.00 D (n = 28), the achieved refraction was within +/-1.00 D of the intended refraction in 27 eyes (96.4%) and within +/-0.50 D in 24 eyes (85.7%). The best corrected visual acuity (BCVA) improved by 1 or more lines in 23 of 32 eyes (71.9%) at 1 year. Two eyes (6.3%) lost 1 line of BCVA.

At 1 year, ICL implantation had good visual and refractive results with excellent biocompatibility.

Menezo et al[53] 2004 evaluated the feasibility and safety of using phakic intraocular lenses (IOLs) to correct high myopia by comparing 3 IOL models: Adatomed, Staar, and Artisan in a prospective comparative study of 217 highly myopic eyes. Fifty-nine eyes received an Adatomed IOL, 21 eyes a Staar IOL, and 137 eyes an Artisan IOL.Anterior cataract formation was higher in the Adatomed group (44.06%) than in the Staar group (9.52%). There was a higher incidence of anterior subcapsular cataract formation in the Adatomed group than in the Staar group.

Pineda-Fernandez et al[54] 2004, did a retrospective study in order to analyze 18 eyes of 12 patients who had implantation of a modified PPC IOL, the implantable contact lens (ICL), for the treatment of high myopia. Four eyes (22.2%) had moderate pigmentary dispersion; two eyes (11.1%) had lens opacification main concerns over potential cataract formation, pigmentary dispersion, and angle-closure glaucoma remain in 2004.

Donoso and Castillo 2006[55] started a prospective study of 53 eyes of 39 patients who received a PRL PIOL.

The mean preoperative BSCVA was 0.50 +/- 0.70 (LogMAR equivalent), and the mean follow-up was 8 +/- 9.4 months. The mean postoperative SE was -0.23 +/- 1.05 D; 71.2% of eyes were within +/-1.00 D. Sixty percent of patients had UCVA of 20/40 or better, and 88.2% of patients had BSCVA of 20/40 or better. Ninety-two percent maintained or gained 1 or more lines of BSCVA; 5.7% lost more than 1 line. There was no significant change in IOP (P = .40), and the mean distance between the crystalline lens and PIOL was 370 micron (ultrasound) and 604 micron (optical coherence tomography). Late complications included 1 case each of retinal detachment and lens subluxation was seen in 36% (45 eyes) at last examination. One eye (0.8%) lost two or more lines of spectacle-corrected visual acuity from a retinal detachment. Posterior chamber phakic IOL implantation with the Staar Collamer plate lens is an effective and safe method for reducing or correcting myopia between –8 and –19 D.

Gierik-Ciaciura et al[56] evaluated the efficacy, predictability and safety of implanting two models of anterior chamber IOLs for high myopia. ICARE in 20 eyes of 12 patients, the Verisyse IOL in 20 eyes of 12 patients. The follow-up period was 12 months. The mean endothelial cell density loss was 6.12% and 6.79% in the ICARE and Verisyse groups, respectively. There were no statistically significant differences regarding the analyzed parameters between the two study groups. The efficacy and safety of surgery for both implanted lens models were very high.

CONCLUSION

We are extremely pleased with the outcomes of surgery using the-**Verisyse Artisan-Veriflex-Artiflex** IOL as a phakic IOL in myopia.

The outcomes using the **Toric version** were also excellent.

A major change and breakthrough was the introduction of the foldable version the **Veriflex-Artiflex lens allowing quasi immediate visual recovery with minimal patient's disturbances.** With this lens the efficacy index postoperative UCVA/preoperative BSCVA was higher than 1(1.01) and the UCVA at day one was extremely good (0.88). In this group only 1 eye needed Lasik enhancement because of existing preoperative astigmatism.

The only **drawback** of using this lens style, on condition that the indications are well met, is the demanding surgery requiring surgical skill. A prerequisite is the adequate training leading towards a short learning curve.

All complications can be avoided by careful surgery. A close follow up of endothelia cell count is also necessary when, practicing this type of surgery. We are convinced that we are not doing any harm to our patient's eyes by using the iris fixation approach.

We are waiting and looking forward to use a foldable toric version that is expected to be on the market very soon.

REFERENCES

1. Sandoval HP, de Castro LE,Vroman DT,et al. Refractive surgery Survey 2004. J Cataract Refract Surg 2005;31:221-33.
2. Duffey RJ,Leaming D. US trends in refractive surgery:2004 ISRS/AAO Survey. J Cataract Refract Surg 2005 21:742-8.
3. Stulting RD, Carr JD, Thompson KP, et al.Complications of laser in situ keratomileusis for the correction of myopia. Ophthalmology1999;106:13-20.
4. Stein R. Photorefractive keratectomy. Int Ophthalmology Clin 2000;40:35-56.
5. Güell JL, Velasco F. Phakic Intraocular Lens Implantation. In: Hannush S, (Ed). Int Ophthalmol Clin 2002;42:119-30.
6. Fyodorov SN, Zyev VK, Tumanyan NR, et al. Clinical and functional follow-up of minus IOL implantation in high grade myopia. Ophthalmosurgery (Moscow) 1993;2:12-7.
7. Zaldivar R, Rocha G. The current status of phakic intraocular lenses. Int Ophthalmol Clin 1996;6:107-11
8. Allemann N, Chamon W, Tanaka HM, Mori ES, Campos M, Schor P, Baikoff G. Myopic angle-supported intraocular lenses: two-year follow-up. Ophthalmology 2000; 107:1549-54.
9. Pitault G, Leboeuf C, Leroux Les Jardins S, Auclin F, Chong-Sit D, Baudouin C. Ultrasound biomicroscopy of posterior chamber phakic intraocular lenses: a comparative study between ICL and PRL models. J Fr Ophthalmol 2005; 28:914-23.
10. Baumeister M, Buhren J, Kohnen T. Position of angle-supported, iris-fixated, and ciliary sulcus-implanted myopic phakic intraocular lenses evaluated by Scheimpflug photography. Am J Ophthalmol 2004 ;138:723-31.
11. Van Der Heyde G.L. Some optical aspects of implantation of an IOL in a myopic eye. A method is given to calculate intraocular lens power in phakic eyes. Eur J Implant Ref Surg 1989;1:244-8.
12. Bechmann M, Ullrich S, Thiel MJ, Kenyon KR, Ludwig K. Imaging of posterior chamber phakic intraocular lens by optical coherence tomography. J Cataract Refract Surg 2002; 28:360-3.
13. Baikoff G, Bourgeon G, Jodai HJ, Fontaine A, Lellis FV, Trinquet L. Pigment dispersion and Artisan phakic intraocular lenses: crystalline lens rise as a safety criterion. J Cataract Refract Surg 2005; 31:674-80.
14. Baikoff G. Anterior segment OCT and phakic intraocular lenses: a perspective. J Cataract Refract Surg 2006; 32:1827-35.

15. Maroccos R, Vaz F, Marinho A, Guell J, Lohmann CP. Glare and halos after "phakic IOL". Surgery for the correction of high myopia. Ophthalmologe. 2001; 98:1055-9.
16. Alio JL, de la Hoz F, Ruiz-Moreno JM, Salem TF. Cataract surgery in highly myopic eyes corrected by phakic anterior chamber angle-supported lenses. J Cataract Refract Surg 2000; 26:1303-11.
17. Menezo JL, Cisneros AL, Rodriguez-Salvador V. Endothelial study of iris-claw phakic lens: four year follow-up. J Cataract Refract Surg 1998; 24:1039-49.
18. Trindade F, Pereira F. Cataract formation after posterior chamber phakic intraocular lens implantation. J Cataract Refract Surg. 1998; 24:1661-3.
19. Moshirfar M, Whitehead G, Beutler BC, Mamalis N. Toxic anterior segment syndrome after Verisyse iris-supported phakic intraocular lens implantation. J Cataract Refract Surg 2006; 32:1233-7.
20. Tahzib NG, Eggink FA, Frederik PM, Nuijts RM. Recurrent intraocular inflammation after implantation of the Artiflex phakic intraocular lens for the correction of high myopia. J Cataract Refract Surg 2006; 32:1388-91.
21. Dick HB, Aliyeva S, Tehrani M. Change in pupil size after implantation of an iris- fixated toric phakic intraocular lens. J Cataract Refract Surg 2005; 31:302-7.
22. Sekundo W, Schneider M, Tietjen A. Influence of incision parameters on astigmatism during implantation of phakic-6-mm-iris-claw intraocular lenses. Ophthalmologe. 2004; 101:246-50.
23. Tehrani M, Dick HB, Schwenn O, Blom E, Schmidt AH, Koch HR. Postoperative astigmatism and rotational stability after artisan toric phakic intraocular lens implantation. J Cataract Refract Surg. 2003; 29:1761-6.
24. Ardjomand N, Kolli H, Vidic B, El-Shabrawi Y, Faulborn J. Pupillary block after phakic anterior chamber intraocular lens implantation. J Cataract Refract Surg 2002; 28:1080-1.
25. Morales AJ, Zadok D, Tardio E, Anzoulatous G Jr, Litwak S, Mora R, Martinez E, Chayet AS. Outcome of simultaneous phakic implantable contact lens removal with cataract extraction and pseudophakic intraocular lens implantation. J Cataract Refract Surg 2006; 32:595-8.
26. Worst JG, van der Veen G, Los LI. Refractive surgery for high myopia. The Worst-Fechner biconcave iris claw lens. Doc Ophthalmol 1990; 75:335-41.
27. Fechner PU, Haubitz I, Wichmann W, Wulff K. Worst-Fechner biconcave minus power phakic iris-claw lens. J Refract Surg 1999; 15:93-105.
28. Landesz M, Worst JG, Siertsema JV, va, Rij G. Correction of high myopia with the Worst myopia claw intraocular lens. J Refract Surg 1995; 11:16-25.
29. Perez-Santonja JJ, Bueno JL, Zato MA. Surgical correction of high myopia in phakic eyes with Worst-Fechner myopia intraocular lenses.J Refract Surg. 1997; 13:2682.
30. Budo C, MD, Hessloehl JC, Milan I, Luyten GPM, Menezo J, MD. Sener BA, Tassignon MJ, Termote H, MD Worst JGF, MD. Multicenter study of the Artisan phakic intraocular lens. J Cataract Refract Surg 2000; 26:1163-71.
31. Maloney RK, MD, Nguyen LH, J John ME. The Artisan Lens Study Group. Artisan Phakic Intraocular Lens for Myopia. Ophthalmology 2002, 109:1631-41.
32. Verisyse Training Course Materials. Advanced Medical Optics, Santa Ana, CA, 2004.

33. Alexander L, John M, Cobb L, et al. U.S. clinical investigation of the Artisan myopia lens for the correction of high myopia in phakic eyes. Report of the results of phases 1 and 2, and interim phase 3. Optometry. 2000;71:630-42.
34. Moshirfar M, Whitehead G, Beutler BC, Mamalis N. Toxic anterior segment syndrome after Verisyse iris-supported phakic intraocular lens implantation. J Cataract Refract Surg 2006;32:1233-7.
35. Lifshitz T, Levy J, Aizenman I, Klemperer I, Levinger S. Artisan phakic intraocular lens for correcting high myopia. Int Ophthalmol 2004; 25:233-8.
36. Benedetti S, Casamenti V, Marcaccio L, Brogioni C, Assetto V. Correction of myopia of 7 to 24 dioptres with the Artisan phakic intraocular lens: two-year follow-up. J Refract Surg 2005; 21:116-26.
37. Saxena R, Landesz M, Noordzij B, Luyten GP. Three-year follow-up of the Artisan phakic intraocular lens for hypermetropia. Ophthalmology 2003; 110:1391-1395.
38. Pop M, Payette Y. Refractive lens exchange versus iris-claw Artisan phakic intraocular lens for hyperopia. J Refract Surg 2004; 20:20-24.
39. Dick HB, Tehrani M, Aliyeva S. Contrast sensitivity after implantation of toric iris-claw lenses in phakic eyes. J Cataract Refract Surg. 2004; 30:2284-89.
40. Nuyts R. Using the Artisan Toric IOL. How to manage postkeratoplasty astigmatism with this lens. Cataract & Refractive surgery today, November/ December 2006.
41. Coullet J, Guëll J, Fourni P,Grandjean H , Gaytan J, Arné JL, MD, PhD, and MalecazeF .Iris-supported Phakic Lenses (Rigid vs Foldable Version) for Treating Moderately High Myopia;Randomized Paired Eye Comparison.Am J Ophthalmol 2006;142:909-16.
42. Artiflex International Study Group 2004.
43. Buhren J, Kasper T, Terzi E, Kohnen T. Higher order aberrations after implantation of an iris claw PIOL (Ophtec Artisan) in the phakic eye. Ophthalmologe. 2004; 101:1194-1201.
44. Tehrani, M, Dick B, MD. Changes in higher-order aberrations after implantation of a foldable iris-claw lens in myopic phakic eyes. J Cataract Refract Surg 2006; 32:250–254.
45. Chandhrasri S, Knorz MC. Comparison of higher order aberrations and contrast sensitivity after LASIK, Verisyse phakic IOL, and Array multifocal IOL. J Refract Surg 2006; 22:231-36.
46. Zaldivar R, Davidorf JM, Oscherow S, Ricur G, Piezzi V. Combined posterior chamber phakic intraocular lens and laser in situ keratomileusis: bioptics for extreme myopia. J Refract Surg 1999; 15:299-308.
47. Guell JL, Vasquez M, Gris O, De Muller A, Manero F. Combined surgery to correct high myopia: iris claw phakic intraocular lens and laser in situ keratomileusis. J Refract Surg 1999; 15:529-37.
48. Guell JL, Vasquez M, Gris O. Adjustable refractive surgery: 6-mm Artisan lens plus laser in situ keratomileusis for the correction of high myopia. Ophthalmology 2001; 108:945-52.
49. Arne JL, Lesueur LC, Hulin HH. Photorefractive keratectomy or laser in situ keratomileusis for residual refractive error after phakic intraocular lens implantation. J Cataract Refract Surg 2003; 29:1167-73.
50. Munoz G, Alio JL, Montes-Mico R, Albarran-Diego C, Belda JI. Artisan iris-claw phakic intraocular lens followed by laser in situ keratomileusis for high hyperopia. J Cataract Refract Surg 2005; 31:308-17.

51. Zaldivar R, Davidorf JM, Oscherow S. Posterior chamber phakic intraocular lens for myopia of -8 to -19 dioptres. J Refract Surg. 1998; 14:294-305.
52. Uusitalo RJ, Aine E, Sen NH, Laatikainen L. Implantable contact lens for high myopia. J Cataract Refract Surg 2002; 28:29-36.
53. Menezo JL, Peris-Martinez C, Cisneros AL, Martinez-Costa R. Phakic intraocular lenses to correct high myopia: adatomed, Staar, and Artisan. J Cataract Refract Surg 2004 ;30:33-44.
54. Pineda-Fernandez A, Jaramillo J, Vargas J, Jaramillo M, Jaramillo J, Galindez A. Phakic posterior chamber intraocular lens for high myopia. J Cataract Refract Surg 2004; 30:2277-83.
55. Donoso R, Castillo P. Correction of high myopia with the PRL phakic intraocular lens. J Cataract Refract Surg 2006 ; 32:1296-1300.
56. Gierek-Ciaciura S, Gierek-Lapinska A, Ochalik K, Mrukwa-Kominek E. Correction of high myopia with different phakic anterior chamber intraocular lenses: ICARE angle-supported lens and Verisyse iris-claw lens. Graefes Arch Clin Exp Ophtalmol, 2004, 24:112-6.

CHAPTER

30

Gerald Schmedinger (Austria)

Diffractive Multifocal Intraocular Lenses

INTRODUCTION

Strategies to overcome postoperative glass dependency like monovision (one eye myopic, the other eye emetropic) and myopic astigmatism using monofocal IOLs have already been developed. However, glass dependency is still high in monovision patients and myopic astigmatism was shown to reduce distance visual acuity.[1-4] In contrast to monofocal IOLs, multifocal intraocular lenses (MIOL) are designed to overcome the postoperative lack of accommodation by dividing the incoming light to two or more focal points (Figs 30.1 and 30.2). One focal point is used for distance vision and one focal point is used for near vision. The increased depth of focus resulting from the additional foci reduces the need of spectacles in daily life.[5-10] The picture of the non-focused image is highly defocused and of very low light intensity and is therefore, usually not recognized. As shown in Figure 30.1, the non-focused image of the near focus overlays the focused image. Under certain circumstances this non focused image can lead to photic phenomena like halos.[6,11]

In case of accurate biometry, MIOLs offer patients a range of good uncorrected vision. Binocular implantation of multifocal lenses was found to lead to better results in visual acuity and spectacle dependence.[12]

The creation of addition foci can be accomplished using refractive optics or diffractive optics. In refractive multifocal lenses, additional

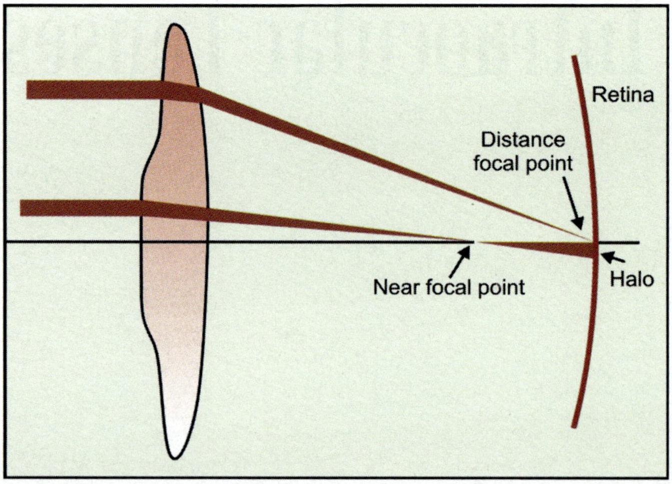

Fig. 30.1: Schematic drawing of a multifocal lens with a central near zone and a peripheral distance zone when looking at a distance object. Light rays passing through the central zone are focused in front of the retina and create a defocused low-contrast image on the retina (halo). Light rays passing through the peripheral zone are focused on the retina

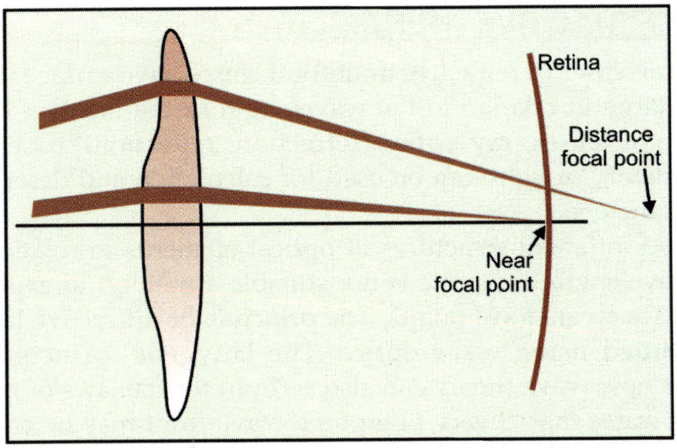

Fig. 30.2: Schematic drawing of a multifocal lens with a central near zone and a peripheral distance zone when looking at a near object. Light rays passing through the central zone are focused on the retina. Light passing through the peripheral zone create a defocused, low-contrast image on the retina

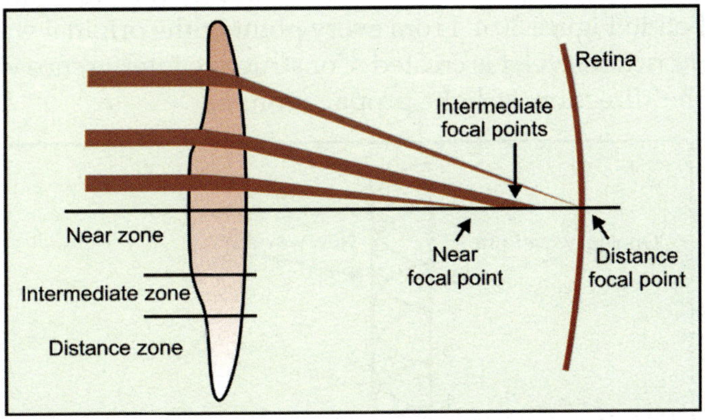

Fig. 30.3: Schematic drawing of a multifocal lens with a central near zone, a peripheral distance zone and a transition zone serving intermediate focal points. The intermediate focal points are usually of lower light energy

foci are created by changes in the curvature of the lens surface. This design uses different zones on the lens surface with different focal powers serving different focal points (Fig. 30.3). It is obvious, that only parts of the optical surface can be used for the creation of each focal point and that the performances of these lenses are highly dependent on pupil size.[13] In contrast to these refractive multifocal intraocular lenses, diffractive multifocal lenses usually use the entire optical zone of the aperture for the creation of the near and the distance focus. Different focal points are created by such lenses using constructive and destructive interference of light rays.

THE DIFFRACTIVE PRINCIPLE

Monofocal lenses or refractive multifocal lenses have surface structures that are large in relation to the wavelength of the incident light. For this type of lenses, ray optics (refraction, reflection), based on the particle theory of light, can be used for calculation and description of lens parameters.

In cases of small structures of optical elements in relation to the lights wavelength, ray optic is not suitable a method to explain how these lenses create focal points. The principle of diffractive lenses can be explained using wave optics. The Huygens´ principle (1670) describes how wave theory can also account for the laws of geometric optics. It states that "Every point on a wave-front may be considered a source of secondary spherical wavelets which spread out in the forward direction at the speed of light. The new wave-front is the tangential surface to all of these secondary wavelets." The principle of wave front propagation in case of an aberration free, plane wave is described in Figure 30.4. From every point of the original wave-front a new spherical wavelet is created. Constructive interference will occur only in the direction of light propagation.

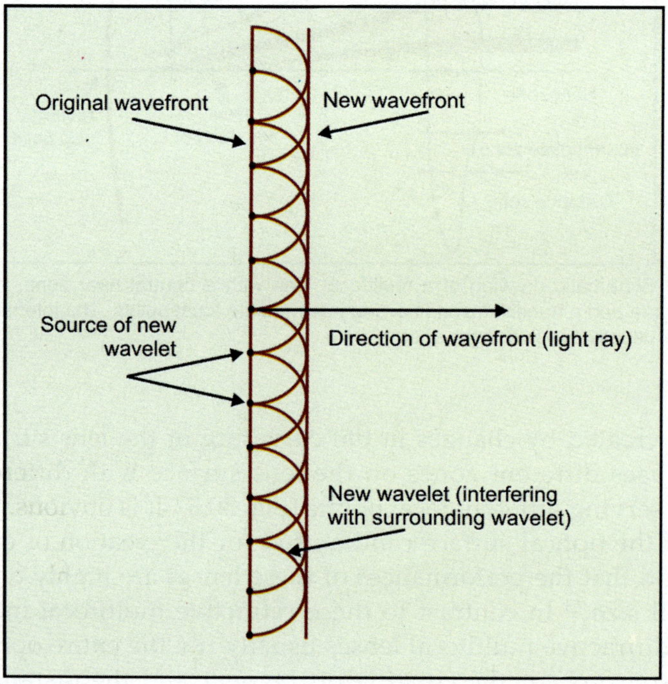

Fig. 30.4: According to Huygens principle the graphic shows the propagation of a planar, aberration-free wavefront from left to right

Modern diffractive lenses usually are a combination of a refractive lens (providing the base power of the lens) and a diffractive optic element creating the additional focal point. Under magnification, the diffractive structures on diffractive multifocal intraocular lenses can easily be recognized as small steps on the anterior or posterior optic surface. If light rays were followed separately through the diffractive zones of the lens, then a focal point would be found half way between the distance focus and the near focus. This is only theory, since in reality no light energy is found at this point, but the light energy is divided between the distance and the near focal point (Fig. 30.5).

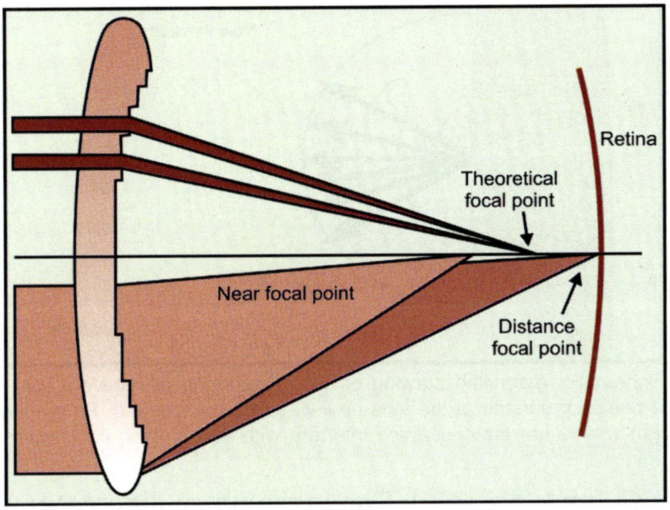

Fig. 30.5: Schematic drawing of a diffractive bifocal lens. The upper half of the lens shows the theoretical focal point, when light rays are followed separately through the diffractive steps. In reality no light energy is found at this focal point. The lower half of the figure shows the actual situation of the light distribution with creation of two focal points

When a light ray hits this lens, it propagates through the lens material at a different speed than in the surrounding media. Since the lens thickness changes from one step of the lens to the next, light passing the lens at thicker steps travels longer than light passing through thinner steps. Therefore, phase differences are created by the different path lengths of light rays passing through the different steps. In bifocal diffractive lenses the height of these steps is about one half of the incident light wavelength, creating a phase delay of half a wavelength. A diffractive lens with a phase delay of one wavelength would create only one focal point (i.e. monofocal diffractive lens).

According to the Huygens´ principle, after passing through the lens, a new wavelet is created on every point on the posterior surface of the diffractive lens. These wavelets interfere with each other and create

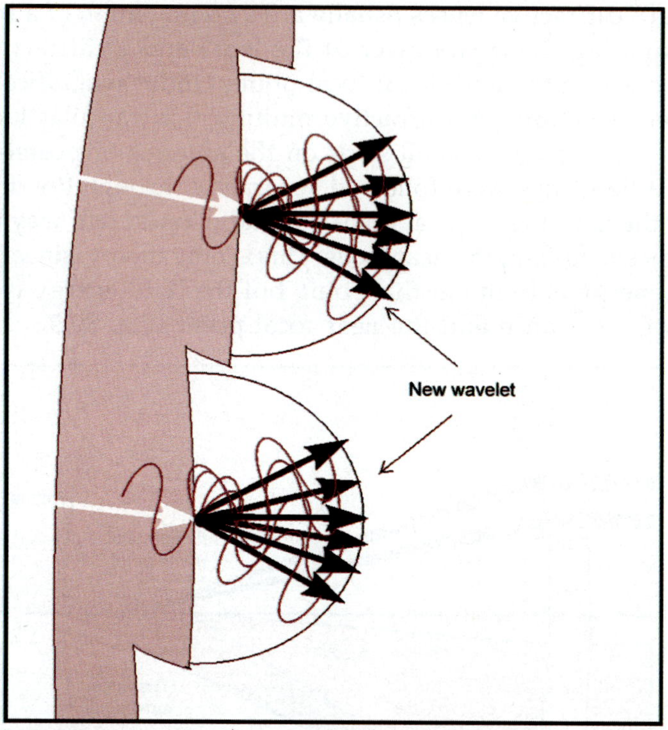

Fig. 30.6: Schematic, magnified drawing of two neighboring diffractive steps. From every point on the posterior surface of the lens new wavelets are created. From these spherical wavelets, light waves are emitted which interfere with surrounding light waves

a new wave-front (Fig. 30.6). Due to the phase differences which are induced by the different path lengths between the steps, destructive interference will occur when the wavelets are 180° out of phase. On the other hand, constructive interference will occur when the wavelets are in phase. Destructive and constructive interference in case of a bifocal diffractive lens is explained in Figure 30.7.

Focal points of higher diffractive orders account for light loss of this lens design. About 18% of the incident light is lost at higher diffractive orders. These higher diffractive orders serve focal points with focal lengths being a multiple of the near additions´ focal length. These focal points are of very low light energy and are therefore of no clinical importance.

The distance between the two focal points, defining the near addition of a bifocal diffractive lens, and the light distribution between the focal points can be calculated and designed by altering the step width and step height of the diffractive elements. Using a diffractive design, two highly defined focal points with a predetermined distance (i.e. near addition) and light distribution can be produced.

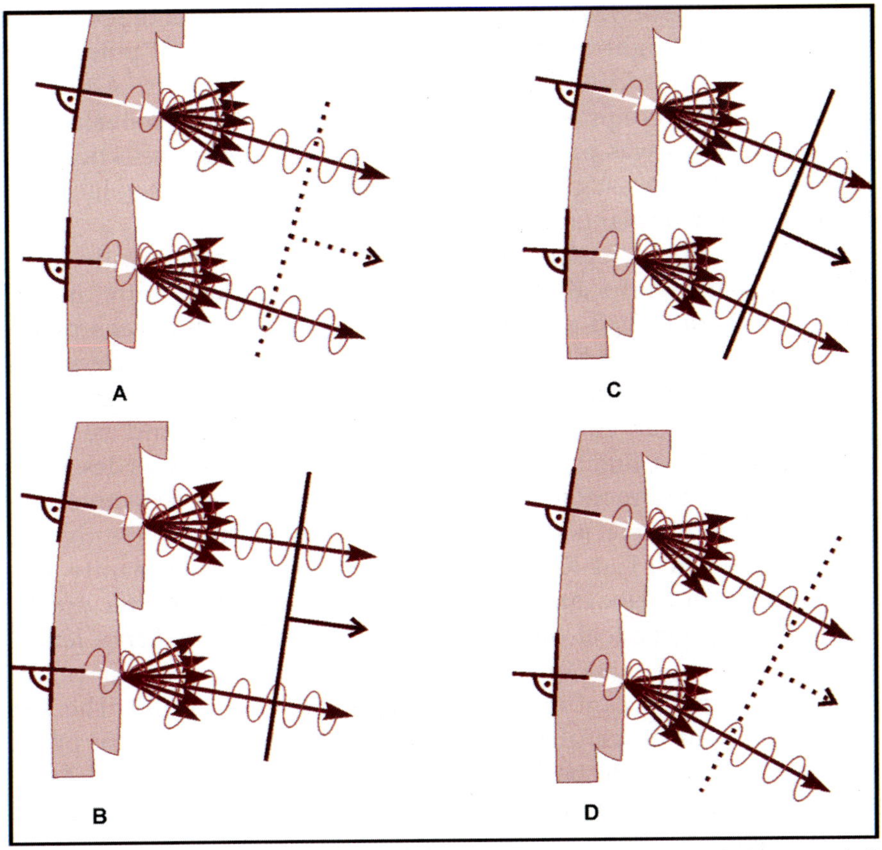

Fig. 30.7: Schematic drawing of a diffractive lens with a step height of about one half wavelengths. In the direction of the theoretical focal point (see Fig. 30.5) a phase difference of one half wavelength leads to destructive interference. Therefore no light energy can be found in this direction of light propagation (A). In the direction of the distance focus the light waves are in phase. This leads to constructive interference and about 41% of the incident light can be found at this focal point (B). The same situation can be found in the direction of the near focal point (C). In every other direction with a phase difference of one half wavelength or an integer multiple of it, not light energy will be found (D). Focal points of higher diffractive orders are not shown

It should be noted, that the commonly used separation between refractive and diffractive multifocal lenses is oversimplified and imprecise. When speaking of "diffractive" or "refractive" multifocal lenses, one should keep in mind that refraction will also play a role in the so called diffractive lenses, and uncontrolled or unwanted diffraction will always occur in so called refractive multifocal lenses due to phase differences between the refractive zones.

DIFFRACTIVE MULTIFOCAL IOL AND CLINICAL RESULTS

One of the first diffractive multifocal intraocular lenses was the 815 LE (3M) lens. This lens was a three piece convex/concave PMMA lens with a 6.0 mm optic. Diffractive structures were placed on the posterior surface and the light distribution between the two focal points was equal. The near addition in lens plane was 3.5 diopters. Although clinical results were promising with this lens,[14, 15] lens removals were described.[16] This was probably due to improper patient selection and high postoperative astigmatism[17] due to the large incisions which had to be used for implantation of a non-foldable lens.

In the European region the Pharmacia 811 E was frequently used. This diffractive bifocal PMMA lens with a 6.0 mm optic and 6° angulated haptics had a near addition of 4.0 diopters at lens plane, resulting in a near addition of about 3.0 diopters in spectacle plane.

Compared to a refractive multifocal intraocular lens, this lens performed better concerning near visual acuity and reading performance.[9,18] A slight reduction in contrast sensitivity was described in comparison to a monofocal IOL.[19] In comparison to a refractive lens, patients with this lens achieved better near visual acuities (Study will be published in J Cat Ref Surg), while distance visual acuity was comparable. In a laboratory setup this lens showed a better optical quality of the near foal point compared the refractive Array lens.[20] Using a model eye, the quality of the near and distance focal points were evaluated by capturing point spread functions (PSF). The PSF shows the light distribution in one meridian at a given focal point. Ideally the PSF should be a narrow and high peak. Testing the Array lens, a broad light distribution in the near focus can be recognized

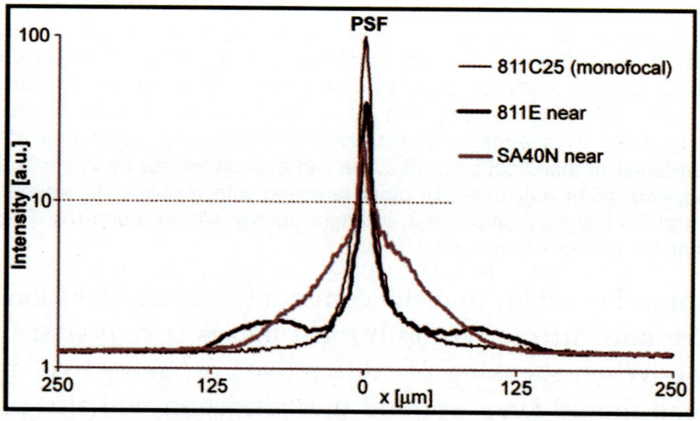

Fig. 30.8: Near focus point spread function (PSF) of a diffractive bifocal (811E), a refractive multifocal (SA40N) and a monofocal IOL (811C25) with near addition. Relative light intensity is shown on the y-axis. The monofocal lens shows a high, steep and narrow PSF congruent with a good image quality. The 811E lens has a narrow peak which is less high (only 41% of the light energy is available for this focal point) then in the monofocal lens. In addition, a halo with distinct separation from the central peak can be found which is created by the distance focus. The SA40N has an even lower central peak which is outshined by intermediate focal points and the distance focus. The broad base of the peak leads to a reduction of the image quality

(Fig. 30.8). This is due to overlying out-of-focus images arising from additional focal points of this multifocal lens. In case of the 811E, a narrower PSF is found with a surrounding halo arising from the second focal point. This clearly shows the advantage of two strictly separated focal points, reducing the blur from additional weak intermediate focal points.

The main disadvantage of the 811E, as for the 3M lens, was the PMMA optic material, necessitating large incisions for lens implantation. In contrast to the refractive Array lens (AMO), these two diffractive lenses were not approved by the FDA. This may explain why these lenses were seldom implanted outside Europe and why there are only few clinical studies available for these lenses.

With upcoming new intraocular lens technology and better manufacturing possibilities, new MIOLs were introduced with the intention to increase optical performance, implantation technique and to reduce side effects like photic phenomena.

The first foldable diffractive intraocular lens was the Acri.Twin lens from Acri.Tec. These lenses are available with silicone optics (737D and 733D), as single piece acrylic lenses (447D and 443D) and as three piece acrylic lenses (527D and 523D). The Acri.Twin lenses always come in pairs, with different light distribution between distance and near focus (Fig. 30.9). One eye is provided with a distance-weighted multifocal intraocular lens and the other eye a near-weighted multifocal lens. This concept of asymmetric light distribution was first described by Jacobi et al.[21, 22] The idea was to further enhance the visual performance of the multifocal lens after binocular implantation. A bilateral implantation results in better binocular visual performance at distance and near focus, with one eye compensating for the other at its stronger focus. The Acri.Twin lenses, consisting of the near-weighted 733D/443D/523D lens and the distance-weighted 737D/447D/527D lens, are bifocal diffractive intraocular lenses. Central thickness of the lens is reduced by the peripheral refractive Fresnel structures. These structures are not responsible for the creation of the near focus. The two focal points are created by diffractive steps on the anterior surface of the lens. These smaller steps can be seen in the central part of the lens in Figure 30.10.

As explained earlier, the distance between the distance focus and the near focus, i.e. the near addition, can be controlled by the radial displacement of the diffractive steps. According to the manufacturer, both lenses have a near addition of four diopters in lens plane. The light intensity of each focus can be regulated by the height of the diffractive steps. The Acri.Tec 733D/443D/523D has a 30 to 70% light distribution between distance and near focus, and the Acri.Tec 737D/447D/527D a 70 to 30% light distribution between distance and near

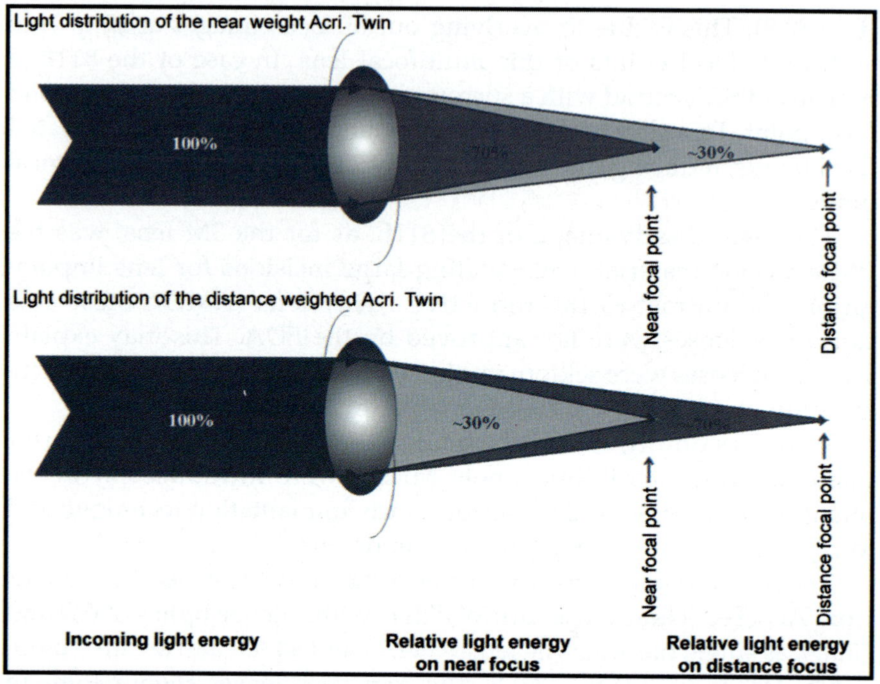

Fig. 30.9: Graphic shows the light distribution of the Acri.Twin lenses not taking in account light loss due to higher diffractive orders. The upper lens is the near weighted lens focusing about 70% of the incoming light on the near focus. The lower lens is the distance weighted lens focusing about 70% of the incoming light on the distance focus

focus, not taking into account the light loss due to higher orders of diffraction (Fig. 30.9). Clinically, these lenses showed excellent distance visual acuities with good near visual acuities. The near weighted lens achieved better near visual acuity than the distance weighted lens, and vice versa. Binocularly, the Acri.Twin lenses had better near visual acuities than patients with the Array lens or the 811 E lens (paper accepted at the J Cat Ref Surg, Schmidinger et al). Interestingly, the Acri.Twin lenses had comparable or even better intermediate visual acuities when compared to the Array lens (Fig. 30.11). Mean intermediate visual acuity did not drop to values lower than 0.1 logMAR (20/25). These results clearly demonstrate that additional intermediate focal points will not necessarily have a beneficial effect on the optical performance of a multifocal lens. In comparison to the 811 E with equal light distribution the Acri.Twin lenses had a better contrast sensitivity function at distance and at reading distance.[23]

Another attempt to increase the optical quality of a multifocal lens was the introduction of the aspheric designed ZM900. The Tecnis ZM900 (formerly named ZM001) is the diffractive bifocal model of the aspheric monofocal Tecnis Z9000 lens. The lens has a negative aspheric

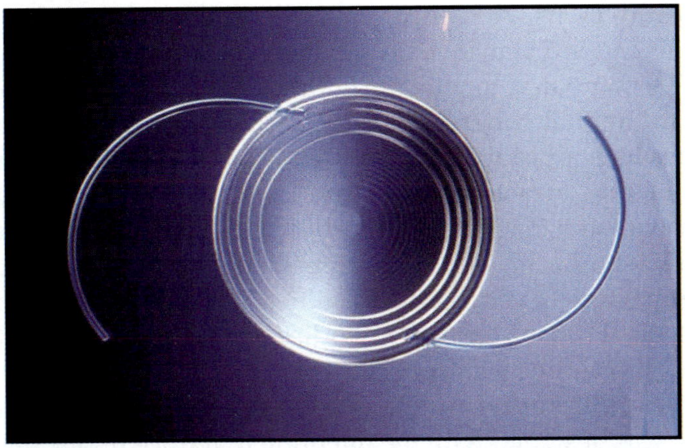

Fig. 30.10: Magnified view of an Acri.Twin silicone three-piece lens. Diffractive structures can be recognized in the center of the lens. The bigger steps in the periphery are Fresnel structures which are used to reduce the central thickness of the lens. These Fresnel structures are not part of the diffractive design

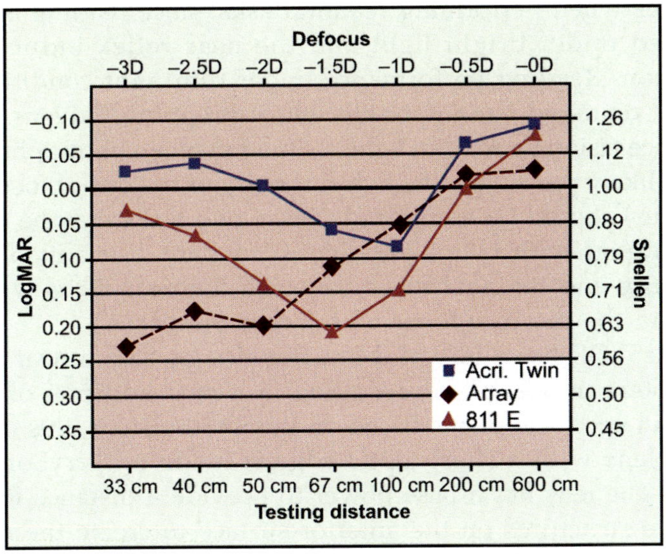

Fig. 30.11: Results of visual acuity measurements under standardized conditions at different distances tested in patients with binocular implantation of the Twin.Set, 811E lenses or Array lenses

anterior surface, which is designed to compensate positive spherical aberrations arising from an averaged human cornea. The silicone optic has a diameter of 6.0 mm and a sharp optic edge design for prevention of PCO. In addition to the aspheric design, the ZM900 has diffractive structures on the posterior surface creating two focal spots. From unpublished laboratory investigations, it is known that this lens is slightly near weighted, meaning that this lens has a stronger near focus than distance focus (Pieh et al.). In a clinical trail, Dillinger et al found significant better distance corrected near visual acuity in patients with the ZM900 compared to patients with an Array lens. In a presentation at the 23rd annual congress of the ESCRS, Ravalico et al presented a study in which a group of patients with the ReZOOM lens (modified version of the refractive Array lens) was compared to a group of patients with the ZM900. It was shown that patients in the ZM900 group had significant better near visual acuities contemporaneously with comparable distance visual acuities. These results are equivalent to the results known from other studies comparing bifocal intraocular lenses with multifocal intraocular lenses.

The latest introduced multifocal lens is the ReSTOR lens from Alcon. This lens was designed with the intention to reduce photic phenomena and increase near optical performance, and was approved by the FDA in 2005. According to Davidson et al[24] the lens design was based on two basic considerations. First, patients are considered to have small pupil sizes when performing reading tasks, since reading is usually performed under bright light and the near reflex induces pupil constriction. Reading performance under dim light conditions was therefore, rendered less important when designing the lens. Second, for distance vision under dim light, a situation when photic phenomena are most likely perceived, the light intensity of the out-of focus image (near focus) should be minimized. These two tasks may be achieved by a lens design with a pupil-size-dependent light distribution between the distance and the near focus, favoring the near focus with small pupils and the distance focus with larger pupils.

The ReSTOR has a bifocal diffractive design with a near addition of 4 diopters in lens plane, resulting in a near addition of about 3 diopters in spectacle plane. Based on the SA60AT lens, this one-piece foldable lens with a sharp optic edge is made of AcrySof (Alcon) material. The lens has a base power to provide a distance focus and diffractive structures on the anterior surface to create the near and distance focus. The diffractive structures cover only the central 3.6 mm of the lens surface. The periphery is of a refractive design serving the distance focal point only (Fig. 30.12).

In contrast to the earlier mentioned diffractive lenses, the diffractive zones on the ReSTOR lens are not of equal height. Higher steps at the center of the lens are getting gradually smaller to the periphery. As explained earlier, a change of the step height results in a change of the light distribution between the two focal points. Therefore, the changing step height results in a pupil size dependent light distribution. With small pupil sizes, about 41% of the incident light is directed to the near focus, with increasing pupil size the light energy serving the

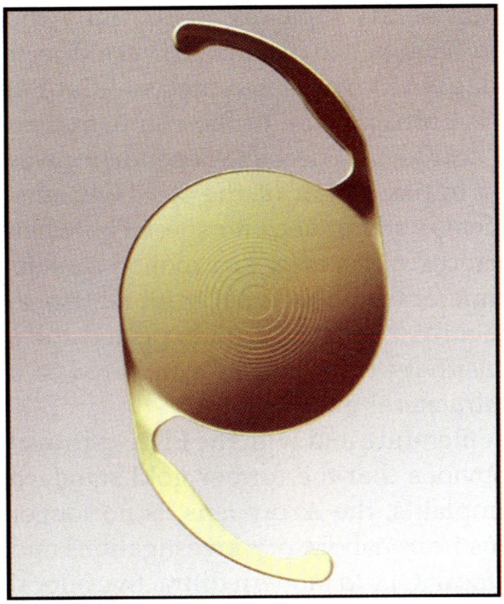

Fig. 30.12: Magnified view of the ReSTOR bifocal diffractive intraocular lens. On this single-piece acrylic lens the diffractive zones are restricted to the central 3.6 mm. In addition to the bifocal design this lens has an incorporated blue light filter known from the SN60AT monofocal lens

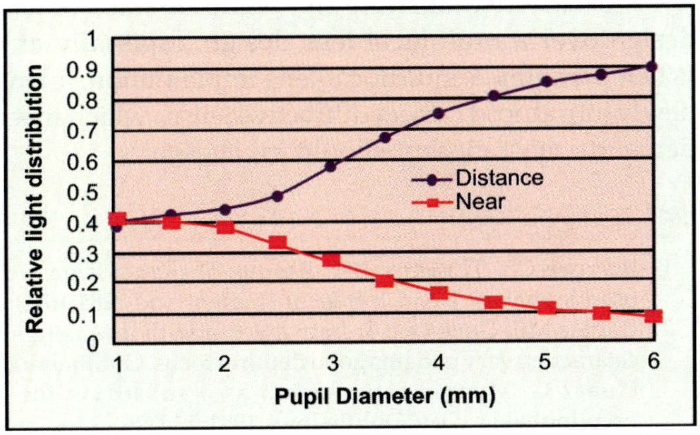

Fig. 30.13: Graphic showing the pupil-size dependent light distribution between the distance focus and the near focus. With increasing pupil diameter the distance focus is provided with more light energy at the expense of the near focus

near focus is getting gradually less (Fig. 30.13). Alcon named the gradual reduction in the step height "apodized diffractive" optic. In the field of optics this term was usually used to describe optic elements which enabled better image quality by the implementation of semi-translucent filters. These filters reduce the light energy in the peripheral parts of the Airy disc, resulting in a better PSF. Concerning the ReSTOR lens, Alcon adopted the term "apodized" to describe the gradual reduction of the height of the diffractive steps towards the periphery.

Clinical results from the FDA trail (using a three-piece design of the lens) showed a mean binocular uncorrected distance visual acuity of 0.04 logMAR and a mean corrected distance visual acuity of –0.05 logMAR. Near visual acuity uncorrected and with best distance correction was 0.09 log MAR and 0.05 logMAR, respectively.[25]

Concerning standardized visual acuity measurements, only the Acri.Twin lenses were shown to have better distance corrected near visual acuities at 33 cm (–0.026 logMAR) (paper accepted in J Cat Ref Surg; Schmidinger et al.). This is probably due to the compensating effect of the lens with a stronger near focus. Spectacle dependency was low in patients with binocular implantation of the ReSTOR lens, resulting in about 85% of the patients without need for spectacles when focusing on objects at close distances. Compared to a monofocal lens distance visual acuity was comparable concomitant with statistical significant better near visual acuity.[26] As it can be expected for a multifocal IOL, the contrast sensitivity was reduced compared to a monofocal IOL or a phakic contralateral eye.[27]

When reading through recent literature and with the FDA approval of the ReSTOR lens, it seems obvious that the former gold-standard in multifocal intraocular lens implants, the Array lens, is no longer unrivalled. Recent multifocal lens trails, laboratory investigations and trails comparing refractive multifocal IOLs to modern diffractive bifocal IOLs, clearly demonstrate the predominance of a bifocal diffractive design over a multifocal lens design, especially at reading distance. When planning a multifocal lens implantation, a lens design from the newly introduced bifocal diffractive lenses which meets the individual's demands most closely should be chosen.

REFERENCES

1. Boerner CF, Thrasher BH. Results of monovision correction in bilateral pseudophakes. J Am Intraocul Implant Soc 1984;10(1):49-50.
2. Datiles MB, Gancayco T. Low myopia with low astigmatic correction gives cataract surgery patients good depth of focus. Ophthalmology 1990;97(7):922-6.
3. Huber C. Myopic astigmatism as a substitute for accommodation in pseudophakia. Dev Ophthalmol 1981;5:17-26.
4. Miranda D, Krueger RR. Monovision laser in situ keratomileusis for pre-presbyopic and presbyopic patients. J Refract Surg 2004;20(4):325-8.
5. Leyland M, Zinicola E. Multifocal versus monofocal intraocular lenses in cataract surgery: a systematic review. Ophthalmology 2003;110(9):1789-98.
6. Leyland MD, Langan L, Goolfee F, et al. Prospective randomised double-masked trial of bilateral multifocal, bifocal or monofocal intraocular lenses. Eye 2002;16(4):481-90.
7. Javitt J, Brauweiler HP, Jacobi KW, et al. Cataract extraction with multifocal intraocular lens implantation: clinical, functional, and quality-of-life outcomes. Multicenter clinical trial in Germany and Austria. J Cataract Refract Surg 2000;26(9):1356-66.
8. Javitt JC, Steinert RF. Cataract extraction with multifocal intraocular lens implantation: a multinational clinical trial evaluating clinical, functional, and quality-of-life outcomes. Ophthalmology 2000;107(11):2040-8.
9. Walkow T, Liekfeld A, Anders N, et al. A prospective evaluation of a diffractive versus a refractive designed multifocal intraocular lens. Ophthalmology 1997;104(9):1380-6.

10. Pieh S, Weghaupt H, Rainer G, Skorpik C. [Visual acuity and use of eyeglasses after implantation of a diffractive multifocal lens]. Klin Monatsbl Augenheilkd 1997;210(1):38-42.
11. Pieh S, Lackner B, Hanselmayer G, et al. Halo size under distance and near conditions in refractive multifocal intraocular lenses. Br J Ophthalmol 2001;85(7):816-21.
12. Shoji N, Shimizu K. Binocular function of the patient with the refractive multifocal intraocular lens. J Cataract Refract Surg 2002;28(6):1012-7.
13. Hayashi K, Hayashi H, Nakao F, Hayashi F. Correlation between pupillary size and intraocular lens decentration and visual acuity of a zonal-progressive multifocal lens and a monofocal lens. Ophthalmology 2001;108(11):2011-7.
14. Slagsvold JE. 3M diffractive multifocal intraocular lens: eight year follow-up. J Cataract Refract Surg 2000;26(3):402-7.
15. Weghaupt H, Pieh S, Skorpik C. Comparison of pseudoaccommodation and visual quality between a diffractive and refractive multifocal intraocular lens. J Cataract Refract Surg 1998;24(5):663-5.
16. Ellingson FT. Explantation of 3M diffractive intraocular lenses. J Cataract Refract Surg 1990;16(6):697-702.
17. Ravalico G, Parentin F, Baccara F. Effect of astigmatism on multifocal intraocular lenses. J Cataract Refract Surg 1999;25(6):804-7.
18. Richter-Mueksch S, Weghaupt H, Skorpik C, et al. Reading performance with a refractive multifocal and a diffractive bifocal intraocular lens. J Cataract Refract Surg 2002;28(11):1957-63.
19. Haaskjold E, Allen ED, Burton RL, et al. Contrast sensitivity after implantation of diffractive bifocal and monofocal intraocular lenses. J Cataract Refract Surg 1998;24(5):653-8.
20. Pieh S, Marvan P, Lackner B, et al. Quantitative performance of bifocal and multifocal intraocular lenses in a model eye: point spread function in multifocal intraocular lenses. Arch Ophthalmol 2002;120(1):23-8.
21. Jacobi FK, Kammann J, Jacobi KW, et al. Bilateral implantation of asymmetrical diffractive multifocal intraocular lenses. Arch Ophthalmol 1999;117(1):17-23.
22. Jacobi KW, Eisenmann D. [Asymmetric multizone lenses—a new concept in multifocal intraocular lenses]. Klin Monatsbl Augenheilkd 1993;202(4):309-14.
23. Schmidinger G, Simader C, Dejaco-Ruhswurm I, et al. Contrast sensitivity function in eyes with diffractive bifocal intraocular lenses. J Cataract Refract Surg 2005;31(11):2076-83.
24. Davison JA, Simpson MJ. History and development of the apodized diffractive intraocular lens. J Cataract Refract Surg 2006;32(5):849-58.
25. Kohnen T, Allen D, Boureau C, et al. European multicenter study of the AcrySof ReSTOR apodized diffractive intraocular lens. Ophthalmology 2006;113(4):584.
26. Souza CE, Muccioli C, Soriano ES, et al. Visual performance of AcrySof ReSTOR apodized diffractive IOL: a prospective comparative trial. Am J Ophthalmol 2006;141(5):827-32.
27. Souza CE, Gerente VM, Chalita MR, et al. Visual acuity, contrast sensitivity, reading speed, and wavefront analysis: pseudophakic eye with multifocal IOL (ReSTOR) versus fellow phakic eye in non-presbyopic patients. J Refract Surg 2006;22(3):303-5.

CHAPTER

31

Ulrich M Klemen (Austria)
Elbland Klinik Radebeul (Germany)

Multifocal Intraocular Lenses

INTRODUCTION

The goal of the cataract surgery is the optimal visual rehabilitation including the correction of the preoperative myopic, hyperopic and astigmatic abnormalities. Based on the optic measurement of the axial length by means of the IOL Master (Zeiss,Germany) and the improved formulas the power of the intraocular lens (IOL) can be exactly evaluated with a tolerance of +/– 0.5 dptrs. postoperatively. The postoperative astigmatisms are much more difficult to correct, we know the difference between the corneal and the total astigmatism and the postoperative induced astigmatisms. So we had to evaluate preoperatively the keratometry and we must decide, what we must do to reduce this abnormality. By means of different techniques of incisions we can neutralize or influence the astigmatisms: by temporal incision it is possible to avoid a postoperative induced corneal astigmatism, depending from the high of the preoperative astigmatism we can reduce the postoperative outcome by opposite clear corneal incisions (up to 1.5 dptrs), by limbal relaxing incisions (up to 2.5 dptrs.), by implantation of toric IOLs (unlimitated) or by bioptics (secondary corneal refractive surgery).

The "golden goal" of each cataract surgery is the complete "spectacle indepence" (life without glasses !) which can only achieved by implantation of multifocal (MIOL)or accommodating IOLs. Since the first introduction of MIOLs 1987 with a diffractive type produced by 3M in Copenhagen (Denmark) at the ESCRS the development of this models was observed in 2 directions: the diffractive and the refractive type of MIOLs. Beside all positive results also a number of problematous side effects were observed: the glare phenomena and the halos and the discussion last until now, which type of MIOL can avoid this problems. Based on a personal experience within the last 2 decades I will prescribe shortly the history, the present situation, the limitations, the patients selection, the results and possible new developments.

HISTORY

As mentioned above the first introduced MIOL was a diffractive type: the principle is very easy to explain: the posterior surface of this IOL is not plane but configurated with multiple, circular, right angular, concentric "steps" so that the incoming light beam is split and produces 2 or more foci on the retina (like a prisma).[24] The sensorium of the patient should select the focus and so it becomes possible to see a far point also like a small letter without additional optic systems. The first descriptions of this model and the results had been very enthusiastic, but more and more also problems were noticed: optic side effects, significant loss of contrast sensitivity, color vision problems, intolerance especially in night-driving[1,2,4,5,7,12,15,16, 25,33,34]— a lot of this implants must be exchanged. This fact was the cause for the development of new styles of MIOLs:[28,35,36] aspheric and multizonal models are introduced, the optic side effects still remained and new problems like the dependence of the pupil size and double images were described and out of all this prototypes only the model of ARRAY was elected for further developments: in contrast to the diffractive type this MIOL is designed with 5 optic zones (3 for far and 2 for near distances) with smooth steps between this optics: the influence of the pupil diameter on to function was not so important as in the other types and additionally approximately 17 % of the incoming light offers also a visual acuity in the intermediate distances which was necessary for computer users: the terminus "multifocal" was new created ! But the refractive types showed also optic side effects and much more problems in reading distances, so that the refractive type was declared as the "far dominant" and the diffractive type as " near dominant".[23,26,40] The cause of the reading problems in the refractive MIOL is the week near addition of +3.5 dptrs, but because of the optic side effects no more addition is possible ! New developments in monofocal IOLs like the sharp right-angular posterior edge, the change from silicone to the hydrophobic acryl and the aberration free or correcting anterior surface were also taken into the MIOLs. The newest ARRAY model, the REZOOM (refractive, AMO) offers a sharp edge configuration with a smooth anterior edge to avoid the edge-glare phenomena, there is a choice of 2 materials (silicone of the last generation or hydrophobic acryl) and optimized optic zones configurations to reduce the optic side effects.

The two other diffractive models are also new designed: the TECNIS ZM Models (AMO) is also a "2-material" type with a prolate surface to correct the aberrations, the ReSTOR (ALCON) has a reduced central diffractive zone (3.6 mm) and the monofocal periphery should be helpful to compensate the near distance dominance, the surface is also prolate and there is a clear and a yellow-tinted hydrophobic acrylic one-piece model.[8,10,13,16,20,25,26,28-30,39]

Based on the fact, that no type of MIOL "fits all expectations" there are new recommendations to combine both models in one patient: The "mix and match" technique recommends depending form the patients expectations the implantation of a near or far dominant model in the leading eye, the "CustomMatch" is the individual decision of the choice of models according to the patients expectation.

The accommodative IOLs showed promising clinical results, objective measurements of the real accommodation (based on the forward-backword movement in the eye) limitated this to a maximum of 1 dptr! The development is still ongoing and the movement seems to be not large enough to offer a reasonable reading visual acuity.

PREOPERATIVE MANAGEMENT

Patients Selection and Explanation

There is only one absolute contraindication for implantation of MIOLS: the patient, who is not allowing an implantation of this type of IOL! All other contraindications are relative and belonging partly to the type of patient as well as to the condition of the eye. The "goal" of the cataract surgery with IOL implantation is the satisfied and happy patient, each depressive and negative patient will not be happy postoperatively, if he will find problems he will find them, also with an UCVA of 20/20 in all distances; on the other hand, you will find optimistic and encouraged patients suffering from many real problems like failure in biometry, reduced postoperative function because of central retinal pathology, corneal edemas, high induced postoperative corneal astigmatism, who are extremely happy!

The personality of the patient is one main criterium for implantation of MIOLs and the second is the subjective expectation: if the expectation is high it is very difficult to be successful. The next item is the life style of the patient: a patient, who is extremely active in driving, in sports and in performing culture like cinema or theater will not be happy with a near dominant MIOL, whereas a "bookworm" is not the candidate for a far dominant MIOL!

The explanation must include the exact information relating optic side effects like halo and glare and their influence on the night driving problems as well as the possible lens exchange.

It is not recommended to promise the patient a "Life without glasses" — it is well known that a high rate of –absolute satisfied-patients use glasses for long time reading ! And there is no absolute prognosis that each patient is able to read without glasses, the neuronal adaption lasts in some patients over a long time.

Biometry

The biometry should be done by the optic method with the IOL master and the target refraction is primarily emmetropia in both types of MIOLs, in refractive MIOLs it was recommended to change the target a little bit into the plus-refraction in order to reduce the postoperative dysphotopsias, but there is no evidence based study for confirmation of this recommendation. And we should not forget, that the near addition of +3.5 dptrs is very low and if you achieve a final far refraction of + 0.5 dptrs. there can be a negative influence on the uncorrected VA for reading ! It is also necessary to check the power of all possible MIOLs and the possibility of a sulcus implantation with an increase of the anterior chamber depth should not be forgotten. A special problems are the eyes after performed corneal refractive surgeries, but the new HAIGIS formula promises a good solution for this problems, as refractive surgeons we should perform in all patients before the refractive operation an exact biometry as well as a record of all datas of the keratometry as well as the topography!

Astigmatism

Preoperative corneal astigmatisms over +1.5 dptrs are relative contraindications for MIOL implantation; it is well known, that this amount of corneal abnormalities leads to problems with the postoperative multifocality, but the criterion is not the pre- but the postoperative amount of the corneal astigmatism. So, it is indicated to compare the values of keratometry with the data of the biometry and the corneal mapping to filter out the corneal from the total astigmatismus ! According to this result you must determine which method for reduction of the corneal astigmatism you choose: opposite clear corneal incisions (up to +1.5 dptrs), limbal relaxing incisions (up to +2.5 dptrs) or a planned corneal refractive surgery with the advantage of correction of possible spherical errors. The patient must be informed concerning the necessity of second operations, especially if you performe an LASIK cut simultaneously with the cataract surgery.[22]

Surgical Technique

The surgical technique is not different to the technique of monofocal IOL implantation; but some items should be pointed out in order reduce the number of postoperative problems.

Incision

To avoid a postoperative induced corneal astigmatism a temporal sclero-corneal tunnel incision should be performed. For reduction of the astigmatisms an opposite clear cornea incision (OCCI) can be performed in the steepest meridian up to +1.5 dptrs. or limbal relaxing incisions (LRI) up to +2.5 dptrs. But do not forget the rotation of the globe in the horizontal position and mark preoperatively the axis on the slit-lamp!

*Capsulotomy:*The continous curvelinear anterior capsulotomy (CCC) is the method of choice, the diameter should be a little bit smaller than the optic diameter in order to overlap completely the optic part of the MIOL, but it should be not too small in diameter to prevent a SOMMERING formation, a shrinkage of the anterior capsular opening. A good centration of the CCC is also recommendable to prevent an ovalization or a dislocation of the MIOL by shrinkage of the capsular bag.

Polishing of the Capsular Bag

A shrinkage of the capsular bag should be avoided to prevent any dislocation of the MIOL, especially in silicon IOLs also the danger of a vaulting is existing. So a complete removal of all visible (and invisible) LECs is recommended. Specific problems of the NdYAG-Lasercapsulotomy will be discussed in "Postoperative Management".

Implantation

For all three types of MIOLs are specific insertes developed which should be used, for the silicone models (REZOOM and TECNIS) the SilverZ and for the acrylic types of these MIOLs the EMERALD EASE injector as well the MONARCH II for the ReSTOR MIOL. All inserters need only an incision length of 2.6 – 2.8 mm, the techniques are easy and there are extremely rare complications. In high power MIOLS (> +28.0 dptrs) sometimes the passage of the IOL is a little bit heavy but possible; measurements of the incision length after implantation showed only small enlargements of 0.1 mm on an average without any negative influence on the postoperative astigmatism (Figs 31.1 to 31.3).[22]

Wound Closure

A self-sealing wound construction is the method of choice, any suturing can influence the postoperative astigmatism and retards the functional rehabilitation; but if suturing is necessary, it should be done very exactly in order to prevent any traction on to the wound lips. Normally this suture can be removed at least one week after surgery.

POSTOPERATIVE MANAGEMENT

The postoperative management after MIOL implantation is almost the same as after monofocal IOLs, but in the follow-up time it becomes necessary to observe the development of the multifocal function, the "remaining" refraction, the corneal topography, the Contrast Sensitivity, the optic side effects, the subjective satisfaction and the

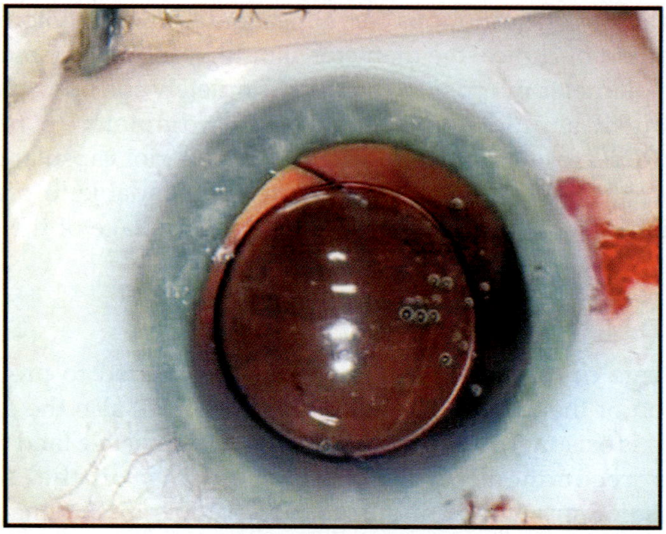

Fig. 31.1: ARRAY 2, hydrophobic acryl, implantation by EMERALD Ease, 2.8 mm incision, one step implantation, excellent self centration

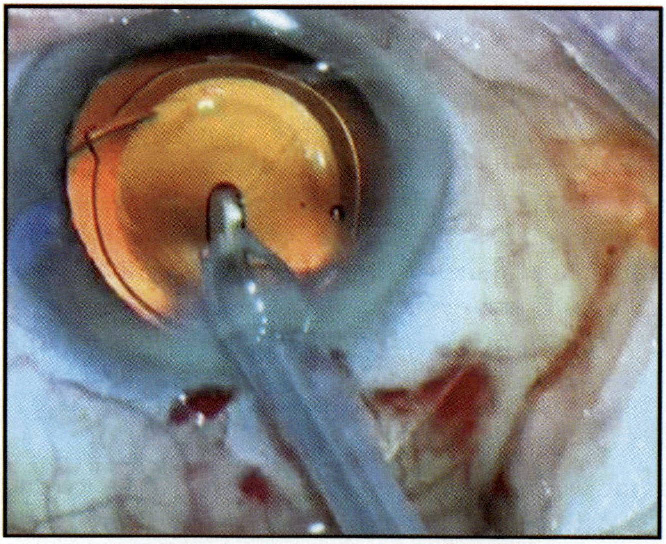

Fig. 31.2: REZOOM, silicone of the last generation, same sizes as ARRAY 2, implantation by Silver Z inserter

"quality of life" situation: the percentage of the time for wearing glasses! A secondary cataract formation disturbs much more the function, especially in reading distance; so the NdYAG Lasercapsulotomy is indicated as soon as the patient notice a decrease of the visual function. The size of the posterior hole should be not too small so that enough zones become clear for multifocality (depending to the type of MIOL) but not too large to "loose" the (silicone) IOL

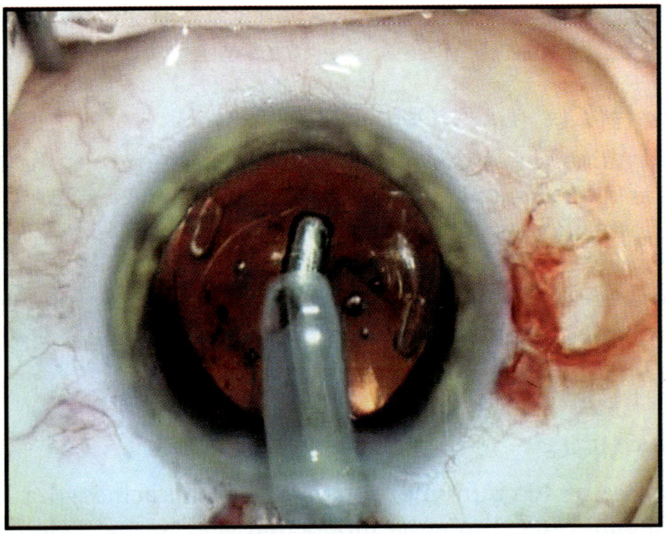

Fig. 31.3: TECNIS ZM 9000, after implantation with Silver Z, excellent centration by the specific haptic configuration, incision size 2.7 mm

into the vitreous cavity ! Lens damages should be avoided because of an additional negative influence on to the optic side effects.[6,27]

RESULTS

Within the last two decades there are more than 1,000 publications regarding the outcome of the function (UCVA and BCVA, contrast sensitivity under different light conditions, color vision), the comparison with monofocal IOLs and the subjective satisfaction of the patients after implantation of MIOLs. A general comparison is very difficult because of the different numbers of patients, the follow-up time and the published results (Snellen and/or Reagan charts, log.mar, Pelli Robson, etc.) Also the exclusions criterias were different, especially the age, the preoperative evaluated prognosted VA, the individual mental condition of the patient and much more, so it is a problem to summarize all the datas from the different publications. We only are able to point out the average outcome of all published studies.

Distance VA

Diffractive MIOLs (TECNIS,ReSTOR)

Monocular three months postoperatively more than 90% of the patients achieved a UCVA of 20/40 or better and after 6 months more than 95%; 95 % of all patients showed a residual refraction in the range of +/- 0.5 dptrs, so the BCVA was not significantly different from the

UCVA. Binocular 92% of all achieved a UCVA of 20/40 or better after 3 months and more than 96% after 6 months.[4,9,15,17,37,38]

Refractive MIOLs (REZOOM)

The far dominance of the refractive MIOLs confirmes the fact, that monocular after 3 months 96% showed an UCVA of 20/40, there is no significant increase after 6 months, and binocular more than 98% of all achieves 20/40 or better after 6 months. The long time of half a year was necessary to choose because of a relatively long period for the neuronal adaptation mentioned above.[22,31,35,40]

Reading Distance

Diffractive MIOLs

In a distance of 40 cmtrs more than 90% of all achieved a UCVA of 20/40 (Regan) after 3 months monocular and an increase up to 98% were observed after 6 months, binocular more than 99% were able to read 20/40 or better half an year after surgery. There was no significant difference between TECNIS and ReSTOR MIOLs and between UCVA and near vision with far distance correction.

Refractive IOLs

Compared with the diffractive MIOLs after 3 months the rate of patients achieving 20/40 or better was reported as 87% with an increase to 89% after 6 months, binocular 94% on an average were found to be able to read 20/40 uncorrected or with far distance correction.

Intermediate Distances

In contrast to the publication relating far and visual acuity there are only few papers relating the VA in intermediate distances, so we will summarize the results of a personal study on 40 patients with binocular REZOOM and TECNIS MIOL implantation. Patients of the REZOOM group achieved in 1 meter distance UCVA of 20/45 on an average (range 20/40–20/50) and the TECNIS group 20/50 (20/40–20/60). In the distance of 60 cmtrs patients with REZOOM MIOLS had seen 20/50 average (20/40–20/80) and patients with TECNIS MIOL 20/55 on an average (20/40 –20/100). This results showed no statistical significance and it was amazing because of the fact, that the light distribution for intermediate distances is 17% in the refractive MIOL and 0 in the diffractive.[19]

Contrast Sensitivity

With any MIOL the division of the incoming light is split in more than one focus and produces physically retinal images of reduced contrast. Compared with monofocal IOLs especially low-contrast acuity was poorer than high-contrast visual acuity (4% contrast less on an average).

But there are no reports of any inconvenience of patients caused by the reduced contrast perception; datas from one of the first FDA studies about the diffractive MIOL (3M) showed only a small contrast sensitivity loss and it was considered clinically insignificant. Comparisons with monofocal IOLs on a representative number of patients are not easy to perform (recommendation for binocular implantation of MIOLs) but the recommended new "mix and Match" technique (in one eye a refractive and in the fellow-eye a diffractive MIOL) will offer us a new chance to compare the contrast sensitivity of two types of MIOL.[1,5,15,16,19,20,33,36]

Optic Side Effects

All reports of optic side effects are subjective and can not be physically measured like the VA and the contrast sensitivity ! At first it is necessary to divide this problem in tolerable and not tolerable complications, and we should not forget, that similar optic side effects are also noticed after monofocal IOL implantation, the only difference is the fact, that no patient wants an exchange of a monofocal IOL with aphacic correction by glasses or contact IOLs. The same problems were tolerated in monofocal but not in multifocal IOLs ! The subjective noticed visual phenomenas were reported in a range from 5 to 40%, by distribution according their violence into mild, moderate, tolerable and not tolerable the percentage of the last group is under 1% ! 5%, however, have severe problems in night-driving, but we have no real rating of those patients with the same problems after monocular IOL implantation. Most of these problems are decreasing after the second eye implantation.[15,19,20,30,38]

Spectacle Independence and Subjective Satisfaction

All publications relating to the frequency of using glasses are depending from the articulation of the questions and the personality of the material ! Patients, who usually like to read over long periods of time need certainly more often glasses as patients who only look at the headlines of newspapers. Generally, -except for long-time reading- the use of glasses is reported as very seldom and the independence of glasses was found in more than 95% of all patients, i.e. that patients do not need any spectacle for their daily life! But, beside of all advantages of the last generation of MIOLS we should not forget, that only 50% of all incoming contrast of a print can be focussed on the retina, and before surgery by means of reading glasses the patient had seen 100% of the print !

Also the evaluation of the patients satisfaction is subjective and difficult to measure, especially in the old population there are sometimes problems in communication and in understanding the questions. The conclusion of all reports showed a relatively high satisfaction, on a scale from 0 (unsatisfied) to 5 (high satisfied) the average level was found between 4 and 5 on an average, but we should not forget, that a group of about 10% are not satisfied, mostly caused by problems in reading distance and by optic side effects, but the rate of patients, in which a lens exchange is necessary is under 1% !

CONCLUSION

1. MIOLs are the ideal implants for a special group of patients – the psychological influence of the surgeon for the decision for this MIOL is important because of the relatively high risks of optic side effects and the costs ! The explanation is time consuming and sometimes difficult bis important to avoid a postoperative unsatisfaction of the patient. We should not promise a "Life without Spectacles", if the patients expectations are to high it will be much more difficult to fullfil. Each patient should know the difference of the types of MIOL, their advatanges and disadvantages as well the optic side effects and the necessity of using glasses in some situations. The expectation of the patient should be realistic, not too optimistic !
2. Under this conditions you can expect a representative group of satisfied and happy patients relating their new increased quality of life; but you also must fear a small group of not satisfied and unhappy individuals because of two main problems: problems with reading and night-driving. The "technique of reading" is complete different from the reading with glasses and must learned by most of the patients by time, the problem of night-driving is not solved until now. Preoperative tests with multifocal contact lenses with the same optic pattern like the MIOL are recommended.
3. If a patient is unsatisfied after the first MIOL implantation do not believe that the problems will be solved by the time alone or after the implantation of an MIOL in the fellow-eye – there are no general rules what is the optimum to do. Personally, I give the decision to the patient, what we should do – it is the eye of the patient, he had to decide, if he tolerate the side effects or not and he must give the decision before the operation of the fellow eye. Out of a total number

of more than 3000 MIOL implantations I overlook 10 patients, in which a lens exchange was necessary - beside very good results, only because of the intolerance of the side effects. One half of these patients were happy (some with minor visual function !) but the rest remained unhappy and reported the same problems with the monofocal exchange IOLs !

4. A lens exchange should not be performed –especially in hydrophobic acrylic MIOL because of the stickening of the optic with the capsule - half a year after the surgery – this time is also necessary for the neuronal adaptation and many immediately after the operation unhappy patients have learned the "new reading technique" or tolerated the side effects.
5. The only absolute contraindication is the patient, who do not want a MIOL implantation; but there are a lot of relative contraindications as well as from the side of the surgeon (astigmatisms management) as from the patient; I believe, that we should give a maximum of all our patients the chance for a spectacle independence, and I have seen a lot of patients who had been unable to read but with a high subjective satisfaction, and I also had to exchange the MIOL in some eyes with UCVA of 20/20 for far distance and reading!

Beside all advantages of the development of the newest introduced models of MIOLs we must not forget, that all these types can only offer a " pseudoaccommodation " The real goal must be the development of a real accommodation by a change of the lens curvatures – all until now offered "accommodating" IOLs offer also only a "pseudo-accommodation" by a backward-forward movement in the eye.

But until the real accommodation could not produced the refractive and diffractive MIOLs of the last generation are the golden standard to give the patient the possibility for a good objective uncorrected visual acuity for far and reading distance as well reasonable outcomes in intermediate distances under toleration of optic side effects and minimal loss of contrast sensitivity.

REFERENCES

1. Akutsu H, Legge GE, Shwoalter M, et al. Contrast sensitivity and reading through multifocal intraocular lenses. Arch Ophthalmol 1992; 1076-80.
2. Akutsu H,Legge GE, Luebker A, et al. Multifocal intraocular lenses and glare, OptomVis Sci 1993; 70: 487-95.
3. Arens B, Freudenthaler N, Quentin CD. Binocular function after bilateral implantation of monofocal and refractive multifocal intraocular lenses. J Cataract Refract Surg 1999; 25:399-404.
4. Belucci R,Scialdone A, Buratto L, et al. Visual acuity and contrast sensitivity comparison between Tecnis and AcrySofSA60AT intraocular lenses. A multicenter randomized study. J Cataract Refract Surg 2005;31(4):712-7.

5. Breitkopf J, Eisenmann D, Jacobi FK. Contrast vision and contrast sensitivity after binocular implantation of multifocal and monofocal intraocular lenses. Ophthalmologe 1997; 94: 519-22.
6. Buehl W, Menapace R, Sacu S, et al. Effect of a silicone intraocular lens with sharp posterior edge on posterior capsule opacification. J Cataract Refract Surg 2004;30: 1661-7.
7. Dick HB, Krummenauer F, Schwenn O, et al. Objective and subjective evaluation of photic phenomena after monofocal and multifocal intraocular lens implantation. Ophthalmology 1999;106:1878-86.
8. Epstein D. Physiological aberration of the cornea. Statistical analysis of 1000 normal eyes. Presented at ASCRS 2003 (in press).
9. Gimbel HV, Sanders DR Raanan MG. Visual and refractive results after multifocal intraocular lenses. Ophthalmology 1991;98:881-8.
10. Guirao A, Tejedor J, Artal P. Corneal aberrations before and after small-incision cataract surgery. Invest Ophthalmol Vis Sci 2004; 45(12): 4312-9.
11. Hayashi K, Hayashi H, Nakao F. Correlation between papillary size and intraocular lens decentration and visual acuity of a zonal-progressive multiofocal lens and a monofocal lens. Ophthalmology 2001;18:2011-7.
12. Holladay JT, Van Dijk H, Land A, et al. Optical performance of multifocal intraocular lenses. J Cataract Refract Surg 1990; 16: 413-22.
13. Holladay JT, Piers PA, Koranyi G, et al. A new intraocular lens design to reduce spherical aberration of pseudophacic eyes. J Cataract Refract Surg 2002;18:683-91.
14. Jacobi FK, Kammann J, Jacobi KW, et al. Bilateral implantation of assymetrical diffractive multifocal intraocular lenses. Arch Ophthalmol 1999;117:17-23.
15. Javitt JC, Steinert RF. Cataract extraction with multifocal intraocular lens implantation: a multinational clinical trial evaluating clinical, functional and quality-of-life outcomes. Ophthalmology 2000;107:2040-8.
16. Kennis H, Huygens M, Callebaut F. Comparing the contrast sensitivity of a modified prolate anterior surface IOL and two spherical IOLs. Bull Soc Belge Ophthalmol 2004;294:49-54.
17. Klemen UM, Hahsel B, Lackinger B. Refractive versus diffractive: a comparison of 4 multifocal intraocular lenses. 19. Kongreß der DGII, Biermann Verlag 2006:345-9.
18. Koch DD, Samuelson SW, Villareal R, et al. Changes in pupil size induced by phacoemulsification and posterior chamber lens implantation: consequences for multifocal lenses. J Cataract Refract Surg 1996;22:579-84.
19. Koch DD, Samuelson SW, Haft EA, et al. Pupillary size and responsiveness: implications for selection of abifocal intraocular lens. Ophthalmology 1991; 98:1030-5.
20. Kohnen T, Kasper T. Incison sizes before and after implantation of foldable intraocular lenses with 6 mm optic using Monarchand Unfolder injector systems. Ophthalmology 2005;112:58-66.
21. 21 Kohnen T, Allen D, Boureau C, et al. European multicenter study of the AcrySof ReSTOR apodized diffractive intraocular lens. Ophthalmology 2006;113:575-84.
22. Liekfeld A, Pham DT, Wollensack J. Functonal results in bilateral implantation of a foldable multifocal posterior chamber lens. Klin Mbl Augenheilkd 1995;207:283-6.
23. Lindtrom RL.Multifocal and bifocal implant Curr Opin. Ophthalmol 1993; 4:3-9.

24. Lindstrom,RL.Food and drug administration study update. One -year results from 671 patients with the 3M multifocal intraocular lens. Ophthalmology 1993;1000:91-7.
25. McBridge DK, Matson W. Assessing the significance of optically produced reduction in braking response time:possible impacts on automotive safety among the elderly. Potomac Institute for Police Studies. April 1,2003.
26. Mester U, Dillinger P, Anterist N. Impact of a modified optic design on visual function: clinical comparative study. J Cataract Refract Surg 2003;29:652-60.
27. Mester U, Fabian E, Gerl R, et al. Posterior capsule opacification after implantation of CeeOn Edge 911A, Phacoflex SI-40NB, and AcrySof MA60BM lenses. J Cataract Refract Surg 2004; 30:979-85.
28. Oshika T, Klyce SD, Applegate RA, et al. Changes in corneal wavefront aberration with aging. Invest Ophthalmol Vis Sci 1999;40:1351-5.
29. Packer M, Fine IH, Hoffmann RS,et al. Improved functional vision with a prolate intraocular lens. J Cataract Refract Surg 2004;30:986-92.
30. Packer M, Fine IH, Hoffmann RS. Maximizing optical quality. Cataract & refractive Surgery Nov/Dec 2006.
31. Pieh S, Lackner B, Hanselmayer G, et al. Halo size under distance and near conditions in refractive multifocal intraocular lenses. Br J Ophthalmol 2001;85:816-21.
32. Pieh S, Marvan P, Lackner B, et al. Quantitative performance of bifocal and multifocal intraocular lenses in a model eye: point spread function of multifocal intraocular lenses. Arch Ophthalmol 2002;120:23-8.
33. Post CT jr. Comparison of depth of focus and low-contrast acuities for monofocal versus multifocal intraocular lens patients at 1 year. Ophthalmology 1992;99:1658-63.
34. Ruther K, Eisenmann D, Zrenner E, et al. Effect of diffractive multi-focal lenses on contrast vision, glare sensitivity and colour vision. Klin Monatsbl Augenheilkd 1994; 204:14-9.
35. Steinert RF, Post CT, Brint SF, et al. A prospective, randomized, double-masked comparison of a zonal –progressive multifocal intraocular lens and a monofocal intraocular lens. Ophthalmology 1992; 99: 853-60.
36. Steinert RF, Aker BL, Trentacost DJ, et al. A prospective comparative study of the AMO ARRAY zonal progressive multifocal silicone intraocular lens and a monofocal intraocular lens. Ophthalmology 199;106:1243-55.
37. Walkow T, Liekfeld A, Anders N, et al. A prospective evaluation of a difrractive versus a refractive designed multifocal intraocular lens. Ophthalmology 1997;104:1380-6.
38. Walkow T, Klemen U. Patients satisfaction after implantation of diffractive designed multifocal intraocular lenses in dependence on objective parameters. Greafes Arch Clin Exp Ophthalmol 2001;239:683-7.
39. Wan I, Dai E, Koch DD, et al. Optical aberrations of the human cornea. J Cataract Refract Surg 2003;29(8):1514-21.
40. Weghaupt H, Pieh S, Skorpik C. Comparison of pseudoaccommodation and visual quality between a diffractive and refractive multifocal intraocular lens. J Cataract Refract Surg 1998;24:663-5.

CHAPTER

32

Paul Rolf Preussner (Germany)

Customized IOLs: Possibilities and Limitations

WHY CUSTOMIZED IOL?

Currently, spherically symmetric IOL are produced normally in steps of 0.5 D for the spherical power (defocus). A few manufacturers also offer toric IOL for the additional correction of astigmatism, in steps of 1-2 D of torical power in addition to the spherical values. Also aspheric IOL came to the market in order to correct spherical aberration, with asphericities fitted to the optical properties of mean eyes. With these mean values, of course many eyes cannot be ideally corrected. Therefore, other manufacturers offer aspheric IOL not to correct the spherical aberration of the whole eye, but which do not produce spherical aberration if they are used as a single optical imaging element, sometimes called "aberration-free" IOL. This term, however, is somewhat ambiguous as it does not define for which condition no spherical aberration is produced. This condition is different for parallel light or for a converging beam as in the human eye behind the cornea.

Let us assume that 6 steps of different asphericities are needed to correct spherical aberration of most individual eyes with sufficient accuracy, further 6 steps with 1 D stepwidth of toric power and, as in most IOL on the market, 41 steps from 10 D to 30 D of spherical power (defocus) with a stepwidth of 0.5 D. Even if this set pattern is still relatively coarse, and some eyes with higher astigmatism or very short or long axis are not covered, it requires already a store of $6 \times 6 \times 41 = 1476$ IOL. Many of these lenses would not be implanted prior to their expiration date. In addition, the step width in the three parameters is higher than the recognition threshold of an ideally corrected human eye, i.e. the corrections with these IOL do not fully achieve the wanted accuracy.

For these reasons, customisation seems to be the better choice for the future. The additional question occurs if perhaps also other optical errors beside defocus, astigmatism and spherical aberration might be correctable in order to further improve the optical quality. This question shall be addressed in the next section.

ARE ALL CORNEAL ERRORS CORRECTABLE BY AN IOL?

The General Problem

It is sometimes suggested to correct all optical errors of the eye on either the cornea by customized corneal ablation or with a customized IOL to achieve an aberration-free optical system. Some theoretical considerations are necessary to understand if this is possible.

If an optical system has only one imaging surface, it is always possible to produce an ideal diffraction-limited image for impinging parallel light, which is a diffraction-blurred "point" in case of monochromatic light.

Different wavelengths always produce chromatic aberration if the imaging surface is the surface of a lens. Only mirrors like in astronomical telescopes do not have chromatic aberration: reflection angles do not depend on wavelength, but refraction angles do, because the refractive index of all materials depends on wavelength.

Extended pictures can never be imaged without distortions. Distortions, however, are negligible if the image size is very small compared to the optical aperture. This condition is matched in the human eye. The relevant retinal (foveal) area is very small compared to pupil size. The neuronal resolution of the eye has a much steeper decay from central fovea to periphery than the decay of optical imaging performance. This is one reason that image distortions are normally not recognized in human visual perception even if they are in fact rather high. This is completely different, e.g. in photography, where the image distortions are relevant and often disturbing, even if they are much smaller than in the eye.

For these reasons the optical errors of the human eye are mostly looked at as the errors of imaging parallel light to a point (or, in finite distance, of imaging a point to a point). Our further considerations shall be restricted to this scenario.

If the eye would consist only of one imaging surface, e.g. the cornea, this surface could be given a shape that it produces an ideal diffraction limited point for monochromatic light, like an astronomical telescope. This shape would be an ideal asphere, already described by Ren´e Descartes and coworkers in the early 17th century.

Therefore, for an aphakic eye, corneal refractive surgery could be performed by calculating such ideal surfaces, and among them, chosing the one which requires least tissue ablation, then performing this ablation and coming out with an ideal eye, at least in theory.

But, what happens if there are more than one refracting surfaces? In fact, there are four in the human eye, two on the cornea and two on the lens, and we are faced here with the problem of finding an ideal lens for a given cornea.

In general, optical errors can be reduced on any of the refracting surfaces. But it is impossible to compensate all optical errors of one surface on another surface, i.e. at another location. Trying to do so, always new errors are induced. A non-trivial example demonstrating that a correction of the errors of one surface is impossible on another surface is shown in Figure 32.1.

It is, however, possible to correct all monochromatic rotationally symmetric optical errors of the human eye on either the cornea or the lens, provided cornea and lens are centered relative to each other. These rotationally symmetric errors are defocus and spherical aberration. But it should be kept in mind that, for a given eye, correction of the defocus on corneal 2 surface produces a different image size than correcting them on the lens, in the sense of the mentioned "induced errors".

The approach to correct non-rotationally symmetric errors is at least critical if the location of the error is different from the location of the correction. It is generally impossible to correct, e.g. corneal errors of higher spatial frequency with an IOL. But already the simplest case of a non-rotationally symmetric error, the astigmatism, cannot be completely corrected as shown in the next section.

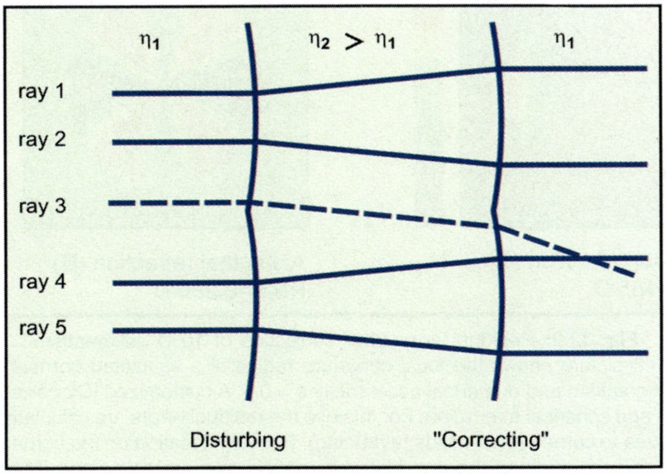

Fig. 32.1: Trial to correct optical errors.
Five parallel rays are impinging on a disturbing surface, and are to be corrected on a second one. The refractive index is higher between the two surfaces than outside. The trial is made to construct a "correcting" surface which compensates the optical errors caused by the first one. Indeed, rays 1,2,4 and 5 are again parallel, but ray 3 fails. It is not possible to construct a surface which corrects all rays. Note that the distances of ray 1 and 2, and of ray 4 and 5 are larger, of ray 2 and 4 smaller after passing the two surfaces than before. In general, the trial to correct optical errors on different surfaces normally causes changes in image sizes, at least in certain directions of the image

Residual Errors after Correcting Astigmatism

Figures 32.2 and 32.3 show the optical performance of an eye with 10 D corneal astigmatism which is corrected by an ideal, customized IOL.

SPHERICAL ABERRATION

We assume in the following that lens and cornea are centered relative to each other. Further, cornea is assumed to be a rotationally symmetric

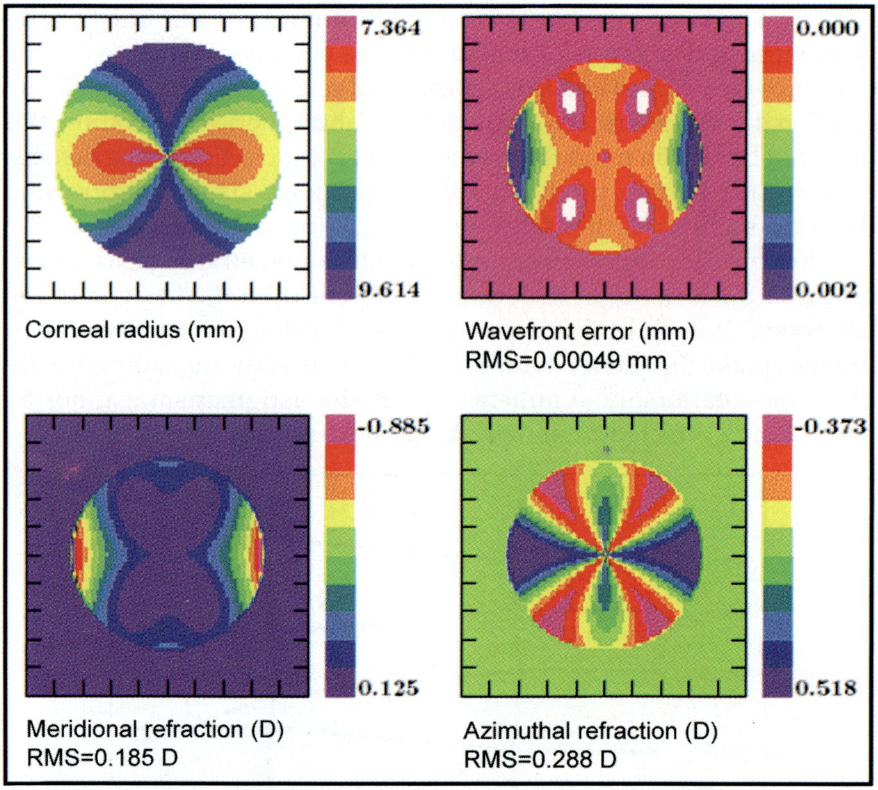

Fig. 32.2: Residual error after correction of 10 D astigmatism.

The upper left picture shows the local curvature radius of a simulated corneal topography with 10D astigmatism and numerical eccentricity e = 0.5. A customized IOL corrects defocus, astigmatism and spherical aberration. For this eye the residual errors are calculated by tracing rays from fovea to cornea (backwards raytracing). For each location on the cornea the optical path length and the angle of the ray relative to optical axis are calculated. The upper right picture shows the error in optical path length, the so-called "wavefront error". The RMS-value of 0.49 μm is more than one order of magnitude higher than the Mar´echal threshold which is 0.0385 μm for a wavelength of 540 nm. For the angles of the rays, the projections in the directions of the corresponding meridians and perpendicular to them are calculated, and the values are then transformed into diopters in order to have a common and comparable measure of quality. The lower left picture shows this meridional refraction error, the lower right the perpendicular component, the azimuthal refraction error which is even larger. Graphically, the non-zero azimuthal error means that it is impossible for a ray to stay exactly in a meridional plane after passing one or more astigmatic surfaces.

The example (10 D !) is exaggerated for better visualization. The residual errors shown here are normally below the recognition threshold of human visual perception for a corneal astigmatism below ≈ 4 D

sphere or asphere. In this case spherical aberration can be fully corrected by a customized IOL. Anterior and/or posterior IOL surfaces have to be aspheres.

How to describe such aspheres? Theoretically, an asphere has to be described by series with many elements. Fortunately, this can be

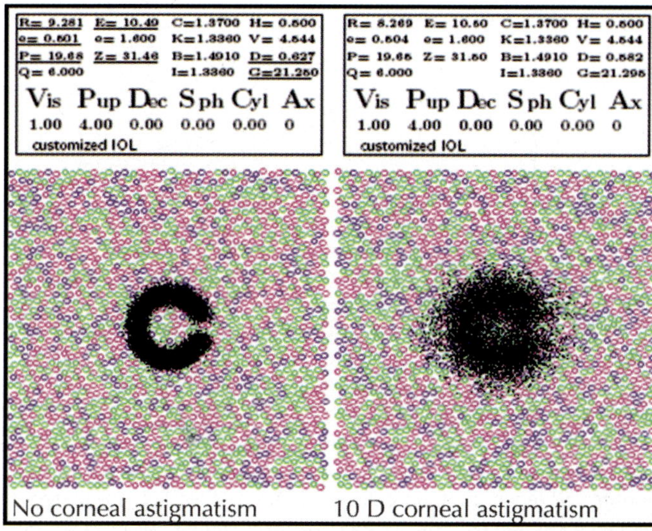

Fig. 32.3: Residual error after correction of 10 D astigmatism. The results of Figure 32.2 are visualized by blurred retinal images. The little colored circles represent the retinal photoreceptors. Landolt's rings of a size corresponding to visual acuity charts of 1.0 (20/20) are calculated.[5-7] Pupil width is 4 mm. The right subimage represents the situation as given in Figure 32.2. Note that the halo is not exactly spherically symmetric, in correspondence to the pattern in Figure 32.2. The left subimage shows the optical performance with a rotationally symmetric cornea and a customized IOL correcting defocus and spherical aberration of this astigmatism-free eye. The little blurring is only caused by diffraction from the pupil aperture. Marechal's criterion is also satisfied here

simplified for the human eye:[8,9] an approximation by conicoids produces residual errors which are normally below the recognition threshold of human visual perception, see also Figure 32.4. Particularly, these residual errors are smaller than the variations of the eye's optical parameters produced by variations of the tear film or by the geometric changes due to variations of intraocular pressure.

The ideal asphericity of the IOL surfaces, mathematically described, e.g. by numerical eccentricity e, is a function of the corneal curvature and asphericity, and of the geometrical properties of the eye, i.e. axial length and IOL position. This ideal asphericity is found by numerical iteration. A solution always can be found beside very long eyes requiring IOL powers below ≈ 5 D. Only in these cases a description of the surface by a series is necessary.

CHROMATIC ABERRATION

IOL normally are manufactured from a single, homogenous material like silicone or acrylates. With these homogeneous materials chromatic aberration is unavoidable. It causes a difference in defocus between violet and red light in the order of 0.5-1D. Exact values depend on the dispersion of the IOL material and on IOL power. With respect to IOL

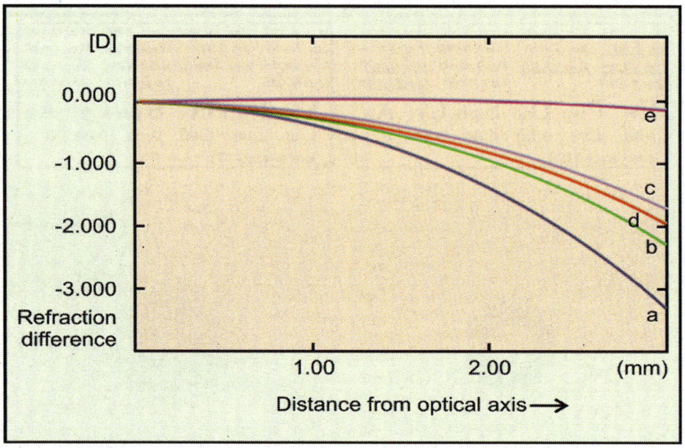

Fig. 32.4: Spherical aberration of different IOL models.
The meridional refraction (D), i.e. the refraction in the direction of the meridians is shown as a function of the distance from the optical axis (mm). Five IOL are compared with each other, all making the eye emmetropic for paraxial rays. The IOL differ in the ratio of anterior to posterior vertex radii Ra/Rp and in the numerical eccentricities of anterior and posterior surface, e_a and e_p. The refraction differences between off-axis and paraxial refraction are a measure of spherical aberration.

a. Ra/Rp = 3/1, $e_a = e_p = 0$
b. Ra/Rp = 1/1, $e_a = e_p = 0$
c. Ra/Rp = 1/3, $e_a = e_p = 0$
d. Ra/Rp = 1/1, $e_a = e_p \approx 1.0$ This IOL has no spherical aberration for impinging parallel light, so-called "aberration-free" IOL
e. Ra/Rp = 1/1, $e_a = e_p \approx 3.0$. This IOL minimizes the spherical aberration of the whole eye, so-called "aberration-correcting" IOL. The very little deviation from a straight line of zero steepness is a result of the conicoidal approximation. The difference, however, is below the recognition threshold of human visual perception

power in the order of 20 D, thus the relative chromatic defocus is in the order of a few percent of IOL power. The influence of chromatic aberration on astigmatic IOL power or on spherical aberration therefore can be neglected.

A particular situation occurs in so-called "diffractive IOL", which in fact are always refractive IOL with powers in the order of 20 D with a diffractive near addition of 3-4 D. A pure diffractive lens has a very high chromatic aberration because the power is directly proportional to wavelength. But the sign of chromatic aberration of the diffractive near addition is inverse to the sign of chromatic aberration of the refractive part of the IOL, thus producing a small resulting chromatic aberration, at least in the mid part of refractive power levels.

SIMULATED OUTCOME OF CUSTOMIZED IOL

The considerations presented so far were given to explain some basic aspects of customized IOL. The question arising now is: what quality can be expected under realistic conditions, and how to fit the IOL data to the data of a given eye?

In the example shown in Figure 32.5 defocus, astigmatism and spherical aberration are corrected. "Higher order" errors are not corrected because they are not correctable, for the reasons described in the previous sections. They are, however, calculated and are responsible for the "residual errors" shown. In order to illustrate the advantages of such customized IOL, the example shown in Figure 32.5 compares the outcome to that of a standard IOL.

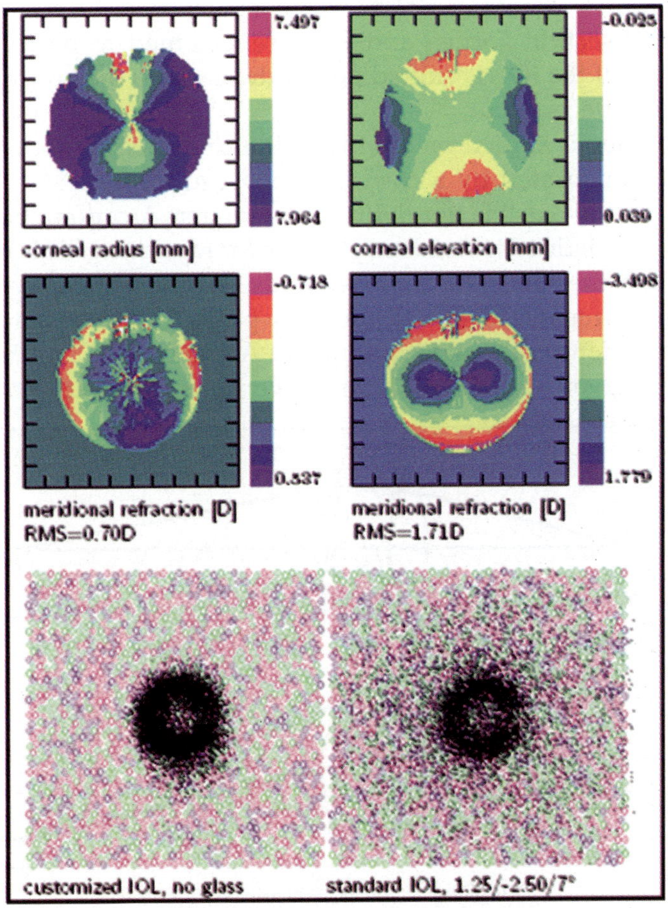

Fig. 32.5: Customized versus standard IOL.
The upper pictures show local corneal curvature radius (left) and local corneal elevation, i.e. height minus best-fitting sphere (right). The mid pictures are the meridional refractions with customized IOL (left) and with a standard model (right). The lower pictures show the retinal images of a Landolt's ring corresponding to a visual acuity chart of 1.0 (20/20) with the customized IOL on the left and with a standard IOL and the best spectacle correction of 1.25/-2.50/7° on the right. Pupil width is 4.0 mm.

THE MISALIGNMENT PROBLEM

All considerations presented so far are related to perfectly aligned IOL. In fact, misalignments cannot be avoided in ocular surgery. The question arises if perhaps misalignments could reduce the advantages of customized IOL or even result in a worse outcome when compared to standard IOL. In order to make the matter more transparent, decentration and rotation are investigated separately. For cataract surgery with in-the-bag implantation, tilt can be neglected, and decentrations are in the order of a few tenths of a mm.[1,2,4]

Decentration

In this subsection cornea and IOL are assumed to be rotationally symmetric. If the IOL is shifted perpendicularly to the optical axis, the following effects occur:

1. The image is shifted on the fovea. But this effect is not recognized but compensated by a corresponding eye movement.
2. An "optical axis" is not defined any longer. A central, bended ray has to be defined instead as reference for raytracing. This ray passes through the center of the fovea and the center of the cornea. It is perpendicular to the tangential plane of the cornea in the intersection point, see Figure 32.6. All refraction and wavefront errors have to be calculated relative to this central ray.

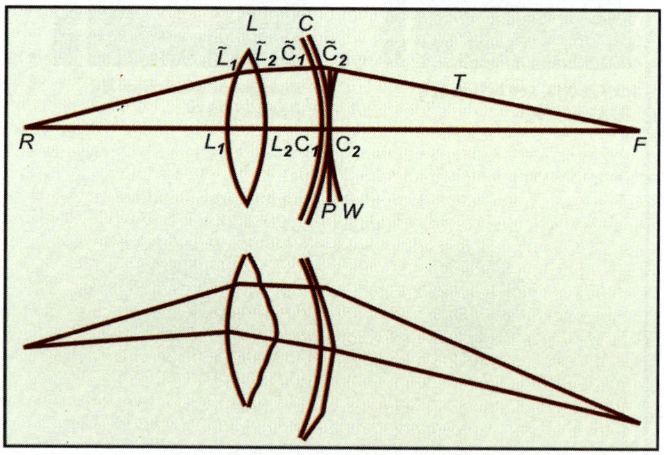

Fig. 32.6: Refraction and wavefront errors.
Upper image: a schematic cross-section of the eye is shown with lens L and cornea C, the optical axis from central retina R to the intersection point F with the off-axis ray r. Wavefront differences are calculated as differences between the optical path lengths of (R,L1,L2,C1,C2, F) and $(R, \tilde{L}_1, \tilde{L}_2, \tilde{C}_1, \tilde{C}_2, F)$. The optical path lengths are the sums over the products of the geometrical lengths and the corresponding refractive indices. The difference between the spherical wave W starting from F and the plane wave P along r has to be added to the path length of r if F is not at infinite distance. The meridional refraction error of r is by definition the reciprocal of the distance from C_2 to F.
Lower image: The IOL can be aspheric and /or bifocal, the cornea irregular and the IOL decentered. For the decenterd IOL the bended ray through central retina and central cornea (which passes cornea perpendicularly to its surface) is calculated first and then used as reference for wavefront and refraction errors instead of the optical axis.

3. The foveal image is blurred in the form of a comet's tail, the dominating error therefore is called "coma".
4. This coma appears somewhat similar to the blurring caused by astigmatism. Therefore, the decentration error normally can be reduced by sphero-cylindrical correction glasses.

Even if the resulting quality with decentered aspheric IOL can be worse than with spherical ones, this is not an issue under realistic conditions. Mostly, the win by reduced spherical aberration dominates. Unfortunately, it is not possible to give a "break-even-point" for the decentration because the results also depend on pupil width. Figure 32.7 shows an example.

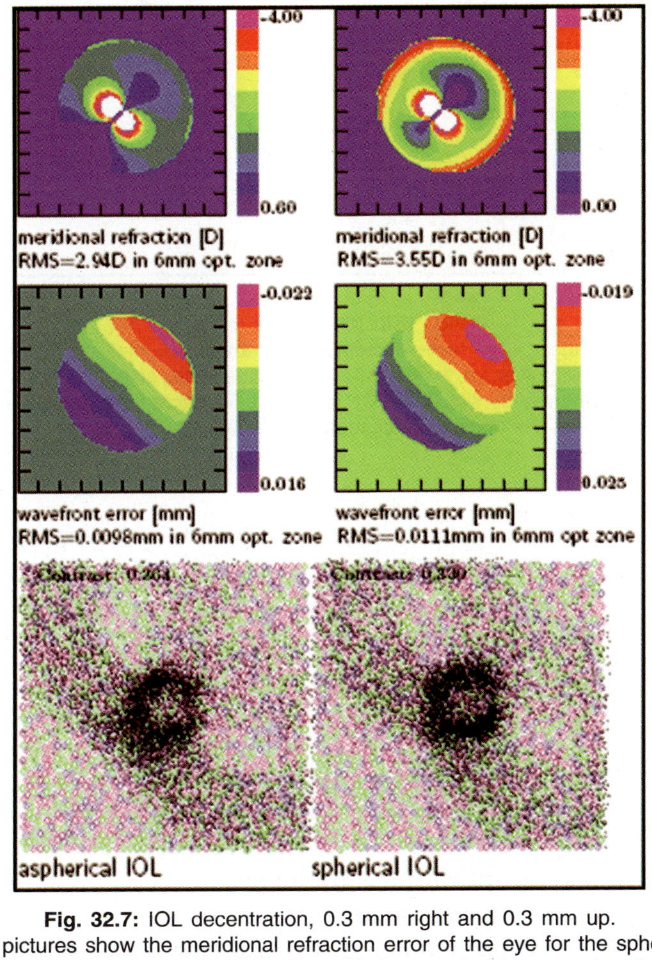

Fig. 32.7: IOL decentration, 0.3 mm right and 0.3 mm up.
The upper pictures show the meridional refraction error of the eye for the spherical (right) and the customized aspherical (left) IOL. The mid pictures give the corresponding wavefront errors. The lower pictures show the retinal images of a Landolt's ring corresponding to a visual acuity chart of 1.0 (20/20) with the customized aspherical IOL on the left and with a standard IOL on the right, both with best correcting spectacle glasses. These glasses are -0.25/-0.25/45° (left) and -0.25/-0.5/45° (right). Pupil width is 2.5 mm

Rotation

The residual error for a rotated astigmatic IOL designed to compensate corneal astigmatism can be approximately understood as the residual refraction caused by the rotation of two astigmatic lenses against each other which have the same astigmatic power. In sofar, the raytracing gives in principle the same results as the analytical formulae first given by Jackson and Stokes already in 19th century, see Figure 32.8.

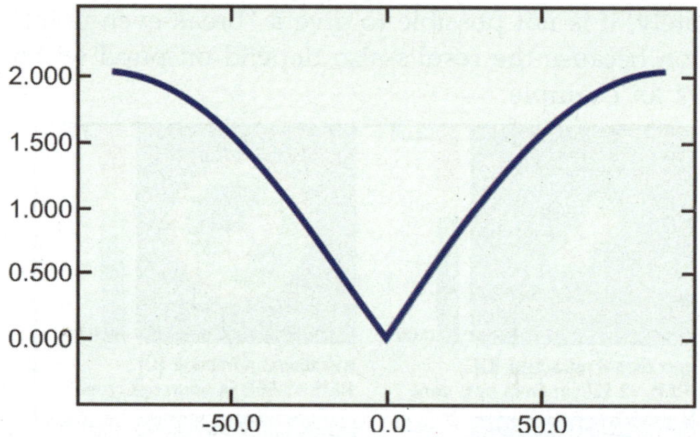

Fig. 32.8: IOL rotation error.
It is assumed that the IOL perfectly compensates corneal astigmatism. For this situation, the relative astigmatic power, i.e. the residul astigmatism in units of the original one, is plotted as a function of the angle by which the IOL is rotated. Note that for a rotation angle of only ≈ 15° already 50% of the originally astigmatic power are lost

Discussion

The data necessary for a customized IOL are the eye's topography, the target refraction and the axial length. With these data, the anterior and posterior IOL surface can be manufactured by lathe cutting, e.g. of dehydrated acrylic material. The optical quality of the outcome depends on the following parameters:

1. The accuracy of axial eye length measurement. Currently, a defocus error in the order of 0.3-0.5 D can be achieved. One major error source cannot be eliminated by future improvements. It is the uncertainty of the parameters of the crystalline lens. The individual sound velocity is unknown in case of ultrasound and the refractive index in case of optical measurements.
2. The accuracy of the corneal topography. In our own measurements we found a reproducibility error in the order of 0.1-0.2 D with respect to defocus and astigmatism. This is below the recognition threshold.
3. The accuracy of IOL manufacturing. Particularly for higher powers, the measuring accuracy decreases. This caused the allowed

tolerances corresponding to ISO 11979 for standard IOL ±0.3 D for powers <15 D, ±0.4 D between 15 D and 25 D, ±0.5 D between 25 D and 30 D and ±1 D above 30 D. Even if the tolerances for customized IOL may fall below 50-30% of the said values, they remain non-negligible.

4. The prediction accuray of postoperative IOL position in axial direction, i.e. the ACD prediction error. It depends on the individually different shrinkage of the capsular bag and causes a defocus error in the order of 0.3D.[3,10]
5. The surgically induced changes in corneal shape. These changes mainly depend on the surgical procedure. A sclero-corneal tunnel causes lower changes than a clear-cornea cut. Also, smaller incision sizes seem advantageous, however, it should be kept in mind that the necessarily smaller IOL sizes may result in a higher error of postoperative ACD.
6. The decentration and rotation of the IOL. Decentration errors are sufficiently small in case of a stable, circular rhexis. If such a rhexis cannot be performed in single cases, no customized IOL should be implanted. The rotational stability depends on haptics design and can be improved by capsular tension rings. Details are subject of current investigations.

Despite these error sources and the higher efford and higher costs of customized IOL their launch seems to be realistic in near future. The higher probability to have spectacle-free patients at least for distant vision is the dominating argument. In addition, one IOL surface can be made bifocal with known techniques in order to allow also spectacle-free reading.

REFERENCES

1. Akkin C, Ozler SA, Mentes J. Tilt and decentration of bag-fixated intraocular lenses: a comparative study between capsulorhexis and envelope techniques. Doc Ophthalmol 1994;87:199-209.
2. Hayashi K, Harada M, Hayashi H, Nakao F, Hayashi F (1997). Decentration and tilt of polymethylmetacrylate, silicone and acrylic soft intraocular lenses. Ophthalmology 1997;104:793-8.
3. Kriechbaum K, Findl O, Preußner PR, K¨oppl C, Wahl J, Drexler W. Determining postoperative anterior chamber depth. J Cataract Refract Surg 2003;29:2122-6.
4. Mutlu FM, Bilge AH, Altinsoy HI, Yumusak E. The role of capsulotomy and intraocular lens type on tilt and decentration of polymethylmetacrylate and foldable acrylic lenses. Ophthalmologica 1998;212:359-63.
5. www.okulix.de
6. Preussner PR, Wahl J. Konsistente numerische Berechnung der Optik des pseudophaken Auges. Ophthalmologe 2000;97:126-41.

7. Preussner PR, Wahl J, Lahdo H, Findl O, Dick B. Ray-tracing for IOL calculation. J Cataract Refract Surg 2002;28:1412-9.
8. Preussner PR, Wahl J, Kramman C. Corneal Model. J Cataract Refract Surg 2003;29:471-7.
9. Preußner PR, Wahl J. Simplified mathematics for customized refractive surgery. J Cataract Refract Surg 2003;29:462-70.
10. Preussner PR, Wahl J, Weitzel D, Berthold S, Kriechbaum K, Findl O. Predicting postoperative anterior chamber depth and refraction. J Cataract Refract Surg 2004;30:2077-83.
11. Preussner PR, Wahl J, Weitzel. Topography based IOL power selection. J Cataract Refract Surg 2005;31:525-33.

CHAPTER

33

Birgit Lackner (Austria)

Clinical Analysis of ICL™-STAAR Posterior Chamber Intraocular Lenses

INTRODUCTION

Poor visual quality of spectacle corrected high ametropia and frequent intolerance to contact lenses justified the introduction of a new technology in the correction of high ametropia.[1-4] The concept of the posterior chamber phakic intraocular lens for the correction of moderate to high myopia carries certain advantages over previous surgical methods, like preservation of accommodation and potential reversibility.[5,6] The STAAR posterior chamber phakic intraocular lens, termed ICL™, was introduced in 1993. This lens, similar to the last generation of Fyodorov lenses, is made of a hydrophilic copolymer of porcine collagen and hydroxyethylmethylacrylate (HEMA). Initial investigations reported excellent efficiency, predictability and peri-operative safety of this design. [5-7]

In some cases eyes are not suitable for anterior phakic IOL implantation, because of relatively flat anterior segments, reduced intraocular space, an increased risk of angle closure glaucoma and uveal effusion.[8]

Clear lens extraction (CLE) has been used with good results in high myopia, but a higher risk of retinal detachment and consequent loss of accommodation must be considered.[9-11]

With longer observation times, it has become obvious that ICL implantation is associated with an elevated incidence of opacifications of the crystalline lens, which can worsen visual outcome after ICL and even necessitate cataract surgery.[12-16]

The introduction of the recent model ICM V4 was therefore followed with considerable expectations due to a improved lens design and vaulting to reduce the risk for cataract formation.

Our clinical experience with the ICM V4 model is herein considered as a report of the outcome of 76 eyes of 46 patients, with a mean patient age of 48.3 ± 7.4 years. In all 76 eyes, the ICL was implanted successfully without the necessity of revisions. Mean and median observation times after ICL implantation were 20.1 months and 24.0 months (± 11.5 months), respectively. The postoperative visual and refractive outcome was excellent. Anterior subcapsular lens opacifications occurred in 11/76 (14.5%) eyes. Eyes with opacifications showed reported difficult surgeries with possible intraoperative microtrauma of the crystalline lens and advanced age over 50 years. We did not observe a correlation between ICL vaulting and the risk of lens opacifications. After onset of lens opacification, 6/11 eyes (55%) showed stable best corrected visual acuity 0.5 lines. The remaining 5 eyes showed progressive opacifications and lost between 3.5 and 0.5 lines compared to the best postoperative values. Three eyes in the progressive group showed best corrected visual acuity loss between 1 and 2 lines compared to preoperative data and subsequently underwent cataract surgery.

PATIENT SELECTION

The candidate for an ICL implant must be subjected to a preselection process to accomplish following criteria: Preoperative refractive error over –5 D of spherical equivalent, age over 21 years, stable refraction for >12 months, corneal diameter >11 mm, and anterior chamber depth (ACD) >2.8 mm, absence of opacifications of the crystalline lens, intraocular pressure in the normal range (10 to 21 mm Hg), absence of iris pigment defect or iris transillumination, absence of retinal breaks or degenerations.

ICL SELECTION AND IMPLANTATION

ICL power is selected based on subjective refraction, keratometry and ACD. Lens power calculations are aimed at emetropia for refractive errors that required ICL powers up to –21.0 D, and at reduction of myopia (after consenting to a residual myopic error) if the necessary correction exceeds the strongest available lens power. ICLs are manufactured in appropriate size (length), which is determined based on horizontal white-to-white corneal diameter measured with a corneal topography system (Orbscan II, Bausch & Lomb), and ACD measured by optical pachymetry (Jaeger II, Haag-Streit). All calculations regarding lens power and size are performed by STAAR Surgical Inc., using a modified vertex formula based on the above parameters.

Two weeks before scheduled ICL implantation, two peripheral neodymium:yttrium-aluminium-garnet laser iridectomies performed at the 10:30 and 1:30 positions are recommended to prevent the possibility of postoperative pupillary block after ICL insertion.

ICL

The STAAR ICL Collamer™ Implantable Contact Lens (ICL™) is a proprietary biocompatible hydrophilic copolymer consisting of hydroxyethyl methylacrylate (HEMA) and porcine collagen. Collamer is a hydrophilic material with high biocompatibilty and permeability to oxygen and metabolites. The lens has a water content of 34%, a light transmission of 99%, and a refractive index of 1.45.

The current ICL model shows a one-piece plate design with a rectangular shape, 7.5 to 8.0 mm wide, available in 4 standard overall lengths (with differences of 0.5 mm between different lengths): 11.5 to 13.5 mm for myopic lenses (ICM) and 11.0 to 13.0 mm for hyperopic lenses (ICH) in order to adapt to eyes of different sizes. The size of the central optic is variable, ranging from 4.65 to 5.5 mm in the ICM, depending on the chosen dioptric power, and constantly 5.5 mm for ICHs. The ICL is supplied in powers ranging from –3.00 to –23.0 D for myopic, and +3.0 D to +21.0 D for hyperopic lenses.

In our department a standardised surgical technique is used under peribulbar anesthesia. After pupil dilation a viscoelastic fluid is instilled into the anterior chamber. The ICL is implanted through a 3.2 mm temporal clear cornea incision (CCI) with the use of an injector cartridge (STAAR Surgical AG Nidau, Switzerland). The ICL is placed in the posterior chamber, anterior to the crystalline lens under protection of the previously applied viscoelastic substance. Viscoelastics were removed with an irrigation/aspiration system and mioticum is instilled. The corneal incision is left sutureless.

During surgery, care should be taken to prevent the surgical instruments from touching the anterior crystalline lens capsule. Postoperatively, non-steroidal antiphlogistic and antibiotic medications should be administered locally 4 times daily over 4 weeks.

COMPLICATIONS

Reports of ICL - induced anterior subcapsular lens opacifications have been described in the literature, but no clear etiology has been established.[12,14,17,18] The genesis of lens opacification after ICL implantation may be multifactorial. Initially, surgical trauma secondary to learning curves associated with surgical skill was proposed to be a main reason for immediate cataract. [17,19]

Earlier studies postulated direct surgical trauma of the crystalline lens to be responsible for the majority of opacifications.[6] Long term studies have revealed a substantial amount of late events (>12 months after surgery), thus arguing against direct trauma having a causative role.[16] Manipulations during implantation surgery may influence the integrity of the lens capsule and can lead to proliferation of subcapsular lens epithelial cells. Other studies do indicate that direct contact between the ICL and the crystalline lens represents a significant risk factor for opacifications.[14,17]

Prolonged subclinical inflammation and induced changes of the blood-aqueous barrier, could also cause metabolic disturbances of the crystalline lens that in turn could trigger a decrease in lens transmittance.[20] These phenomena have also been observed after the implantation of angle-fixated anterior chamber phakic lenses.

A relationship between ICL vaulting and cataract formation is subject of discussion.

A lens to lens contact could induce metabolic changes in the crystalline lens caused by alteration of the lens nutrition and reduced aqueous flow. The myopic ICL lens has a convex-concave optic zone, which allows for the presence of a central space between the ICL and the crystalline lens that is occupied by aqueous humor. The vaulting of the anterior capsule of the crystalline lens and posterior surface of the ICL influence the central distance between these two structures. Given the natural convex shape of the anterior crystalline lens surface, the vaulting is reduced peripherally. But during pupillary activity and accommodation there is a potential risk of ICL lens touch at the rim of the shoulder, which is the thickest part of the posterior ICL surface.

The most recent ICL model V4 has higher inherent vaulting and is designed to provide a larger distance to the crystalline lens. However, the ratio of ICL length/posterior chamber width is difficult to reliably predict due to the inaccuracy of the approximation of the posterior chamber width (calculated from the corneal white-to-white distance).[21]

The well positioned ICL does not rest on the zonules and is not in contact with the crystalline lens, allowing a continuous flow of aqueous humor. Given the good biocompatibility to uveal structures of Collamer it seems that the suspected disrupted blood-aqueous barrier is caused by microtraumas due to the constant friction between the posterior iris surface on the ICL or its haptic on the ciliary sulcus.

In individual cases also biocompatibility has to be discussed. Individual sensitiveness of the crystalline lens may also be an explanation of bilateral developed opacifications. Moreover, the age of the patients is of some importance, because in older and female patients opacifications tended to occur earlier.[16]

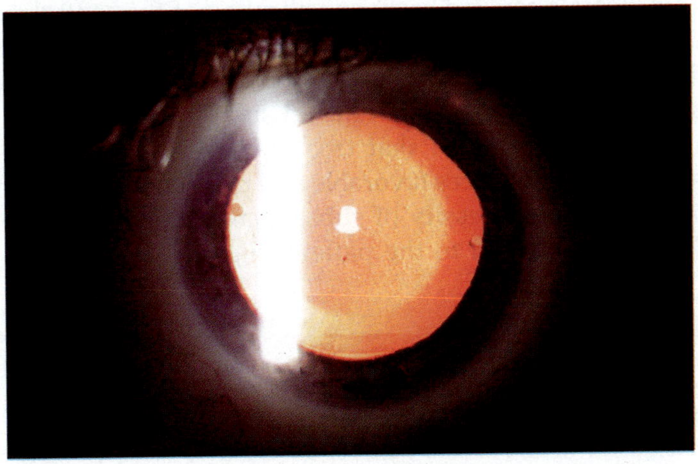

Fig. 33.1: Opacification

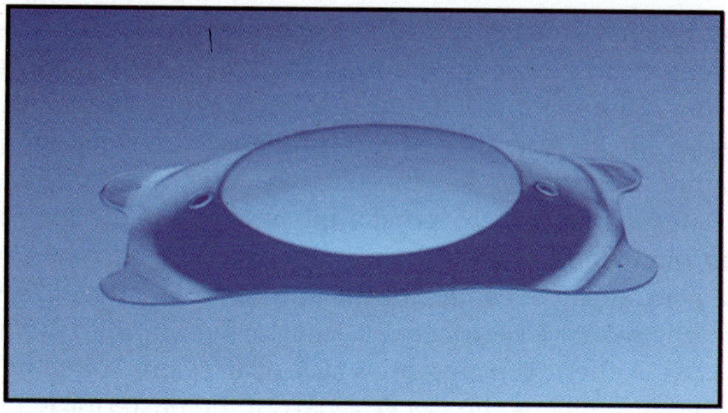

Fig. 33.2: ICM 3D

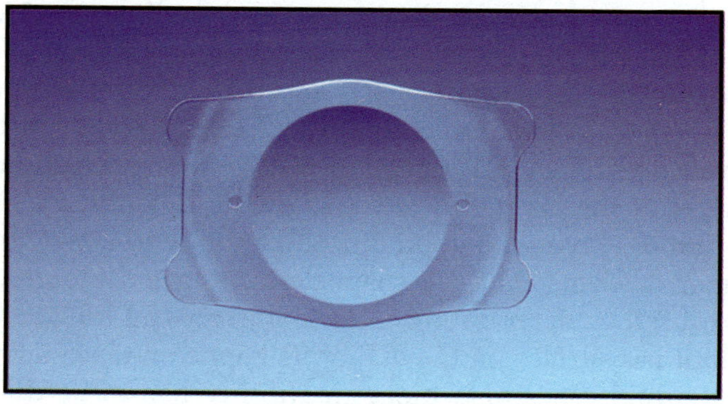

Fig. 33.3: ICM flat

In our patient collective, perioperative complications were low. The only severe complication is the formation of opacifications of the crystalline lens.

Old age, female sex and early opacification of the contralateral eye after ICL implantation are independent significant risk factors for early formation of opacifications, whereas previous surgery, different ICL models or degree of ametropia had no significant effect.

Our experience suggest that treatment with the ICL of severe myopia is feasible, produces favorable and predictable results, but also a certain risk of the necessity of subsequent cataract surgery, which has to be communicated to the patient (Figs 33.1 to 33.3).

REFERENCES

1. Applegate RA, Howland AC. Magnification and visual acuity in refractive surgery. Arch Ophthalmol 1993;111:1335-42.
2. Lovisolo CF, Pesando PM, (Eds). The Implantable Contact Lens (ICL™) and Other Phakic IOLs. Fabiano Editore, Canelli (AT) Italia, 1999:315-8.

3. Colin J, Mimouni F, Robinet A, Conrad H, Mader P. The surgical treatment of high myopia: comparison of epikeratoplasty, keratomileusis and minus power anterior chamber lenses. Refract Corneal Surg 1990;6:245-51.
4. Baikoff G Joly P. Comparison of minus power anterior chamber intraocular lenses and myopic epikeratoplasty in phakic eyes. Refract Corneal Surg 1990;6:252-60.
5. Rosen E, Gore C. Staar Collamer posterior chamber phakic intraocular lens to correct myopia and hyperopia. J Cataract Refract Surg 1998; 24:596-606
6. Zaldivar R, Davidorf JM, Oscherow S. Posterior chamber phakic intraocular lens for myopia of –8 to –19 diopters. J Refract Surg 1998; 14:294-305.
7. Assetto V, Benedetti S, Pesando P. Collamer intraocular contact lens to correct high myopia. J Cataract Refract Surg 1996; 22:551-6.
8. Davidorf JM, Zaldivar R, Oscherow S. Posterior chamber phakic intraocular lens for hyperopia of +4 to +11 diopters. J Refract Surg 1998;14(3):306-11.
9. Goldberg MF. Clear lens extraction for axial myopia: An appraisal. Ophthalmology 1987;94:571-82.
10. Siganos DS, Siganos CS, Pallikaris IG. Clear lens extraction and intraocular lens implantation in normally sighted hyperopic eyes. J Cataract Refract Surg 1994;10:117-24.
11. Lyle WA, Jin GJ. Clear lens extraction for the correction of high refractive error. J Refract Corneal Surg 1994;20:273-6.
12. Fink AM, Gore C, Rosen E. Cataract development after implantation of the Staar Collamer posterior chamber phakic lens. J Cataract Refract Surg 1999; 25:278-82.
13. Zaldivar R, Oscherow S, Ricur G. The STAAR posterior chamber phakic intraocular lens. Int Ophthalmol Clin 2000; 40:237-44.
14. Gonvers M, Bornet C, Othenin-Girard P. Implantable contact lens for moderate to high myopia: Relationship of vaulting to cataract formation. J Cataract Refract Surg 2003; 29:918-24.
15. Jimenez-Alfaro I, Benitez del Castillo JM, Garcia-Feijoo J, et al. Safety of posterior chamber phakic intraocular lenses for the correction of high myopia: anterior segment changes after posterior chamber phakic intraocular lens implantation. Ophthalmology 2001; 108:90-9.
16. Lackner B, Pieh S, Schmidinger G, et al. Outcome After Treatment of Ametropia with Implantable Contact Lenses. Ophthalmology 2003;
17. Sanchez-Galeana CA, Smith RJ, Sanders DR, et al. Lens opacities after posterior chamber phakic intraocular lens implantation. Ophthalmology 2003; 110:781-85.
18. Trindade F, Pereira F. Cataract formation after posterior chamber phakic intraocular lens implantation. J Cataract Refract Surg 1998; 24:1661-3.
19. Sanders DR, Vukich JA, Doney K, et al. US Food and Drug Administration Clinical Trial of the Implantable Contact Lens for moderate to high myopia. Ophthalmology 2003; 110:255-66.
20. Jimenez-Alfaro I, Benitez del Castillo JM, Garcia-Feijoo J, et al. Safety of posterior chamber phakic intraocular lenses for the correction of high myopia: anterior segment changes after posterior chamber phakic intraocular lens implantation. Ophthalmology 2001;108(1):90-9.
21. Gonvers M, Othenin-Girard P, Bornet C, et al. Implantable contact lens for moderate to high myopia: Short-term follow-up of 2 models. J Cataract Refract Surg 2001; 27:380-8.

CHAPTER

34

Ashok Garg (India)

Pearls of Multifocal Refractive Lenses

INTRODUCTION

Multifocal Refractive Lens Technology offers a greater benefits for the patients. The elimination of a presbyopic condition and restoration of normal vision by simulating accommodation greatly enhances the quality of the life for most of the patients. The advantages of astigmatically neutral clear corneal surgery have allowed for increased utilization for multifocal technology in lens-based refractive surgery. It will allow surgeons to offer multifocal technology to their patients with better visual outcome.

The loss of accommodative ability following cataract surgery has been overcome to an extent by the development of intraocular lenses with multifocal optics. The different types of multifocal IOLs are the diffractive type, which provides distance vision by refraction and near vision by diffraction from a series of phase controlled concentric slopes on the posterior lens surface, the refractive aspheric type and the two or three zone refractive type.[1] The last mentioned IOL design is now obsolete because of extensive side effects that affected the quality of vision and will not be discussed further in this discussion.

Another option available nowadays for the correction of post-operative presbyopia is accommodative IOLs.[2,3] These lenses are based on the focus shift principle, which involves movement of the IOL within the capsular sac. The hinged design allows the lens to move forward as the eye attempts to focus on near objects restoring some amount of accommodative function. Accommodative lenses have plate haptics which when placed into the capsular bag, vaults anteriorly upon contraction of the ciliary body, akin to the natural physiology of the crystalline lens and the ciliary body. The extensive use of multifocal intraocular lens has been limited till now because of certain inherent problems associated with these IOLs in the form of decreased contrast sensitivity and severe visual symptoms like discomfort at night, halos, and glare. The newer designs incorporating aspheric optics and asymmetrical light distribution, decreases many of these problems, ensures satisfactory intermediate vision, and thus offers better quality of vision.

MULTIFOCAL IOLs

Multifocal IOLs work on the principles of simultaneous imaging of two optical systems at least 3 D apart. The brain interprets the two images as separate images, selects the more focused image and suppresses the other. The optical performance of multifocal intraocular lenses has improved over the last few years. The clinical results have also improved due to the application of the astigmatically neutral small incision surgery. However, the system-inherent characteristics of multifocal lenses, namely a severe loss in the contrast visual acuity as well as disturbing scattering of light have persisted and form a limiting factor for larger-scale standard application of these IOLs. The reason for this is that in the older variety of refractive-diffractive lenses, the light distribution in both the main foci being 50% each, resulted in reduced light intensity and contrast visual acuity as compared to monofocal lenses. Furthermore, the dependence of contrast visual acuity on the pupil width and perfect centration of the IOL resulted in accentuation of symptoms of reduced contrast, haloes and glare.

The different types of multifocal IOLs are:

Diffractive IOLs

The diffractive IOLs provide distance vision by refraction and near vision by using diffraction from series of phase controlled concentric slopes on the posterior lens surface. Since these concentric rings for near and distance are present in the center of the lens itself, decentration of the IOL or the pupillary size does not affect vision. One of the main disadvantages of these IOLs has been the compromise in the resolution of the image when the contrast of the focused image is reduced by the out of focus images due to incomplete cortical suppression.

Nonfoldable diffractive multifocal IOLs are available by Pharmacia in both PMMA (CeeOn 811E) and silicone (Z9000M), and by Alcon in acrylic (MA60D3).

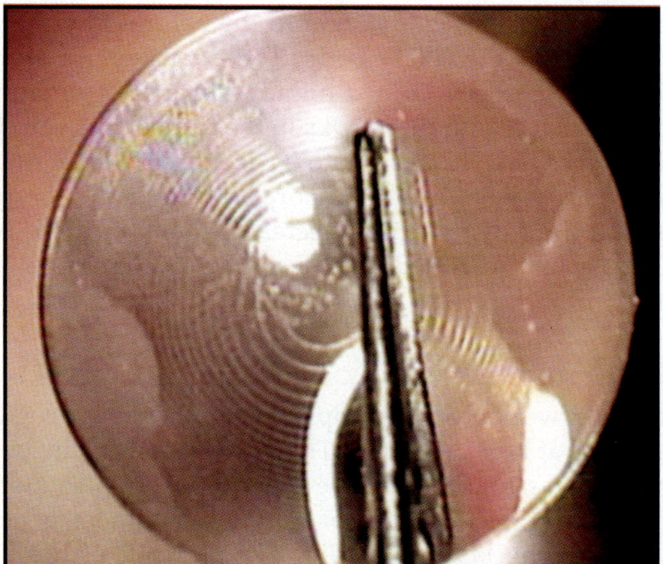

Fig. 34.1: Diffractive multifocal IOL

With the increasing need to adapt multifocal IOLs to smaller incisions, diffractive multifocal IOLs are available now as foldable lenses (Acri. Tec GmbH, Munich). This is a 3-piece foldable silicone IOL with a 6 mm optic. It is biconvex, aspheric with Fresnel zones available from +0.00 D to +40.00 D which has been used with good results in terms of patient satisfaction. These bifocal intraocular lenses are characterized by an asymmetrical light distribution. The dominant eye is implanted with a bifocal lens with light distribution of 70% for the far focus and 30% for the near focus. The accompanying eye receives an intraocular lens with a light distribution of 70% for the near focus and 30% for the far focus. As a result, with planned bilateral implantation of the IOL, considerable improvement of the contrast can be achieved. The contrast visual acuity is such a case is only reduced by a factor of 1.4 as compared to a factor of almost 2 with multifocal lenses with symmetrical bifocal intraocular lenses. These lenses are reported to have extremely low secondary cataract rate, hold a firm and steady position in the capsular bag, demonstrate no vaulting, bending or decentration of the IOL. The smaller incision is more stable, shows lesser astigmatism and faster wound healing.

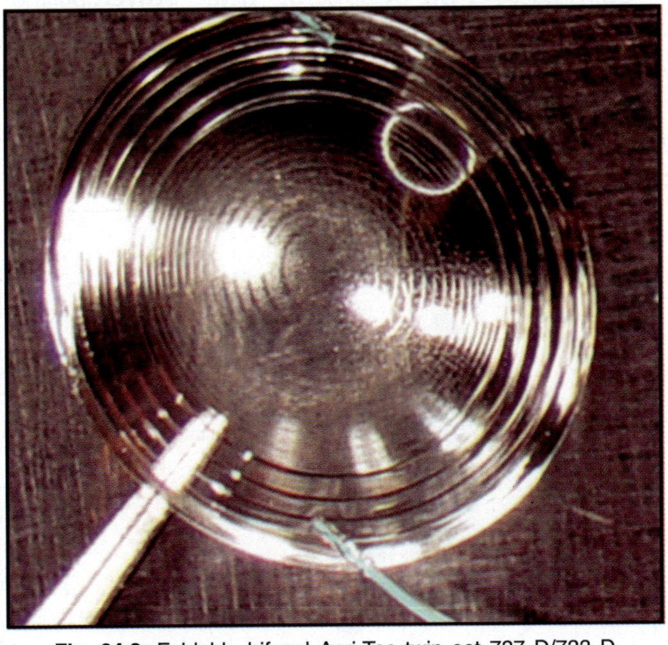

Fig. 34.2: Foldable bifocal Acri.Tec twin set 737 D/733 D

Refractive Multifocal IOL Implant

The Array Multifocal IOL Implant is a silicone IOL of the refractive multifocal type. This lens incorporates in its surface concentric rings

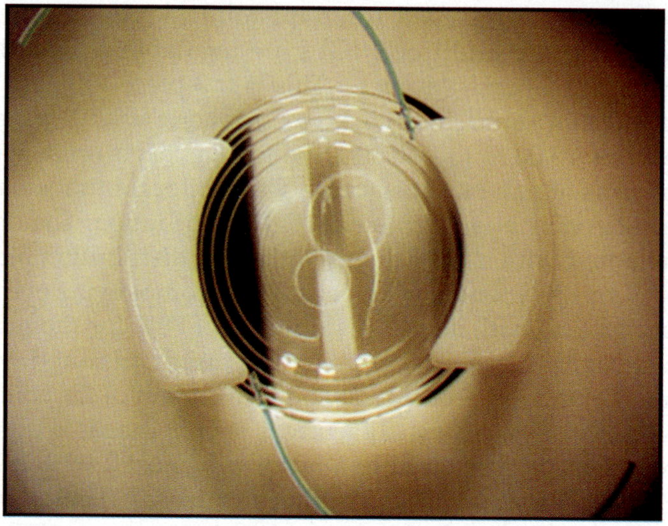

Fig. 34.3: A 38 D bifocal foldable Acri.Tec IOL showing Fresnel zones

of varying power around a central power for distance. This central power is dominant over the peripheral "near" power. 50% of the IOL is dedicated to distance vision, 36% to near vision and the remaining 14% to intermediate vision. Good contrast sensitivity is maintained in this IOL due to the asymmetric light distribution. A bothersome side effect especially associated with the use of this particular type of IOL is haloes around lights especially at night. The reason for the same is

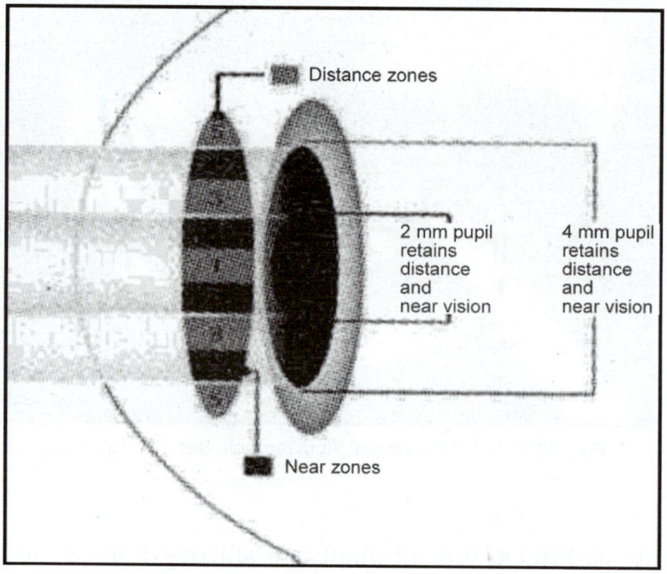

Fig. 34.4: Optics of the refractive array multifocal IOL

not clear. However, this side effect needs to be explained to the patient prior to surgery.

Older Models

The older models of two or three zone refraction type of IOL as has been used previously are no longer in use because of the subjective deterioration of the quality of vision caused by them in the form of decreased contrast sensitivity, glare, haloes etc. Hence, they have not been discussed further in this chapter.

Accommodative IOLs

Certain newer types of IOLs have been developed that take into account the normal physiological interplay of the ciliary body with the crystalline lens (replaced by the capsular bag containing the IOL post-operatively). These accommodative IOLs like the Human Optics Accommodative 1 CU IOL are designed to transform the contracting forces of the ciliary muscle into anterior movement of the IOL optic. The pseudo-phakic accommodation by this method has been measured between 1.3 D to 1.7 D as the lens performs an anterior focus shift of about 0.65 mm.[2-4]

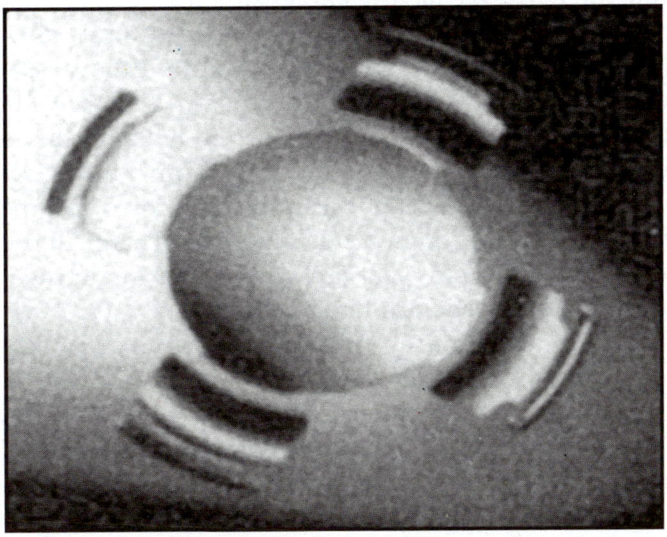

Fig. 34.5: Accommodative IOL

The principle of these lenses are that when the haptic plates are placed in the capsular bag, the anterior capsule fibroses and applies pressure on the haptics which vault posteriorly such that the optic lies next to the vitreous face. With the contraction of the ciliary muscle and its subsequent pressure on the vitreous face, the optics move forward resulting in pseudo-phakic accommodation. These lenses are larger lenses available as both non-foldable and foldable IOLs. Crystalens was the first accommodative IOL available for use in the US. Another accommodating IOL, the AT-45 silicone accommodative intraocular lens is undergoing the initial phases of the FDA trial.[4]

MULTIFOCAL IOLs AND MICRO-INCISION CATARACT SURGERY

Technology runs forward in leaps and bounds. Starting from the Ridley IOLs to modern day micro-incision cataract surgery IOLs has been a long journey spanning over half a century. As the desire for perfection increases, the unwanted effects of the older procedures, equipments or implants are modified so as to increase the benefits derived from the same procedure, equipment or implants. Sometimes, one technology may advance faster than other complementary technologies. To cite an example, phacoemulsification became a routine procedure for performing cataract extraction much before the advent of foldable IOLs. Thus though the procedure could be performed through a 3 mm incision, the incision had to be increased to a minimum of 5.5 mm to incorporate the IOLs. We have a similar situation again, when cataract extraction can be performed through incisions as small as 1 mm, but the IOL technology is just beginning to explore the possibilities of inserting IOLs through that small incision and simultaneously maintaining the optical quality of the inserted IOLs. Thus the ongoing research not only has to evaluate the long term benefits, results and efficacy of these newer IOLs but also the associated technique of its appropriate insertion through a microincision. This includes designs for newer injecting systems that are safe and maintain the quality of the IOL while the insertion is taking place.

Another dream remains the amelioration of postoperative presbyopia. Most new models of multifocal IOLs incorporate special aspherical designs with asymmetrical light distribution that takes into account the spherical aberration of the cornea and the loss of contrast due to symmetrical light distribution in the two foci for distance and near. Due to the rotational symmetry of these new lenses, the image is also independent of the diameter of the pupil. Thus many problems of the yesteryears have been taken care of. Multifocal IOLs are now available as foldable IOLs and trials are on to assess the long term results of these newer generation IOLs. These IOLs thus facilitate both, the non-distortion of a small, astigmatically neutral incision and the amelioration of postoperative presbyopia thus simulating or at times bettering the preoperative visual status in the immediate postoperative period. These could be of specific use in the pediatric age group where amblyopia is a major concern. Being able to correct vision for both distance and near would be of immense benefit in these cases.

Pseudo-accommodation has been a feature of many lenses, both silicone and acrylic, that have been used for microincision cataract surgery. This has been hypothesized to be due to the ultra-thin thickness of these lenses which aids the normal physiological accommodative response of the capsular bag upon contraction of the ciliary muscle. Longer trials are required to authenticate these hypotheses.

The symbiosis and subsequent syntheses of the newer generation IOLs incorporating larger lenses with accommodative and multifocal optics and the ultra-thin lenses with the quality of pseudo-accommodation for use in micro-incision cataract surgery remains a dream today. But just as the dreams of yesterday have become realities today in our continuous quest for perfection, there is no reason to think that true accommodative and multifocal IOLs that can be incorporated through a micro-incision of 1 to 1.5 mm will not become a viable reality tomorrow.

REFERENCES

1. Montes-Mico R, Alio JL. Distance and near contrast sensitivity function after multifocal intraocular lens implantation. J Cataract Refract Surg 2003; 29:703-11.
2. Findl O, Kiss B, Petternel V, Menapace R, Georgopoulos M, et al. Intraocular lens movement caused by ciliary body contraction. J Cataract Refract Surg 2003; 29:669-76.
3. Kuchle M, Seitz B, Langenbucher A, Gusek-Schneider GC, Martus P, et al. The Erlangen Accommodative Intraocular Lens Study Group. Comparison of 6 month results of implantation of the 1 CU accommodative intraocular lenses with conventional intraocular lenses. Ophthalmology 2004; 111:825-34.
4. Humming JS, Slade SG, Chayet A, AT-45 Study Group. Clinical evaluation of the model AT-45 silicone accommodating intraocular lens: Results of feasibility and the initial phase of the FDA Clinical Trial. Ophthalmology 2001;108: 2005-10

Section 4

Complications and their Management

CHAPTER

35

Maria I Kalyvianaki, Ioannis G Pallikaris (Greece)

Phakic Refractive Lens (PRL™): Precautions and Complications

INTRODUCTION

Posterior chamber phakic intraocular lenses (PIOLs) are reported to be an effective, predictable, stable and safe technique for the treatment of high myopia and hyperopia.[1-10] After posterior chamber PIOL implantation uncorrected visual acuity has been reported to improve, while refractive results are stable after the first postoperative month.[8-10] A common finding in the previous studies is the postoperative improvement in best-corrected visual acuity.[1-3,6,7,9,10] Phakic Refractive Lens (PRL™) is a silicone posterior chamber lens, which has no anatomical fixation sites and is supposed to float in the posterior chamber having no contact with the anterior capsule of the crystalline lens. Despite its reported encouraging results, not all myopic and hyperopic eyes are suitable for PRL implantation, while this implantation may lead to complications. Some of these complications can be prevented and most of them can be managed with no visual consequences. In this chapter we are going to deal with the precautions and complications of PRL implantation.

PRECAUTIONS

For a phakic refractive lens to be inserted anterior chamber depth has to be greater than 3 mm. This is rarely a problem in myopic eyes, but needs careful evaluation in hyperopic eyes. Of great importance is the method of anterior chamber depth estimation. A-scan biometry is the most used method, but its accuracy is highly examiner-dependent. Therefore, non-contact methods, such as immersion ultrasound, Orbscan Topography[11] or IOLMaster,[12] might be preferable for anterior chamber depth calculations.

An exclusion criterion for PRL™ implantation is cataract. In these cases cataract extraction is performed. Glaucoma is also a contraindication for this kind of surgery, as well as pigment dispersion syndrome. Additionally, in case of an endothelial dystrophy an intraocular surgery had better be avoided. Retinal lesions are not an absolute contraindication for PRL implantation, but especially the symptomatic ones should be treated before the surgery. However, it is suggested[13] that more important than the prophylactic treatment of myopic lesions is the postoperative careful fundus examination. A thorough preoperative examination is mandatory in all candidates for PRL implantation.

Ultrasound biomicroscopy (UBM) is also a useful tool for the selection of the proper model of phakic lens for each eye and for the postoperative estimation of the exact intraocular position of posterior chamber PIOLs. The implant model is most often chosen based on the white-to-white measurement with the use of a calliper. However, only high-frequency ultrasound biometry can give an accurate measurement of the sulcus-to-sulcus diameter. In a recent study of PRL-implanted eyes ultrasound microscopy demonstrated that haptics of the PRL were in the zonules, in the ciliary sulcus, or in the ciliary body.[14] The difference between the PRL diameter and the sulcus diameter causes different positions of the implant. Relatively small implants rest on the zonules, while relatively larger PRLs fit in the sulcus, while intermediate sizes may adopt mixed positions; that is one haptic of the implant on the sulcus and the other in the ciliary body, or one haptic on the sulcus and the other in the zonula. Rotation of the lens is common (even in 75% of the cases)[3] when its haptics rest on the zonules. A positioning in the sulcus can lead to pigment dispersion and inflammation. Therefore, in order to find the correct model of the posterior chamber PIOL that has to be inserted in each case, the sulcus-to sulcus diameter would be more preferably measured, instead of the white-to-white diameter, while the existence of more PRL models may be necessary as well.

Except for the patient and the model selection, the surgery requires very gentle manipulations. The surgeon has to avoid any contact of the implant or his instruments with the endothelium or the crystalline lens. Moreover, any damage of the fragile implant should lead to its replacement, while special care should be taken for the placement of the phakic lens in its upright position and not upside down.

COMPLICATIONS

A serious concern after implantation of a posterior chamber lens is cataract formation, which can occur during surgery or postoperatively.[15-20] A touch of the crystalline lens during surgery or even surgical iridectomy[2] (Fig. 35.1) can lead to anterior capsule opacification. To avoid this complication, gentle manipulations are required during surgery. The use of viscoelastic in the posterior chamber before placing the lens under the iris widens the space for the implant to be inserted and protects the crystalline lens. When cataract occurs during surgery, the operation has to be converted to crystalline lens extraction. If the opacity is clinically insignificant and not progressing during the follow-up, no further treatment is needed.[1,2] Moreover, postoperative contact or inadequate space between the phakic and the crystalline lens[9,15,16,18] may provoke cataract. For the implant to keep safe distance from the crystalline lens, the appropriate model for each eye has to be selected.[18] Although PRL is available only in two models for myopic and one for hyperopic corrections, no

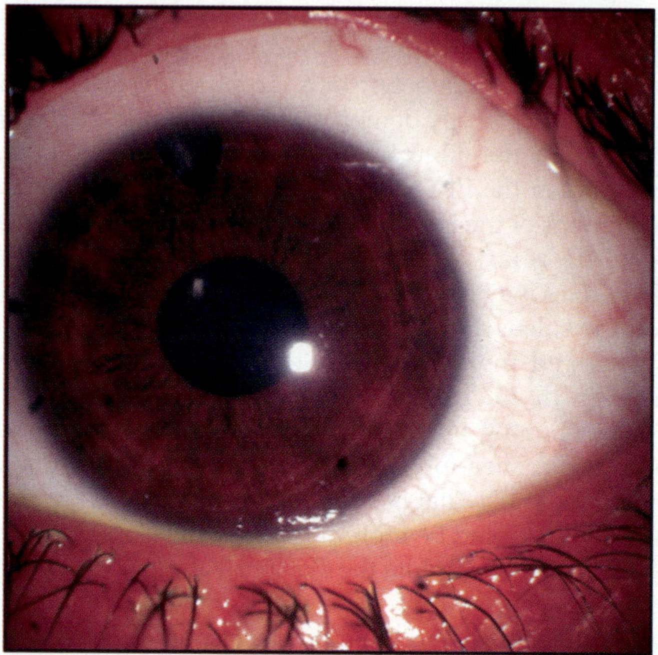

Fig. 35.1: Slit lamp photograph of a PRL-implanted eye six months after the surgery. The anterior capsule opacification occurred during surgical iridectomy with the probe of a vitreotome. The opacity remained focal and did not require any further treatment

postoperative cataract formation irrelevant to surgical trauma has been reported, perhaps due to the hydrophobic material of the implant. However, in case of progressive cataract that causes decrease of visual acuity, the phakic lens has to be explanted and cataract extraction has to be performed.[20] In our series of PRL-implanted eyes no postoperative cataract has occurred during a 6-year follow-up period.

Iris atrophy is another complication (Fig. 35.2), which can occur intraoperatively due to surgical manipulations or postoperatively due to touch of the PRL and the posterior surface of the iris.[3] Iris chafing can cause pigment dispersion inside the eye. Pigment dispersion has been reported to be induced by posterior chamber lenses,[1,7,21] due to contact of the latter with the posterior surface of the iris. The main reason for this event is the implantation of a large phakic lens for the specific eye, and it is more common in hyperopic eyes. Bleeding can occur during surgical iridectomy but usually ceases in few minutes with no further consequences.

The evaluation of intraocular pressure is very important after PRL implantation, as well as the correlation of the findings to the preoperative values, in order to early estimate any IOP changes due to the presence of the phakic lens. During the first postoperative days

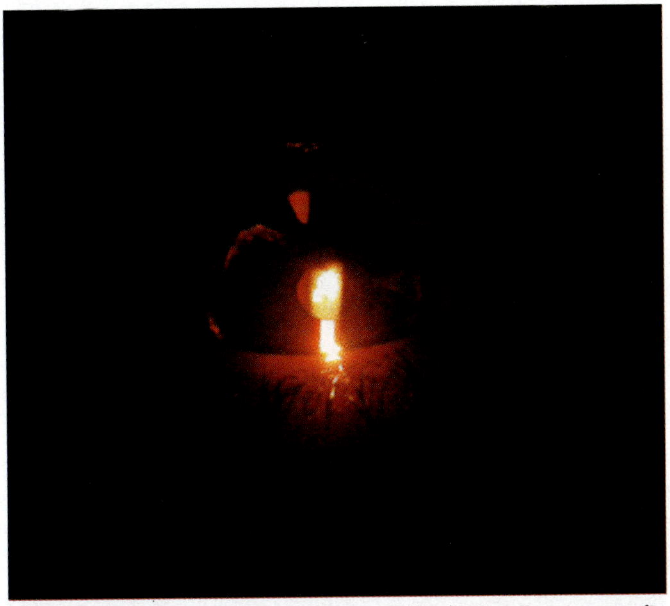

Fig. 35.2: Iris chafing was apparent by retroillumination three years after PRL implantation in a hyperopic eye perhaps due to contact of the implant and the posterior surface of the iris

residual viscoelastic is the most probable cause. During the first month IOP increases mostly due to corticosteroid-response,[2] which is frequent in high myopic patients. In these cases intraocular pressure returns to normal levels after discontinuation of steroid drops. Another cause of IOP increase in hyperopic eyes more frequently is closed iridectomies, that may lead to pupillary block glaucoma.[1,3,19] Further iridotomies can solve this problem.

The proper placement of the implant is very important. In case of inverse placement of the PRL™ pigment dispersion and peripheral anterior iris-endothelium synechias occur (Figs 35.3A and B), which provoke IOP increase. This problem is managed with PRL removal, which must be decided soon after the recognition of the problem, as it may lead to permanent glaucoma due to the peripheral anterior synechias.

A study[3] reported endothelial cell loss more evident one week after PRL implantation. Because no statistically significant difference in endothelial cell density was found between one week and one year after surgery, the endothelial cell loss might be attributed to the surgical trauma.

According to the study and the used questionnaire a percentage of patients from 20[2] to 53%[9] complained of glare and halo during night postoperatively. These night phenomena could be explained by the

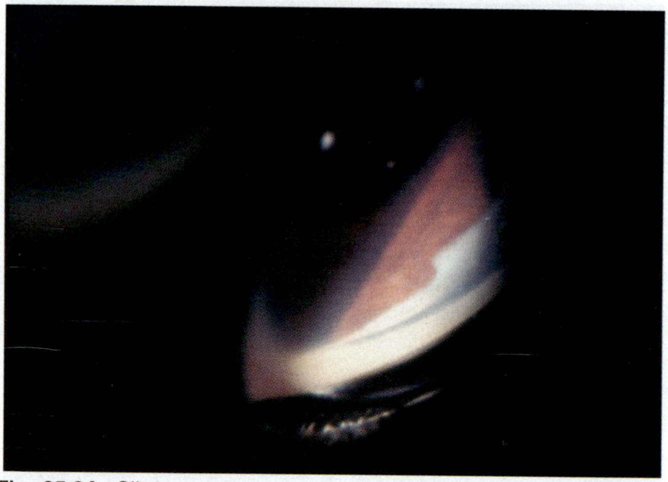

Fig. 35.3A: Slit lamp photograph of the anterior chamber angle of a myopic eye two years after inverse PRL implantation. Peripheral anterior iris-endothelium synechias are apparent

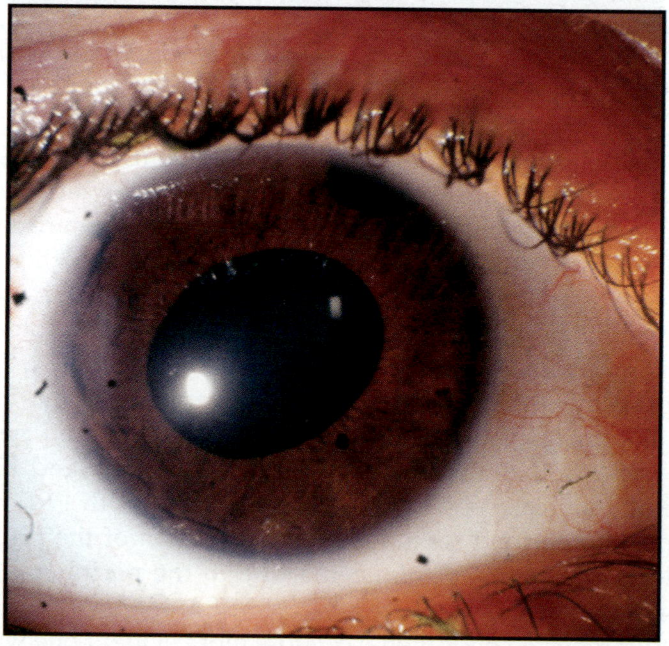

Fig. 35.3B: Slit lamp photograph of the eye of Figure 35.3A. The synechias caused high intraocular pressure and ovalization of the pupil

patients' large pupils, 6 and 7 mm at scotopic conditions, while the optical zone of the implant is 5 to 5.5 mm. Because not all patients with large pupils experience these phenomena, perhaps other factors besides the size of the pupil, such as a small residual refractive error, contribute to their existence.

Decentration of the PRL can occur if its size is not appropriate (too short) for the specific eye. Two recent studies[22,23] reported three cases of dislocation of PRL into the vitreous cavity two, four and twenty-two months after surgery. A pars plana vitrectomy had to be performed in all cases to remove the implant. This dislocation could be attributed to preoperative zonular weakness, which is common in high axial myopic eyes. Previous ocular trauma that might have caused zonular defects or Marfan's syndrome or other systemic diseases with zonular weakness should be considered as contraindications for a posterior chamber PIOL implantation. Other causes for the dislocation could be a surgical damage of the zonular fibers during the positioning of PRL haptics into the posterior chamber and/or postoperative rotation of the PRL in cases of zonule-haptic contact. It is also hypothesized[24] that implants of intermediate size that have one haptic resting on the sulcus, which is a resistant surface, and the other in the zonula, which is a fragile surface, may favor the transmission of the elastic force of the PRL toward the zonules. Although we have not experienced a PRL dislocation, a decentration occurred in one myopic eye 3 years postoperatively (Fig. 35.4). The patient experienced a sudden decrease in visual acuity and glare at night. The lens was removed immediately with no further complications.

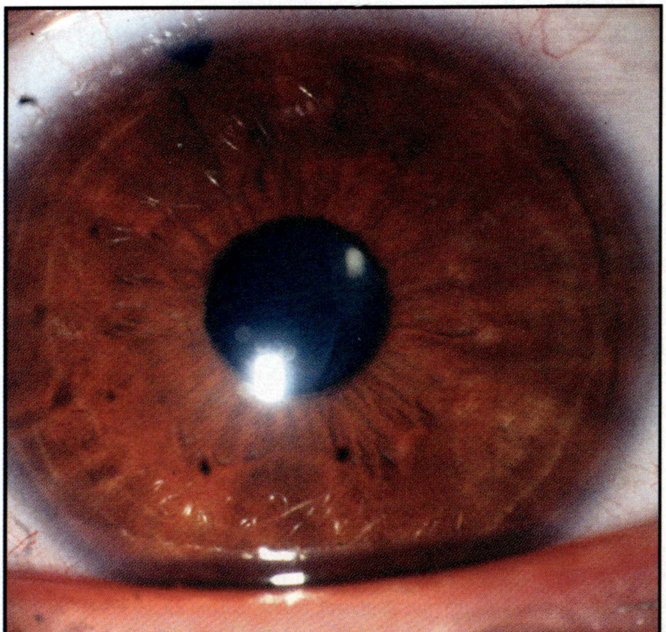

Fig. 35.4: Decentration of the PRL occurred three years after its implantation in a myopic eye

In conclusion the implantation of a Phakic Refractive Lens requires careful preoperative and postoperative evaluation. Selection of PRL candidates is mandatory in order to avoid some of the postoperative problems, while the early recognition of complications could lead to their successful management.

REFERENCES

1. Hoyos JE, Dementiev DD, Cigales M, Hoyos-Chacon J, Hoffer KJ. Phakic refractive lens experience in Spain. J Cataract Refract Surg 2002; 28:1939-46.
2. Pallikaris IG, Kalyvianaki MI, Kymionis GD, Panagopoulou SI. Phakic refractive lens implantation in high myopic patients: One-year results. J Cataract Refract Surg 2004; 30:1190–7.
3. Koivula AM, Petrelius A, Zetterström C. Clinical outcomes of phakic refractive lens in myopic and hyperopic eyes: 1-year results. J Cataract Refract Surg 2005; 31:1145-52.
4. Pesando PM, Ghiringhello MP, Tagliavacche P. Posterior chamber Collamer phakic intraocular lens for myopia and hyperopia. J Refract Surg 1999; 15: 415-23.
5. Zaldivar R, Davidorf JM, Oscherow S. Posterior chamber phakic intraocular lenses for myopia –8 to –19 diopters. J Refract Surg 1998; 14:294-305.
6. The Implantable contact lens in treatment of myopia study group. US Food and Drug administration clinical trial of the Implantable contact lens for moderate to high myopia. Ophthalmology 2003; 110:255-66.
7. Asseto V, Benedetti S, Pesando P. Collamer intraocular contact lens to correct high myopia. J Cataract Refract Surg 1996; 22:551-6.
8. Rosen E, Gore C. Staar collamer posterior chamber phakic intraocular lens to correct myopia and hyperopia. J Cataract Refract Surg 1998; 24:596-606.
9. Arne LA, Leseur LC. Phakic posterior chamber lenses for high myopia: Functional and anatomical outcomes. J Cataract Refract Surg 2000; 26:369-74.
10. Jimerez-Alfaro I, Benitez del Castilo JM, Garcia-Feijoo J, Gil de Bernabe JG, Serrano de la Iglesia JM. Safety of posterior chamber phakic intraocular lenses for the correction of high myopia-anterior segment changes after posterior chamber phakic intraocular lens implantation. Ophthalmology 2001; 108:90-9.
11. Auffarth GU, Tetz MR, Biazid Y, et al. Measuring anterior chamber depth with Orbscan Topography System. J Cataract Refract Surg 1997; 23:1351-5.
12. Nemeth J, Fekete O, Pesztenlehrer N. Optical and ultrasound measurement of axial length and anterior chamber depth for intraocular lens power calculation. J Cataract Refract Surg 2003; 29:85-8.
13. Martinez-Castillo V, Boixadera A, Vertugo A, et al. Rhegmatogenous retinal detachment in phakic eyes after posterior chamber phakic intraocular lens implantation for severe myopia. Ophthalmology 2005; 112:580-5.
14. Garcia-Feijoo J, Hernandez-Matamoros JL, Castillo-Gomez A, et al. Ultrasound biomicroscopy of silicone posterior chamber phakic intraocular lens for myopia. J Cataract Refract Surg 2003; 29:1932–9.
15. Fink AM, Gore C, Rosen E. Cataract development after implantation of the Staar Collamer posterior chamber phakic lens. J Cataract Refract Surg 1999; 25:1278-82.

16. Trindade F, Pereira F. Cataract formation after posterior chamber phakic intraocular lens implantation. J Cataract Refract Surg 1998; 24: 1661-3.
17. Sanchez-Galeana CA, Smith RJ, Sanders DR, et al. Lens opacities after posterior chamber phakic intraocular lens implantation. Ophthalmology 2003; 110:781-5.
18. Gonvers M, Bornet C, Othenin-Girard P. Implantable contact lens for moderate to high myopia; relationship of vaulting to cataract formation.J Cataract Refract Surg 2003; 29:918-24.
19. Sanders DR, Vukich JA. Incidence of lens opacities and clinically significant cataracts with the Implantable Contact Lens: Comparison of two lens designs; the ICL in Treatment of Myopia (ITM) Study Group. J Refract Surg 2002; 18:673-82.
20. Morales AJ, MD, Zadok D, Tardio E, et al. Outcome of simultaneous phakic implantable contact lens removal with cataract extraction and pseudophakic intraocular lens implantation. J Cataract Refract Surg 2006; 32:595-8.
21. Brandt JD, Moskovac ME, Chayet A. Pigmentary dispersion syndrome induced by a posterior chamber phakic refractive lens. Am J Ophthalmol 2001; 131:260-3.
22. Martinez-Castillo V, Elies D, Boixadera A, et al. Silicone posterior chamber intraocular lens dislocated into the vitreous cavity. J Refract Surg 2004; 20: 773-7.
23. Eleytheriadis H, Amoros S, Bilbao R, Teijeiro MA. Spontaneous dislocation of a phakic refractive lens into the vitreous cavity. J Cataract Refract Surg 2004; 30:2013-6.
24. Garcia-Feijoo J. Phakic refractive lenses and vitreous dislocation. J Cataract Refract Surg 2005; 31:2245-6.

CHAPTER

36

Antonio A Marinho (Portugal)

Complications of Iris-supported Phakic IOLs

CORE MESSAGES

a. Artisan is available from –23.00 to +12.00.
b. Toric Artisan is available from –2.00 to –7.50 and from +2.00 to +7.50.
c. Artisan/Artiflex is independent of the internal dimensions of the eye ("one size fits all").
d. Good selection of patients and good surgical technique are the keys to avoid complications.
e. Very few complications are associated with these phakic IOLs.

INTRODUCTION

In this chapter, we will try to show the possible complications associated with implantation of iris supported phakic Iols. As many of the complications found are related not to the lenses themselves, but to poor selection of the candidates for implantation or to somewhat rough surgery, we will cover briefly both of these aspects after presenting the available models of iris supported phakic IOLs.

IRIS SUPPORTED PHAKIC INTRAOCULAR LENSES

The concept of implantation of an intraocular lens supported by the mid-periphery of the iris was developed by Jan Worst, for aphakia in 1979. The great success and safety of this implant led Jan Worst and Paul Fechner[15, 16] to implant the first iris supported phakic Iol for myopia in 1986. It was originally a biconcave lens, that was sometimes too close to the corneal endothelium possibly causing damage. In 1991 the phakic IOL was redesigned to a safer plano-concave shape. This IOL has been renamed "ARTISAN" in 1997. We will now describe in summary the different available iris supported phakic Iols pointing to their material,optic diameter and powers. All these lenses have in common the following characteristics:[1,5,7,8,10,12,14,23]

a. Anterior chamber lenses consisting of an optic and two haptics.
b. The haptics are in the form of a "claw" (lobster claw) to receive the enclavation of iris tissue.
c. The overall size of these lenses is 8.5 mm for all eyes (except for a very rarely used pediatric model), so it is independent of the size of the anterior chamber. This what we call "one size fits all".
d. All these lens are manufactured by OPHTEC (Netherlands) and distributed worldwide by OPHTEC (Artisan/Artiflex) and AMO (USA) under the brand names of Verysize/Veryflex.

CHARACTERISTICS OF DIFFERENT MODELS OF IRIS SUPPORTED PHAKIC IOLs

a. Model 206: Artisan Myopia 5/8.5 mm
   Material: PMMA; Optic: 5.0 mm; Power: -3.00 to -23.50 (Fig. 36.1)
b. Model 204: Artisan Myopia 6/8.5 mm
   Material: PMMA; Optic: 6.0 mm; Power: -3.00 to -15.50 (Fig. 36.2)
c. Model 203: Artisan Hyperopia 5/8.5 mm
   Material: PMMA; Optic: 5.0 mm; Power: +1.00 to +12.00 (Fig. 36.3)
d. Artisan Toric 5/8.5mm
   Material: PMMA; Optic: 5.0 mm; Power: cylinder from –2.0o to – 7.50 and +2.00 to +7.50. Both negative and positive cylinders are available at 0º (type A) and 90º(type B) (Figs. 36.4 and 36.5).

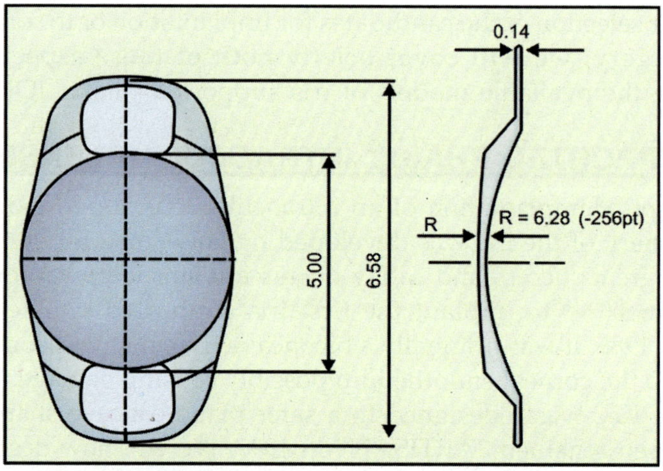

Fig. 36.1: Artisan Model 206 (Myopia PMMA 5.0 mm)

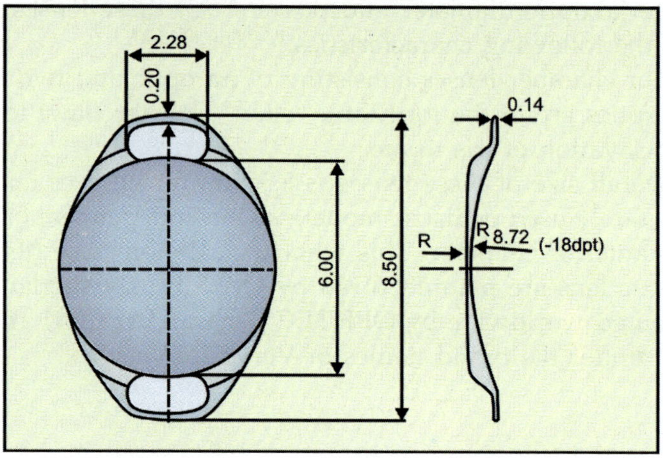

Fig. 36.2: Artisan Model 204 (Myopia PMMA 6.0 mm)

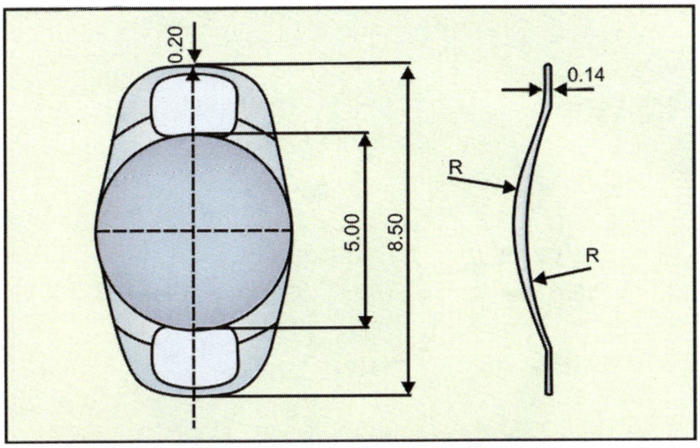

Fig. 36.3: Artisan Model 203 (Hyperopia PMMA 5.0 mm)

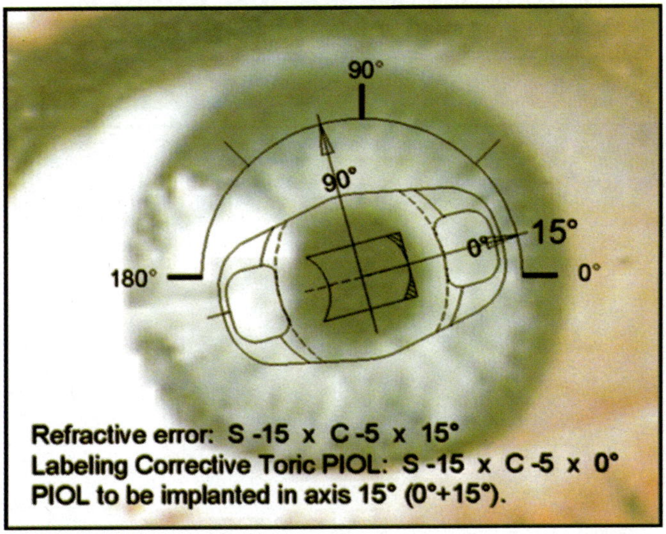

Fig. 36.4: Toric Artisan (Type A)

e. Artiflex Myopia 6/8.5 mm
   Material: Polysiloxane (silicone) optic / PMMA haptics; Optic: 6.0 mm; Power: –3.00 to –14.50 (Fig. 36.6).

SELECTION OF PATIENTS

The selection of candidates for implantation of Artisan/Artiflex follows the general rules of refractive surgery, like 18 years minimum age (exception in pediatric anisometropia) and a stable refraction. Absence of intraocular vascular (diabetes) or inflammatory (uveitis) diseases are also mandatory. As the IOL is going to be implanted in the anterior chamber it is very important to be sure that no damage is inflicted to

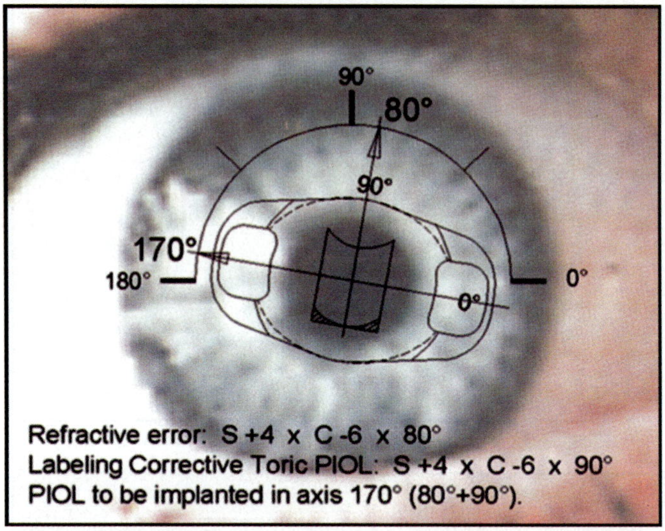

Fig. 36.5: Toric Artisan (Type B)

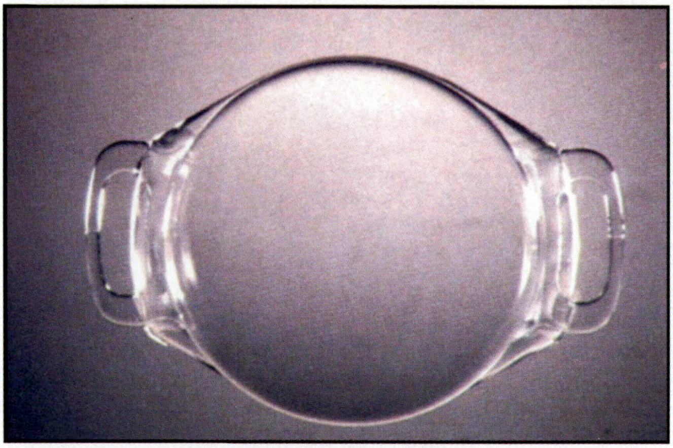

Fig. 36.6: Artiflex (Foldable)

the corneal endothelium. The anterior chamber depth must be carefully measured. Classically it was stated that an anterior chamber depth (from endothelium to natural lens) should be at least 2.8 mm. However, the central anterior chamber depth is not the main issue, as because of the shape of the cornea (dome-shaped) and the greatest thickness of the lens in periphery (myopia lens), the critical distance between the Iol and the endothelium must be 1.5 mm (Fig. 36.7).[1]

This measurement is not available by ultrasound biometry or Orbscan (B&L USA). Although there are tables, that can extrapolate this distance from the central anterior chamber depth and the power of the Iol to implant is much safer today to simulate the implantation

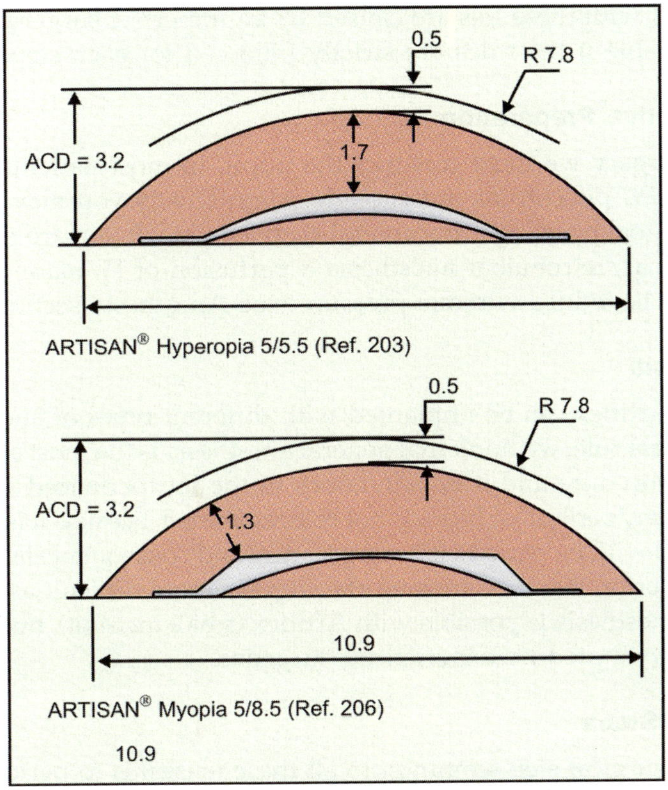

Fig. 36.7: Critical distances to the endothelium in myopia (bottom) and hyperopia (top)

and actually measure the distances using devices like the anterior chamber OCT (Visante, Zeiss Germany). This device will certainly be clinical routine in the near future.

Despite the safety of these lenses to the corneal endothelium, we must not implant Artisan/Artiflex in eyes with endothelial disease. Endothelial cell count of at least 2400 cells/mm and absence of significant polymegatism and polymorphism are criteria for implantation (except in eyes after penetrating keratoplasty, where lower counts can be accepted).

One last very important point concerning the inclusion/exclusion criteria for implantation of Artisan/ Artiflex deals with the shape of the iris. Eyes with a convex iris (mostly hyperopes) should not be implanted with this kind of phakic IOL.[6,17]

SURGERY

It is very important to review in detail the surgical technique of implantation of Artisan/Artiflex, because many of the complications associated with these Iols are caused by an imperfect surgery, and so are avoidable if the rules are strictly followed for each step.[4]

Preoperative Preparation

Before surgery we must constrict the pupil. In most patients, 2 or 3 drops of 2% pilocarpine are enough. Alternatively you may achieve the same goal by using intracameral acetylcholine. If you are planning a peribulbar/retrobulbar anesthesia a perfusion of IV mannitol may be useful to reduce vitreous pressure (see Anesthesia section).

Anesthesia

Artisan/Artiflex can be implanted with different types of anesthesia. As a general rule, we think that general anesthesia is the most adequate for the procedure and it is mandatory to the inexperienced surgeon. Retrobulbar/peribulbar block is not recommended, because it is usually associated with increased vitreous pressure and consequent shallowing of the anterior chamber, turning the surgery more difficult and risky. Topical anesthesia is possible with Artiflex (small incision), but should only be attempted by experienced surgeons.

Surgical Steps

The first surgical step (common to all these lenses) is to perform two side ports. These side ports are classically done at 10 and 2 o'clock positions (assuming the main incision is at 12 o'clock), but their location can change according to the desired position of the Iol. This side ports must be 1.5 mm wide. After completing the sideports the anterior chamber is filled with cohesive viscoelastic material. Dispersive viscoelastics should never be employed. The next step is the main incision. When using PMMA IOLs the incision is 5.2 mm or 6.2 mm according to the model. The incision can be clear corneal, sclerocorneal or scleral, with or without a tunnel. The importance of the location of the incision relates to the possible induction of astigmatism with these large incision. In most hands slightly posterior incisions give better results.

When implanting Artiflex a clear cornea 3.2 mm incision is the rule.[7,8] The IOL is then introduced in the anterior chamber and rotated to the desired position. This position is critical when implanting Toric Artisan.[4,10,12,14] In this case we must define the axis of implantation, by marking the the limbus with a surgical pen (preferably in the sitting to avoid cyclotorsion). In all the other models the axis of implantation is irrelevant. Once the Artisan/Artiflex is in the proper position we proceed to the most critical point of the surgery—the enclavation. In

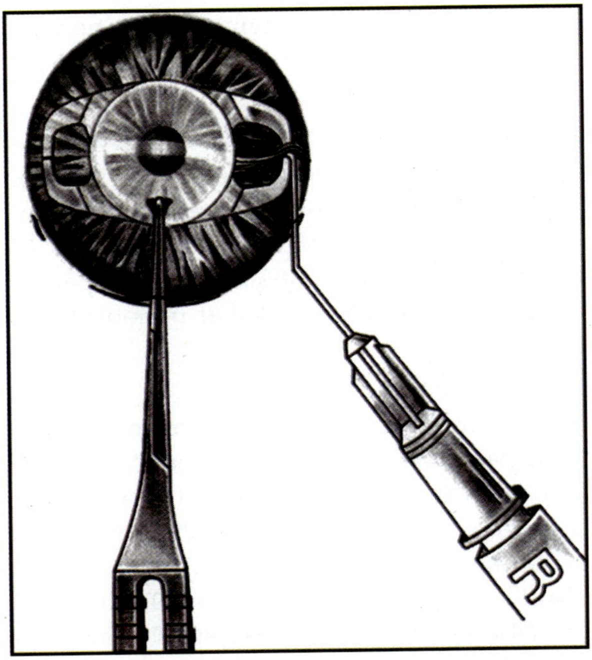

Fig. 36.8: Fixating the IOL to the iris (enclavation using the needle)

this step the Artisan/Artiflex is fixated to the mid periphery of the iris. We achieve this fixation by a bimanual technique (Fig. 36.8). One hand holds the IOL with a forceps. In Artisan the foceps holds the optic of the lens,[4] while in Artiflex, as the optic is soft, special forceps were designed to hold the haptics.[7,8] With the other hand a blunt "needle" is introduced through the side port and introduce (enclavate) a sufficient amount of iris tissue in the claw of the haptic. This is repeated in both haptics. It is very important at this stage to check the correct the perfect centration of the Artisan/Artiflex with the pupil. In this type of phakic IOLs the centering of the IOL is of exclusive responsibility of the surgeon. The next step consists of performing a small iridotomy or iridectomy (this can also be done with YAG preoperative). After completing the iridotomy/iridectomy the viscoelastic material must be completely removed. We usually use passive irrigation to achieve this goal. The last step of the surgery is the suture of the incision for Artisan and simply hydration of the wound for Artiflex (sutureless surgery).

Postoperative Care

At the end of the surgery, a subconjuntival injection of antibiotic and steroids is recommended. The postoperative regimen consists of topical ofloxacin and topical prednisolone acetate 4×/day for two weeks. Oral prednisolone for a week is recommended in patients with heavily pigmented eyes.

COMPLICATIONS

The complications related to the implantation of iris supported phakic IOLs can be divided in three groups. Short-term complications are those found during surgery or in the first post-operative days. Medium-term complications occur during the first 3 weeks postoperative and long-term complications are those beyond that period of time.[3,9,18]

Short-term Complications

The most common complications found during implantation of Artisan are the iris prolapse and the loss of anterior chamber depth.[3] These problems are related to the large incision (5.2 mm or 6.2 mm) and mostly to high vitreous pressure. This high vitreous pressure is related mostly to patient anxiety and high volume of retrobulbar/peribulbar anesthetic. This loss of anterior chamber makes the surgery very difficult and usually leads to other complications. The best way to avoid it, is to use general anesthesia, and if peribulbar is needed, association of preoperative mannitol can help. In the presence of iris prolapse, an iridectomy/ iridotomy should be performed immediately and usually the eye calms down, and the surgery may continue. These two complications are very rarely observed with Artiflex as the small incision (3.2 mm) allows us to work in a closed system.[7,8,23]

Bleeding can occur during surgery. If the iris is pulled too vigorously during the enclavation process, we can observe some bleeding from the root of the iris. Also, when performing iridectomy bleeding is possible. Generally, this complication is avoided with gentle surgery, and if bleeding does occur, it is usually easily stopped putting some viscoelastic in the bleeding site. Postoperative hyphema is exceptional.

Centration of the IOL and sufficient amount of iris tissue enclavated in the haptic (grasp) are very important, and failure to do so will lead to later complications. The suture, when needed (Artisan) must astigmatic free. Corneal edema may be present in the first day after surgery. It usually caused by a traumatic surgery with excessive manipulation. It is a more common complication during the learning curve of the procedure, or if the surgical conditions of the eye were not perfect (loss of anterior chamber). This edema generally goes away in a matter of days, but later damage to the endothelium is possible. It is easily avoidable with good surgery and adequate surgical conditions.

Another complication seldom seen, but possible in the first days postoperative is a flat anterior chamber with possible touch of the Iol to the cornea. This flat anterior chamber can occur in two different settings. We can observe a flat anterior chamber with low ocular pressure or with high ocular pressure. In the first case it is due to inadequate closure of the surgical incision. In this case the suture must be fixed. More serious is the situation of flat anterior chamber with high ocular pressure. This can be related to retained viscoelastic,but more often to not patent iridectomy. In this situation, we must act immediately to avoid the risk of a permanent dilated pupil (Urrets-Zavalia syndrome). Yag laser iridotomy usually solves the problem. The most feared complication in the first days postoperative is the infectious endophthalmitis. In this exceptional event (common to every intraocular surgery) routine endophthalmitis treatment (systemic and intravitreal) must be used.

Medium-term Complications

In the first 3 months after the surgery, some complications may occur. As we are going to see they are mostly related to poor surgery or failure to follow the guidelines for patient selection.

During the first two weeks postoperative sometimes a high ocular pressure is present. This is due to the topical steroids. Suspension of the steroids brings the pressure to normal levels and no further treatment is needed.

However, the most important complications on this period are optical and inflammatory. The most common optical complication is the complain of halos and glare. This is more frequent if the optic is small (5.0 mm) or the pupil is large. Decentration of the IOL (even slight) (Fig. 36.9) may cause a lot of halos and glare, specially if the lens is decentered superiorly. To avoid (or to minimize) this problem, centration of the IOL must be carefully done and we should not implant patients with mesopic pupil larger than the optic of the Artisan/ Artiflex.[3,9] If we find a decentred IOL with symptoms in the post-op surgical recentering of the lens is advised. Although halos and glare may be present in patients with perfect surgeries and normal pupils, these symptoms tend to wane over time and it is exceptional (never done it personally) to have to explant the lens.

Another optical problem we may find is the induction of astigmatism. This can occur with Toric Artisan if the IOL is not implanted in the right axis or in Artisan if the suture is poorly constructed. Doing slightly posterior incisions (avoiding clear cornea) reduces the risk. It also very important in Toric Artisan to mark

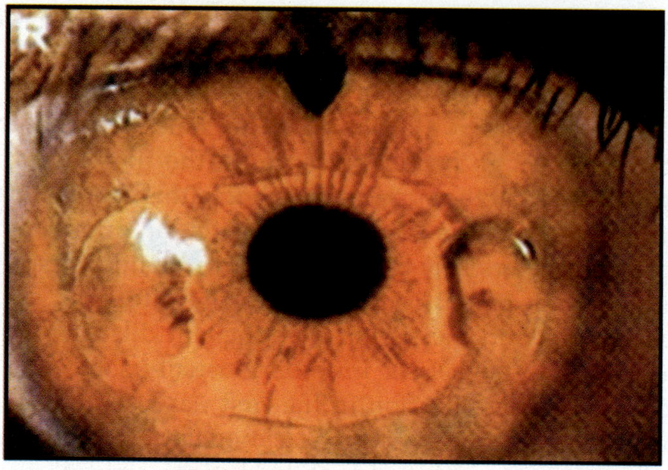

Fig. 36.9: Decentered Artisan

carefully (sitting position) the axis of implantation. To manage this complication, we may try to do a new suture, but most often more reliably, we manage the residual astigmatism with laser corneal surgery (if corneal conditions allow). With Artiflex we never observed any significant change in astigmatism.[7,8,23]

However, the most feared complications in the first 3 months after surgery are the inflammatory.[6,17] Acute uveitis immediately after surgery is a rare event and is almost always associated with a very traumatic surgery.

Standard uveitis treatment solves the problem. Pigment deposits on the surface of the lens are commonly observed between two weeks and three months. These pigment deposits are asymptomatic, tend to disappear with time and do not require treatment. These pigment deposits are seen in both Artisan and Artiflex lenses. Giant cell deposits have also been observed in some eyes implanted with Artiflex (Fig. 36.10). In these cases there is normally a decrease of visual acuity, with only very mild inflammatory signs. In our personal series of 120 eyes implanted with Artiflex these giant cell deposits have been observed in 4 eyes.[7,8,23] To avoid this complication, we suggest the subconjuntival injection of steroids at the end of the surgery. If these deposits occur, topical and oral steroid treatment lead to full recovery.

Late onset uveitis (after 3 weeks of surgery) associated with cyclitic membranes and posterior synechiae have been described mostly in hyperopic eyes. This is due to special anatomic conditions of the iris (convex iris).[6,17] As it was stated above (patient selection), this form of the iris is a contraindication for the implantation of these lenses. In the presence of such a situation aggressive therapy with oral and topical

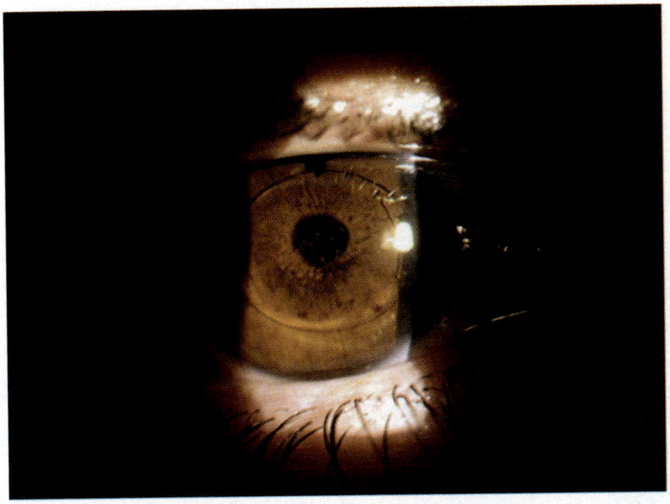

Fig. 36.10: Artiflex with pigment deposits

steroids and topical be implemented. If the treatment does not succeed or the situation recurs, explantation is recommended.

Long-term Complications

One possible complication observed later than 3 months after surgery (may also be seen sooner) is the luxation of the IOL.[3,9] This means that one (Fig. 36.11) (exceptionally both) haptic of the IOL became free from the iris tissue, leading to the luxation of the IOL. This is always due to insufficient amount of iris tissue enclavated in the claw of the lens (weak grasp). A good grasp definitively avoids this problem. In the event of a luxation of an iris supported phakic IOL, surgical reposition must be done immediately, as the loose lens may damage the corneal endothelium.

The relationship between phakic IOLs (mostly anterior chamber) and corneal endothelium has been widely discussed. Several studies concerning the impact of Artisan implantation and endothelial cell loss have been done. The most complete study is the European Multicenter Study published in 2000,[13] where 518 eyes implanted with Artisan showed a loss of endothelial cell count of 4.8% at 3 months (surgically induced) but only a further loss of 1.7% at 2 years and a 0.4% at 3 years. Most other published studies (however much smaller) show similar results.[2,14,19,20,23]

A classic paper by Perez Santonja et al[22] in 1996 stated important losses endothelial cells in eyes implanted with Artisan. In this paper however, there is no relationship of these losses with power of the implanted IOLs and the anterior chamber depths. Of course if the

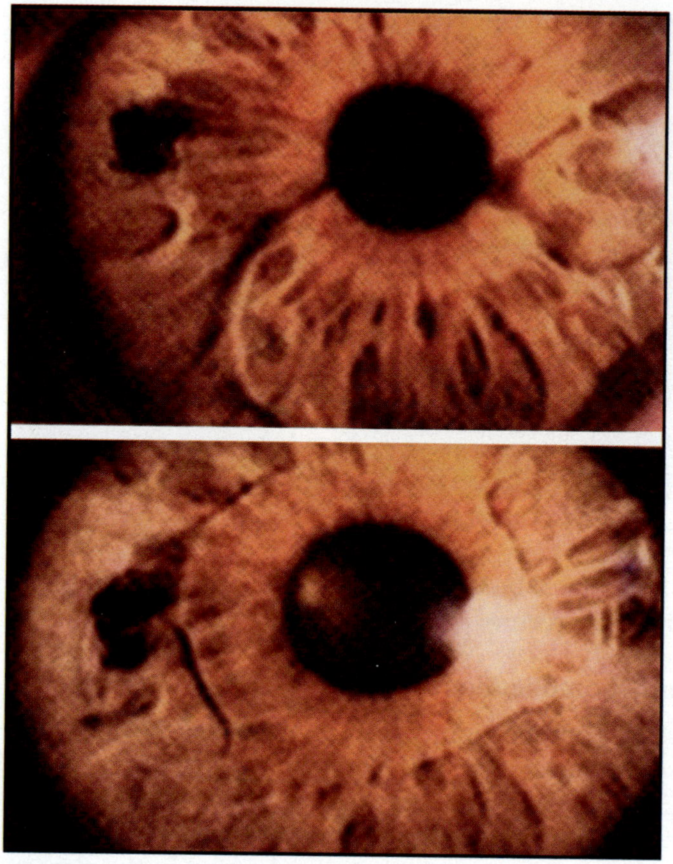

Fig. 36.11: Luxation of Artisan (top) and after management (bottom)

anterior chamber is not deep enough, endothelial cell loss will occur.

Personal data show that Artisan/Artiflex are safe for the corneal endothelium as long as the selection criteria for implantation are met.[7-9]

Nevertheless, it is advised to check the corneal endothelium yearly after surgery and to explant if endothelial cell count or shape (polymorphism, polymegatism) degrades significantly.

Being at a safe distance from the natural lens, the iris supported phakic IOLs do not induce anterior subcapsular cataract, as the posterior chamber phakic IOLs. However, some nuclear cataracts have been observed in eyes implanted with Artisan. These nuclear cataracts are age related, but in implanted eyes tend to be present at younger age (late forties, early fifties). The reason for this is not clear, but it has been suggested that the opening of the eye during surgery or the misdirection of the aquous humor (due to the iridectomy) may account for the earlier development of nuclear cataracts.[11,18,21]

CONCLUSIONS

Like any surgery, the implantation of iris supported phakic IOLs can be associated with many complications. What is important at this point is to differentiate the complications related to the IOL itself, from those arising from other factors such as the selection of candidates for implantation or the surgical technique.

As we clearly see from the presentation of possible complications, most of them are not related to the IOL, but to other factors. Let us summarize the most frequent complications relating them with their origin:

a. Complications due to incorrect surgery (or anesthesia)
   1. Iris prolapse.
   2. Hyphema.
   3. Endothelial touch (corneal edema; endothelial cell loss).
   4. IOL decentration (Glare).
   5. Induced astigmatism (Artisan).
   6. IOL luxation (weak grasp).
   7. Acute uveitis .
b. Complications due to bad selection of candidates for implantation
   1. Late onset uveitis with posterior synechia (convex iris).
   2. Endothelial cell loss (shallow anterior chamber).
   3. Glare and halos (large pupils).

This clearly shows that a good selection of candidates and a gentle and precise surgical technique allows us to implant iris supported phakic IOLs with almost no complications. Artisan/Artiflex are the safest phakic IOLs available in the market.

Take Home Pearls

1. Good selection of candidates is the first key to avoid complications with Artisan/Artiflex.
2. A perfect surgery is the second key.
3. The surgeon (not the IOL) is the only responsible for perfect position of the lens.
4. With Artisan/Artiflex "one size fits all".
5. There are very few (if any) complications related to the IOL.

REFERENCES

MONOGRAPHS

1. Lens Power Calculation and Critical Distance. Artisan Phakic IOL training Manual. Ophtec BV The Netherlands, 2004.

BOOK CHAPTERS

2. Budo C. Clinical Results.In Budo C (Ed): The Artisan Lens. Highlights of Ophthalmolgy, Panama, 2004.
3. Budo C. Complications. In Budo C (Ed): The Artisan Lens. Highlights of Ophthalmolgy, Panama, 2004.
4. Budo C. Surgical procedures.In Budo C (Ed): The Artisan Lens. Highlights of Ophthalmolgy, Panama, 2004.
5. Budo C. Types of lens and applications.In Budo C (Ed): The Artisan Lens. Highlights of Ophthalmolgy Panama, 2004.
6. Izak M Izak A. Inflammatory reaction associated to artisan phakic refractive IOL Implantation. In Budo C (Ed): The Artisan Lens. Highlights of Ophthalmolgy Panama, 2004.
7. Marinho A Artiflex: a new phakic IOL. In Garg A, Pandey S, Chang D, et al (Eds): Advances in Ophthalmology 2. Jaypee Brothers New Delhi, 2005.
8. Marinho A Artiflex: A New Phakic IOL. In Garg A, Alio J, Marinho A, et al (Eds): Lens Based Refractive Surgery (Phakic IOLs). Jaypee Brothers: New Delhi, 2005.
9. Marinho A, Salgado R, Complications of phakic IOLs . In Garg A, Alio J, Marinho A, et al (Eds): Lens Based Refractive Surgery (Phakic IOLs). Jaypee Brothers: New Delhi, 2005.
10. Marinho A, Salgado R, Toric Phakic IOLs. In Garg A, Alio J, Marinho A, et al (Eds): Lens Based Refractive Surgery (Phakic IOLs). Jaypee Brothers: New Delhi, 2005.

JOURNALS

11. Alio J, et al. Phakic anterior chamber lenses for the correction of myopia: a 7 year cumulative analysis of complications in 263 cases. Ophthalmology 1999; 106(3):458-66.
12. Bartels M, Santana N, Budo C, et al. Toric phakic intraocular lens for the correction of hyperopia and astigmatism. J Cataract Refract Surg 2006; 32(2):243-9.
13. Budo C, Hessloehl J, Izak M. Multicenter study of the Artisan phakic intraocular lens. J Cataract Refract Surg 2000; 26(8):1163-71.
14. Dick H, Alio J, Bianchetti M, et al. Toric phakic intraocular lens:European multicenter study. Ophthalmology 2003; 110:150-62.
15. Fechner P, van der Hejde G, Worst J The correction of myopia by lens implantation into phakic eyes. Am J Ophthal 1989; 107:659-63.
16. Fechner P, Wichman W. Correction of myopia by implantation of minus optic (Worst iris claw) lenses in the anterior chamber of phakic eyes. Eur J Imp Ref Surg 1993; 5.
17. Izak M. Surgical Trauma not lens design is responsible for myopia claw IOL irritation. Ocular Surgery News 1998; 9:38.
18. Marinho A. Phakic IOLs: what could go wrong? Ophthalmol Times 2006; 2(6):29-33.
19. Menezo JL, Cisneros A, Cervera M, et al. Iris claw phakic lens immediate and long term corneal endothelial changes. Eur J Implant Refract Surg 1994; 6(8):195-9.
20. Menezo JL, Cisneros A, Rodriguez-Salvador V. Endothelial study of iris claw phakic lens. Four-Year Follow-up. J Cataract Refract Surg 1998; 24(8):1039-49.

21. Menezo JL, Peris-Martinez C, Cisneros A, et al. Rate of cataract formation in 343 highly myopic eyes after implantation of three types of phakic intraocular lenses. J Refract Surg 2004; 20:317-24.
22. Perez-Santonja J, Iradier M,Sanz-Iglesias L, et al Endothelial changes in phakic eyes with anterior chamber intraocular lenses to correct high myopia. J Cataract Refract Surg 1996; 22(10):1017-22.
23. Tehrani M, Dick H. Short term follow-up after implantation of a foldable iris-fixated intraocular lens in phakic eyes. Ophthalmology 2005; 112(12):2189-95.

CHAPTER

37

Claes Feinbaum (Poland)

Pitfalls of Phakic IOLs: How to Avoid Them?

INTRODUCTION

Intraocular lenses have been used since 1999 for correcting larger errors in myopic (near-sighted), hyperopic (far-sighted), and astigmatic eyes. This type of IOL is also called PIOL (phakic intraocular lens), and the crystalline lens is not removed.

More commonly, aphakic IOLs (that is, not PIOLs) are implanted via Clear Lens Extraction and Replacement (CLEAR) surgery. During CLEAR, the crystalline lens is extracted and IOL replaces it in a process that is very similar to cataracts surgery: both involve lens replacement, local anesthesia, both last approximately 30 minutes, and both require making a small incision in the eye for lens insertion. People recover from CLEAR surgery 1-7 days after the operation. During this time, they should avoid strenuous exercise or anything else that significantly raises blood pressure. They should also visit their ophthalmologists regularly for several months so as to monitor the IOL implants. CLEAR has a 90% success rate (risks include wound leakage, infection, inflammation, and astigmatism). CLEAR can only be performed on patients ages 40 and older. This is to ensure that eye growth, which disrupts IOL lenses, will not occur post-surgery.

Once implanted, IOL lenses have three major benefits. First, they are an alternative to LASIK, a form of eye surgery that does not work for people with serious vision problems. Effective IOL implants also entirely eliminate the need for glasses or contact lenses post-surgery. IOL implants prevent cataracts from forming later in life.

Most PIOLs have not yet been approved by FDA, but many are under investigation, and some of the risks that FDA have been found so far during a three year study of the Artisan lens, produced by Ophtec USA Inc, are:

- A yearly loss of 1.8% of the endothelial cells,
- 0.6% risk of retinal detachment,
- 0.6% risk of cataract (other studies has showed a risk of 0.5 - 1.0%), and
- 0.4% risk of corneal swelling.

Other risks include:

- 0.03 - 0.05% eye infection risk, which in worst case can lead to blindness. This risk exists in all eye surgery procedures, and is not unique for IOLs.
- Glaucoma,
- Astigmatism,
- Remaining near or far sightedness,
- Rotation of the lens inside the eye within one or two days after surgery.

One of the causes of the risks above is that the lens can rotate inside the eye, because the PIOL is too short, or because the sulcus has a slightly oval shape (the height is slightly smaller than the width).

Special types of Phakic IOLs (PIOLs) are available in patients requiring IOL implantation without removal of crysalline human lens, particularly useful in refractive surgery for high myopia. For this, the eye surgeon has to determine the size of the PIOL. If the lens is of incorrect length, then it can rotate inside the eye, causing astigmatism, and/or damage to the natural lens. It can also block the natural flow of fluid inside the eye, causing glaucoma. The size is usually estimated, by measuring white-to-white, and estimating the ciliary sulcus diameter. However, the surgeon can perform 3D ultrasound biomicroscopy with, for example, Artemis for a completely accurate measurement. 3D ultrasound is to traditional 2D ultrasound as computer assisted tomography is to X-ray. Therefore, 3D ultrasound examination is strongly recommended, since the white-to-white guesstimate does not have a strong correlation with sulcus-to-sulcus - neither for myopic, nor for hyperopic. About 1% of sulcus-to-sulcus estimates based on white-to-white are so wrong that serious complications can arise. This type of phakic lens has to be ordered from the manufacturer, requiring a number of weeks before the surgery. However, on the other hand, the routine posterior chamber IOLs (PC-IOLs) used for routine cataract surgical cases are available with the surgical suite or doctor's office, and the cataract surgery can usually be performed without delay once the patient is cleared for surgery.

Phakic IOLS (PIOLs) can be either spheric or toric — the latter is used for astigmatic eyes. The difference is that toric PIOLs has to be inserted in a specific angle, or the astigmatism will not be fully corrected, or it can even get worse.

According to placement site in the eyes phakic IOLs can be divided to:

- Angle supported PIOLs: Those IOLs are placed in the anterior chamber. They are notorious for their negative impact on the corneal endothelial lining, which is vital for maintaining a healthy dry cornea.
- Iris supported PIOLs: This type is gaining more and more popularity. The IOL is attached by claws to the mid peripheral iris by a technique called enclavation. It is believed to have a lesser effect on corneal endothelium.
- Sulcus supported PIOLs: These IOLS are placed in the posterior chamber in front of the natural crystalline lens. They have special vaulting so as not to be in contact with the normal lens. The main complications with this type is their tendency to cause cataracts and/or pigment dispersion.

IOL MANUFACTURERS

There are many different manufacturers of intraocular lenses.

Acrylic

- Hoya manufacturers high quality hydrophobic acrylic IOLS, distributed by Spectrum
- ERILENS produces hydrophilic acrylic lenses
- Medennium produces the Matrix Acrylic™ IOL, distributed by Medennium.
- Ophtec produces the Artisan® lens, distributed by Spectrum
- OII Intraocular Lenses produces hydrophilic acrylic IOLs.

Silicone

- AMO (Advanced Medical Optics) produces the Verisyse™ lens.
- Tekia Inc. produces the Kelman Duet lens.
- The Vision Membrane phakic IOL is produced by Vision Membrane Technologies Inc., Apollo Optical Systems LLC, and Millennium Biomedical Inc.
- The PRL™ Phakic Refractive Lens is produced by Medennium, distributed by IOLTech.

Other

- Staar produces the Visian ICL™ lens, in a material called Collamer®.

MYOPIA

Compared to the corneal procedures, the intraocular procedures suffer from one glaring handicap, i.e. patients with the lens implants have to be under careful supervision of the ophthalmic surgeon throughout their lives to prevent or to treat any adverse development. The role of microtrauma or macrotrauma as a result of blinking, squeezing, and minor rubbing during the waking hours and involuntary hard rubbing during some phases of sleep, in producing tissue changes, cannot be overemphasized.

The future of phakic IOLs shall be determined by the newer techniques of corneal refractive surgery, especially the wave-guided ablations. Phakic IOLs cannot take care of preexisting astigmatism. Surgery might introduce astigmatism of its own. Also, with the passage of months and years, patients with phakic IOLs tend to miss detailed follow-up examinations. Situations do exist where phakic IOLs and corneal procedures can be combined to provide the best refractive results. Whether a phakic myopia IOL in a young patient will be a problem in future decades is still unknown.

Myopia is a common refractive error, which exists from a young age. A unilateral myopia, with or without amblyopia, might remain undiscovered for a long time. The treatment of unilateral myopia is not easy. Since the vision is very good in the other emmetropic eye, the child is not impressed by the glass or the contact lens for the affected eye because the child prefers to use the nonaffected eye. Most parents give up all efforts out of sheer frustration, and the magnitude of wasted sight is immense.

While there is some experience with these new and promising modalities, such as the excimer laser for use as PRK or LASIK and newly designed phakic IOLs, these have been used in adult patients, and there is little or no experience in the group of young patients who need the treatment. Slight or moderate myopia is hardly a problem as far as the vision is concerned. These patients do extremely well with glasses or contact lenses. However, high myopes do experience serious handicaps, both cosmetic and visual, for which surgery becomes a matter of importance.

Myopia is not merely a refractive problem. The importance of regular retinal examination should not be overlooked.

Patient Manifestation

- Defective uncorrected vision
- Defective corrected vision — myopic retinal degeneration and deprivation amblyopia
- Strabismus
- Nystagmus
- The eyeball may be normally placed, prominent, or deeply set.
- The cornea may have a normal diameter, or some degree of microcornea or megalocornea may be present.
- Axial length — 20 mm to greater than 30 mm
- Keratometry reading — 38-50 D
- Depth of the anterior chamber — 2.5-4 mm
- Myopia may be moderate or severe, even going beyond — 20.0 D.
- IOP should be normal, and the patient should not be under treatment for any kind of glaucoma.
- Strabismus
- Nystagmus
- Fundus examination may show various degrees of lattice degeneration, with or without one or more holes. The macular area may show disturbed macular reflex, chorioretinal atrophy, or posterior staphyloma.
- Visual field defects of myopia may be present.

Patient Examination

- All patients should undergo a complete ophthalmic examination.
- Manifest and cycloplegic refraction
- Uncorrected visual acuity
- Spectacle and/or contact lens corrected visual acuity
- Slit lamp examination of the anterior segment and ocular adnexa
- IOP
- Pupil size measurement under scotopic conditions
- Corneal endothelial cell count with specular endothelial microscopy
- Biometry to calculate axial length of the eyeball and the anterior chamber
- White-to-white corneal diameter measurement, if contemplating angle-supported or posterior chamber implants
- Videokeratography and keratometry
- Fundus examination by indirect ophthalmoscopy
- Field charting.

Surgical Indications

Indications include unilateral or bilateral, moderate or severe myopia; cosmetic needs; and professional requirements.

- What is the minimum age at which the lens is to be implanted?
- What is the minimum or the maximum refractive error to be treated?
- What should be the lowest limit for anterior chamber depth?
- What is the lowest corneal diameter at which lens implantation will be refused?
- How accurate is the white-to-white diameter on the basis of which the length of an implant lens is to be derived?
- What is the smallest size of the lens available?
- How can the risk of complications be minimized? What are those complications? What are the chances of occurrence?

The final decision to do lens implantation comes after a discussion with the patient, stressing the need for a life-long follow-up.

Surgical Contraindications

- Myopia other than axial
- Evidence of nuclear sclerosis or developing cataract
- History of uveitis
- Presence of anterior or posterior synechiae
- Corneal dystrophy
- Glaucoma or IOP higher than 20 mm Hg
- Personal or family history of retinal detachment
- Diabetes mellitus
- Anterior chamber depth less than 2.75 mm

HYPEROPIA

Today, the quality of corneal refractive procedures is improving. However, lens-related procedures are getting more popular. They include phakic intraocular lenses and a procedure like clear lens extraction with high-plus power lens implantation. Clear lens extraction causes a loss of accommodation but is preferred if the patient is older than 45 years or has any degree of cataract.

Hyperopia is a common refractive error that exists from a young age. A unilateral hyperopia, with or without amblyopia, might remain undiscovered for a long time. The treatment of unilateral hyperopia is not easy. The child does not notice the correction by the glass or the contact lens for the affected eye, since the other eye is so much better. Most parents give up all efforts at an early stage, and the childs eye is wasted as a result, since the parents do not see any improvement.

Numerous innovative corneal procedures have been tried. All have been discontinued because of the difficult nature of these procedures, the serious flaws, and the complications.

Two new and promising modalities have appeared: the excimer laser for use as PRK or LASIK and newly designed phakic IOLs. While some experience with these modalities exists in adult patients, little or no experience exists in the group of young patients who need the treatment.

The optic-mechanical solution to the problem of hyperopia is only one side of the story. The prevention and management of amblyopia is equally important, and efforts in these areas are being made but the outcomes are with variable results so far.

Patient Manifestation

The following ranges of the eye are:

- Axial length — 15-23 mm
- Keratometry reading — 38-50 D
- Depth of the anterior chamber — 2.5-4 mm
- Hyperopia — A low of +2 D or +3 D to as high as +18 D

The intraocular pressure (IOP) should be normal, and the patient should not be under treatment for glaucoma. In addition, unilateral moderate or severe hyperopia cases usually have amblyopia in the affected eye. The patient may have strabismus, nystagmus, or both.

When planning for an IOL implant in phakic hyperopes, consider the following:

- What is the minimum age at which the lens is to be implanted?
- What is the minimum or the maximum refractive error to be treated?
- What should be the lowest limit for anterior chamber depth?

- What is the lowest limit for the diameter of the cornea beyond which there will be a refusal to perform surgery?
- How accurate is the white-to-white diameter on the basis of which the length of a length is to be derived?
- What are the smallest available lenses of the 2 types (i.e., posterior chamber lens, iris claw lens)?
- How can the risk of complications be minimized? What will those complications be? What will be the chances of occurrence?

The final decision to do lens implantation comes after discussion with patient or the parents of the patient and it must be stressed that follow-ups will be necessary for life.

Complications

Precrystalline Lens Phakic Implant

Early problems can develop within 24 hours of the operation. Pupillary block glaucoma may develop because of the blockage of previous laser iridotomies or viscoelastic material residue in the posterior chamber. Red eye, corneal edema, shallow anterior chamber, dilated pupil, and a marked rise in IOP can occur.

If the condition does not respond to systemic therapy with acetazolamide, hyperosmotic agents, local miotics, and beta-blockers, opening the eye under general anesthesia to explant the lens is recommended. In 2-3 weeks, the eye might regain the earlier corrected vision.

Specular endothelial microscopy may reveal a substantial loss of endothelial cells. The closure of the peripheral iridotomies and pupil block glaucoma can occur after 1 or more weeks. Such cases may be treated by a repeat laser iridotomy, surgical peripheral iridectomy, or a lens explantation.

Late Complications

An anterior subcapsular cataract may form due to contact with the natural lens. A small IOL has greater chances of having direct contact with the crystalline lens. Uveitis also can occur in an acute or a chronic form. Pigment dispersion may be seen on the artificial lens or the natural lens. Late glaucoma may occur because of crowding of the angle and pigment deposits in the angle. In some cases, the pupil may become partially dilated and not respond to the usual miotics. The implanted lens may dislocate due to the dissolution of the zonular fibers.

Iris Claw Lens

Early dislocation is due to inadequate fixation. Early or late anterior uveitis can occur. If a patient compulsively rubs the eyes and produces recurrent endothelial touch, late corneal decompensation can occur. Postoperative endophthalmitis has not been reported; however, since it is an intraocular procedure, the possibility cannot be excluded.

ENDOPHTHALMITIS

Endophthalmitis is an inflammatory reaction of intraocular fluids or tissues. Infectious endophthalmitis is one of the most serious complications of ophthalmic surgery. Occasionally, infectious endophthalmitis is the presenting feature of an underlying systemic infection. Successful management of infectious endophthalmitis depends on timely diagnosis and institution of appropriate therapy.

ESCRS study of prophylaxis of postoperative endophthalmitis after cataract surgery: Preliminary report of principal results from a European multicenter study.

- **Barry P,**
- **Seal DV,**
- **Gettinby G,**
- **Lees F,**
- **Peterson M,**
- **Revie CW,**
- **ESCRS Endophthalmitis Study Group**.

European Society of Cataract and Refractive Surgeons, Dublin, Ireland. escrs@agenda-comm, i.e.

Purpose

To report results in the European Society of Cataract and Refractive Surgeons (ESCRS) multicenter study of the prophylaxis of endophthalmitis after cataract surgery.

Setting

Twenty-four ophthalmology units and eye clinics in Austria, Belgium, Germany, Italy, Poland, Portugal, Spain, Turkey, and the United Kingdom, with an administrative office in Ireland, coordinating center in England, and data management and statistical unit in Scotland.

Methods

This partially masked randomized placebo-controlled multinational clinical study to evaluate prospectively the prophylactic effect of intracameral cefuroxime injection and/or perioperative levofloxacin eyedrops on the incidence of endophthalmitis after phacoemulsification cataract surgery began in September 2003 and was terminated early in January 2006. The study used random allocation of patients in a 2 × 2 factorial design.

Results

By the end of 2005, complete follow-up records had been received for 13 698 study patients. Such a clear beneficial effect from the use of intracameral cefuroxime had been observed that it was agreed it would be unethical to continue the study and to wait for the completion of all follow-up procedures before reporting this important result. If total reported cases of endophthalmitis are considered, the incidence rate observed in those treatment groups not receiving cefuroxime prophylaxis (23 cases in 6862 patients) was almost 5 times as high (odds ratio [OR], 4.59; 95% confidence interval [CI], 1.74-12.08; P = .002) as that in the groups receiving this treatment (5 cases in 6836 patients). If only cases proved to be due to infection are considered, the rate was more than 5 times as high (OR, 5.32; 95% CI, 1.55-18.26; P = .008) in the treatment groups not receiving cefuroxime. Although the use of perioperative levofloxacin eyedrops as prophylaxis was also associated with a reduction in the observed incidence rate of postoperative endophthalmitis, this effect was smaller and was not statistically significant, whether total reported cases or only cases proven to be due to infection are used in calculating the rates. As not all follow-up procedures are complete, it is possible that further cases of endophthalmitis may be reported; however, it is not expected that this will alter the main conclusion. Nevertheless, it is anticipated that successful completion of follow-up procedures in all patients will increase the total number in the study to approximately 16,000.

Conclusion

Intracameral cefuroxime administered at the time of surgery significantly reduced the risk for developing endophthalmitis after cataract surgery.

OPTICAL QUALITY

Negative spherical aberration of the young crystalline lens balances positive spherical aberration of the cornea

- The young eye has very little spherical aberration (Fig. 37.1)
- Light is sharply focused on the retina, producing a quality image and good functional vision
- In older patients, function vision is reduced as the aging crystalline lens loses the ability to compensate for corneal spherical aberration
- The cornea and lens, which worked well together in a youthful eye, become out of balance
- The aging eye has positive spherical aberration (Fig. 37.2)

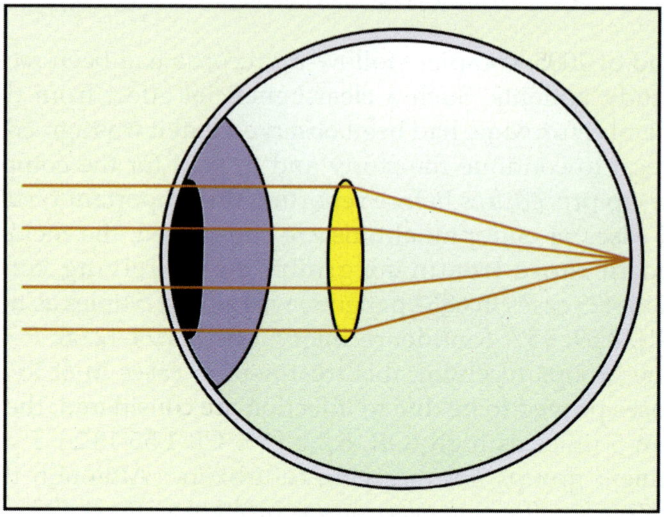

Fig. 37.1 The young lens

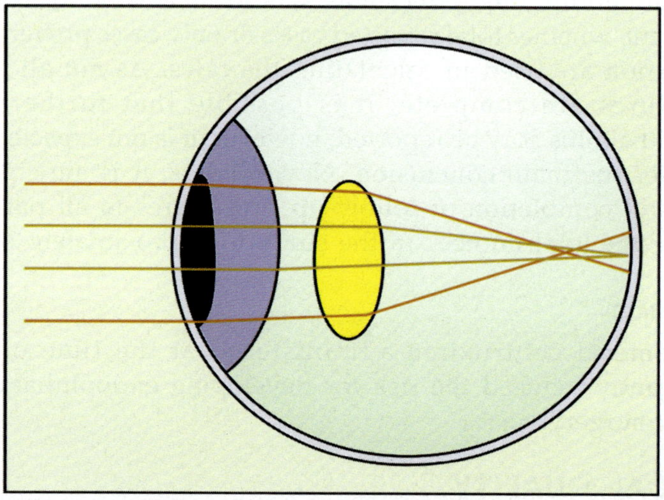

Fig. 37.2 : Aberration in the aging lens

- Aberrations cause blurred vision and reduce contrast sensitivity and functional vision
- Onset of a cataract exacerbates the problem

- Traditional spherical IOLs may add positive spherical aberration, to a level more like that found in the aging natural lens (Fig. 37.3)
- Therefore, while Snellen visual acuity may be good after implantation, functional vision may still be poor.

Objective Assessment of Optical Quality

Wavefront aberrometry measures aberrations over the entire eye, in that it takes into account not only spherocylindrical refractive error,

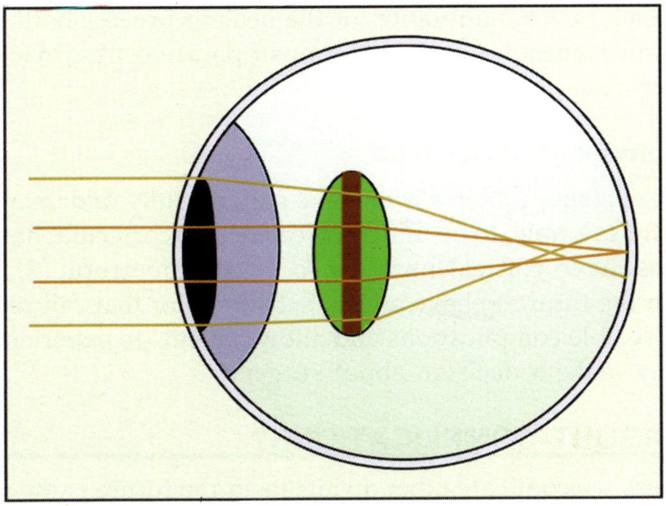

Fig. 37.3: Aberration with traditional spherical IOLs

but also spherical aberration, trefoil, coma, secondary astigmatism, and several other "higher order" aberrations described by Zernike polynomials. Such higher order aberrations are thought to contribute to over 20% of the total number of aberrations in a normal eye, and may contribute to a much greater percentage of aberrations in eyes with diseases such as keratoconus or those that have undergone previous surgery.

WHAT IS FUNCTIONAL VISION?

Functional vision: the ability to see clearly while performing daily activities in varying levels of light: Snellen does not take into account "real world" situations of low contrast and of low light.

Trends

Refractive surgery is a relatively young subspecialty of ophthalmology but its rate of growth in terms of the number of practitioners and patients, and its rate of development in terms of new technologies and techniques, is very **dramatic.**

Exciting Developments

The wound healing response of the cornea is one of the most important factors affecting the outcome of corneal refractive surgery, both in terms of topography and of complications like corneal haze. It is likely our understanding of this process, will increase dramatically just as it has done with wound healing in trabeculectomy surgery, and this will allow a much better modulation of the healing process both through advances in technique and in the postoperative pharmacological manipulation.

Patient Information/Education

One of the current problems is to make patients fully understand what it means, for example, to be undercorrected, overcorrected, have glare, have halos, have corneal haze, or to be anisometropic. It may be possible in the future to have a head set simulator that can reproduce all these possible complications and allow patients to experience them before they make a decision about surgery.

WHAT ABOUT COMPLICATIONS?

Another less welcome area that awaits us in the future is the problem of long term complications. Many of the procedures described above have a relatively short track record, and thus the long term effects on the health and stability of the ocular tissues are unknown.

Other Question Marks

The possibility of underrecording intraocular pressure in an eye that has reduced corneal thickness due to previous refractive surgery, and the effect of previous refractive surgery on IOL power calculations. These problems may be compounded in years to come when a patient forgets to mention, and is not asked, about refractive surgery performed 20 or more years before.

FURTHER READING

1. Alio JL, de la Hoz F, Ismail MM. Subclinical inflammatory reaction induced by phakic anterior chamber lenses for the correction of high myopia. Ocular lenses for the correction of high myopia. In Ocular Immunology and Inflammation. Vol 1. Swets & Zeitlinger 1993; 219-23.
2. Asano-Kato N, Toda I, Hori-Komai Y. Experience with the Artisan phakic intraocular lens in Asian eyes. J Cataract Refract Surg 2005; 31(5): 910-5.
3. Assetto V, Benedetti S, Pesando P. Collamer intraocular contact lens to correct high myopia. J Cataract Refract Surg 1996; 22(5): 551-6.
4. Baikoff G, Arne JL, Bokobza Y, et al. Angle-fixated anterior chamber phakic intraocular lens for myopia of –7 to –19 diopters. J Refract Surg 1998; 14(3): 282-93.
5. Baikoff G, Colin J. Intraocular lenses in phakic eyes. Ophthalmol Clin North Am 1992; 5: 789-95.
6. Bron AJ, Tripathi RC, Tripathi BJ. In Wolff's Anatomy of the Eye and Orbit. 8th ed. London: Chapman & Hall Medical; 1997: 322-5, 350-1.
7. Fechner PU, Haigis W, Wichmann W. Posterior chamber myopia lenses in phakic eyes. J Cataract Refract Surg 1996; 22(2): 178-82.

8. Fechner PU, Singh D, Wulff K. Iris-claw lens in phakic eyes to correct hyperopia: preliminary study. J Cataract Refract Surg 1998; 24(1): 48-56.
9. Fechner PU, van der Heijde GL, Worst JG. The correction of myopia by lens implan-tation into phakic eyes. Am J Ophthalmol 1989 Jun 15; 107(6): 659-63.
10. Fechner PU, Wichmann W. Correction of myopia by implantation of minus optic (Worst iris claw) lenses into the anterior chamber of phakic eyes. Eur J Implant Surg 1993; 5: 55-9.
11. Fechner PU. Cataract formation with a phakic IOL. J Cataract Refract Surg 1999; 25(4): 461-2.
12. Fechner PU. Intraocular lenses for the correction of myopia in phakic eyes: short-term success and long-term caution. Refract Corneal Surg 1990; 6(4): 242-4.
13. Fyodorov SN, Zuew VK, Tumanyan NR, Suheil AJ. Clinical and functional follow-up of minus IOL implantation in high grade myopia. Oftalmochirurgia 1993; 2: 12-7.
14. Kashani AA. Phakic posterior chamber intraocular lenses for the correction of high myopia. J Refract Surg 1996; 12(4): 454-6.
15. Krumeich JH, Daniel J, Gast R. Closed-system technique for implantation of iris-supported negative- power intraocular lens. J Refract Surg 1996; 12(3): 334-40.
16. Landesz M, Worst JG, Van Rij G, Houtman WA. Opaque iris claw lens in a phakic eye to correct acquired diplopia. J Cataract Refract Surg 1997; 23(1): 137-8.
17. Menezo JL, Avino JA, Cisneros A, et al. Iris claw phakic intraocular lens for high myopia. J Refract Surg 1997; 13(6): 545-55.
18. Menezo JL, Cisneros A, Hueso JR, et al. Long-term results of surgical treatment of high myopia with Worst-Fechner intraocular lenses. J Cataract Refract Surg 1995; 21(1): 93-8.
19. Menezo JL, Martinez MC, Cisneros AL. Iris-fixated Worst claw versus sulcus-fixated posterior chamber lenses in the absence of capsular support. J Cataract Refract Surg 1996; 22(10): 1476-84.
20. Menezo JL, Peris-Martinez C, Cisneros AL: Phakic intraocular lenses to correct high myopia: Adatomed, Staar, and Artisan. J Cataract Refract Surg 2004; 30(1): 33-44.
21. Perez-Santonja JJ, Bueno JL, Zato MA. Surgical correction of high myopia in phakic eyes with Worst-Fechner myopia intraocular lenses. J Refract Surg 1997; 13(3): 268-81; discussion 281-4.
22. Perez-Santonja JJ, Hernandez JL, Benitez del Castillo JM, et al. Fluorophotometry in myopic phakic eyes with anterior chamber intraocular lenses to correct severe myopia. Am J Ophthalmol 1994; 118(3): 316-21.
23. Perez-Santonja JJ, Iradier MT, Benitez del Castillo JM, et al. Chronic subclinical inflammation in phakic eyes with intraocular lenses to correct myopia. J Cataract Refract Surg 1996; 22(2): 183-7.
24. Perez-Santonja JJ, Iradier MT, Sanz-Iglesias L, et al. Endothelial changes in phakic eyes with anterior chamber intraocular lenses to correct high myopia. J Cataract Refract Surg 1996; 22(8): 1017-22.
25. Perez-Torregrosa VT, Menezo JL, Harto MA, et al. Digital system measurement of decentration of Worst-Fechner iris claw myopia intraocular lens. J Refract Surg 1995; 11(1): 26-30.

26. Pesando PM, Ghiringhello MP, Tagliavacche P. Posterior chamber collamer phakic intraocular lens for myopia and hyperopia. J Refract Surg 1999; 15(4): 415-23.
27. Rosen E, Gore C. Staar Collamer posterior chamber phakic intraocular lens to correct myopia and hyperopia. J Cataract Refract Surg 1998; 24(5): 596-606.
28. Sanders DR, Brown DC, Martin RG, et al: Implantable contact lens for moderate to high myopia: phase 1 FDA clinical study with 6 month follow-up. J Cataract Refract Surg 1998; 24(5): 607-11.
29. Sanders DR, Martin RG, Brown DC, et al. Posterior chamber phakic intraocular lens for hyperopia. J Refract Surg 1999; 15(3): 309-15.
30. Trindade F, Pereira F, Cronemberger S: Ultrasound biomicroscopic imaging of posterior chamber phakic intraocular lens. J Refract Surg; 14(5): 497-503.
31. Verma A, Singh D. Active vision therapy for pseudophakic amblyopia. J Cataract Refract Surg 1997; 23(7): 1089-94.
32. Wiechens B, Winter M, Haigis W, et al: Bilateral cataract after phakic posterior chamber top hat-style silicone intraocular lens. J Refract Surg 1997; 13(4): 392-7.
33. Zaldivar R, Davidorf JM, Oscherow S, et al. Combined posterior chamber phakic intraocular lens and laser in situ keratomileusis: bioptics for extreme myopia. J Refract Surg 1999; 15(3): 299-308.
34. Zaldivar R, Davidorf JM, Oscherow S. Posterior chamber phakic intraocular lens for myopia of -8 to -19 diopters. J Refract Surg 1998; 14(3): 294-305.
35. Zaldivar R, Rocha G. The current status of phakic intraocular lenses. Int Ophthalmol Clin 1996 Fall; 36(4): 107-11.

CHAPTER

38

José M Ruiz-Moreno, Javier A Montero (Spain)

Retinal Complications of Intraocular Phakic Anterior Chamber Lenses

RETINAL COMPLICATIONS OF HIGH MYOPIA

The most important fact regarding retinal disease and refractive surgery is probably the consideration whether refractive surgery may increase or precipitate the apparition of vitreoretinal complications. Vitreoretinal disorders in myopic eyes undergoing refractive surgery are usually related to two different factors. Firstly, retinal disorders are more frequent in myopic eyes than among general population. Secondly, we may hypothesize whether refractive surgery might induce one or more iatrogenic factors increasing the frequency of vitreoretinal conditions.

Retinal detachment (RD) and choroidal neovascularization (CNV) are the most outstanding, sight-threatening disorders of the myopic eye. The incidence of RD is higher among myopic eyes, and the risk of RD ranges between 0.71% and 3.2%.[1,2] The incidence of RD has been estimated in 0.015% for eyes with a spherical equivalent (SE) $\leq$ –4.75D; 0.07% for eyes with SE ranging –5.00D to –9.75D; and 0.075% for eyes with SE $\geq$ –10.00 D.[3] The chances of going through an RD are 15 to 110 higher among myopic patients with SE $\geq$–15 to –20D than among the general population.[2] According to Burton, the risk of RD caused by retinal atrophic holes rises when an SE $\geq$–5.00 D is associated with lattice degeneration, especially during the 2nd to 4th decade of life.

Early posterior vitreous detachment in patients with peripheral retinal degenerative changes and low to moderate myopia may increase the risk for RD among patients in the 5th to 6th decade of life.[4] Peripheral chorioretinal degenerative changes are the most significant factors favoring RD in myopic eyes.[5]

High myopia (HM), as defined by an SE >–6D, is the 7th cause of blindness in the USA,[6] affecting 0.5% of the European population,[7] and 2% of the myopic patients.[8] The pathogenesis of the degenerative changes in HM remains unknown, but axial elongation seems to be an important factor.

The relationship between CNV and HM has been reported.[10] CNV is frequently associated with Bruch's membrane and retinal pigment epithelium (RPE) defects,[9, 11, 12] as can be seen in 82% of myopic eyes with CNV.[10] Bruch's membrane and RPE defects as well as other degenerative changes in HM are believed to be caused by a progressive mechanic retinal and choroidal thinning in the posterior staphyloma.[13] The formation or growth of a defect in Bruch's membrane frequently causes macular hemorrhages which may or not be connected with CNV. These small, round hemorrhages are caused by the tight anatomical relationship formed by Bruch's membrane, RPE and choriocapillaris, and usually disappear spontaneously and do not cause visual impairment.

From a theoretical point of view, ruptures in Bruch's membrane might allow the growth and progression of CNV from the choriocapillaris.[10] According to Curtin, Bruch's membrane may be defective in myopic eyes, and ruptures in Bruch's membrane are always necessary to permit the development of CNV, since Curtin considers that the reduced choriocapillaris blood flow and the low metabolic needs of myopic retina by themselves are not enough to induce the appearance of new vessels.

Two different mechanisms have been proposed to explain the growth of CNV in highly myopic eyes. Firstly, choroidal thinning causes stromal loss and vessel obliteration affecting choroidal hemodynamics. Secondly, the elongation of the eye is associated with Bruch's membrane ruptures allowing CNV ingrowths.[14]

CNV may appear in 4 to 11% of highly myopic eyes.[11, 15-17] Myopia seems to be a predisposing factor when SE is higher than –6D.[18] HM is the leading cause of CNV (62%) among young patients.[18] The higher the SE, the more frequently RPE defects and CNV may appear[19] though there is not a complete agreement on the subject.[10]

According to most of the authors, CNV appear most frequently under the fovea (58-74%),[20, 21] followed by the juxtafoveal location (27-33%).[10]

CNV is part of the disorders affecting eyes associated with Fuchs' spot. Förster-Fuchs´ spot was described by Förster as a hemorrhagic lesion,[22] and later studied by Fuchs as a pigmented lesion.[23] It is formed by an evagination of choroidal fibrovascular tissue and RPE proliferation.[24] According to Gass, two definite phases may be differentiated in the formation of Fuchs' spot: in the first phase an acute serous or hemorrhagic detachment appears; in the second phase the hemorrhage is joined by RPE proliferation.[24]

RETINAL DETACHMENT IN HIGHLY MYOPIC PATIENTS CORRECTED BY PIOL

RD in myopic eyes undergoing PIOL implantation may be caused by HM itself, as is the case of any other refractive surgery. However, the doubt arises whether PIOL implantation may increase this risk.

RD in highly myopic patients after refractive surgery by PIOL implantation (Fig. 38.1) is a severe complication which was first reported by Alio et al in 1993.[25] This complication was later described by other authors in short series: Fechner reported 1 case of RD after 125 surgeries (0.8%),[26] Pesando 1 case after 19 surgeries (5.3%),[27] and Zaldivar 1 case after 124 surgeries (0.8%).[28]

Our group has reported eight cases of RD after 168 surgeries (4.8%),[29] and 12 cases after 294 surgeries (4.08%) in a subsequent paper with a greater group of patients and longer follow-up.[30]

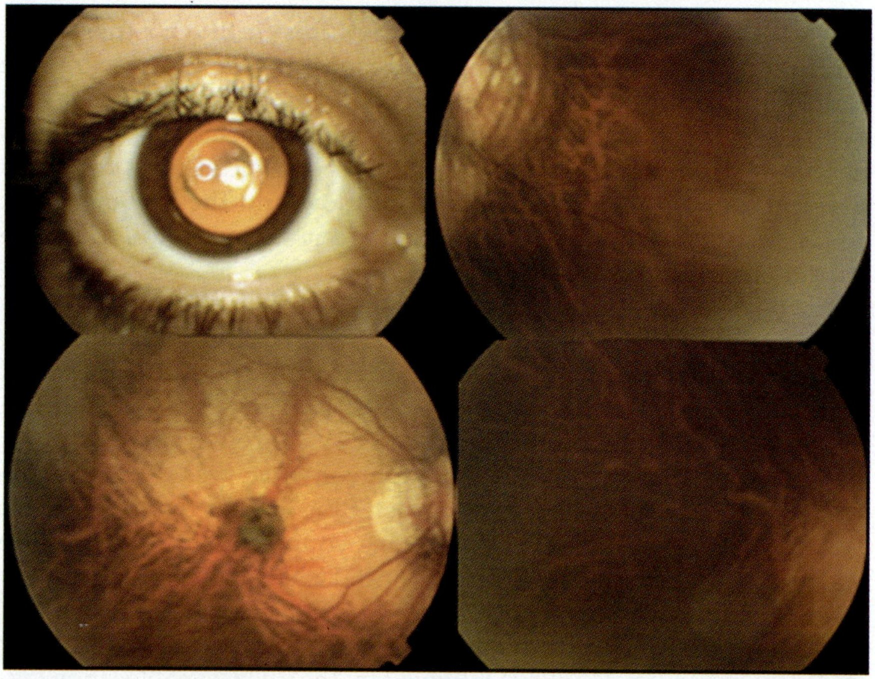

Fig. 38.1: (A) Phakic intraocular lens (PIOL) implanted to correct high myopia. (B) Retinography of the same patient shows rhegmatogenous retinal detachment. (C) Retinal posterior pole and (D) Periphery after surgery. The detachment was successfully repaired by pars plana vitrectomy. The patient had a previous Fuchs´ spot

The last series reported by our group described a frequency of 2.87% after 522 surgeries.[31] In this paper the occurrence of RD after PIOL implantation was described in 522 consecutive eyes from 323 patients averaging 32.1±7.3 years-of-age (range, 18 to 52) and an average SE –18.1±5.0 D (range, –7 to –38). Mean follow up was 60.4±39.1 months (range, 12 to 145).

RD occurred in 15 eyes (2.87%), nine males and six females. The lapse between PIOL implantation and RD was 24.4±24.4 months (range, 1 to 92). No complications arose during PIOL implantation in any of these cases. Two eyes had received argon laser photocoagulation for predisposing lesions to retinal breaks. In these two cases RD was not related to the treated lesions.

The incidence of RD among eyes with SE –6 to – 12 D (145 eyes), was 0%; it was 4.1 % (6 cases) among eyes with SE –12 a –18 D (145 eyes); and it was 3.8% (9 cases) among eyes with SE higher than –18 D (232 eyes). The highest incidence occurred among eyes with higher SE.

The risk of RD in highly myopic patients corrected by PIOL implantation was calculated using the Kaplan-Meier test since there was no control group. The cumulative risk of RD in these patients was 0.57% at three months, 0.96% at 8 months, 2.14% at 25 months, 3.44% at 52 months and 4.06% between months 92 and 145.

The group of patients with RD after PIOL implantation was compared with the whole group of highly myopic patients corrected by PIOL. No statistically significant differences were found for age, initial best corrected visual acuity (BCVA), initial SE, follow up or type of PIOL implanted. No differences were found between patients treated or not with prophylactic laser photocoagulation. However, statistically significant differences were found regarding axial length (P=0.028).

Multiple logistic regression confirmed the statistically significant difference for axial length (P=0.029). There was a statistically significant difference of RD risk considering two groups of patients with axial length shorter or greater than 30.24 mm. We are able to confirm that the risk of RD in highly myopic eyes corrected by PIOL is highest among eyes with axial length greater than 30.24 mm.

The previously reported incidences of RD 5.3%,[27] 4.8%,[29] and 4.08%[30] were higher than our present study. Zaldivar was the only author to report an incidence lower than ours (0.8%).[28] Similarly, these frequencies are higher than those reported for myopias over –6 D (3.2%).[1] However, the value of these reports is limited by the shorts series and follow up.

Comparing the risk of RD in our series with the reported incidence of highly myopic patients with SE higher than –10.00D in the literature (0.075%),[3] a much higher risk is found in the former. In our series the risk is 0.96% at the first year, 1.64% at the second year and 3.44% at the third year.

The prevalence of RD in our series (2.87%) is similar to that of non operated highly myopic patients (3.2%); however, the risk of RD is higher when follow up is longer. We must consider that RD is more probable in our series of highly myopic patients corrected by PIOL than among non operated highly myopic population, and a longer follow up of this series would imply a higher prevalence of RD. Nevertheless, we should also take into consideration that our series is formed by very highly myopic patients (average SE –18.18D), invalidating direct comparison.

The alternative refractive surgery for these highly myopic patients might be transparent lens removal. The reported frequency of RD in highly myopic patients undergoing transparent lens removal varies according to different authors. Fernandez-Vega reported a 2.10% risk of RD in a group of 190 eyes undergoing phacoemulsification for transparent lens removal, with an average 4.78 years follow up.[32] Pucci reported 4.0% RD in the eyes with SE higher than -12 D undergoing transparent lens renoval,[33] Cashtang reported 6.1%,[34] Barraquer 7.3%[35] and Colin reported 8.1%.[36]

These results cannot be compared with those of cataract removal in highly myopic patients, which are much lower. This fact is probably attributable to the changes induced in the vitreous by lens surgery, increasing retinal traction.[37]

Colin suggests that the risk of RD in patients with transparent lens removal may increase with time, reporting increasing RD frequency with longer follow up: 0% at 12 months, 1.9% at 48 months and 8.1% at 84 months.[36,38,39]

CHOROIDAL NEOVASCULARIZATION IN HIGHLY MYOPIC PATIENTS CORRECTED BY PIOL

The inflammatory reaction induced by refractive surgery may affect CNV growth. Pollack et al have reported that progression in hemorrhagic macular degeneration is more frequent in operated eyes than in fellow eyes.[40] Blair et al suggested that surgery may induce hemodynamic changes in the choriocapillaris which might cause pre-existing new vessels to grow or bleed, or induce the formation of CNV in predisposed eyes.[41]

Intraocular inflammation associated with surgery might explain the acceleration of myopic maculopathy. Furthermore, the pro-angiogenic factors released by macrophages may induce neovascularization.[42] This seems to occur in eyes with predisposing lesions, such as drusen and/or Bruch´s membrane injuries (Fig. 38.2).[43,44]

The first study performed by our group reported 5 cases (1.70%) with myopic CNV (Fig. 38.3) on 294 eyes with an average SE –18.5±5.8D and 50.6±32.8 months follow up.[45]

A subsequent paper based on the same series of patients averaging 32.6±7.3 years-of-age (range, 18 to 50 at the time of surgery) and longer follow up (56.7±31.7 months, and more than 12 months in all the cases) reported CNV in 7 eyes (2.38%), five females and two males. The average lapse between refractive surgery and the appearance of CNV was 49.0±33.5 months (range, 1.5 to 87).[30] CNV appeared in none of 25 eyes with SE –6 to –12D (0%), three of 125 eyes with SE –12 to –18D (2.40%) and four of 144 eyes with SE higher than –18D (2.77%).

Kaplan-Meier survival test for cumulative risk of CNV was 0.77% at 18 months, 2.91% at 64 months and 6.25% at 87 months.

In the latest report from our group CNV appeared in 2.29% of the eyes in a greater series of highly myopic patients corrected by PIOL implantation (522 eyes from 323 patients) averaging 32.1±7.3 years-of-

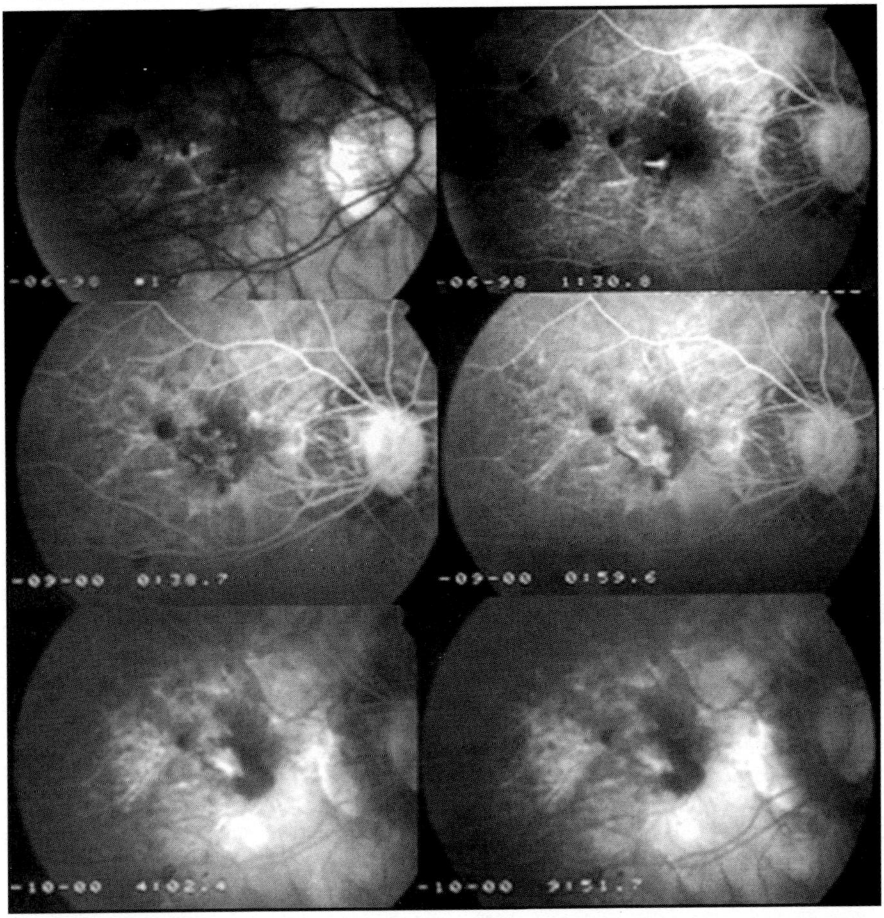

Fig. 38.2: (A) Red-free fundus photography and (B) Middle phase fluorescein angiogram (FA) of a highly myopic eye corrected by PIOL implantation with lacquer cracks. (C) Early and (D) Middle phase FA show a classic subfoveal choroidal neovascularization (CNV) in the same eye two years later. (D) Middle and (E) Late phase FA show CNV closure after photodynamic therapy

age (range 18 to 52) with a mean follow up of 60.4±39.1 months (range 12 to 145).[46] This series was formed by highly myopic patients (mean SE -18.1±5.0D, range, –7.0 to –38.0D), with a male to female ratio of 40%/60% in which most of the eyes (487 eyes) were corrected by PIOL implantation with anterior chamber four-point angle-support lenses. Three eyes were implanted with phakic anterior chamber three-point angle support lenses, 24 eyes with iris grasp lenses and nine eyes with phakic posterior chamber lenses.

Myopic CNV appeared in 12 eyes (2.29%) during follow up, (six females, five males), after an average lapse of 33.7±29.6 months (range, 1 to 87). One eye in 145 eyes (0.68%) with SE –6 to –12D, six in 145

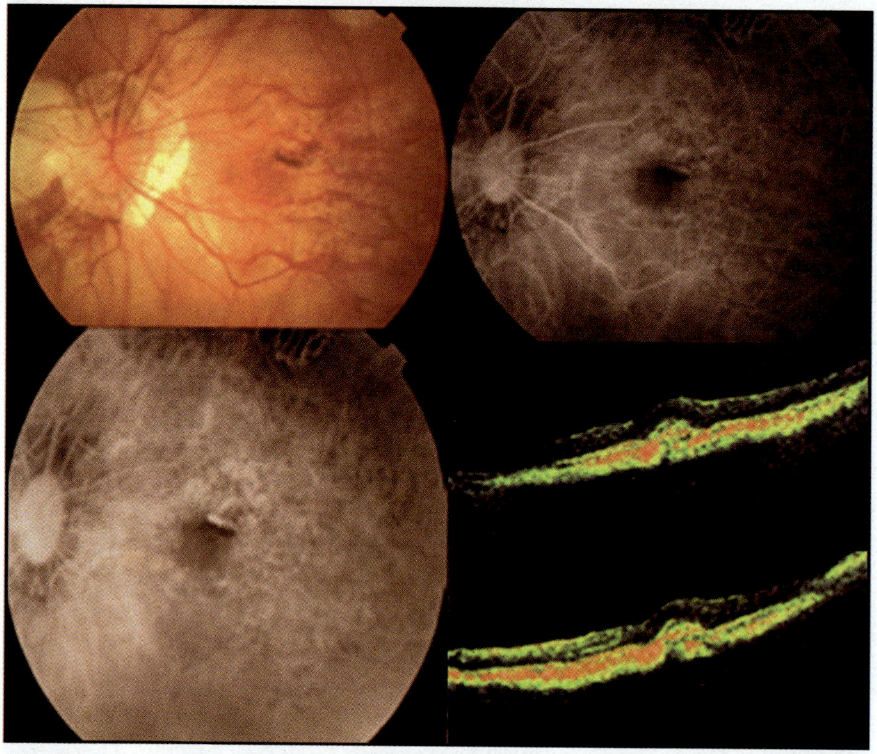

Fig. 38.3: Retinography (A) and early (B) and middle phase (C) FA with a classic subfoveal CNV in one highly myopic patient after PIOL implantation. (D) Vertical and horizontal optical coherence tomography (OCT) scans before treatment. (E) Vertical and horizontal OCT scans after one single injection of an antiangiogenic drug achieving CNV closure

eyes (4.1%) with SE –12 to –18D and five in 232 eyes (2.1%) with SE higher than -18.0D developed myopic CNV. CNV followed uneventful PIOL implantation in all cases. CNV was subfoveal in most of the eyes (eight eyes, 66%) and predominantly classic (11 eyes, 92%), as usually happens in myopic CNV.[20, 21]

A Kaplan-Meier survival test was performed in order to calculate the cumulative risk of developing myopic CNV, since there was no similar control group formed by myopic patients with equivalent SE –18.1±5.0. The cumulative risk for CNV was 0.57% at 5 months, 0.81% at 18 months, 2.63% at 63 months and 3.72% at 87 to 145 months.

No statistically significant differences were found for age, axial length, SE, follow up and type of PIOL implanted between the group of patients developing myopic CNV and those who had not developed it. The differences were almost statistically significant for initial BCVA (P=0.085; ANOVA one factor test). This fact might suggest that myopic CNV could be associated with the degenerative changes induced by HM in the posterior pole. Even though CNV appeared sooner than six months after surgery in three cases, and this might suggest that refractive surgery had played a role in it, the other data did not support this association.

The results of these two series regarding the risk of myopic CNV are similar, supporting the idea that PIOL implantation to correct HM does not imply an increased risk of CNV. However, these data should be carefully considered in the absence of a control group.

CONCLUSION

We may conclude that PIOL implantation to correct HM does not imply an increased risk of retinal diseases. We have demonstrated that the risk for RD is higher in eyes with axial length greater than 30.34 mm. A controlled study with similar non surgical highly myopic patients and similar follow up should be performed in order to validate the data reported so far.

REFERENCES

1. Schepens CL, Marden D. Data on the natural history of retinal detachment: further characterization of certain unilateral non traumatic cases. Am J Ophthalmol 1966;61:213-26.
2. Kaluzny J. Myopia and retinal detachment. Polish Medical Journal 1970;9: 1544-49.
3. Michels RG, Wilkinson CD Rice TA. Retinal detachment. St Louis: Mosby, 1990;83-4.
4. Burton TC. The influence of refractive errors and lattice degeneration on the incidence of retinal detachment. Trans Am Ophthalmol Soc 1990;87:143-55.
5. Curtin BJ. Physiologic vs pathologic myopia: genetics vs environment. Ophthalmology 1979;86:681-91.
6. National Society for the Prevention Blindness. NSFB Fact Book; Estimated Statistics on Blindness and Vision Problems. New York; National Society for the Prevention of Blindness, 1996; 44.
7. Strömberg E. Über Refraction und Achsenlänge des menschlichen Auges. Acta Ophthalmol 1936;14:281-93.
8. Michaels DD. Visual optics and refraction; a clinical approach. 2nd Ed. St Louis: CV Mosby, 1980;513.
9. Curtin BJ. Myopia. In: Yannuzzi LA, Gitter KA, Schatz H, eds. The macula: a comprehensive text and atlas. Baltimore: Williams and Wilkins, 1979; 232-42.
10. Hotchkiss ML, Fine SL. Pathologic myopia and choroidal neovascularization. Am J Ophthalmol 1981;91:177-83.
11. Curtin BJ. The posterior staphyloma of pathologic myopia. Trans Am Ophthalmol Soc 1977;75:67-86.
12. Johnson DA, Yannuzzi LA, Shakin JL, Lightman DA. Lacquer cracks following laser treatment of choroidal neovascularization in pathologic myopia. Retina 1998;18:118-24.
13. Luna JD, Artal MN, Juarez CP. Retinal detachment in myopic eyes after laser in situ keratomileusis. Am J Ophthalmol 2000;130:259-60.

14. Stafford WR. Degeneration and atrophy of the choroid. In: WT and EA J eds. Duane's Clinical Ophthamology. Philadelphia. Lippincot Co. 1982;1-15.
15. Curtin BJ, Karlin DB. Axial length measurements and fundus changes of the myopic eye. Am J Ophthalmol 1971;71:42-53.
16. Blatt N. Augenhintergrundveränderungen bei hochgradiger Myopie. Klin Monatsbl Augenheilkd 1965;146:391-411.
17. Grossniklaus HE, Green WR. Pathologic findings in pathologic myopia. Retina 1992;12:127-33.
18. Cohen SY, Laroche A, Leguen Y, Soubrane G, Coscas G. Etiology of choroidal neovascularization in young patients. Ophthalmology 1996;103:1241-44.
19. Fried M, Siebert A, Meyer-Schwickerath G, Wessing A. Natural history of Fuchs's spot: a long-term follow-up study. Doc Ophthalmol Proc Ser 1981;28:215-21.
20. Hampton G, Kohen D, Bird A. Visual prognosis of disciform degeneration in myopia. Ophthalmology 1983;90:923-26.
21. Soubrane G, Pison J, Bornet P, Perrenoud F, Coscas G. Néo-vaisseaux sous-rétiniens de la myopie degenerative: résultats de la photocoagulation. Bull Soc Opht France 1986;86:262-72.
22. Foerster R. Ophthalmologische Beitrage. Berlin. Enslin 1862; 55.
23. Fuchs E. Der zentrale schwarze Fleck bei Myopie. Z Augenheilkd 1901;5:171-78.
24. Gass JDM. Stereoscopic atlas of macular diseases: Diagnosis and treatment. St Louis. Mosby Co. 1997; 126-29.
25. Alió JL, Ruiz-Moreno JM, Artola A. Retinal detachment as a potential hazard in surgical correction of severe myopia with phakic anterior chamber lenses. Am J Ophthalmol 1993; 115:145-48.
26. Fechner PU, Strobel J, Wicchmann W. Correction of myopia by implantation of a concave Worst-iris claw lens into phakic eyes. Refract Corneal surg 1991;7:286-98.
27. Pesando PM, Ghiringhello MP, Tagliavacche P. Posterior chamber collamer phakic intraocular lens for myopia and hyperopia. J Refract Surg 1999;15:415-23.
28. Zaldivar R, Davidorf JM, Oscherow S. Posterior chamber phakic intraocular lenses for myopia of –8 to –19 diopters. J Refract Surg 1998;14:294-305.
29. Ruiz-Moreno JM, Alió JL, Pérez-Santonja JJ, de la Hoz F. Retinal detachment in phakic eyes with anterior chamber intraocular lenses to correct severe myopia. Am J Ophthamol 1999;127:270-75.
30. Ruiz-Moreno JM, Alió JL. Incidence of retinal diseases following refractive surgery in 9239 eyes. J Refract Surg 2003;19:534-47.
31. Ruiz-Moreno JM, Montero J, de la Vega C, Alió JL, Zapater P. Retinal detachment in myopic eyes after phakic intraocular lens implantation. J Refract Surg 2006;22:247-52.
32. Fernandez-Vega L, Alfonso JF, Villacampa T. Clear lens extraction for the correction of high myopia. Ophthalmology 2003;110:2349-54.
33. Pucci V, Morselli S, Romanelli F, et al. Clear lens phacoemulsification for correction of high myopia. J Cataract Refract Surg 2001;27:896-900.
34. Cashtang P, Ruellan YM, Rozembaum JP et al. Phakoémulsification à visée réfractive sur cristallin clair; a propos de 33 yeux myopes fortes. J Fr Ophtalmol 1998;21:560-66.
35. Barraquer C, Cavelier C, Mejía LF. Incidence of retinal detachment following clear-lens extraction in myopic patient; retrospective analysis. Arch Ophthalmol 1994;112:336-39.

36. Colin J, Robinet A, Cochener B. Retinal detachment after clear lens extraction for high myopia: seven-year follow-up. Ophthalmology 1999;106:2281-85.
37. Ravalico G, Michieli C, Vattovani O, Tognetto D. Retinal detachment after cataract extraction and refractive lens exchange in highly myopic patients. J Cataract Refract Surg 2003;29:39-44.
38. Colin J, Robinet A. Clear lensectomy and implantation of a low-power posterior chamber intraocular lens for the correction of high myopia. Ophthalmology 1994;101:107-12.
39. Colin J, Robinet A. Clear lensectomy and implantation of a low-power posterior chamber intraocular lens for the correction of high myopia: four-year follow-up. Ophthalmology 1997;104:73-7.
40. Pollack A, Marcovich A, Bukelman A, Oliver M. Age-related macular degeneration after extracapsular cataract extraction with intraocular lens implantation. Ophthalmology 1996;103:1546-54.
41. Blair CJ, Ferguson JJr. Exacerbation of senile degeneration following cataract extraction. Am J Ophthamol 1979;87:77-83.
42. Werb Z. How the macrophage regulates the extracellular environment. Am J Anat 1983;166:237-56.
43. Sarks SH. Ageing and degeneration in the macular region: a clinico-pathological study. Br J Ophthalmol 1976;60:324-41.
44. Grindle CFJ, Marshall J. Aging changes in Bruch's membrane and their functional implications. Trans Ophthalmol Soc UK 1978;98:172-75.
45. Ruiz-Moreno JM, de la Vega C, Ruiz-Moreno O, Alió JL. Choroidal neovascularization in phakic eyes with anterior chamber intraocular lenses to correct high myopia. J Cataract Refract Surg 2003;29:270-74.
46. Ruiz-Moreno JM, Montero J, de la Vega C, Alió JL, Zapater P. Macular choroidal neovascularization in myopic eyes after phakic intraocular lens implantation. J Refract Surg 2006;22:689-94.

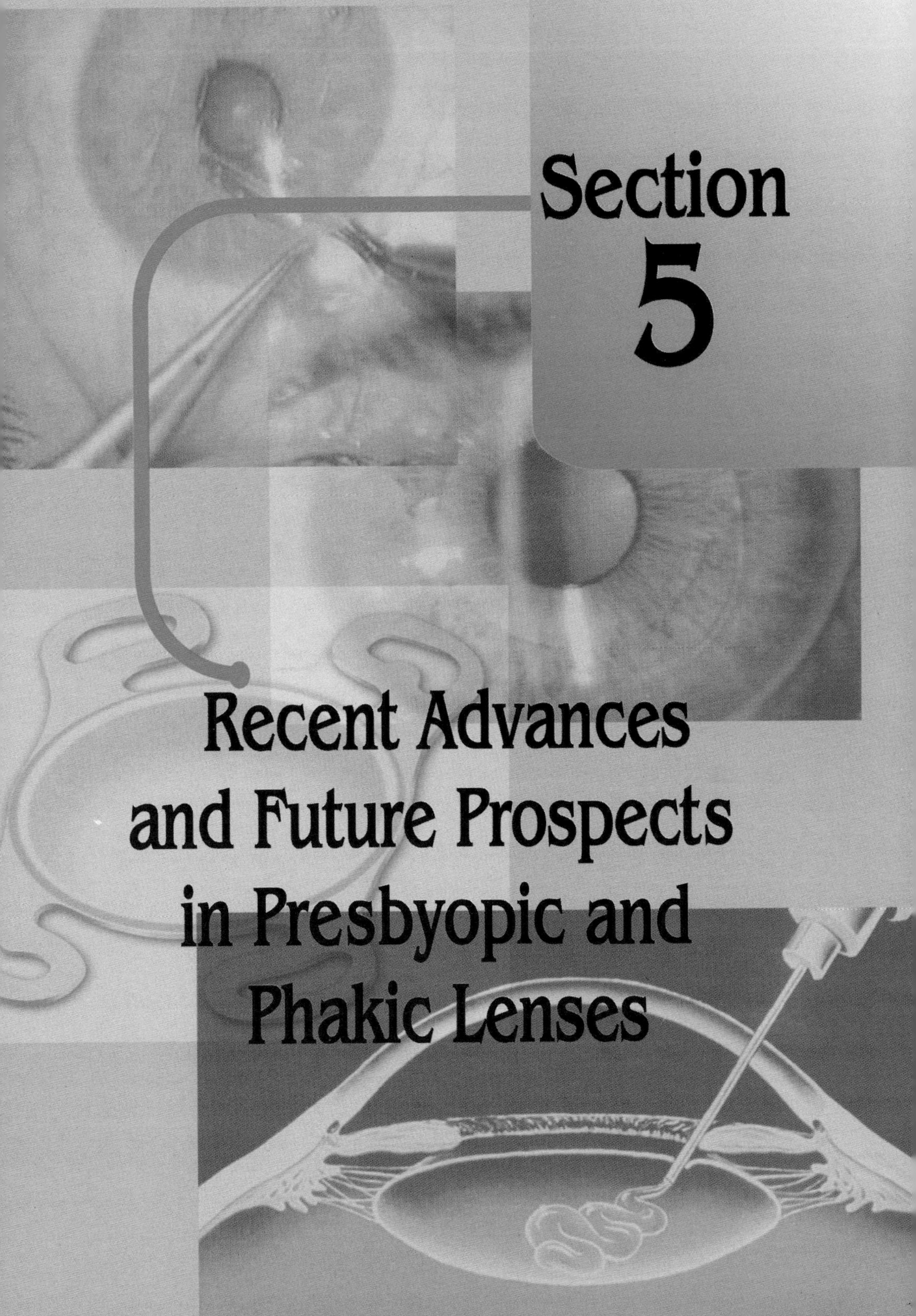

Section 5

Recent Advances and Future Prospects in Presbyopic and Phakic Lenses

CHAPTER

39

Dimitrii Dementiev (Italy)

Implantation of Phakic Refractive Lenses (PRL) in Pediatric/Myopic Eyes Associated with Scleral Reinforcement Surgery

INTRODUCTION

High myopia in early childhood can impede development of normal binocular vision and cause irreversible amblyopia. Myopic anisometropia, a condition in which there is more than 2-2.50 diopters (D) of difference between the refractive power of two eyes induces anisoconia resulting in difference of retinal image size. Left untreated, the perfect fusion of the two images is impossible, causing loss of binocular vision and deep amblyopia. The amount of amblyopia is usually correlated with the amount of anisometropia. Several times strabismus easy occurs in these patients. It is well-known that amblyopia cannot be treated in adult age. That is why the correct treatment of anisometropia in childhood is important for the prevention of amblyopia and strabismus. Current modalities to treat high ametropia in pediatrics are limited. At present, the refractive amblyopia in children is treated with spectacles or contact lenses associated with occlusive patching of the dominant eye. Various surgical treatments used successfully in adults as RK, LASIK or PRK have limited use in pediatric cases due to irreversibility of these refractive procedures, as well as the need for further refractive correction of progressive ametropia. However, significant impairment of life quality exists in this group of patients, as early intervention to prevent development of amblyopia is critical, especially in cases of unilateral myopia.

Phakic refractive lenses to treat ametropia have been in evolution since 1986. Current designs include anterior chamber lenses: iris-fixated,[1-6] angle-supported[7-12] and posterior chamber lenses.[13-33] The benefit of phakic refractive lenses in pediatrics is reversibility of the procedure. The potential concerns include lack of long-term information on complications, especially on cataractogenesis, iridocyclitis, glaucoma and retinal detachment.

Refractive procedures used in pediatric patients have included RK, PRK, LASIK and ICL posterior chamber lens implantation.[39-49]

The posterior chamber Phakic Refractive Lens (PRL™) has been used extensively in our practice in over 800 adult patients to treat high myopia and hyperopia. Results have included accuracy and stability of refraction, good vision quality and a low incidence of complications in these cases. The objective of this series was to evaluate the use of the PRL, following scleral reinforcement surgery to retard/prevent progression of axial myopia and to prevent/reversal of amblyopia in a small series of pediatric cases.

PATIENTS AND METHODS

Patients

Implantation of the PRL was performed in 11 eyes of 11 pediatric patients. The mean age of the 7 females and 4 males was 9.5 years (range 7 to 12 years). The preoperative mean spherical equivalent was –10.6 diopters (D) ranging from –7.0 D to –17.5 D. The refractive goal was emmetropia. The mean follow-up was 22.2 months.

Inclusion criteria were: All the patients had unilateral (anisometropic) axial myopia, amblyopia with the BCVA not less than 20/60 and not more than 20/40, strabismus was observed in 5 cases, progressive axial myopia were observed in all cases. Only the eyes with the clear media and no macular changes were chosen for this study. In all patients, all methods of amblyopia therapy had failed.

Unsuccessful occlusion therapy was observed partially due to high anisometropia and partially due to the psychological factors, 6 of the patients refused the occlusion and it was impossible to be sure that the eyes were patched in a right way. No prior procedures were performed to correct strabismus before the implantation of phakic implant.

Anterior chamber depth was 3.85 mm (+/– 0.42); in all the eyes the anterior chamber angle was seen open during the gonioscopy examination.

The exclusion criteria were: Shallow anterior chamber (less than 3.0mm), chronic inflammation, significant amblyopia with low BCVA and no potential for visual improvement, maculopathy, and persistent eye ipertension-glaucoma.

Preoperative evaluation included:
The best spectacle-corrected visual acuity (BSCVA) using Snellen chart, cycloplegic refraction, keratometry, tonometry (Tonopen), slit lamp examination, axial length and anterior chamber depth with A-scan method, gonioscopy, specular microscopy and fundus examination.

Six months after the first visit the AXL measurements and cycloplegic refraction examination were repeated to verify the progress of myopia.

The surgical procedure and its possible complications were explained to the parents, who signed the informed consent.

Surgical Procedure

The PRL *(IOLTECH /CARL ZEISS MEDITECH, FRANCE)* Figures 39.1 and 39.2 are a posterior chamber silicone lens for treatment of high myopia and hyperopia. The high refractive index (1.46) enables a slim optic profile and flexible design. The PRL dioptric power required for

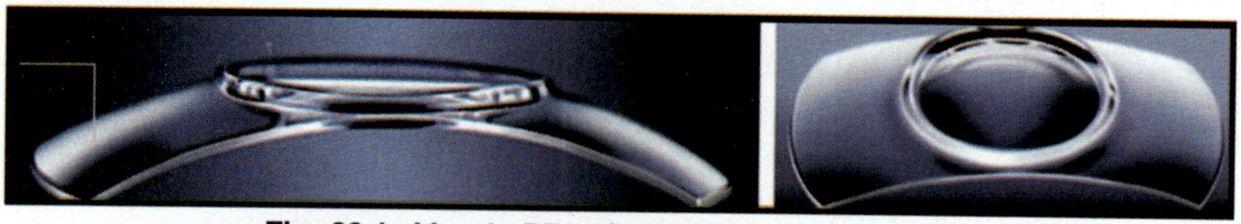

Fig. 39.1: Myopic PRL IOLtech/Carl Zeiss meditec

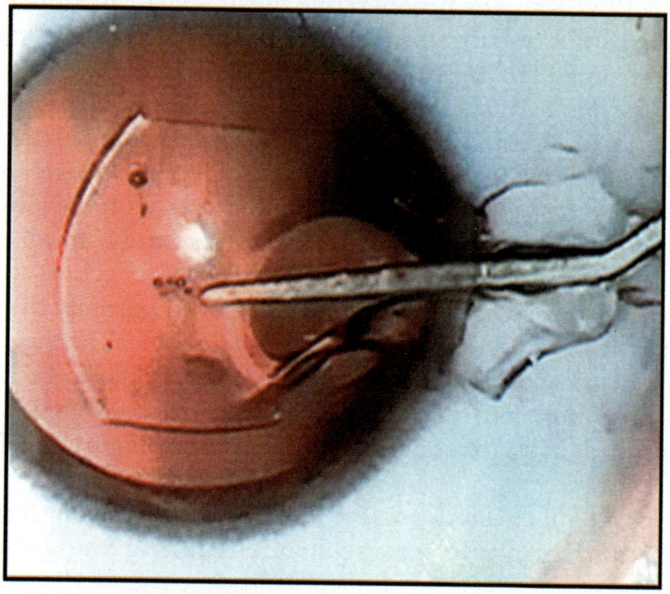

Fig. 39.2: PRL insertion with the forceps

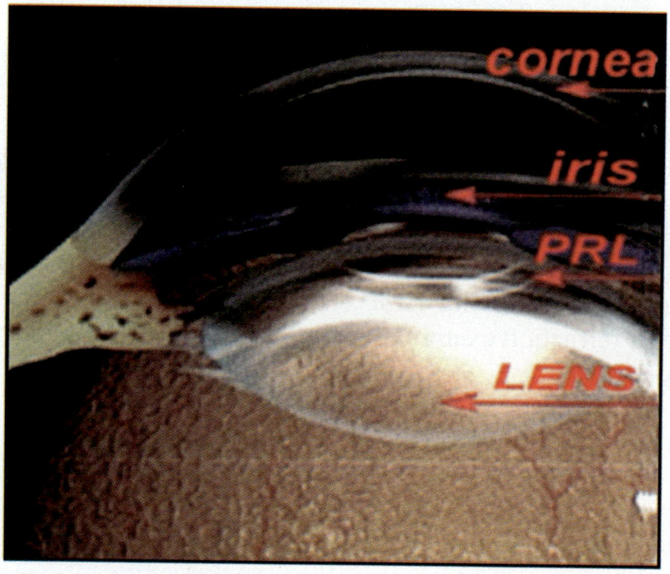

Fig. 39.3: Implant is floating in the posterior chamber, no sulcus fixation

each case was determined using formulas developed that incorporate the patient's refraction and vertex distance. The length of the implant was 11.3 mm, the width was 6.0 mm, and the optic center diameters were different: from 4.5 to 5.0 mm, according to the optic power of the implant. The lens is not fixed in the sulcus straightly, but "floats" in the posterior chamber touching the zonule with the distal and proximal edge. Being manufactured from the hydrophobic material the aqueous humor can move it easy towards the iris avoiding the contact with the anterior capsule of the crystalline lens (Fig. 39.3). Space between PRL and lens is well-seen during slit lamp examination and Ultrasonic Biomicroscopy (UBM), (Figs 39.4 to 39.6). I believe that free aqueous circulation in the posterior chamber even in presence of the PRL permits to maintain the normal lens metabolism and not to create its opacification.

Prior to implantation of the PRL, all the patients underwent unilateral scleral reinforcing surgery (scleroplasty)[34-38] in highly myopic eye to prevent or at least strongly retard progression of axial myopia.

All surgeries were performed under general anesthesia. No complications were noticed. In the period of 1-3 months after the scleroplasty all the patients underwent the next step of the treatment-PRL implantation for the correction of myopia.

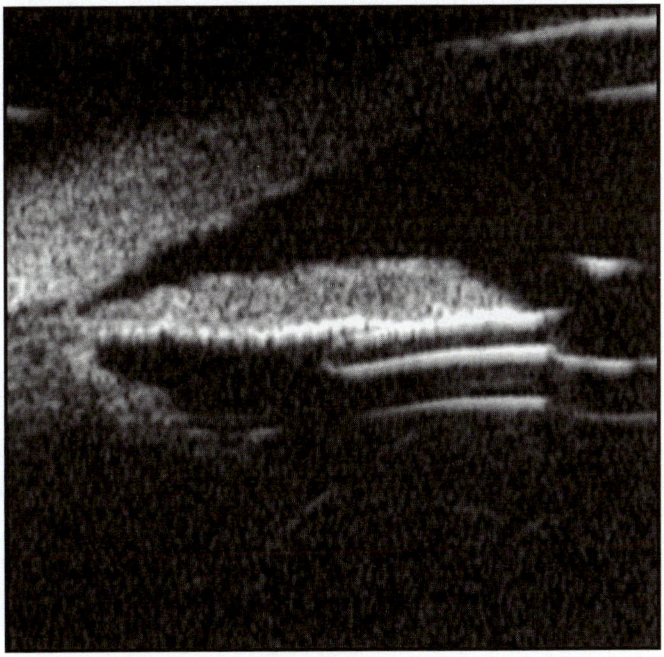

Fig. 39.4

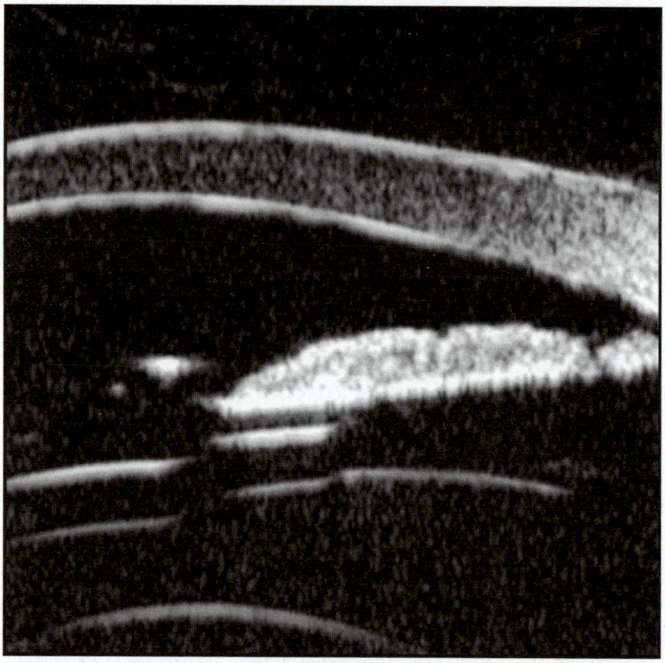

Fig. 39.5

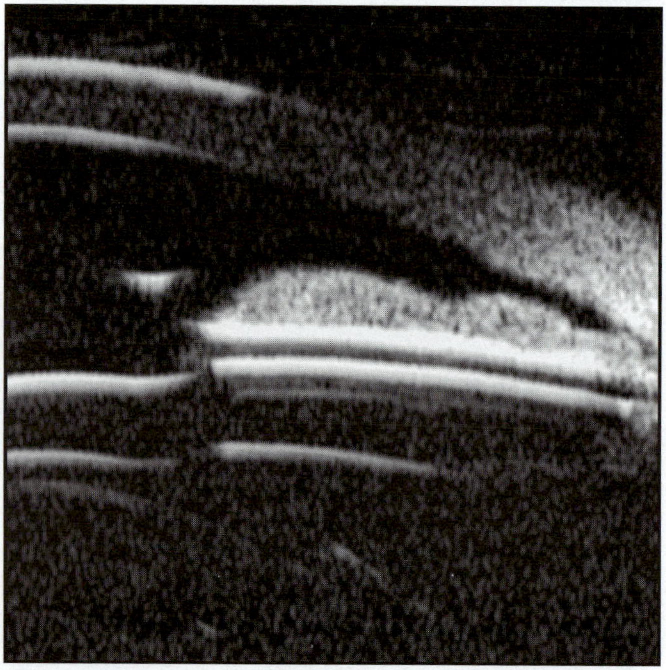

Fig. 39.6

UBM picture, evidence of the free space between PRL and anterior capsula, aqueous easy passes, no voulting is seen, floating in the posterior chamber

Every patient started to install the antibiotics drops (Tobramicin) 3 days before the surgery; the pupil was dilated (min. 8.0 mm) with midriacyl and fenelefrin 20 minutes before the procedure.

The PRL implantation was also performed under general anesthesia.

The clear cornea 3.0 mm incision was performed with *PRL Dementiev trapezoid blade (Rumex International, USA)* temporally, following injection of viscoelastic (Ophtaline® Ciba Vision), the paracentesis 1.0mm large was done at 12.00 in order to have the second access in AC for implant manipulation and peripheral iridectomy performance. The PRL was inserted through a temporal 3.0 mm. Clear corneal incision (see Fig. 39.3) using *Dementiev PRL forceps (Janach, Italy)* specially designed to insert the implant. Haptics were positioned posteriorly to the iris with a *Dementiev PRL manipulator (Janach, Italy)* and the PRL was centered. After viscoelastic removal with irrigation only and pupil constriction *(Miochol®),* a surgical iridectomy was performed through the previously created paracentesis at 12.00. No stitches were applied to the incision.

Tobradex and **pilocarpin** drops with the eye patching were the final steps of the surgery.

The postoperative regimen included:

1. Eye patched for one night.
2. Diamox 250 mg two times a day for 2 days
3. Tobradex drops 5-6 times a day for 10-12 days
4. Midriacyl 0.5 % drops 2 times a day for 3 days
5. Voltaren ofta drops 3 times a day for 7 days starting from the 10th day after procedure.
6. Patch occlusion of the fellow eye for the amblyopia treatment was starting from the 3rd day after the surgery.

Follow-up examinations were scheduled at 1, 3, 7 and 14 days, and at 1, 2, 3, 6 and 12 months, and thereafter as needed. Postoperative evaluations included slit lamp biomicroscopy, ocular symptomatology, BCVA, cycloplegic refraction at 14 days, 6 month and 1 year visits, IOP, anterior chamber depth all the visits, specular microscopy 6 months and 1 year visits, keratometry and gonioscopy 1 month and 1 year visits. AXL measurement at 1 year visit. Binocular vision testing 3 months, 6 months and 1 year visits.

Pre- and postoperative outcomes at the most recent visit are provided in Tables 39.1 and 39.2.

RESULTS

No surgical complications of PRL surgery were experienced. Three eyes developed increased IOP at 3 days postoperatively. Antiglaucoma

Table 39.1: Preoperative parameters

Patient/ Sex (F/M)	Age (years)	Cycloplegic spherical equivalent (D)	BCVA [or BSCVA]	Endothelial cell count	IOP (mm Hg)	AC depth (mm)
1/F	8	– 11.0	20/50	3475	14	3.87
2/F	11	– 10.0	20/50	3340	16	3.68
3/F	9	– 7.0	20/40	3105	14	3.69
4/F	10	–14.50	20/60	2980	18	3.90
5/F	8	– 9.0	20/40	3578	14	3.84
6/F	7	– 17.50	20/60	3160	16	3.95
7/F	11	– 10.0	20/50	3014	16	4.01
8/M	12	– 9.0	20/40	3246	17	3.81
9/M	10	– 8.75	20/50	3437	16	3.90
10/M	9	–13.00	20/50	3349	14	3.85
11/M	9	– 7.50	20/40	3298	15	3.90

Table 39.2: Postoperative parameters

Patient/ Sex (F/M)	Age (years)	Cycloplegic spherical equivalent (D)	BCVA [or BSCVA]	Endothelial cell count	IOP (mm Hg)	AC depth (mm)
1/F	8	– 0.50	20/40	3365	14	3.67
2/F	11	– 0.25	20/40	3150	17	3.57
3/F	9	0	20/20	2978	14	3.48
4/F	10	– 1.0	20/40	2847	16	3.70
5/F	8	– 0.50	20/20	3429	14	3.61
6/F	7	– 1.0	20/50	3051	17	3.73
7/F	11	0	20/40	2989	16	3.89
8/M	12	+ 0.25	20/20	3104	15	3.65
9/M	10	0	20/20	3321	16	3.80
10/M	9	– 1.0	20/40	3189	14	3.69
11/M	9	+ 0.50	20/40	3127	15	3.64

medications including diamox, trusopt, timoptol 0.5% were administered, and IOP returned to preoperative status by the 2-4 days after the treatment began. The implants remained centered throughout the follow-up examination period, and anterior chamber depth was maintained.

All patients improved their best corrected visual acuity and uncorrected visual acuity. Eight patients experienced an improvement of at least 4 lines by 3 months postoperatively. Additionally, 6 patients with the preoperative BCVA more than 20/50 developed binocular vision three months postoperatively and after 3 months of occlusion therapy of fellow eye.

Two patients improved 2 lines after 3 months of occlusion therapy. One patient improved only one line the first day after the surgery and it remained stable BCVA even after 3 months of occlusion therapy without further improvement.

Endothelial cell loss was not more than 4.0% in all the eyes, and no progress was noticed in the period from the 3rd months till the 6th months and 1.5 year visits.

Improvement of UCVA was in all the eyes from the first day after the surgery and was improving with the occlusion therapy till 6th months. At 1 year and 2 years control visit the same UCVA like 6 months control visit was noticed, except one eye of the youngest patient (age 9 YO during last visit) in which the UCVA is improving every visit. This patient is still under occlusion therapy daily 2 hours a day. Strabismus was improved in all 5 eyes of previously strabic patients. No any additional strabismus surgery was necessary. The progress of myopia was not noticed in all the period of follow-up, the measurement of AXL remained the same like after the scleroplasty procedure. Postoperatively, mean refraction was –0.5 D, and ranged from +0.5 to –1.0 D. Gonioscopy revealed open angles. No cataractogenesis was observed, and the status of the crystalline lens remained unchanged throughout the postoperative follow-up period.

DISCUSSION

To date refractive surgery in children remains controversial. The treatment of high anisometropic myopia and the resulting ambyopia however often fails. Current methods used are correction with contact lenses or glasses associated with eye patching. Often the wearing of contact lenses is not well-tolerated or the compliance is poor especially if the need for contact lens is for one eye only. Children who have myopic anisometropia and who refuse the conventional therapy are at risk of developing greater amblyopia when left without treatment. In these cases refractive surgery has been proposed. The procedures considered an option for refractive correction in adults in children might be the only way to treat amblyopia in children.

Radial keratotomy has been performed in some cases with poor results and many limits treating not more than 4-5 diopters.[39]

The use of excimer laser has been reported in children. Singh[40] reported PRK results in 10 children, 5 of whom were myopic. The results were good but 2 patients developed corneal haze. Nano[41] evaluated the results of PRK in 5 children with myopic anisometropia with 40% of haze incidence.

Aliò[42] reported results of 5 PRK treatments in myopic anisometropia having one case of severe corneal haze.

The destruction of Bowman's layer during PRK initiates a heavy healing response that is stronger in children than in adults. This process is responsible for the instability of refraction, regression of refractive effect and development of corneal haze. The need of using corticosteroids drops for several months after the procedure can cause a secondary rise of intraocular pressure.[43]

Also the LASIK procedure has been proposed in pediatric patients. Khaled[44] reported results of LASIK treatment of 14 eyes with myopic anisometropia and amblyopia (mean SE –7.87 D) with BSCVA improved in all eyes. The follow-up was of one year with spherical equivalent manifest refraction from 0 to –1.50 D at that time.

Niteen[7] described the results of three months of follow-up in 3 pediatric eyes of 3 anisometropic amblyopes treated with LASIK with satisfactory outcomes and relative stability.

Performing LASIK in children the progression of myopia after the surgery must be taken into account and the long term safety and predictability need further evaluation.

Our experience with highly myopic adults treated with implantation of Phakic Refractive Lens convinced us of the superiority of phakic IOLs in these cases. After the treatment of 11 pediatric eyes we feel completely satisfied with the results obtained with the PRL even in children. We had several reasons for preferring PRL to treat anisometropic myopia. The procedure is completely reversible; the phakic lens can be exchange to another one of different power in case of axial myopia progression or wrong power calculation. The quality of vision is often better and there is no fear of corneal haze or ectasia. The surgery is simple and fast. The only transitory postop adverse effect was transient IOP increase. There is no risk of corneal endothelial cell loss or pigment dispersion as it may happen with anterior chamber phakic lenses using the children rub their eyes. No anatomic complications were observed and BSCVA improved in all eyes implanted with PRL. 6 patients developed binocular vision. During the follow-up no cases of lens opacification, glaucoma or uveitis were noticed. The endothelial cell loss was about 4%, what is considered in the physiological range.

Scleral reinforcement surgery to prevent or limit the progression of axial myopia associated with subsequent PRL implantation to treat anisometropic amblyopia is an effective way to limit the handicap of highly myopic children. The functional outcomes are very satisfying and a marked progress in the child's quality of live was reported us by the parents. Encouraged by the results we are convinced that the procedure is safe and predictable to correct progressive myopia and amblyopia resulting from myopic anisometropia. Additional cases and longer follow-up observation are needed to evaluate the full extent of benefits of this technique in children.

REFERENCES

1. J.Worst. Phakic high myopia correction, ASCRS meet 1997 Boston
2. Landesz M., Worst JGF, Siertsema JV, Van Rij G."Correction of High Myopia with the Worst Myopia Claw Intraocular lens" XXVIII International Congress Ophtalmology, June 1998, Amsterdam, Holland.
3. Gelender H. "Corneal Endothelial Cell Loss, Cystoid Macular Edema, and iris- suported intraocular lenses. Ophtalmology 1984;91: 841-6.
4. JGF Worst. "Iris Anatomy and its Surgical Implications" XXVIII International Congress of Ophtalmology, June 1998,Amsterdam, Holland.
5. Izak M. "Worst Myopia Iris Claw IOL implantation" ASCRS annual meeting, april 1997 Boston, USA.
6. JGF Worst. "Recent improvements in phakic refrative correction with Iris Claw Lens" ASCRS annual meeting 1998, San Diego, USA.
7. Baikoff G, Arne JL, Bokobza Y, et al. Angle fixated anterior chamber phakic intraocular lens for myopia of –7 to –19 D. J Refract Surg 1998;14:282-93.
8. Menezo JL, Avino JA, Cisneros A, et al. Iris claw phakic intraocular lens for high myopia. J Refract Surg 1997;13:545-55.
9. Refractive Baikoff Anterior Chamber Lenses Implantation, U.Kariger ASCRS 1997.
10. Baikoff G, Colin J. "Intraocular Lenses in Phakic Patients" Ophtalmol Clin North Am.1992;5.
11. Saragoussi JJ,et al. "Damage to the corneal endothelium by minus power anterior chamber intraocular lenses." Refract Corneal Surg. 1991;7.
12. Fechner PU. Intraocular lenses for the correction of myopia in phakic eyes: Short long success and long term caution. Refract Corneal surgery 1990; 6:242-4.
13. Tumanian E. "Surgical correction of high myopia by the method of implantation of negative phakic IOL."In Russian, Diss. Kand. Medic 1989; 158-64.
14. Fyodorov, Zuev, Aznabaev. "Intraocular correction of high myopia with negative posterior chamber lens." Ophtalmosurgery 1991;3:57-8.
15. Fyodorov,Zuev, Tumanian,Suheil. Clinical and functional follow up of minus IOL implantation in high grade myopia. Ophtalmosurgery 1993;2:12-17).
16. E Tumanian, VK Zuev, TV Koslova. "Hydrodynamics before and after implantation of negative IOL in highly myopic phakic eye". Ophtalmosurgery, 4:1997, 50-6.
17. Grabby,Deitz,Fyodorov. Staar implantable contact lens(ICL) in: Martin RG, Dills JP, Sanders DR. Eds, Foldable Intraocular Lenses. Slack, INC, Thorafare, NJ 1993,pp 251-5.
18. Asseto, Benedetti, Pesando. "Collamer intraocular contact lens to correct high myopia, J Cataract Refract Surg,1996;22.
19. Luger MHA. "The Staar Collamer phakic posterior chamber IOL to correct myopia and hyperopia," XXVIIIth ICO, Amsterdam 1998.

20. DJ Apple. Complications of Phakic IOL,s AAO annual meet 1998 New Orleans.
21. R. Zaldivar, J Davidorf, S Osheraw. "Intarocular Contact Lens" in LASIK 2000 of L.Buratto. M.Ferrari.Fabiano Editore, Belbo(CN), 1998.pp 359-75.
22. J M Davidorf, R Zaldivar, S Oscherow "Posterior Chamber Phakic Intraocular Lenses for Hyperopia of +4 to +11 Diopters " and " Posterior Chamber Phakic Intraocular lenses for Myopia of –8.0 to –19.0 Diopters" J. Refract Surg. May/June 1998, Vol.14, N.3.
23. D Dementiev. Comparison of tree generations of Posterior Chamber Phakic Lenses for the Correction of high myopia and hypropia, ASCRS 1997, Boston,USA..
24. A Hatsis. Phakic Posterior IOLs for the correction of high Hyperopia and high Myopia, ASCRS 1997, Boston,USA.
25. G Rozakis, D Dementiev, A Hatsis, G Avalos. Complications of silicon phakic posterior chamber lenses for the correction of high ammetropia. ASCRS 1998, San Diego. USA.
26. A Tereschenko. "Complications of minus silicone Posterior Chamber Phakic Lenses":ASCRS annual meet. 1997,Boston,Usa.
27. D Dementiev, G Rozakis, A Hatsis, K Hoffer, G Sborgia, P Marucchi. "The 5 Years Experience in the Phakic Refractive Posterior Chamber I.O.L. Implantation for the correction of High Ametropia" Binkhorst Symposium during XXVIII International Congress of Ophtalmology, 1998 June,Amsterdam, Holland.
28. G Avalos. " Comparison Between LASIK and Phakic Posterior Chamber Intraocular Lenses in High Myopia and High Hyperopia" ASCRS annual meet., april 1998, San Diego, USA.
29. D Dementiev. "Silicone Phakic Posterior Chamber Intraocular Lens (P-PCIOL) and the management of pediatric Anisometropia." ASCRS annual meeting apr 1998, San Diego, USA.
30. G Avalos. "Silicone Posterior Chamber Intraocular Lens(P-PCIOL) in the management of LASIK complications."ASCRS annual meet. April 1998, San Diego, USA.
31. A Hatsis. "Silicone Posterior Chamber Intraocular Lens (P-PCIOL), American Blind Eye Study." ASCRS annual meet. April 1998, San Diego, USA.
32. G Rozakis, D Dementiev, G Avalos, A Hatsis "Complications of silicone phakic posterior chamber intraocular lens (P-PCIOL) for the Correction of High Ametropia." ASCRS annual meet. Apr1998, San Diego, USA.
33. Holladay JT. Refractive power calculation for intraocular lenses in the phakic eye. Amer J Ophthalmol 1993; 116:63-6 (24)
34. Kanski J. Clinical Ophthalmology. Butterworth Ltd., 1989, 360,Woo GC., Wilson MA. Current methods of treating and preventing myopia. Optometry and vision science. 1990;67(9):719-27.
35. Sosnier Z. Evaluation of the effect of Synder-Thompson scleroplasty based on the behavior of the axial dimension of the eye ball. Klin. Oczna. 1989 Jan;91:19-20.
36. Tratta E, Shamlokova E. An analysis of the late results of scleroplasty in progressive myopia. Ophthal Zh.1989; (4):204-7.
37. Tarutta E, Saksanova E. Peripheral segments of the fundus oculi in highly myopic patients after scleroplasty. Vestn Opht 1991 Jul-Aug;107 (4):19-23.
38. Zaikova M, Molokova N. Scleroplasty results in progressive myopia with use of allogenic. Vestn. Opht 1990 May-June;106(3):16-9).

39. Von Norden GK, Bleik JH. Controversies in Ophthalmology- Radial keratotomy for the reduction of myopic anisometropia in children. Middle East J Ophthalmol 1993;1;81.
40. Singh D. Photorefractive keratectomy in pediatric patients. J Cataract Refract Surg 1995;21:630-2.
41. Nano HD Jr, Muzzin S, Irigaray F. Excimer laser photorefractive keratectomy in pediatric patients. J Cataracr Refract Surg 1997;23:736-9.
42. Aliò JL, Artola A, Claramonte P, et al. Photorefractive keratectomy for pediatric myopic anisometropia. J Cataract Refract Surg 1998;24:327-30.
43. Morale J, Good D. Permanent glaucomatous visual loss after photorefractive keratectomy. J Cataract Refract Surg 1998;24:715-8.
44. Khaled M Rashad. Laser in situ Keratomileusis for myopic anisometropia in children. J Refract Surg 1999;15:429-35.
45. Niteen C, Dedhia, Seema Behl. Laser in situ keratomileusis for anisometropic amblyopia. J Refract Surg 2000;16: S264-67.
46. F. Lavery. "Laser in situ Keratomilesusis for Myopia" Jornal of Refractive Surgery, apr 1998.
47. E K Vorotnikova, V V Kurenkov, G S Polunin. "Retreatment of Regression after Photorefractive Keratectomy for Myopia." Jornal of Refractive Surgery, apr.1998 Vol 14, N.2 (supl.).
48. Y Wang, K Zhao, H Wang. "Histopatoplgy of corneal wound healing after PRK in rabbit eyes"- Journal of Refractive Surgery, Apr 1998 Vol 14, N.2 (supl.).
49. A Chatterjee, S Shah "Predictability of spherical PRK based on initial refraction"-Journal Refractive Surgery, Apr 1998 Vol 14, N.2 (supl).

CHAPTER

40

Keiki R Mehta, Cyres K Mehta (India)

Multifocal IOLs in Children: A Long-term Analysis

PEDIATRIC CATARACT SURGERY

Most challenging surgery, not only in ophthalmic speciality but in any branch of surgery. It needs follow up for the rest of life. It has changed considerably in last 20 years, because of early intervention and immediate optical correction.

Though intraocular implants in children are a well-established entity, it required the efforts of McClatchey & Hofmesiter (1997, 1998, 2000, 2005) who demonstrated that after the age of 6 months, the intraocular power calculation follows a virtual linear logarithmic pattern thus proving that the refractive status of the eye can be predicted with a high level of accuracy.

Coupled with the ability to achieve this level of accuracy are the advent of the newer more sophisticated computer controlled machines and the availability of alternative modalities to ultrasound like neosonx and aqualase

Until the availability of mutifocal IOLs one had to be content wth monofocal IOL for children the most popular being the Alcon single piece and multipiece AcrySof IOL. The material, thanks to its bioadhesive ability and the restriction of capsular growth due to the square edged design made it a very [popular IOL in infants and children .

All was good except that the child had, for practical purposes very limited near vision and since, for children, their proximal horizon accounts for more than 80% of their daily activities, it became extremely problematical. There is nothing sadder than to see a little child with reading glasses or wearing bifocal trying to move his head to focus. It placed a great deal of restrictions on the daily activities and in many ways was psychological reminder to both the children and the parents that the child was a visually deficient.

Stein 2004, critically analyzed and brought out three salient factors which need consideration a) Critical period of visual maturation completes in 3 to 4 months period. b) Upto the age of 8 months the visual apparatus goes on developing at a very rapid rate, and perhaps the most important c) The ability to see near and distance important for the child to be able to develop depth perception and enhance visual development.

Jacobi PC; Dietlein TS2001 from the University of Cologne, Cologne, Germany, evaluated implantation of a zonal-progressive multifocal intraocular lens (IOL) in children. Thirty-five eyes of 26 pediatric patients aged 2 to 14 years with multifocal IOL implantation at one institution with more than 1 year of follow-up using a multifocal IOL

(Array SA40-N; Allergan, Irvine, CA) implantation in all eyes. Their results were very encouraging . Twenty-six patients (35 eyes) had an average follow-up of 27.4 +/– 12.7 months (range, 12-58 months). At last follow-up, best-corrected distance visual acuity improved significantly (P = 0.001), 71% of eyes with a visual acuity of 20/40 or better and 31% of eyes with a visual acuity of 20/25 or better. In the 9 bilateral cases, spectacle dependency was moderate, with only 2 children (22%) reporting the permanent use of an additional near correction. The remaining children were either using distance-correction only (4 patients; 44%) or no glasses at all (3 patients; 33%). Stereopsis also improved significantly after multifocal IOL implantation (P = 0.01. concluded: Multifocal IOL implantation is a viable alternative to monofocal pseudophakia in this age group.

With all the above factors described started a thought towards the use of multifocal implants in infants and children. In the earlier days, the Array (AMO) had the problems of decentrage, typical to silicone based IOLs. The newer hydrophobic acrylic material, the allergen ReZoom ReStor, do not suffer from that problem.

CAN CHILDREN AND INFANTS MANAGE MULTIFOCALITY?

The Institute runs a well-established contact lens clinic However for many years, fitting contact lenses in small children has been a labor of love. Unfortunately the success rates with contact lenses even in the best of hands has been poor. Implants were the obvious answer and were implanted in all cases unless contraindicated with nystagmus, microphthalmos, uncontrolled glaucoma. It has been a practice that following implantation that the children were always fitted with varifocal glasses. Children adapt to varifocality very easily . There is never the problems of adaptation. Even a 4-year-old once he perceives the obvious benefits will wear his glasses. Not having separate reading glasses or having glasses with a bifocal segment obvious, makes wearing of the glasses easier with no social stigma attached to them.

Considering how easily children accept varifocality, and with the encouraging results in the ophthalmic literature we had decided on the concept of multifocal IOL for all children over the age of 2 years. An additional small power could be worn over as single vision glasses, in those whom we had calculated as an excess, which would over time, with the myopic shift achieve emmetropia in adulthood. Naturally as the reading addition in the implants sufficed for all.

MULTIFOCAL IOLs IN CHILDREN

We commenced multifocal IOLs in 2002 February. The one good IOL available was the Allergan Array IOL. A year later came the Preziol which was a three zone refractive IOL made by the CareGroup.

The results were immediate. The children were very contented and there was no immediate problem. The long-term problem of the Array was the tendency to shift out from the center (decenter) due to eccentric bag contraction typical of silicone IOLs.

In 2005 came the newer ReZoom, 5 zone multifocal and in early 2006 came the ReStor IOL made by Alcon, the first 2 infants were implanted with the ReStor in India in March and June of 2006. Implantation of a zonal-progressive multifocal IOLs in pediatric cataract patients provides a high level of distance-corrected far, intermediate and near vision, reduced spectacle dependence and improved binocular vision

Again the acceptability was very good. The ReZoom and the ReStor gave good intermediate vision which was very gratifying.

At present we have restricted ourselves to the ReZoom and the ReStor while the Preziol has been kept for those who cannot afford the otherwise,extremely (for India) costly IOLs. Interestingly, though the Preziol is a 2 stage IOL, still some intermediate vision is existent too and the patients even with the more economical implant are quite satisfied.

The AcrySof ReSTOR ® intraocular lens has a patented optic design using apodization, diffraction and refraction technologies.

Apodization is a gradual reduction or blending of the diffractive step heights. The apodized diffractive optic design gives it the ability to focus light correctly on the retina for images at various distances without mechanical movement of the lens.

Apodization optimally manages light energy delivered to the retina because it distributes the appropriate amount of light to near and distant focal points, regardless of the lighting situation.

Apodization based diffractive optics are designed to improve image quality while minimizing visual disturbances. The result is an increased range of quality vision that delivers a high level of spectacle freedom.

The ReZoom™ multifocal lens has a patented lens design called *Balanced View Optics*™ technology. This lens design creates multiple focal points so patients can see well at a variety of distances, be it near, mid-distance, or far.

The ReZoom™ multifocal lens has carefully proportioned visual zones that provide it with the ability to provide patients with vision at varying distances.

Each ReZoom ™ multifocal lens is divided into five different zones with each zone designed for different light and focal distances.

Unlike other earlier multifocal lens designs,(Array) the ReZoom™ multifocal lens has proportioned the size of its zones to provide for good vision in a range of light conditions

PERIOPERATIVE ROUTINE AND SELECTION OF ANESTHETIC AGENTS

There is no need to separate children and parents as this is a very trying time for both. Too early an separation leads to a distraught mother and a crying unhappy non-cooperative child. Ideally children may receive clear liquids 4 hr before surgery without increasing the risk of aspiration.

Though many institutions routinely use premedication for young children (between 18 months and 5 years of age) before ophthalmic procedures we have never found it necessary.

Both inhalational and intravenous general anesthetic techniques have been used successfully for pediatric cataract surgery. However, with the exception of a history of malignant hyperthermia, most general anesthesia in young children undergoing cataract surgery is done with an inhalational agent. Isoflurane has widely replaced halothane as the induction agent of choice in children. It possesses a less offensive odor than other volatile agents, is less stimulating to the airway, and lacks the arrhythmogenic properties of halothane.

Nitrous oxide, traditionally used with volatile anesthetics, may increase postoperative nausea and vomiting. The cause-and-effect relationship between nausea/vomiting and nitrous oxide remains controversial.

Propofol is the intravenous induction agent of choice for cataract surgery in older pediatric patients and those with preoperative intravenous access. Propofol is an isopropyl phenol that has a rapid onset and offset of action. It is used for the induction and maintenance of anesthesia or sedation. Intravenous injection of a therapeutic dose of propofol produces hypnosis rapidly with minimal excitation. Propofol is also believed to have antiemetic properties. It effectively produces hypnosis of short duration with minimal "hangover."

We usually combine it with ketamine hydrochloride, a dissociative anesthetic that can be used for the induction and maintenance of anesthesia. However, ketamine hydrochloride does causes an increase in IOP, which should be kept in mind when following patients with glaucoma.

During anesthesia, even in patients whose IOP is usually normal, an increase in pressure can produce catastrophic effects. And may lead to prolapse of the iris and lens and loss of vitreous. Therefore, proper control of IOP is critical. We usually supplement the anesthesia with a1.5 cc sub tenon block and let the eye soften for 3 minutes which obviates much of the risk of inhalation or inject able anesthesia.

Bell's phenomenon is an useful indicator an can be seen at any time during anesthesia when the patient's depth of anesthesia has changed. It manifests as upward (or sometime downward) movement of the eye. It is usually a sign of being light, although the patient is not awake. It is an indicator that the anesthesiologist should be prepared to "deepen" the anesthesia to facilitate surgery.

OCULOCARDIAC REFLEX

The oculocardiac reflex is stimulated by pressure on the globe and/ or by traction on the extraocular muscles, the conjunctiva, or the orbital structures. The afferent limb is trigeminal and the efferent limb is vagal. Although the oculocardiac reflex is commonly associated with bradycardia, virtually any dysrhythmia, including ventricular tachycardia and asystole, may be seen.

It must be remembered that children have increased vagal tone and, therefore, are more likely to present with the reflex. If a dysrhythmia appears, the surgeon to cease the manipulation and check that the depth of anesthesia and ventilatory status are adequate. Usually, the heart rate and rhythm return to baseline within 20 sec. If the reflex becomes a problem, atropine should be given intravenously.

SURGICAL TECHNIQUE

A well-made surgical tunnel is mandatory for babies and young children. It is important that the tunnels be made-well. The first step is to make two 0.8 mm tunnels at 9.00 o'clock and 2.00 o'clock. The tunnels are made by applanating the scleral surface so that the tunnels are longer than they are broad. The next step is to fill the eye with an OVD (Ophthalmic Viscosurgical Device). The best in the opinion of the authors is Viscoat By Alcon. The next best is Healon 5. The most economical is methylcellulose which unfortunately runs out freely. If Methylcellulose is to be utilized it should be frozen (kept under the freezer) . Methylcellulose increases its viscosity by a factor of 3 if frozen and does not run out at all. However, once it warms up it runs again freely.

The next step is to carefully 'construct' the corneal incision . Refill OVD. Once again taking a 2.8 mm diamond blade (ideal for children) applanated it to the sclera and then advance. Only enter the tunnel after the length is more than the breadth. *Be careful when removing the blade not to incise the sides of the tunnel.*

Rhexis in young children is best commenced with a sharp bent 27 G needle as the capsule is tough and does not give way easily and then continue the rhexis with a capsule forceps refilling the OVD at regular intervals. Do remember in children that the tendency is for the rhexis to increase. So plan for a 5 mm rhexis, and it invariably becomes bigger. If the eye is soft, after a block, rhexis is far easier. To do a rhexis in a tight eye is foolish as it will run away.

Hydrodissection under the rhexis is done with a blunt tipped side ported 24 G cannula. That way accidental injury to the capsule is avoided if the chamber suddenly shallows. The Hydrodissection is started at the 7 o'clock position and fliuid injected slowly in all the clock hours . Usually the nucleus will tumble out if the cataract is soft.

The authors use the Alcon AquaLase which uses bursts of warmed water as a routine in children. It has a polymer blunt ti p which protects the capsule. It is essential not to increase the suction too much. Usually all the cortex can be easily removed with the AquaLase but if any is left behind it can be easily removed with a I/A bimanual system.

AquaLase polishing if the capsule is essential. It leaves a very clean capsule. If not available than manual polishing of the capsule is compulsory.

Refill the chamber with the OVD of your choice and inject in the IOL.

The intraocular implant is [placed in its folder being careful to be sure that it is properly sited and then injected into the eye using the proprietary injector. The 2.8 mm incision is more than adequate for both the Rezoom and the ReStor IOL and even the Preziol which has its own disposable injector.

The pupil is narrowed with a miotic (Intracameral pilocarpine 1% with no preservative works well.) The pupil must be brought down to less than 4 mm prior leaving the case as in a child any sudden pressure will lead to the IOL being captured in the iris.

Up to the age of 4 years we do a posterior rhexis, but that to only after implanting the IOL, after ascertaining that the pressure and the anesthesia is very stable. The PCCC is followed by a short core anterior vitrectomy. The vitrectomy is an essential part of the procedure. Reports mention almost 63% of PCCC close by secondary membrane formation if core vitrectomy is not carried out. Usually following the AquaLase polishing the capsules are very clear. We prefer to delay doing the Posterior capsulotomy if the conditions are not ideal and prefer to enter via after 3 months when the IOL has had a good chance to stabilize.

After the age of 4 we prefer to simply do a Yag capsulotomy as a more stable procedure.

The chamber following surgery must reform with saline, and stay formed on the table. If the chamber immediately flattens, it is prudent to take a single 10/0 Vicryl buried stitch at the site of the corneal incision.

An exceptional cleaning of the anterior chamber should be done. Meticulous removal of even slight traces of blood from anterior chamber at the end of surgery is must.

Epithelial cell metaplasic activities uses the intact anterior vitreous face, as well as surface of IOL as scaffolding, also RBCs are source of fibrosis.

Postoperative treatment is fairly simple. We do not permit the mother to handle a infant or even a small child's eyes under any circumstance. The mother is taught to place the drops in the inner corner of the eye and simply pat the child on the abdomen gently and wait. The moment the eye opens the drops go in. The child lids are very tight and very closely apposed to the eye . Any forcible effort only leads to the drops being literally "wipered" off. Previously we used to use tobramycin, now replaced by moxifloxacin eye drops tid with prednisolone eye drops tid.

It is coupled with oral steroids. Oral drops of betamethasone, 10 drops, bid for children under 3 years of age, tid for upto 5 years of age and qid for over for a month. This usually takes care of any inflammation. We do not use mydriatics, but prefer to use a drop of 1% pilocar once a day for a month. In this regime, we never get lens capture, get perfectly centered pupils and do not have any inflammation.

POSTERIOR RHEXIS AND VITRECTOMY

There have been many publications since the time that Gimbel taught that a PCCC with a optic capture is the way to go. If the eye is soft, and the child is under GA with a positive pressure insufflations, doing a PCCC is easy. However, if the anesthesia is not perfect and the eye is a bit tight, an attempt at PCCC often leads to a tear with vitreous in the A/C which means that the stability of the IOL is immediately at risk.

Statistics

We have done, 157 eyes, 65 are bilateral, 27 are unilateral of over the last 41/2 years starting from February of 2002. The results have been very gratifying. The maximum multifocal IOLs have been with the Array with the next highest, the Preziol. The only reason being that they were available earlier. We have nor restricted ourselves to the Rezoom and the Restor with the Preziol for the unaffording.

The visual results have been excellent in the bilateral group with 88% of them achieving 6/12 or better with the maximum correction and N8 easily. The unilateral group consisted of some who are bilateral but have not yet had the surgery done in the other eye. Again the results are excellent but the unilateral cataract with no or negligible cataract in the second eye have all achieved an maximum result of 6/18, 4 of whom are 6/24 which is reasonable considering that unilateral cataracts invariably do not do as well due to a latent amblyopia. Interestingly, the near vision is N8 which shows the near vision seems to be better than the distance in these unilateral cataracts. 9 eyes had to be re-operated to center the IOL (Tables 40.1 to 40.4).

Table 40.1: Multifocal IOLs implanted

Unilateral or bilateral				
Unilateral	*%*	*Bilateral*	*%*	*Total children*
27	29.3	65	70.7	92

Total eyes 27 + 130 (65*2) = 157 eyes

Table 40.2: Age at implantation

Age at implantation	*No*	*%*
2-3 years	27	17.2
4-6 years	47	29.9
7-9 years	38	24.2
10-12 years	45	28.7

Table 40.3: Complications n = 157

Complication	*No*	*%*
Corneal abrasion	03	1.9
Shallow A/C	11	7.0
Iritis mild	12	7.6
Iritis severe	03	1.9
Raised IOP ..Temp	15	9.6
Raised IOP .needed surgery	02	1.3
Hyphema	07	4.4
IOL decentrage requiring surg.	09	5.7

Table 40.4: Types of IOL implanted

Type of IOL implanted	*Manufacturer*	*No*	*%*
Preziol	(Care Group)	40	25.4
Array	(AMO)	74	47.2
ReZoom	(AMO)	36	23.0
ReStor	(Alcon)	7	4.4

CONCLUSION

It would seem from a 41/2 years study which we are still evaluating that a primary Multifocal IOL is the way to go in infants and your pediatric cataracts.

- Regrettably children are brought too late, parents and doctors are not aware of cataract. There are still too many opinions regarding whether an IOL should be placed in a small child, let alone a multifocal IOL, and invariably the parents are skeptical about surgery.
- Too many opinions, wastes precious time. Equally unfortunate is the concept in India of waiting till the cataract is mature to the level that one cannot see one's finger in adults.. It is this concept which they apply to the child not realizing that it will, in the long run affect the rehabilitation of the child.
- It is also important to calculate the power as precisely as possible and if there is residual ametropia… correct with glasses or contact lenses as may prove necessary and consider the option of doing an Excimer laser at a later date after the child grows up.

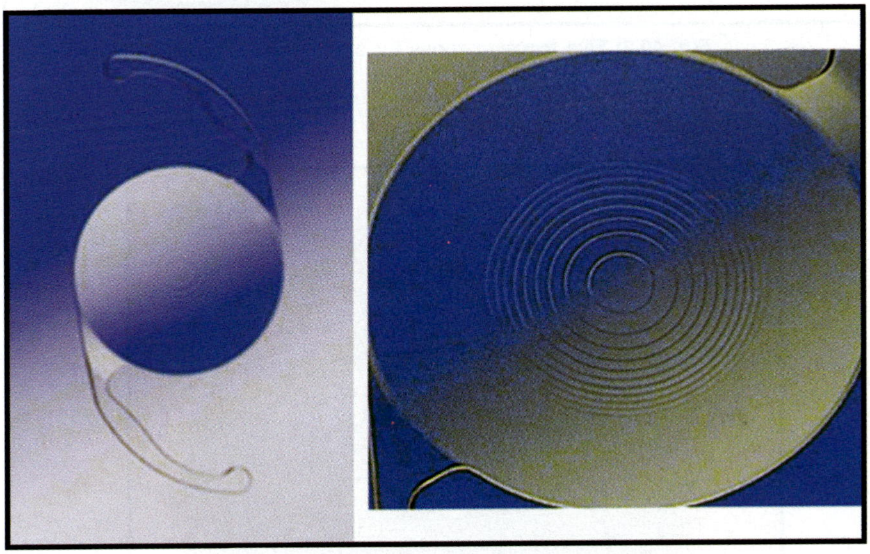

Fig. 40.1: ReStor IOL

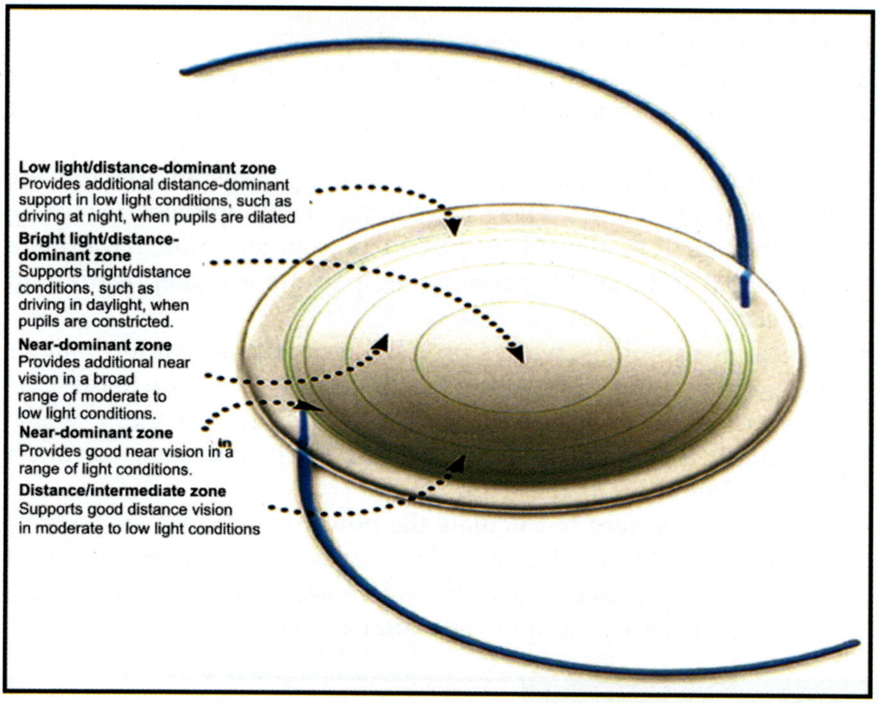

Fig. 40.2: Five focusing zones for a full range of vision

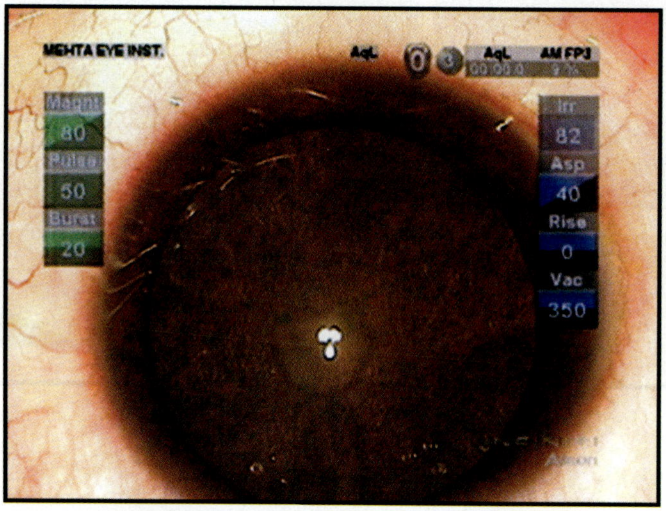

Fig. 40.3: Central cataract in a 6-year-old child

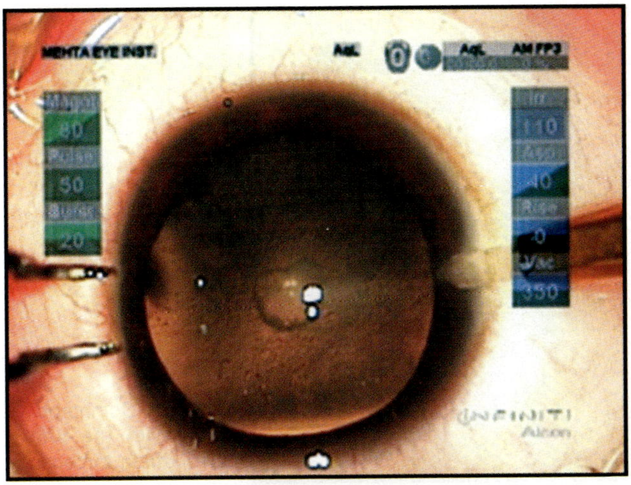

Fig. 40.4: A 0.8 mm diamond side port at 9 o'clock

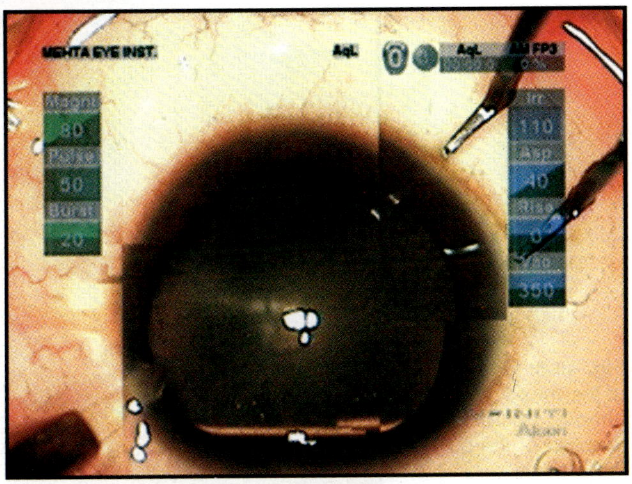

Fig. 40.5: A 0.8 mm diamond side port at 2 o'clock

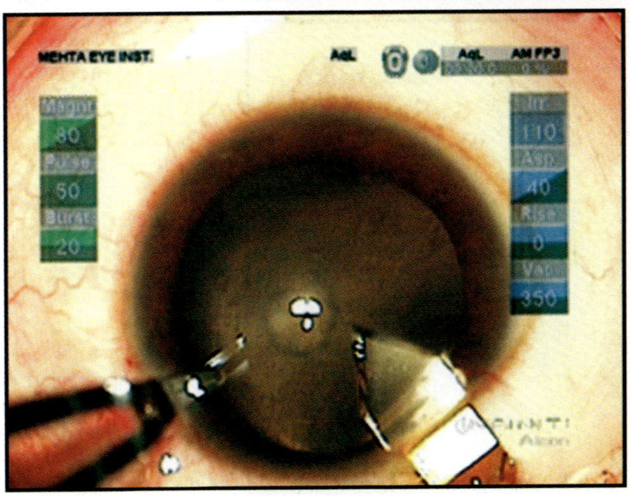

Fig. 40.6: A 2.8 mm tunnel is made . Not the length of the square tunnel

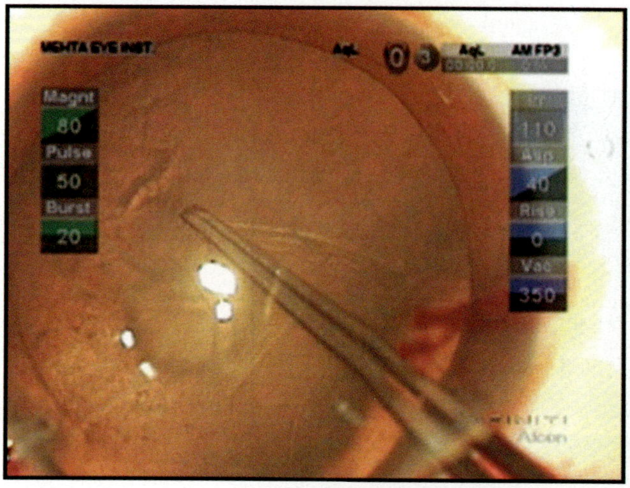

Fig. 40.7: Commencing rhexis with the sharp tipped Utrata forceps

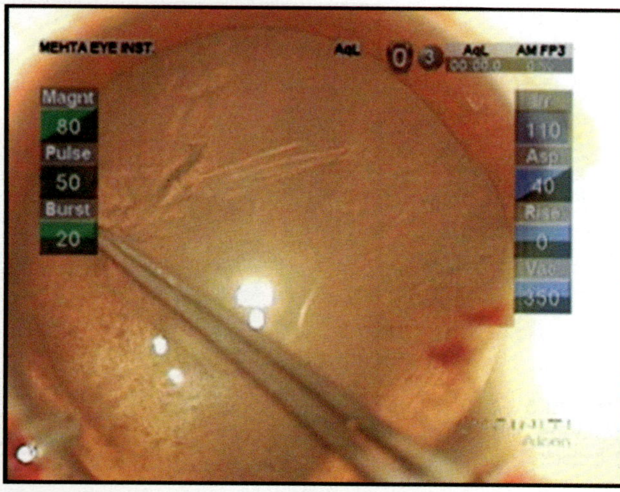

Fig. 40.8: Completion of the rhexis. Note the almost 90 degrees direction of the pull on the capsule

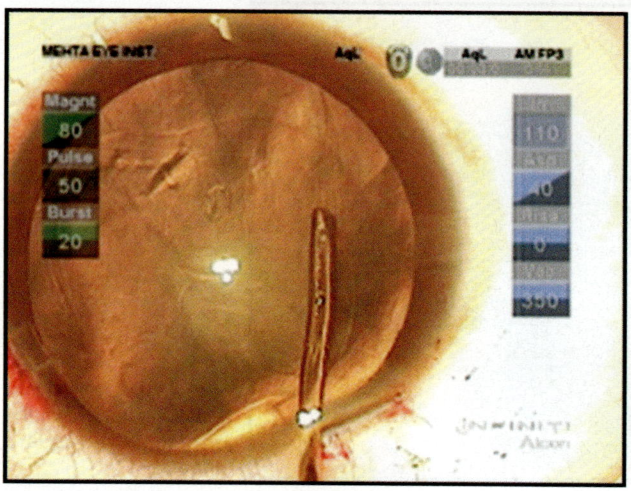

Fig. 40.9: Application of the viscoelastic. Since AquaLase will be utilized, the hydrodissection is not done

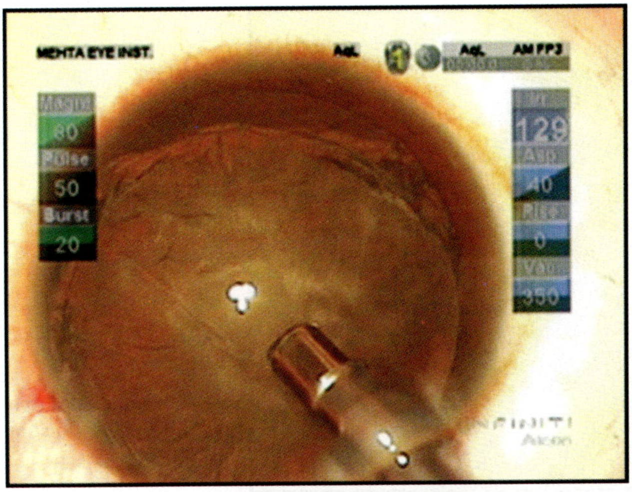

Fig. 40.10: AquaLase grooving off the nuclear mass in the center

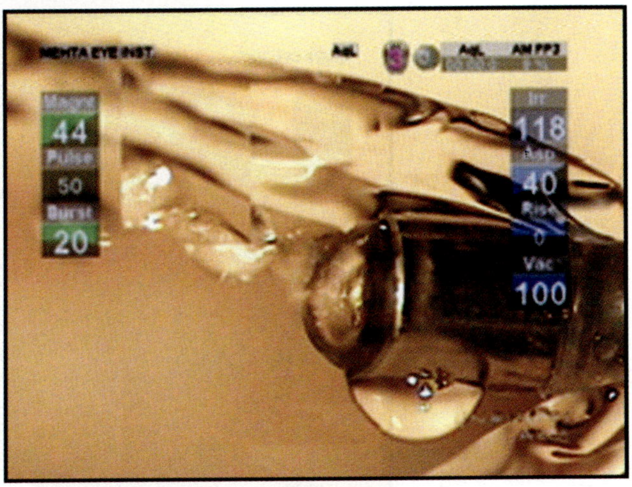

Fig. 40.11: The AquaLase tip showing the polymer tip and the pulsed fluid flow

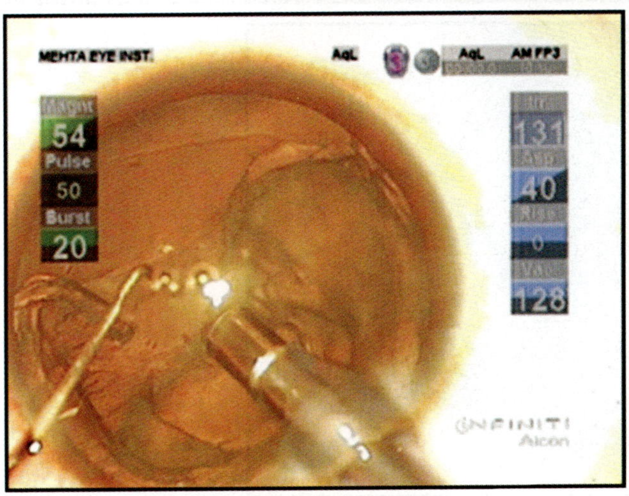

Fig. 40.12: Note the nuclear mass enfolded and being AquaLased off

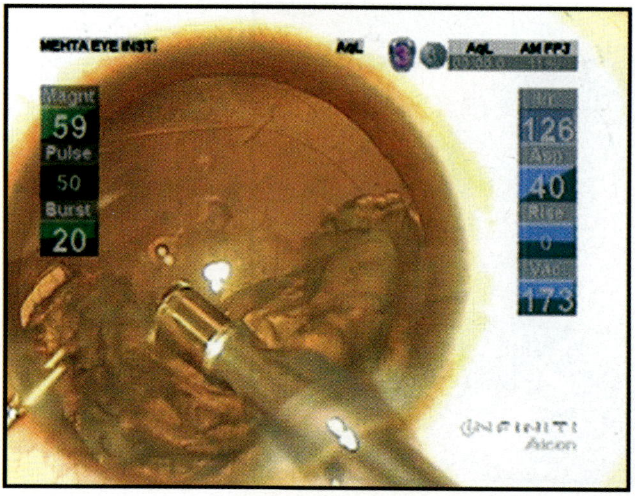

Fig. 40.13: AquaLase working on the nuclear fragments

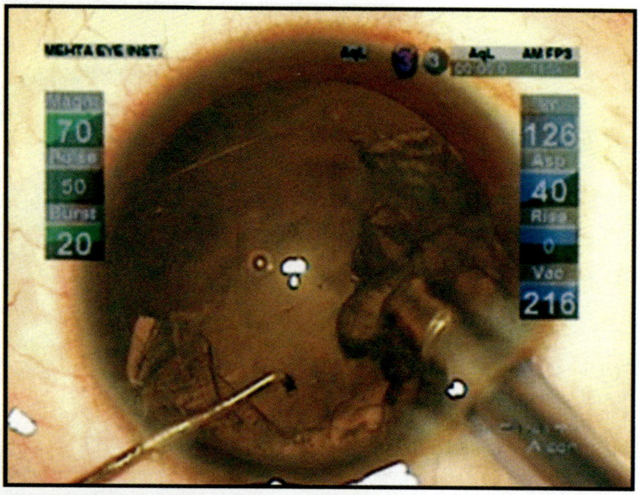

Fig. 40.14: AquaLasing the final remnants

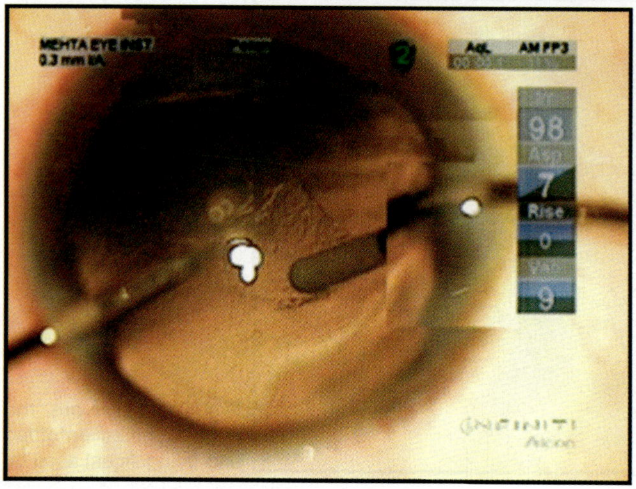

Fig. 40.15: Polishing the posterior capsule

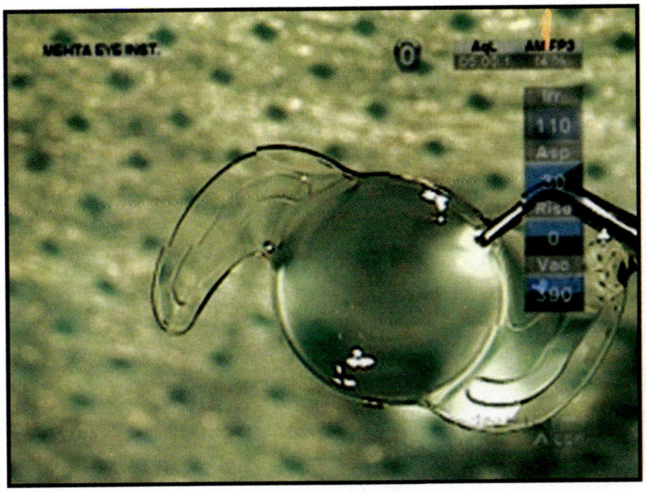

Fig. 40.16: Preziol IOL (Care Group) . Note the two zone optics

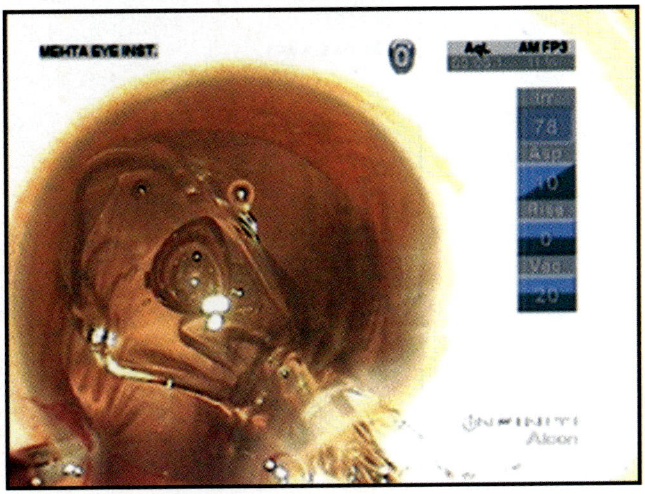

Fig. 40.17: Lens being injected into the eye. Note the smooth slow entry , slipping under the edge of the rhexis

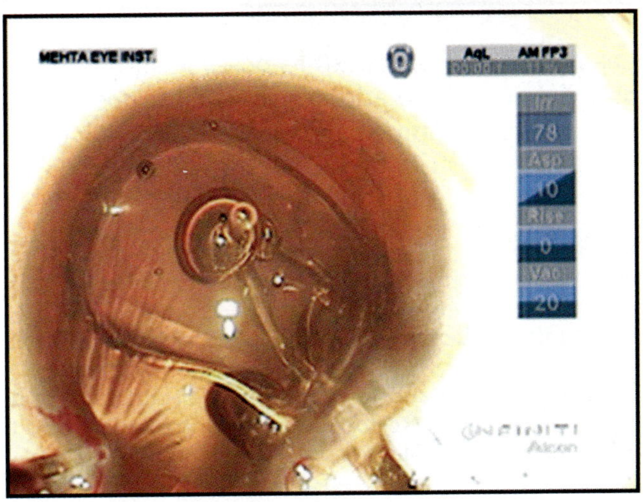

Fig. 40.18: IOL injected using the sleeve and injector

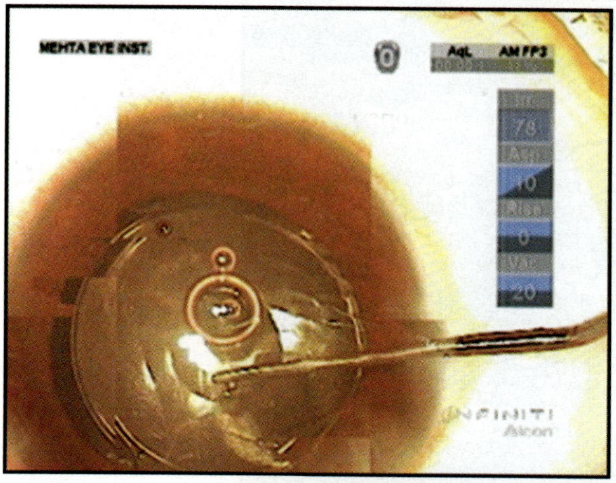

Fig. 40.19: IOL rotated into place

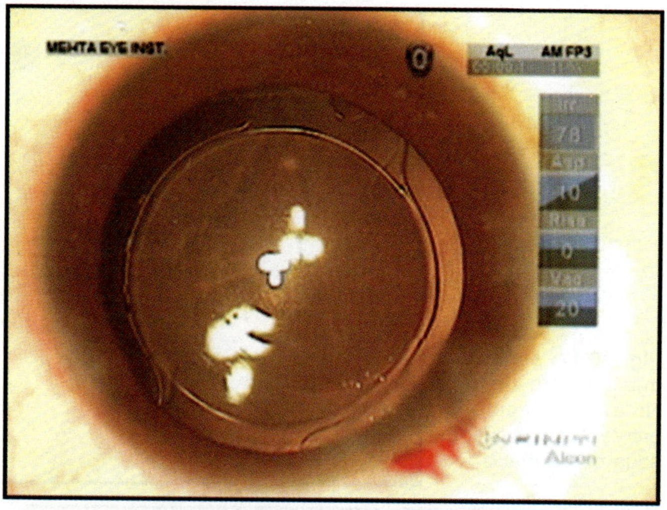

Fig. 40.20: The final picture with the IOL well centered

The aim is to get as perfect a visual result as possible and to make the child achieve good vision with no additional visual props which would affect the child's ability to compete in the world of today (Figs 40.1 to 40.20).

BIBLIOGRAPHY

1. Ahmadieh H, Javadi MA. Intraocular lens implantation in children. Curr Opin Ophthalmol 2001; 12(1):30-4.
2. Bellucci R. Multifocal intraocular lenses. Curr Opin Ophthalmol 2005; 16(1):33-7.
3. Blaylock JF, Si Z, Vickers C. Visual and refractive status at different focal distances after implantation of the Restor multifocal intraocular lens. J Cataract Refract Surg 2006; 32(9):1464-73.

4. Chiam PJ. Chan JH; Aggarwal RK; Kasaby S. Restor intraocular lens implantation in cataract surgery: quality of vision. J Cataract Refract Surg 2006; 32(9):1459-63.
5. Crouch ER, Crouch ER, Pressman SH. Prospective analysis of pediatric pseudophakia: Myopic shift and postoperative outcomes. J AAPOS 2002; 6(5):277-82.
6. Jacobi PC, Dietlein TS, Jacobi FK. Scleral fixation of secondary foldable multifocal intraocular lens implants in children and young adults. Ophthalmology 2002; 109(12):2315-24.
7. Jacobi PC, Dietlein TS, Konen W. Multifocal intraocular lens implantation in pediatric cataract surgery. Ophthalmology 2001; 108(8):1375-80 (ISSN: 0161-6420).
8. Jacobi PC, Dietlein TS, Lueke C, Jacobi FK. Multifocal intraocular lens implantation in patients with traumatic cataract.Ophthalmology 2003; 110(3):531-8.
9. McClatchey SK, Dahan E, et al. A comparison of the rate of refractive growth in pediatric aphakic and pseudophakic eyes. Ophthalmology 2000; 107(1): 118-22.
10. Menezo JL, Taboada J. Assessment of intraocular lens implantation in children. J Am Intraocul Implant Soc 1982 Spring;8(2):131-5.
11. Moore BD. Pediatric aphakic contact lens wear: Rates of successful wear J Pediatr Ophthalmol Strabismus 1993;30(4):253-8.
12. Ozmen AT, Dogru M, Erturk H, Ozcetin H. Trans-sclerally fixated intraocular lenses in children Ophthalmic Surg Lasers 2002; 33(5):394-9.
13. Pavlovic S. Cataract surgery in children Med Pregl. 2000;53(5-6):257-61.
14. Peterseim MW, Wilson ME. Bilateral intraocular lens implantation in the pediatric population. Ophthalmology 2000;107(7):1261.
15. Speeg-Schatz C, Flament J, Weissrock M. Congenital cataract extraction with primary aphakia and secondary intraocular lens implantation in the ciliary sulcus. J Cataract Refract Surg 2005;31(4):750-6.

CHAPTER

41

Donald R Sanders (USA)

Clinical Trial of the Implantable Collamer Lens (ICL) for Moderate to High Myopia

ABSTRACT

ICL in Treatment of Myopia (ITM) Study Group

Purpose: To report on 3-year postoperative safety and efficacy outcomes with the myopic Implantable Collamer Lens (ICL).

Design: Prospective nonrandomized clinical trial.

Participants: Five hundred twenty-six eyes of 294 patients with between 3.0 and 20.0 diopters (D) of myopia participating in the United States Food and Drug Administration clinical trial of the ICL for myopia.

Intervention: Implantation of the ICL.

Main Outcome Measures: Uncorrected visual acuity (VA), refraction, best spectacle-corrected VA (BSCVA), adverse events, operative and postoperative complications, lens opacity analysis, subjective satisfaction, and patient symptoms.

Results: At 3 years, 59.3% had 20/20 or better VA, and 94.7% had 20/40 or better uncorrected VA if BSCVA was 20/20 and patients were targeted for emmetropia; 67.5% of patients were within 0.5 D and 88.2% were within 1.0 D of predicted refraction. The mean improvement in BSCVA ranged between 0.5 and 0.6 lines. At 3 years postoperatively, 3 eyes (0.8%) decreased by $\geq$2 lines of BSCVA, in contrast to 40 eyes (10.8%) that improved by a similar amount. Contrast sensitivity improved postoperatively. Cumulative 3-year corneal endothelial cell loss was under 10%. Early largely asymptomatic, presumably surgically induced anterior subcapsular opacities (trace or greater) were seen in 14 eyes (2.7%), with only >2 being clinically significant. Five eyes (0.9%) of 3 patients developed nuclear opacities of grade <2 at 2 to 3 years postoperatively. Three (0.6%) ICL removals with cataract extraction and IOL implantation have been performed. Only 0.6% reported dissatisfaction; 97.1% of patients reported they would choose ICL implantation again. Incidences of patient symptoms, glare, halos, double vision, night vision problems, and night driving difficulties decreased or remained unchanged after ICL surgery.

Conclusion: Three-year results from this standardized, multicenter clinical investigation support the safety, efficacy, and predictability of ICL surgery to treat moderate to high myopic refractive errors. *Ophthalmology* 2004;111:1683-92 by the American Academy of Ophthalmology.

INTRODUCTION

A previous report by the authors concerning clinical outcomes from the United States Food and Drug Administration (FDA) multicenter STAAR Myopic Implantable Contact Lens (STAAR Surgical, Monrovia, CA) clinical investigation demonstrated the safety and effectiveness of the Myopic Implantable Contact Lens in the treatment of moderate to high myopia (with up to 2 years follow-up in less than half of the eyes studied).[1] This earlier US Investigational Device clinical trial experience, in conjunction with clinical outcomes from a number of international series,[2–12] has documented that an implantable posterior chamber phakic intraocular lens may be a viable alternative to existing refractive laser surgical treatment options for the correction of myopia. The FDA has requested that the term *Implantable Contact Lens* be changed to avoid confusion with corneal contact lenses. Because the Implantable Contact Lens is made of a material referred to as Collamer, a proprietary hydrophilic porcine collagen (<0.1%)/hydroxyethyl copolymer containing an ultraviolet chromophore, STAAR Surgical has changed the name to Implantable Collamer Lens (ICL) to retain the ICL acronym, which is well recognized. Common observations with the Myopic ICL include a high level of best-corrected vision preservation and even improvement relative to preoperative values, a reduction in patient symptoms in combination with a high patient satisfaction rating, and minimal operative and postoperative complications, with a rapid improvement in uncorrected acuity and refraction that is stable over time.

The purpose of this article is to provide an update on the long-term follow-up through 3 years after ICL implantation from the US Myopic ICL multicenter clinical investigation with the ICL lens design currently under consideration for commercial approval in the US. In comparison to our earlier analysis, data are stratified by degree of preoperative myopia in addition to data from the 3-year examination.

PATIENTS AND METHODS

Study Design

The US STAAR Myopic ICL clinical study was designed as a prospective, 2-year, multicenter, nonrandomized clinical trial intended to evaluate the safety and efficacy of the ICL to treat moderate to high myopia. The FDA Ophthalmic Devices Advisory Panel, at a recent meeting (August 2, 2002), however, recommended atleast 3-year follow-up for all phakic IOLs before Premarket Approval Application (PMA) submission, so the current study was extended until over 350 eyes had reached the 3-year follow-up window. Assessment of ICL outcomes was based on a comparison of preoperative and postoperative values and the achieved versus expected refractive outcomes postoperatively in conjunction with a complete analysis of adverse events or complications.

Study Outcome Parameters

The primary outcomes parameters for this multicenter clinical study were uncorrected visual acuity (UCVA), refraction, best spectacle-corrected visual acuity (BSCVA), operative and postoperative adverse events and complications, lens opacity analysis (Lens Opacity Classification System III)[13], and subjective patient satisfaction and symptoms.

An endothelial cell density substudy was performed using Emory University as the photographic reading center. The design and protocol for the substudy have been described elsewhere, as have been the results,[14] which will only be briefly summarized. A contrast sensitivity substudy was performed at 2 of the study centers. The tests were performed under mesopic conditions using the Stereo Optical Optec X 1600 F2 Vision Tester (Stereo Optical, Inc., Chicago, IL). Testing was performed with best spectacle correction before and after the operation using light levels of 3 candelas/m^2 after 10 minutes of dark adaptation, with and without a glare source of 10 lux. Testing was performed at 1.5, 3, 6, 12, and 18 cycles per degree.

RESULTS

Patient Population

A detailed description of the myopic ICL study cohort, which is comprised of 526 eyes of 294 study subjects (3 eyes of 3 patients have been added to the cohort since the previous report[1]) with preoperative myopia (manifest refraction spherical equivalent [MRSE]) between –3.00 diopters (D) and –20.0 D, was previously reported by the authors.1 Implantable collamer lens implantations took place at 14 US clinical investigational sites between November 1998 and December 2002. All eyes received the current ICL design version (version 4) that is presently under consideration by the FDA for commercial marketing approval.

Of the 294 study subjects, 178 were female (60.3%) and 84.7% were Caucasian. Mean age at the time of implantation (primary eye in bilateral subjects) was 36.5±5.8 years (range, 22–45). Preoperative MRSE for this study cohort averaged –10.06±3.74 D. Only 21.3% of eyes had a preoperative myopia of ≤7.0 D, 33.1% had one of >7.0 D but ≤10 D, 35.7% had one of >10 D but ≤15 D, and 9.9% had one of >15 D.

Subject compliance with postoperative follow-up visit requirements was extremely high. The percent accountability was ≥89% at all prospective study visits through the 2-year visit (89.7– 100%) and 77.2% at the additional 3-year follow-up period. The FDA currently recommends a follow-up of 70% at 3 years as acceptable in their Refractive Implant Guidance document. At 2 years postoperatively, 454 eyes were examined, and 369 eyes were examined at 3 years postoperatively.

Fifteen eyes (2.9%) underwent LASIK procedures after ICL implantation. Although the pre-LASIK refractive data were included, the post-LASIK refractive data were not included in the Table 41.1.

Effectiveness Outcomes: Total and Stratified by Preoperative Manifest Refraction Spherical Equivalent

Uncorrected Visual Acuity

Effectiveness outcomes at 3 years postoperatively for the myopic ICL PMA cohort for the entire group and ≤7-D, >7- to 10-D, and >10-D preoperative MRSE groups are summarized in Table 41.1.

Uncorrected visual acuity at 3 years postoperatively for the entire population was 20/20 or better in 40.8% of eyes and 20/40 or better in 81.3%. The uncorrected visual results in this "all eyes" group must be put in the context that only 67.6% of these eyes had BSCVA of 20/20 or better at baseline. Furthermore, only 52.1% of the eyes examined at 3 years postoperatively had a BSCVA of 20/20 or better preoperatively and were targeted for emmetropia (±0.5 D). As anticipated, UCVA for the overall myopic ICL PMA cohort was better with lower levels of preoperative myopia. In the ≤7-D group, 97.2% of eyes had UCVA of 20/40 or better, and 68.1% of eyes had UCVA of 20/20 or better. In the >7- to 10-D group, the proportion of eyes with UCVA 20/40 or better was 86.3%, and 48.9% were 20/20 or better at 3 years. In the high myopia group (>10 D), 70% of eyes had UCVA of 20/40 or better, and 21.9% had UCVA of 20/20 or better.

At 3 years after ICL surgery, in the subset of eyes with good visual potential (BSCVA of 20/20 or better at baseline), the proportion of eyes 20/20 or better uncorrected was 51.6%, and the proportion of eyes 20/40 or better was 88.8%. For the stratified groups, the ≤7-D (98.4%) and >7 to 10-D (86.9%) groups exceeded the FDA recommended target value of 85% of eyes 20/40 or better. Of the high myopes in the myopic ICL PMA cohort (>10 D), 83.8% reported UCVA of 20/40 or better, a proportion substantially higher than the FDA laser refractive target for >7-D myopes (75%). Predictability outcomes for all 3 stratified groups combined were better than the FDA's overall predictability target values.

As would be expected, an analysis of the subset with a preoperative BSCVA of 20/20 or better where emmetropia was targeted (±0.5 D) shows an even greater improvement in postoperative UCVA outcomes. Uncorrected visual acuity of 20/20 or better occurred in 59.3% of cases, and 94.7% were 20/40 or better. At 3 years postoperatively, 57.5% of patients could see uncorrected postoperatively as well as or better than they could with their best-corrected spectacle correction preoperatively. In the stratified groups, UCVA of 20/40 or better was reported at 3 years postoperatively for 98.3% in the ≤7-D group, 92.8% in the >7- to 10-D group, and 93.8% in the >10-D group. Incidences of UCVA of 20/20 or better were 72.4% in the ≤7-D group, 62.7% in the >7 to 10-D group, and 37.5% in the >10-D group (Fig 41.1).

Table 41.1: Summary of key efficacy variables stratified by preoperative spherical equivalent (SE)*

		Preoperative SE			
		≤7-D Myopia	*>7 to 10-D Myopia*	*>10-D Myopia*	*Total (3–20 D)*
Uncorrected visual acuity	20/20 or better	68.1%	48.9%	21.9%	40.8%
	20/40 or better	97.2%	86.3%	70%	81.3%
UCVA (if BSCV≥20/20)	20/20 or better	71.4%	54.2%	32.5%	51.6%
	20/40 or better	98.4%	86.9%	83.8%	88.8%
UCVA for patients with preoperative BSCVA	20/20 or better	72.4%	62.7%	37.5%	59.3%
≥20/20 (for eyes targeting emmetropia)	20/40 or better	98.3%	92.8%	93.8%	94.7%
Predictability: attempted vs. achieved	± 0.50 D	84.7%	71%	56.9%	67.5%
	± 1.00 D	97.2%	93.1%	80%	88.2%
	±2.00 D	100%	100%	95.6%	98.1%
Patient satisfaction	Unsatisfied	0%	0%	1.4%	0.6%
	Fairly/moderately satisfied	4.2%	5.7%	10.2%	7.3%
	Very/extremely satisfied	95.8%	94.3%	88.4%	92.1%

BSCVA—Best spectacle-corrected visual acuity; D – diopters; UCVA – Uncorrected visual acuity.
*Data from 3 years postoperatively.

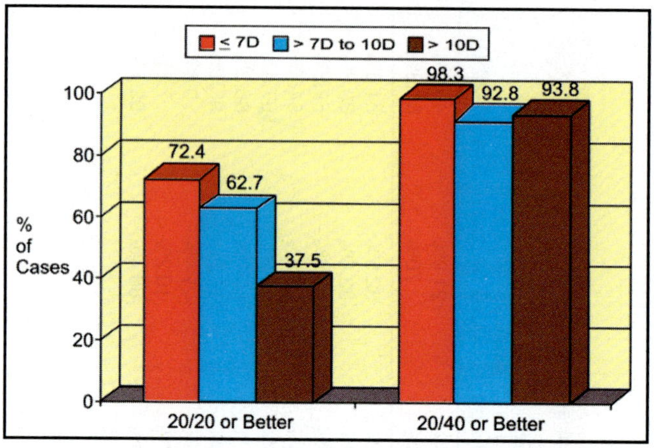

Fig. 41.1: Three-year postoperative uncorrected visual acuity stratified by preoperative myopia in the subset of patients with preoperative best spectacle-corrected visual acuity of 20/20 or better and in those targeted to within 0.5 diopters (D) of emmetropia

Predictability of Manifest Refraction (Attempted versus Achieved)

Myopic lenses were available from –3.0 D to –20.0 D. It is noteworthy that not all eyes were targeted for emmetropia, as discussed previously, because 9.5% of eyes required a ≥20-D implant power and were therefore intentionally undercorrected. Thus, the following predictability outcomes provide a more accurate assessment of refraction accuracy than the postoperative MRSE outcomes. At 3 years postoperatively, 67.5% of eyes were within 0.50 D and 88.8% within 1.0 D of attempted correction. In the stratified groups, attempted versus achieved outcomes were within 1.0 D in 97.2% of the ≤7-D group, 93.1% of the >0.7 to 10-D group, and 80% of the >10-D group; this compares very favorably with the overall FDA target of 75% within 1.0 D and >7-D refractive laser target of 60% (Fig. 41.2). For the myopic ICL PMA cohort, 84.7% of the ≤7-D group, 71.0% of the >7 to 10-D group, and 56.9% of the >10-D group achieved at 3 years a refractive outcome within 0.50 D of the intended correction. This compares favorably with the FDA refractive implant target of 50% within 0.5 D for all eyes and 30% for eyes with >7 D of refractive error for refractive lasers.

Subjective Assessments

At 3 years postoperatively, 92.1% reported that they were very or extremely satisfied with the results of their surgery, 7.3% were moderately to fairly satisfied, and only 0.6% reported that they were unsatisfied. Three years after ICL surgery, 97.1% of patients reported that they would choose ICL implantation again. Subjective patient satisfaction was excellent for all 3 preoperative MRSE groups, with

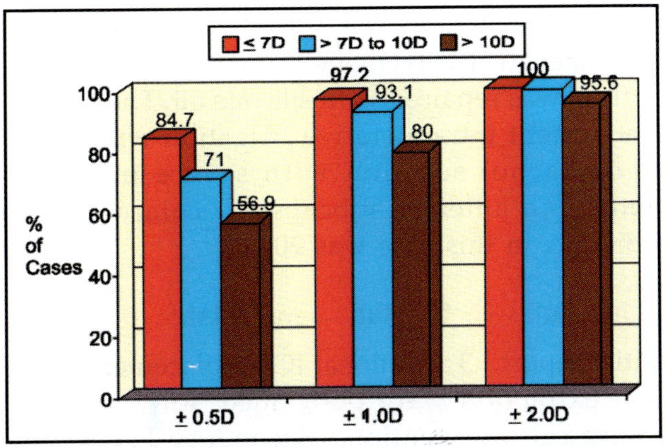

Fig. 41.2: Attempted versus achieved correction (±0.5 diopters [D], ±1.0 D, and ±2.0 D) at 3 years postoperatively stratified by preoperative myopia

slightly lower values in the highest myopia group (>10 D). Patients were very or extremely satisfied for 95.8% of eyes in the ≤7-D group, 94.3% in the >7- to 10-D group, and 88.4% in the high myopia group (>10 D). In both the low and middle myopic groups, no patients reported being unsatisfied, and dissatisfaction was reported for only 2 eyes (1.4%) in the high myopia group.

Best Spectacle-corrected Visual Acuity

Best Spectacle-corrected Visual Acuity Over Time

Best spectacle-corrected visual acuity in the study cohort improved after ICL implantation over preoperative levels. At the 2- and 3-year follow-up windows, 82.3% and 84.8% of eyes, respectively, had BSCVA of 20/20 or better, an improvement over the baseline level of 67.7%. Further, BSCVA 20/40 or better values were 98.2% and 98.6% at 2 and 3 years postoperatively, compared with 97.0% preoperatively.

Change in Best Spectacle-corrected Visual Acuity

Overall, there was an improvement in BSCVA at all follow-up visits over preoperative levels. The mean improvement in BSCVA ranged between 0.5 and 0.6 lines between 1 and 3 years postoperatively. At 3 years after ICL implantation, 3 eyes (0.8%) decreased by ≥2 lines, in contrast to 40 eyes (10.8%) that improved by a similar amount.

Best spectacle-corrected vision was well preserved after ICL surgery, with only 5 eyes (1%) losing ≥ 2 lines atlast visit with the ICL in place. Three of the 5 eyes were associated with nuclear opacities that developed during follow-up (between 1 and 3 years postoperatively). One of these eyes had undergone cataract extraction, with a final

BSCVA of 20/25 (pre-ICL BSCVA, 20/30). The fourth eye lost vision as a result of macular involvement and cataract formation; a retinal detachment (RD) was repaired with silicone oil. The fifth case was the result of inadvertent intraoperative irrigation with a preservative-containing carbachol solution with severe inflammation and development of an anterior subcapsular cataract. After cataract extraction, BSCVA in this case was 20/20.

Secondary Implantable Contact Lens-related Surgeries

Since the initial report,[1] 3 additional ICL replacements and 1 removal with cataract extraction were performed, for a total of 16 (3.0%) secondary surgical interventions. Secondary ICL related surgical procedures had little or, for the most part, no effect on either safety or efficacy final outcomes at last visit. Of the 16 eyes that underwent secondary surgical procedures, only 1 had a decrease in BSCVA at last visit (1 line loss), 1 eye gained 2 lines, 8 eyes (50%) gained 1 line of BSCVA, and 6 eyes (37.5%) had no change in BSCVA. Only 3 eyes underwent cataract surgery (0.6% of the entire cohort). These 3 eyes had a mean preoperative spherical equivalent of 15.8 D (12.8–18 D). The remaining 13 eyes (81%) remained phakic; 12 of 13 (92%) kept their ICL. Uncorrected acuity in these 12 eyes with the ICL in place was 20/40 or better in 83% of eyes.

Postoperative Complications

Since the initial report,[1] 2 additional RDs were reported, for a total of 3 in the entire series (0.6%; 95% confidence interval, 0.4%– 0.8%). The average preoperative myopia in these eyes was 14.5 D.

Lens Opacity Classification System III Opacities

Nuclear Opacities

Since the previous report,[1] a total of 5 eyes (0.9%) of 3 patients developed nuclear opacities of grade >2 at 2 to 3 years postoperatively. The first patient, a 42-year-old Hispanic female with a preoperative spherical equivalent of –16.25 D, had a clear lens until 31 months postoperatively, when an RD involving the macula developed. Repair was achieved with silicone oil. Six months after silicone oil had been in contact with the crystalline lens, the patient had >4 nuclear color, >4 nuclear opalescence, and a >4 posterior subcapsular opacity. Final visual acuity was counting fingers.

The second patient was a 32-year-old Hispanic female with preoperative spherical equivalents of –16.75 D in the first eye and –14 D in the secondary eye. The crystalline lens was completely clear in each eye at the 2-year postoperative visit; however, the patient presented at the 3-year postoperative visit with bilateral >2.5 nuclear opalescence, and a loss of 2 and 3 lines of BSCVA in the primary (right) and secondary (left) eye, respectively.

The third patient was a 40-year-old male with preoperative spherical equivalents of –16.75 D and –16.63 D in the primary and fellow eyes, respectively. The patient presented with a >0.5 nuclear opacity preoperatively in both eyes, and a >0.5 anterior subcapsular opacity was observed at 3 months postoperatively in the primary eye; this remained stable through the 1-year postoperative visit. Surgery was performed in the fellow eye 1 year after ICL placement in the primary eye. The fellow eye was observed to have the same >0.5 anterior subcapsular opacity preoperatively as was observed in the primary eye at the 3-month postoperative visit. This opacity in the fellow eye was not present a year earlier when the primary eye underwent surgery. Two years after the primary eye's operation and 1 year after the fellow eye's, both eyes had a >1.5 nuclear opacity and a >1 anterior subcapsular opacity. Thirty-one months after the primary eye's operation and 19 months after the fellow eye's, both eyes demonstrated a >3 nuclear opacity and the development of a >1 cortical change. The primary eye also presented with a progression of an anterior subcapsular opacity (>1.5), and the development of a posterior subcapsular opacity (>1) associated with significant glare symptoms and cataract extraction was planned. Cataract extraction had already been performed on the fellow eye, resulting in a 1 line improvement in BSCVA from before the operation, 20/30 to 20/25. The average preoperative myopia of the eyes with nuclear opacities was 16 D (range, –14 to –16.75 D).

Posterior Subcapsular Opacities

Only 2 posterior subcapsular opacities of trace or greater were observed at any of the postoperative visits. They were both associated with nuclear opacities already described.

Anterior Subcapsular Opacities

Since the initial report,1 no additional anterior subcapsular opacities greater than or equal to trace were reported. At the last available visit in the 14 eyes with anterior subcapsular opacities, 2 eyes lost 1 line of BSCVA (20/ 20–20/25 and 20/15–20/20), 9 eyes had no change in BSCVA, 2 eyes had an improvement of 1 line of BSCVA, and 1 eye had an improvement of 2 lines of BSCVA.

The overall incidence of anterior subcapsular opacities of trace or more in this series was 14/526 (2.7%). Nine of 19 investigators reported anterior subcapsular opacities; 1 investigator reported 6 opacities, and 8 investigators reported 1 each. Although the investigator reporting 6 opacities implanted only 12% of the ICLs (64/526), these opacities represent 43% of the anterior subcapsular opacities graded trace or greater. Although the incidence of opacities at this site was 6/64 (9.4%), the remainder of the investigators had a total of 8 events in 462 eyes, or 1.7% ($P - 0.003$). This investigator also reported both of the clinically significant anterior subcapsular cataracts. The incidence of clinically significant anterior subcapsular cataract at this site was 2/64 (3.1%), whereas there were no reports at the other sites ($P - 0.01$).

Subjective Symptom Assessment

The incidence of glare, halos, double vision, night vision problems, and night driving difficulties decreased or remained unchanged from before the operation after ICL surgery (Table 41.2). There was no marked increase in any of these patient symptoms after ICL implantation.

Table 41.2: Change in subjective patient symptoms (before to 3 years after the operation)

	Glare		*Halos*		*Double Vision*		*Night Vision*		*Night Driving*	
	n	%	n	%	n	%	n	%	n	%
Improved 2 categories	10	2.8	8	2.3	0	0	11	3.1	12	3.6
Improved 1 category	32	9.1	24	6.9	4	1.1	31	8.9	34	10.1
No change	275	78.3	278	79.4	341	97.2	266	76.0	255	76.1
Worsened 1 category	30	8.5	30	8.6	6	1.7	34	9.7	25	7.5
Worsened 2 categories	4	1.1	10	2.9	0	0	8	2.3	9	2.7

Endothelial Cell Substudy

Endothelial cell density measurements were obtained in over 200 eyes at each of the preoperative and 3-month, 1-year, 2-year, and 3-year postoperative visits; 67 eyes were also evaluated at 4 years postoperatively. Cumulative cell loss over the first 3 postoperative years was 8.4 to 9.7%, depending upon the method of analysis. There were 57 eyes that were examined at both 3 and 4 years postoperatively; the mean endothelial cell densities were 2354 cells/mm^2 and 2355 cells/mm^2, respectively. The 3 to 4-year percentage cell loss was a 0.1% gain (90% confidence intervals, –1.4–1.6%). There was no decrease in percentage hexagonality or increase in coefficient of variation at any interval studied.

Contrast Sensitivity Substudy

Figure 41.3 demonstrates the mesopic contrast sensitivity results without glare, demonstrating no loss of contrast at any spatial

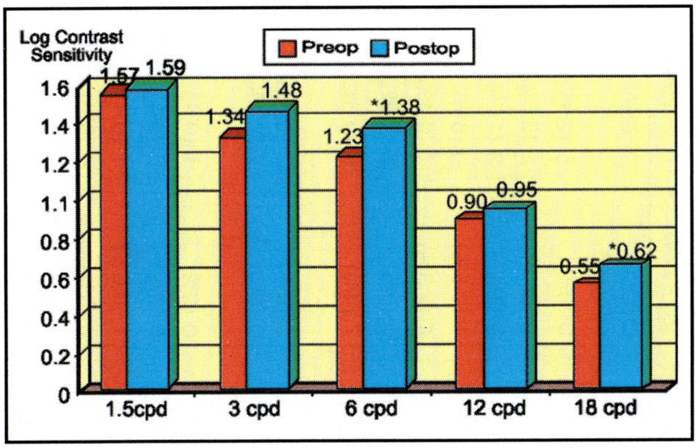

Fig. 41.3: Log contrast sensitivity under mesopic illumination (3 candelas/ m^2) without a glare source. cpd – cycles per degree. *Statistically significantly different at a level of 0.05

frequency and a statistically significant improvement in contrast value at 6 and 18 cycles per degree. Contrast sensitivity with glare (Fig. 41.4) demonstrated a significant improvement in contrast sensitivity at 4 of the 5 spatial frequencies tested (except 1.5 cycles per degree).

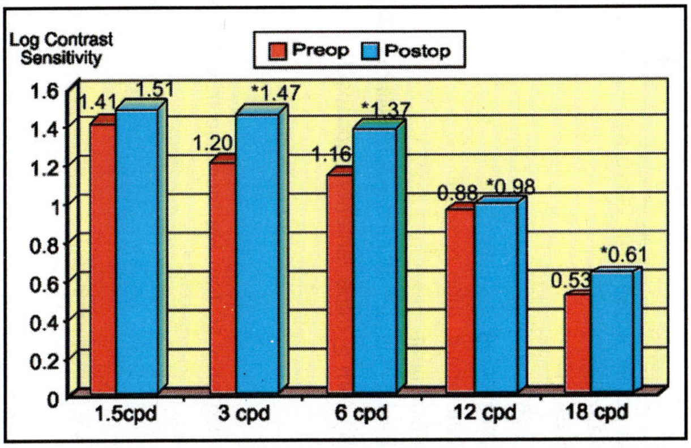

Fig. 41.4: Log contrast sensitivity under mesopic illumination (3 candelas/ m^2) with a glare source (10 lux). cpd – cycles per degree. *Statistically significantly different at a level of 0.05

Summary of Key Safety Variables Stratified by Preoperative Manifest Refraction Spherical Equivalent

As shown in Table 41.3, in general, the higher the degree of preoperative myopia (MRSE), the greater the incidence of complications or adverse events. Specifically, all 5 of the eyes with persistent loss of ≥2 lines

Table 41.3: Summary of key safety variables stratified by preoperative spherical equivalent (SE)

Safety events	*Preoperative SE*			*Total*
	≤ 7 D (n – 112)	*>7–10 D (n – 174)*	*>10 D (n – 240)*	*(3–20 D) (n = 526)*
Best spectacle-corrected visual acuity worse than 20/40 at 1–3 yr postoperatively (if 20/20 or better preoperatively)	0 (0%)	0 (0%)	0 (0%)	0 (0%)
Loss of ≥2 lines BSCVA (persistent)	0 (0%)	0 (0%)	5 (2.1%)	5 (1.0%)
Increase > 2 D cylinder (3 yr postoperatively)	0 (0%)	0 (0%)	2 (0.8%)	2 (0.4%)
Implantable Collamer Lens repositioning	1 (0.9%)	0 (0%)	3 (1.2%)	4 (0.8%)
Implantable Collamer Lens replacement, then removal	0 (0%)	1 (0.6%)	0 (0%)	1 (0.2%)
Implantable Collamer Lens replacement	3 (2.7%)	4 (2.3%)	1 (0.4%)	8 (1.5%)
Implantable Collamer Lens removal/cataract extraction/with/without IOL	0 (0%)	0 (0%)	3 (1.2%)	3 (0.6%)
Lens Opacities Classification System ≥ trace, anterior subcapsular	1 (0.9%)	7 (4%)	6 (2.5%)	14 (2.7%)
Clinically significant cataract*				
Anterior subcapsular	0 (0%)	0 (0%)	2 (0.8%)	2 (0.4%)
Nuclear	0 (0%)	0 (0%)	5 (2.1%)	5 (1.0%)
Intraocular pressure > 25 mm Hg or > 10 mm Hg Increase from before the operation (atlast visit†)	0 (0%)	0 (0%)	1 (0.4%)	1 (0.2%)
Endophthalmitis	0 (0%)	0 (0%)	0 (0%)	0 (0%)
Increased IOP on medications	0 (0%)	1 (0.6%)	1 (0.4%)	2 (0.4%)
Corneal haze/edema (after 1 wk postoperatively)	0 (0%)	0 (0%)	0 (0%)	0 (0%)
Retinal detachment	0 (0%)	1 (0.6%)	2 (0.8%)	3 (0.6%)

BSCVA – best spectacle-corrected visual acuity; D – diopters; ICL – Implantable Collamer Lens; IOP – intraocular pressure; LOCS – Lens Opacities Classification System.

*Any anterior subcapsular/posterior subcapsular score of trace or more at any postoperative visit with increase in glare, ≥ 2-line loss BSCVA, or nuclear opalescence ≥ 2.0 also symptomatic.

†Includes IOP from unscheduled visit 3 mos or more after the operation.

of BSCVA occurred in the >10-D group. In addition, both cases of a >2-D increase of cylinder at 3 years postoperatively also occurred in the high myopic individual (>10-D myopia) group. Consistent with these outcomes, all of the cataract extractions and 3 of 4 of the ICL repositionings occurred in the >10-D myopia group. Anterior opacities were observed in 6 eyes (2.5%) in the >10-D group, 7 eyes (4%) in the >7- to 10-D group, and in only 1 case (0.9%) in the ≤7-D group. All clinically significant cataracts, both nuclear and anterior subcapsular, occurred in the >10-D myopic individual group (7 of 7 eyes). The only eye with an intraocular pressure (IOP) of >25 mm Hg (last visit) or an increase in IOP from baseline of 10 mm Hg (last visit) was in the >10-D group, with no eyes (0%) in either the ≤7-D or the >7- to 10-D subsets. One eye with increased IOP on medication was in the >7- to 10-D group, and 1 was in the >10-D subset. Two of the 3 reported patients with an RD occurred in the >10-D group, and the third case was a –9.5-D myopic individual.

DISCUSSION

The FDA granted the ICL file "expedited review" status for high myopia. The FDA's guidance document on expedited review[15] states, "Expedited review will generally be considered when a device offers a potential for clinically meaningful benefit as compared to the existing alternatives (preventative, diagnostic, or therapeutic) or when the new medical device promises to provide a revolutionary advance (not incremental advantage) over currently available alternative modalities." On October 3, 2003, the Ophthalmic Devices Advisory Panel to the FDA determined that the ICL for myopia of –3 D to –20 D was approvable for commercial use in the United States. If approved by the FDA, this will be the first IOL of any kind to be approved for patients younger than 60 years, the first phakic IOL approved in the US, the first intraocular device and procedure approved for a refractive indication, the widest range of myopia approved for any refractive procedure, and the first refractive procedure to be approved for patients with myopia of ≥15 D.

Since the first report describing this series of patients, 2 types of late complications have been reported with greater frequency: clinically significant nuclear opacities in 5 eyes of 3 patients (none reported previously) and 2 additional RDs (one reported previously).

With regard to nuclear opacities, in one eye the nuclear opacity was first observed 6 months after RD repair with silicone oil, which is known to induce lens opacities.[16,17] The other 2 nuclear opacities were observed to occur bilaterally in 2 patients with preoperative myopia of ≥14 D in all 4 eyes. A number of epidemiologic studies have documented a direct relationship between the development of nuclear opacities and myopia.[18–21] The average age of our study population was 36.5 years (range, 22–45). The development of lens opacities or the progression of myopic retinopathy may differ in an older population, and our results may not be applicable to that older group.

With regard to the RD, the 3 eyes in this series had preoperative myopia of –9.50 D, –16.25 D, and –17.75 D. Perkins[22] has estimated that the expected risk of RD in phakic myopes is as high as 0.68% per year. Given the current follow-up of this reported series of high myopes, as many as 9 RDs would be expected, whereas only 3 were observed. Thus, it is unlikely that the ICL caused this particular complication. Interestingly, one of these detachments involved the only patient with severe nonreversible visual loss in the entire reported series.

With regard to anterior subcapsular opacities, in the previous report of this series, 14 opacities of trace or more, 2 of which were clinically significant, were observed. These numbers have remained unchanged despite a 2-year follow- up on an additional 196 eyes and a previously unreported follow-up on 369 eyes at 3 years postoperatively.

Myopic ICL results to date have compared favorably with clinical outcomes with the latest refractive laser surgical treatments. A recent comparative analysis of the safety and effectiveness outcomes from this FDA multicenter ICL clinical study with clinical study results using LASIK for 8- to 12-D myopes demonstrated that every index of BSCVA, UCVA, predictability of refraction, and stability favored the ICL over the LASIK procedure.[23] The ICL was also equivalent or better by every parameter in a separate series of 4- to <8-D myopes.[24]

In the previous report we compared the results of the ICL series to FDA clinical trials of photorefractive keratectomy and LASIK with preoperative myopia of >6 D or >7D, because the ICL series had a mean preoperative myopia of >10 D. In this report, we stratified the data by preoperative myopia so that it might be instructive to compare corneal refractive surgery (LASIK) to ICL outcomes in the ≤7-D preoperative myopia group, a range generally accepted to be optimum for excimer refractive procedures.

Comparison of Implantable Collamer Lens with Approved LASIK ≤7-Diopter Myopia Clinical Trials

We compared the efficacy outcomes in the FDA ICL clinical study for myopia with the effectiveness data available for FDA-approved LASIK investigational device clinical studies. The excimer refractive surgery outcomes reported here were all published by the FDA in the summaries of safety and effectiveness data of the approved Premarket Approval Applications through the Freedom of Information Act.[25–33] We chose the FDA clinical trials of LASIK to compare with the ICL because they are the most well controlled and monitored studies available.

Table 41.4 is an overview of the primary efficacy variables for all myopic or myopic astigmatism LASIK clinical investigations in which the data have been stratified by the level of preoperative MRSE to allow an evaluation of low myopia outcomes (≤7 D). The goal of this overall analysis was to assess the value of the ICL at the present time for the potential refractive surgical candidate seeking a permanent correction of his or her low to moderate myopia.

The LASIK studies required the patients to be followed-up with the end point being the point of refractive stability, the demonstration of which required meeting strict criteria developed by the FDA. In 6 of the 9 LASIK series, refractive stability was demonstrated at 6 months postoperatively; in 2 series, at 3 months postoperatively; and in 1 series, at 12 months postoperatively. As expected, the ICL demonstrated refractive stability early in the postoperative course, between 1 and 3 months postoperatively. We used 6-month ICL data for this comparison to LASIK so that the duration of follow-up would be similar; however, once refractive stability occurred, there was little difference in outcome. The LASIK and ICL series are comparable with regard to baseline patient age, with all series' populations having an average age in the late 30s or early 40s. Although all series, ICL and LASIK, had <7 D of myopia, the average spherical equivalent was higher in the ICL series (–5.3 D), whereas the LASIK series averaged between –3.2 D and –3.9 D. If anything, this difference tends to bias the comparison of visual and refractive outcomes in favor of the LASIK series because it is widely accepted that refractive procedures are more predictable as one decreases the amount of preoperative myopia.

Effectiveness of the STAAR Implantable Collamer Lens versus LASIK

Uncorrected visual acuity represents the primary efficacy variable for the ICL clinical study and the majority of refractive laser surgery clinical investigations. The dramatic improvement in UCVA after ICL surgery in the subset of eyes with low myopia exceeded all FDA targets and was better than or comparable to all approved LASIK clinical study results (Table 41.5). The proportion of eyes in the ICL study with 20/

Table 41.4: Comparison of the STAAR Implantable Collamer Lens (ICL)

Sponsor	*STAAR*	*Nidek**	*Autonomous†*	*Summit‡*
Procedure	Myopia	Myopia/astigmatism LASIK	Myopia/astigmatism LASIK	Myopia/astigmatism LASIK
Device	ICL	Nidek EC-5000	LADARVision Apex	Apex plus
Study population	N = 112 (≤7 D)	N = 664 eyes (<7 D)	N – 153 eyes (<7 D; sphere only)	N – 176 eyes at 6 (≤–7 D; sphere only)
Mean age (yrs)	37.9	42.4	39.8	38.8
Mean preoperative SE (D)	–5.3	Not reported	–3.4	Not reported
Preoperative BSCVA	20/100 or better	20/40 or better	20/40 or better	Criteria not reported
Target correction	UCVA analysis only of eyes with emmetropia target; target *not* emmetropia in all eyes	Target *not* emmetropia in all eyes	UCVA analysis only of eyes with emmetropia target; target *not* emmetropia in all eyes	Not reported
Postoperative time reported	6 mos	6 and 12 mos	3 mos	6 mos
UCVA 20/20 or better	70.5%‡‡	Not reported	64.2%	69.1%
UCVA 20/40 or better	98.9%‡‡	Not reported	93.4%	95.4%
MRSE ±0.5 D	88.8%	67.1% (6 mos)	81.3%	70.9%
MRSE ±1.0 D	99%	90.0% (6 mos) 89.7% (12 mos)	94.5%	89.7%
MRSE ±2.0 D	100%	99.6% (6 mos) 100% (12 mos)	100%	98.2%

*US Food and Drug Administration, Center for Devices and Radiological Health. Premarket Approval Application (PMA) summary of safety and available at: http://www.fda.gov/cdrh/pdf/p970053s002.html. Accessed April 27, 2004.

†US Food and Drug Administration, Center for Devices and Radiological Health. Premarket Approval Application (PMA) summary of safety and available at: http://www.fda.gov/cdrh/pdf/p970043s002.html. Accessed April 27, 2004.

‡US Food and Drug Administration, Center for Devices and Radiological Health. Premarket Approval Application (PMA) summary of safety and Radiological Health; 1999. Available at http://www.fda.gov/cdrh/pdf/p930034s013.html. Accessed April 27, 2004.

§US Food and Drug Administration, Center for Devices and Radiological Health. Premarket Approval Application (PMA) summary of safety and primary myopia with and without astigmatism. Rockville, MD: Center for Devices and Radiological Health; 1999. Available at: http://www.fda.gov/cdrh.

¶US Food and Drug Administration, Center for Devices and Radiological Health. Premarket Approval Application (PMA) summary of safety and at: http://www.fda.gov/cdrh/pdf/p990027.html. Accessed April 27, 2004.

¶US Food and Drug Administration, Center for Devices and Radiological Health. Premarket Approval Application (PMA) summary of safety and at: http://www.fda.gov/cdrh/pdf/p990010.html. Accessed April 27, 2004.

#US Food and Drug Administration, Center for Devices and Radiological Health. Premarket Approval Application (PMA) summary of safety and http://www.fda.gov/cdrh/pdf/p970049.html. Accessed April 27, 2004.

**US Food and Drug Administration, Center for Devices and Radiological Health. Premarket Approval Application (PMA) summary of safety and Radiological Health; 2002. Available at: http://www.fda.gov/cdrh/pdf/p970043s010.html. Accessed April 27, 2004.

††US Food and Drug Administration, Center for Devices and Radiological Health. Premarket Approval Application (PMA) summary of safety and 2001. Available at http://www.fda.gov/cdrh/pdf/p980008s005.html. Accessed April 27, 2004.

‡‡BSCVA 20/20 or better.

Table 41.5 Food and Drug Administration (FDA) trial to FDA LASIK clinical trials

Photomed§	*Bausch & Lomb*	*Visx¶*	*Dishler#*	*Alcon***	*LaserSight††*
Myopia/astigmatism	Myopia/astigmatism	Myopia/astigmatism	Myopia/astigmatism	Myopia/astigmatism	Myopia/astigmatism
LASIK	LASIK	LASIK	LASIK	LASIK	LASIK
Kremer excimer laser	Technolas 217A	STAR S2	Dishler excimer laser	LADARVision-Wavefront	LaserScan LSX
N = 476 eyes (<7 D)	N = 110 eyes (<7 D; sphere only)	N = 267 eyes (≤7 D sphere only)	N = 367 eyes (<7 D sphere only)	N = 139 eyes	N = 109 eyes (≤6 D)
Not reported	36.8	42.0	40.0	38.1	39.8
−3.9	−3.9	Not reported	Not reported	−3.2	Not reported
Criteria not reported	20/40 or better	20/40 or better	20/40 or better	20/25 or better	20/25 or better
Undercorrection allowed; target not emmetropia in all eyes	Target not emmetropia in all eyes	Undercorrection allowed; target not emmetropia in all eyes	UCVA analysis only eyes with emmetropia target; target not emmetropia in all eyes	Emmetropia in all eyes	UCVA analysis only eyes with emmetropia target; target not emmetropia in all eyes
6 mos	3 mos	6 mos	6 mos	6 mos	12 mos
36.3%	90%	58.6%	58.6%	79.9%	51.8%
86.6%	100%	97.0%	87.9%	98.6%	97.6%
66.4%	50.0%	77.8%	70.7%	74.8%	67.9%
84.2%	80%	94.4%	87.5%	95.7%	86.8%
98.1%	100%	99.8%	100%	Not reported	96.8%

effectiveness data (PMA P970053/S002). Nidek EC-5000 excimer laser system. Rockville, MD: Center for Devices and Radiological Health; 2000.
effectiveness data (PMA P970043/S005). LADARVision excimer laser system. Rockville, MD: Center for Devices and Radiological Health; 2000.
effectiveness data (PMA P930034/S013). SVS Apex Plus excimer laser workstation, emphasis "M" discs. Rockville, MD. Center for Devices and
effectiveness data (PMA P970005). Kremer excimer laser system serial no. KEA940202 for laser in situ keratomileusis (LASIK) for the correction of
pdf/p970005.html. Accessed April 27, 2004.
effectiveness data (PMA P990027). Technolas 217A excimer laser system. Rockville, MD: Center for Devices and Radiological Health; 2000. Available
effectiveness data (PMA P990010). Visx STAR S2 excimer laser system. Rockville, MD: Center for Devices and Radiological Health; 1999. Available
effectiveness data (PMA P970049). Dishler excimer laser system. Rockville, MD: Center for Devices and Radiological Health; 1999. Available at:
effectiveness data (PMA P970043/S010). Alcon Laboratories, Inc. LADARVision 4000 excimer laser system. Rockville, MD: Center for Devices and
effectiveness data (PMA P980008/S005). LaserSight LaserScan LSX excimer laser system. Rockville, MD: Center for Devices and Radiological Health;

20 or better UCVA at 6 months after ICL implantation if BSCVA was 20/20 or better was 70.5%, compared with the low myopia LASIK study 3- to 6-month outcomes (36.3%, 51.8%, 58.6%, 58.6%, 64.2%, 69.1%, 79.9%, and 90%). At 20/40 or better, the ICL (98.9%) continued to show long-term results comparable to or better than the early 3- to 6-month LASIK values (range, 86.6%–100%).

Predictability outcomes were excellent during the ICL for Myopia clinical study and, specifically, for the subset of eyes with myopic refractive errors of ≤7 D. Predictability with the ICL was better at all values when compared with currently approved LASIK devices. The proportion of eyes within 0.50 D in the approved LASIK studies ranged from 50.0 to 81.3% (50.0%, 66.4%, 67.1%, 67.9%, 70.7%, 70.9%, 74.8%, 77.8%, and 81.3%), falling short of the 88.8% 6-month outcome reported with the ICL. Predictability within 1.0 D showed a similar trend with the ICL result (99%), exceeding all LASIK outcomes (80.0%, 84.2%, 86.8%, 87.5%, 89.7%, 90.0%, 94.4%, 94.5%, and 95.7%).

The efficacy of the ICL procedure has been shown to be superior to that of LASIK for myopia between –8 and –12 D.[22] These data suggest that the ICL should be given serious consideration for use in eyes with ≤7 D of myopia.

Clinical study outcomes presented in this study substantiate the overall safety of the myopic ICL in this moderate to high myopia patient population. The low incidence of complications or adverse events reported with the myopic ICL should be taken in the context of the potential alternative refractive surgical procedures available to myopes with between –3.0- and –20.0-D refractive errors. In general, the greater the level of preoperative myopia, the higher the incidence of complications or adverse events. In particular, for the highest myopia group (>10 D), lack of safe and efficacious alternative refractive surgery options combined with the low overall incidence of safety events with the myopic ICL results in a risk–benefit ratio that supports the use of the myopic ICL across this full patient population.

APPENDIX: THE ITM STUDY GROUP

The participants in the ITM Study Group, as of October 2003, are as follows:

Writing Committee: Donald R. Sanders, MD, PhD,* Kimberley Doney, Monica Poco.

Davis Duehr Dean Medical Center, Madison, Wisconsin: John A. Vukich, MD*; Center for Clinical Research, Chicago, Illinois: Donald R. Sanders, MD, PhD,* Kimberley Doney; The Barnett Dulaney Eye Center, Phoenix, Arizona: Ronald Barnett, MD, David Dulaney, MD, Scott Perkins, MD; Rowen Laser Vision & Correction Center, Towson, Maryland: Sheri L. Rowen, MD; Advance Sight Medical Group, Los Angeles, California: Douglas Steel, MD; Houston Microsurgery Center,

Houston, Texas: Ralph Berkeley, MD, Michael Caplan, MD, Paul Mann, MD; Shepard Eye Center, Santa Maria, California: Stephen Bylsma, MD; Carolina Eye Associates, Southern Pines, North Carolina: R. Gale Martin, MD; Eye Centers of Florida, Fort Myers, Florida: David C. Brown, MD; Sarasota Cataract Institute, Sarasota, Florida: Harry Grabow, MD; Williamson Eye Center, Baton Rouge, Louisiana: Charles H. Williamson, MD; Shepherd Eye Center, Las Vegas, Nevada: John R. Shepherd, MD; Oregon Eye Surgery Center, Eugene, Oregon: I. Howard Fine, MD; Kraff Eye Institute, Chicago, Illinois: Manus Kraff, MD; Pacific Eye Institute, Upland, California: Robert Fabricant, MD; Advanced Vision Correction Centers, Burbank, California: Alan Berg, MD; STAAR Surgical, Monrovia, California: Helene Lamielle, MD, Monica Poco, Darcy Smith; Endothelial Microscopy Reading Center, Emory University, Atlanta, Georgia: Henry Edelhauser, MD.

*Paid consultants to STAAR Surgical.

REFERENCES

1. Implantable Contact Lens in Treatment of Myopia (ITM) Study Group. US Food and Drug Administration clinical trial of the Implantable Contact Lens for moderate to high myopia. Ophthalmology 2003;110:255-66.
2. Arne JL, Lesueur LC. Phakic posterior chamber lenses for high myopia: functional and anatomical outcomes. J Cataract Refract Surg 2000;26:369-74.
3. Gonvers M, Othenin-Girard P, Barnet C, Sickenberg M. Implantable contact lens for moderate to high myopia: short-term follow-up of 2 models. J Cataract Refract Surg 2001;27: 380-8.
4. Menezo JL, Peris-Martinez C, Cisneros A, Martinez-Costa R. Posterior chamber phakic intraocular lenses to correct high myopia: a comparative study between STAAR and Adatomed models. J Refract Surg 2001;17:32-42.
5. Pesando PM, Ghiringhello MP, Tagliavacche P. Posterior chamber collamer phakic intraocular lens for myopia and hyperopia. J Refract Surg 1999;15:415-23.
6. Assetto V, Benedetti S, Pesando P. Collamer intraocular contact lens to correct high myopia. J Cataract Refract Surg 1996;22:551-6.
7. Zaldivar R, Davidorf JM, Oscherow S. Posterior chamber phakic intraocular lens for myopia of –8 to –19 diopters. J Refract Surg 1998;14:294-305.
8. BenEzra D, Cohen E, Karshai I. Phakic posterior chamber intraocular lens for the correction of anisometropia and treatment of amblyopia. Am J Ophthalmol 2000;130:292-6.
9. Fink AM, Gore C, Rosen E. Cataract development after implantation of the Staar Collamer posterior chamber phakic lens. J Cataract Refract Surg 1999;25:278-82.
10. Jimenez-Alfaro I, Benitez del Castillo JM, Garcia-Feijoo J, et al. Safety of posterior chamber phakic intraocular lenses for the correction of high myopia: anterior segment changes after posterior chamber phakic intraocular lens implantation. Ophthalmology 2001;108:90-9.
11. Kaya V, Kevser MA, Yilmaz OF. Phakic posterior chamber plate intraocular lenses for high myopia. J Refract Surg 1999; 15:580-5.
12. Rosen E, Gore C. Staar Collamer posterior chamber phakic intraocular lens to correct myopia and hyperopia. J Cataract Refract Surg 1998;24:596–606.
13. Chylack LT Jr, Wolfe JK, Singer DM, et al. Longitudinal Study of Cataract Study Group. The Lens Opacities Classifi- cation System III. Arch Ophthalmol 1993;111:831-6.

14. Edelhauser HF, Sanders DR, Azar R, et al. Corneal endothelial assessment after ICL implantation. J Cataract Refract Surg 2004;30:576-83.
15. US Food and Drug Administration, Center for Devices and Radiological Health. Guidance for industry and FDA staff: expedited review of premarket submissions for devices. Available at: http://www.fda.gov/cdrh/mdufma/guidance/108.html. Accessed March 18, 2004.
16. Abu El-Asrar AM, Al-Bishi SM, Kangave D. Outcome of temporary silicone oil tamponade in complex rhegmatogenous retinal detachment. Eur J Ophthalmol 2003;13:474-81.
17. Scott IU, Flynn HW Jr, Azen SP, et al. Silicone oil in the repair of pediatric complex retinal detachments: a prospective, observational, multicenter study. Ophthalmology 1999;106:1399-407.
18. Leske MC, Wu SY, Nemesure B, Hennis A, Barbados Eye Studies Group. Risk factors for incident nuclear opacities. Ophthalmology 2002;109:1303-8.
19. Wong TY, Klein BE, Klein R, et al. Refractive errors and incident cataracts: the Beaver Dam Eye Study. Invest Ophthalmol Vis Sci 2001;42:1449-54.
20. Younan C, Mitchell P, Cumming RG, et al. Myopia and incident cataract surgery: the Blue Mountain Eye Study. Invest Ophthalmol Vis Sci 2002; 43:3625-32.
21. Leske MC, Chylack LT Jr, Wu SY. The Lens Opacities Case-Control Study. Risk factor for cataract. Arch Ophthalmol 1991;109:244-51.
22. Perkins ES. Morbidity from myopia. Sight Sav Rev 1979;49:11-9.
23. Sanders DR, Vukich JA. Comparison of Implantable Contact Lens and laser assisted in situ keratomileusis for moderate to high myopia. Cornea 2003;22:324-31.
24. Sanders DR, Vukich JA. Comparison of the Implantable Contact Lens (ICLTM) and laser assisted in situ keratomileusis (LASIK) in low myopia. Cornea. In press.
25. US Food and Drug Administration, Center for Devices and Radiological Health. Premarket Approval Application (PMA) summary of safety and effectiveness data (PMA P970053/ S002). Nidek EC-5000 excimer laser system. Rockville, MD: Center for Devices and Radiological Health; 2000. Available at: http://www.fda.gov/cdrh/pdf/p970053s002.html. Accessed November 1, 2003.
26. US Food and Drug Administration, Center for Devices and Radiological Health. Premarket Approval Application (PMA) summary of safety and effectiveness data (PMA P970043/ S005). LADAR Vision excimer laser system. Rockville, MD: Center for Devices and Radiological Health; 2000. Available at: http://www.fda.gov/cdrh/pdf/p970043s002.html. Accessed November 1, 2003.
27. US Food and Drug Administration, Center for Devices and Radiological Health. Premarket Approval Application (PMA) summary of safety and effectiveness data (PMA P930034/ S013). SVS Apex Plus excimer laser workstation, emphasis "M" discs. Rockville, MD. Center for Devices and Radiological Health; 1999. Available at: http://www.fda.gov/cdrh/pdf/p930034s013.html. Accessed November 1, 2003.
28. US Food and Drug Administration, Center for Devices and Radiological Health. Premarket Approval Application (PMA) summary of safety and effectiveness data (PMA P970005). Kremer excimer laser system serial no. KEA940202 for laser in situ keratomileusis (LASIK) for the correction of primary myopia with and without astigmatism. Rockville, MD: Center for

Devices and Radiological Health; 1999. Available at: http://www.fda.gov/cdrh/pdf/p970005.html. AccessedNovember 1, 2003.

29. US Food and Drug Administration, Center for Devices and Radiological Health. Premarket Approval Application (PMA) summary of safety and effectiveness data (PMA P990027). Technolas 217A excimer laser system. Rockville, MD: Center for Devices and Radiological Health; 2000. Available at: http://www.fda.gov/cdrh/pdf/p990027.html. AccessedNovember 1, 2003.
30. US Food and Drug Administration, Center for Devices and Radiological Health. Premarket Approval Application (PMA) summary of safety and effectiveness data (PMA P990010). Visx STAR S2 excimer laser system. Rockville, MD: Center for Devices and Radiological Health; 1999. Available at: http://www.fda.gov/cdrh/pdf/p990010.html. AccessedNovember 1, 2003.
31. US Food and Drug Administration, Center for Devices and Radiological Health. Premarket Approval Application (PMA) *ITM Study Group´* US FDA Clinical Trial of the ICL for Moderate to High Myopia 1691 summary of safety and effectiveness data (PMA P970049). Dishler excimer laser system. Rockville, MD: Center for Devices and Radiological Health; 1999. Available at: http:// www.fda.gov/cdrh/pdf/p970049.html. Accessed November 1, 2003.
32. US Food and Drug Administration, Center for Devices and Radiological Health. Premarket Approval Application (PMA) summary of safety and effectiveness data (PMA P970043/ S010). Alcon Laboratories, Inc. LADARVision 4000 excimer laser system. Rockville, MD: Center for Devices and Radiological Health; 2002. Available at: http://www.fda.gov/cdrh/ pdf/p970043s010.html. Accessed November 1, 2003.
33. US Food and Drug Administration, Center for Devices and Radiological Health. Premarket Approval Application (PMA) summary of safety and effectiveness data (PMA P980008/ S005). Laser Sight Laser Scan LSX excimer laser system. Rockville, MD: Center for Devices and Radiological Health; 2001. Available at: http://www.fda.gov/cdrh/pdf/ p980008s005.html. Accessed November 1, 2003.

CHAPTER

42

Donald R Sanders, David Schneider,
Robert Martin, David Brown, David Dulaney,
John Vukich, Stephen Slade, Steven Schallhorn
(USA)

Toric Implantable Collamer Lens (ICL™) for Moderate to High Myopic Astigmatism

ABSTRACT

Purpose: To assess the efficacy of the Toric Implantable Collamer Lens (ICL™) to treat moderate to high myopic astigmatism.

Design: Prospective non-randomized clinical trial.

Participants: 210 eyes of 124 patients with between 2.38 and 19.5 diopters (D) of myopia (spherical equivalent) and 1 to 4 D of astigmatism participating in the US FDA clinical trial of the Toric ICL.

Intervention: Implantation of the Toric ICL.

Main outcome measures: Uncorrected visual acuity (UCVA), refraction, best spectacle corrected visual acuity (BSCVA), adverse events and postoperative complications.

Results: At 12 months postoperative, the proportion of eyes with 20/20 or better UCVA (83.1%) was identical to the proportion of eyes with preoperative 20/20 or better BSCVA (83.1%); 76.5% had postoperative UCVA better than or equal to preoperative BSCVA. The mean manifest refractive cylinder dropped from 1.93 D (± 0.84) at baseline to 0.51 D (± 0.48) postoperatively, a 73.6% decrease in astigmatism. While only 21.0% of eyes had 1 D refractive cylinder preoperatively (none less), 91.4% of cases had 1D or less of cylinder postoperatively. Furthermore, 65.6% had ≤ 0.5 D and 40.9% had ≤ 0.25 D of refractive cylinder postoperatively.

The mean manifest refraction spherical equivalent (MRSE) improved from –9.36 D (± 2.66) preoperatively to 0.05 D (± 0.46) postoperatively. A total of 76.9% of eyes were accurately predicted to within ± 0.5D, 97.3% to within ± 1.0D and 100% to within ± 2.0D of predicted MRSE.

Postoperatively, 37.6% of eyes had a BSCVA of 20/12.5 or better; compared to a preoperative level of 4.8%. Furthermore, BSCVA 20/20 or better occurred in 96.8% postoperatively compared to 83.1% preoperatively. The mean improvement in BSCVA was 0.88 lines; there were three cases (1.6%) that lost ≥ 2 lines of BSCVA after 12 months postoperative while 18.9% of cases improved by ≥ 2 lines. A total of 76.4% of cases gained ≥ 1 line of BSCVA while only 7.5% of cases lost the equivalent amount.

Three ICL removals were performed without significant loss of BSCVA and one clinically significant lens opacity was observed.

Conclusion: The results support the efficacy and predictability of Toric ICL implantation to treat moderate to high myopic astigmatism. Important safety concerns were not identified.

INTRODUCTION

Astigmatic correction has become a long-standing topic of debate, from the traditional use of spectacles and contact lenses, to the era of keratotomy and laser *in situ* keratomileusis (LASIK). A recent alternative for astigmatic management is the toric phakic intraocular lens (IOL). Phakic intraocular implants overcome the disadvantages of corneal refractive surgeries, and have been shown to successfully correct for ametropia with astigmatism.[1-11]

The first toric Implantable Collamer Lens (ICL, STAAR Surgical, Monrovia, CA) was performed in 1999 by Thomas Neuhann, MD, in Munich, Germany (unpublished data); in 2002, the first implant in North America was reported by Gimbel and Ziémba.[1]

Several studies have recently been published on an anterior chamber iris-fixated toric phakic IOL, manufactured from Perspex CQ-UV poly (methyl methacrylate) (PMMA) and termed the Artisan (now Verisys) phakic IOL.[2-11] The results of these studies demonstrated that a toric phakic IOL is capable of correcting low to high astigmatism, as well as mild to high ametropia. The largest study was reported by Dick et al[9], in which 70 eyes underwent phakic IOL implantation for the correction of myopia (up to –19 diopters (D)) or hyperopia (up to 8D) with astigmatism of up to –7.25 D. Spherical errors and astigmatism were significantly reduced in all cases. In the myopic group, the mean refractive astigmatism was reduced from 3.74 +/– 1.09 D to 0.63 +/ – 0.53 D. In the hyperopic group, the mean refractive astigmatism was reduced from 3.70 +/– 1.05 D to 0.77 +/– 0.64 D.[9]

Toric phakic IOLs have also been shown to correct astigmatism in complicated cases, in which keratorefractive techniques were not necessarily a good or viable option. Tahzib et al[4] described the effective reduction of postkeratoplasty astigmatism in 36 eyes from –7.06 +/– 2.01 D preoperatively to –2.0 +/– 1.53 D at last follow-up. Bartels et al[6] used toric lenses to correct for high astigmatism (7D) in a patient with marginal corneal degeneration, and Nuijts et al[7] used a toric phakic lens to treat mixed astigmatism in an eye complicated by flap decentration after LASIK.

Although several studies have demonstrated effective treatment of astigmatism using the iris-fixated toric phakic IOL,[2-11] concerns still exist over the level of endothelial cell loss associated with anterior chamber and iris-fixated lenses, and the extent of surgically induced astigmatism by implantation of the rigid PMMA lens through a 5.3 mm corneal incision.[2,4]

The Visian spherical ICL was first used in humans in 1995 for the correction of moderate to severe myopia, with the hydrophilic collamer material proving to be highly biocompatible. Reports relating to the US Food and Drug Administration (FDA) ICL™ for myopia study[12-14] in combination with international series[15-25] demonstrated impressive results, including high levels of best corrected vision preservation or improvement, minimal intraoperative/postoperative complications, a reduction in subjective patient symptoms, early and stable improvements in vision and high degrees of predictability in this refractive treatment for moderate to high myopia. All of these reports studied

ICLs with spherical optics. The US FDA Toric ICL clinical study for myopic astigmatism was initiated in May of 2002. The primary objective of this paper is to provide the clinical outcomes of this FDA trial.

PATIENTS AND METHODS

The US multi-center FDA clinical study of the toric ICL for myopic astigmatism was designed as a 125 patient, 1 year duration, non-randomized clinical trial intended mainly to evaluate the efficacy of the ICL to treat moderate to high myopic astigmatism. Sample size was calculated to evaluate efficacy while safety of the phakic intraocular lens (IOL) was chiefly based upon the larger study (526 eyes of 294 patients) of the spherical version of the ICL[13,14] which was otherwise identical with the exception of the incorporation of a toric optic in the current study. Most FDA device trials require a sample size of 300 in order to detect low incidence complications (on the order of 0.1%); an observed rate of 1.0% is the minimum rate detectable as statistically significantly greater than the 0.1% expected rate with 80% power. Allowing for sampling error, the maximum number of subjects with this adverse event would be 1. Any greater number of subjects with this adverse event in a group of 300 subjects would be statistically significantly greater than the expected rate of 0.1%. (Draft Standard on Phakic IOLs, American National Standards Institute 4/25/04).

The enrollment criteria for the toric ICL study were identical to that for the spherical ICL study except that in the spherical ICL study patients were required to have ≤ 2.5 D of refractive cylinder while in the toric study, patients had between 1 and 4 D of refractive cylinder. In the toric study, the spherical component of the refraction in plus cylinder form was between –3 to –20 D, while in the spherical ICL study this was the range of allowed spherical equivalent. In addition, the spherical ICL study allowed patients with best spectacle corrected visual acuity (BSCVA) of better than or equal to 20/100 while the toric ICL study required BSCVA of 20/40 or better. Seven (7) clinical sites across the US enrolled 210 eyes of 124 patients in the toric ICL study that fulfilled the enrollment criteria, and 186 eyes (88.5%) have been examined at 1 year postoperatively.

The toric ICL is a posterior chamber phakic intraocular lens (IOL) designed to vault anteriorly to the crystalline lens and intended to have minimal contact with the natural lens. The toric ICL was manufactured from hydrophilic porcine (scleral tissue) collagen based biocompatible material, identical to that used for the spherical ICL.[13,14] It features a plate-haptic design with central convex/concave optical zone, and cylinder in a specified axis location as required, to address each patient's astigmatic condition. The toric ICL haptic design is identical to the spherical ICL in terms of size, thickness and configuration.[13,14]

ICL power calculation for the toric ICL was performed using the astigmatic decomposition method described by Sarver and Sanders.[26] This formula calculates the appropriate ICL cylinder using the patient's manifest refractive cylinder.

Toric ICLs were manufactured to minimize rotation and required the surgeon to rotate the ICL not more than 22.5° (3/4 of a clock hour) from the horizontal meridian. Each toric ICL was sent to the surgeon with a guide demonstrating the amount and direction of rotation from the horizontal axis required of the ICL to exactly align the ICL cylinder axis to the patient's required cylinder correction. With the exception of the requirement to mark the horizontal axis and rotate some of the toric ICL cases, the surgical technique was the same as in the spherical ICL study.[13,14] To control for potential cyclotorsion upon laying supine, the surgeons marked the zero horizontal axis at a slit lamp while the patient was sitting upright. The surgeon also used a Mendez ring to measure required rotation from horizontal during the operative procedure. In summary, each patient received two peripheral iridectomies within 2 weeks of the surgery using a Nd:YAG laser. On the day of surgery, patients were administered dilating and cycloplegic agents, after which an anesthetic of the surgeon's choice was applied to the operative eye. The toric ICL was inserted through a horizontal temporal 3 mm corneal incision (which has been shown to have a negligible effect on postoperative astigmatism)[27], then injected through the incision into the anterior chamber and allowed to slowly unfold. With the Vukich ICL manipulator (ASICO LLC, Westmont, IL) in contact with the footplate, the proper motion was gentle posterior pressure combined with slight rotation of one clock hour or less. This maneuver was repeated over each corner of the implant until all four footplates were posterior to the iris plane. Adjustment of the implant, if necessary, was accomplished by a gentle movement touching the ICL at the junction of the haptic and optic. Correct positioning of the ICL in the center of the pupillary zone was verified before intraocular miotic was used to decrease pupil size. Any remaining viscoelastic was irrigated out of the anterior chamber with balanced salt solution. Postoperative management was the same as in the spherical ICL study.[13,14] Slit lamp evaluation of alignment of the ICL was also performed at all visits postoperatively recorded as the clock hour of the long axis of the lens. Changes in axis alignment from 1 visit to the next were reported with a clockwise change being assigned as a plus rotation and counterclockwise change as a minus rotation.

Assessment of toric ICL outcomes was based on a comparison of preoperative to postoperative values, and the achieved versus expected refractive outcomes postoperatively in conjunction with a complete analysis of adverse events/complications. The primary outcome parameters for this multi-center clinical study were uncorrected visual acuity (UCVA), manifest refraction spherical equivalent (MRSE), refractive cylinder, best spectacle-corrected visual acuity (BSCVA), and adverse events and complications.

RESULTS

Patient Population

Of the 124 study subjects, 69 were female (55.6%) and 82.3% were Caucasian. Mean age at the time of implantation (primary eye in bilaterally implanted subjects) was 36.4 (± 7.4) years with a range of 21 to 45 years. Preoperative MRSE for this study cohort averaged –9.36D ± 2.66. Only 17.6% of eyes had a preoperative myopia ≤7.0 D, 45.7% had >7.0 D, but ≤10 D, and 36.7% had >10 D. Preoperative cylinder for this study cohort averaged 1.93 D ± 0.84. Only 21.0% of eyes had a preoperative cylinder of 1.0 D, 35.2% had >2.0 D, and 11.4% had >3D.

The number of eyes examined at each visit were as follows; 200 (95.2%) at 1 week, 195 (92.8%) at 1 month, 188 (89.5%) at 3 months, 175 (83.3%) at 6 months and 186 (88.6%) at 12 months postoperatively. We report on the efficacy data of the cases examined at 12 months postoperatively and the safety data on all cases implanted.

Effectiveness Outcomes

Preoperative Best Spectacle Corrected Acuity (BSCVA) vs Postoperative Uncorrected Visual Acuity (UCVA)

Figure 42.1 provides a comparison of preoperative best spectacle corrected visual acuity values to 12 months postoperative follow-up uncorrected acuity values. When comparing the proportion of eyes with 20/12.5 or better, only 4% of eyes had this level of BSCVA before ICL surgery compared to 20% of eyes having this level of UCVA at 12 months postoperatively. Similarly, at the 12 months exam, 55% of eyes had 20/16 or better UCVA compared to 40% BSCVA at baseline. The proportion of eyes with 20/20 or better UCVA at the 12 months visit was identical to the proportion of eyes with pre-operative 20/20 or better BSCVA (83% BSCVA *vs.* 83% UCVA). For 20/25 or better, 92% of eyes achieved 12 months UCVA while 94% of eyes had 20/25 or better BSCVA preoperatively. Seventy-six and one half percent

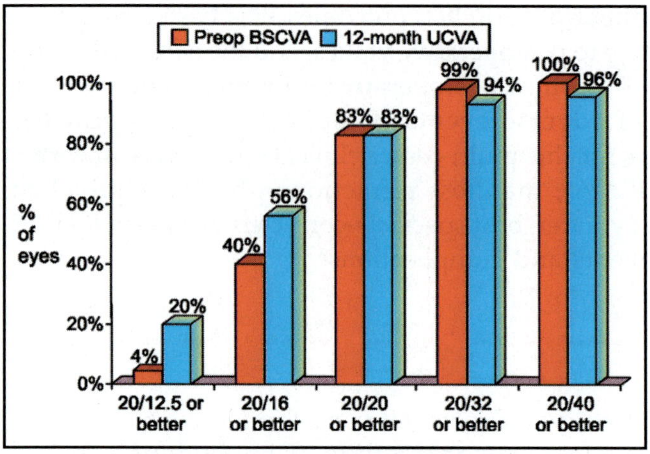

Fig. 42.1: Cumulative visual acuity

of cases had 12 months postoperative UCVA equal to or better than preoperative BSCVA.

Manifest Refraction Cylinder

Table 42.1 and Figure 42.2 present the manifest refractive cylinder prior to ICL implantation compared to the 12-month visit outcomes. While only 21.0% of eyes had 1 D refractive cylinder preoperatively (none

Table 42.1: Manifest refraction cylinder: the Toric ICL

Cylinder	*Preoperative n/N (%)*	*12 Months n/N (%)*
<= 0.25D	0/186 (0%)	76/186 (40.9%)
<= 0.50D	0/186 (0%)	122/186 (65.6%)
<= 1.00D	39/186 (21%)	170/186 (91.4%)
<= 1.50D	83/186 (44.6%)	180/186 (96.8%)
<= 2.00D	122/186 (65.6%)	185/186 (99.5%)
<= 3.00D	164/186 (88.2%)	186/186 (100%)
<= 4.00D	186/186 (100%)	186/186 (100%)
Mean	1.93	0.51
STD	0.84	0.48
Range	1 to 4	0 to 3
TOTAL	186	186

*pairwise cohort of cases
STD: Standard Deviation

less), 91.4% of cases had 1D or less of cylinder at the 12-month follow-up visit. Furthermore, no eyes (0.0%) preoperatively had refractive cylinder of 0.50 D while 65.6% had ≤ 0.5 D and 40.9% had ≤ 0.25 D of refractive cylinder at the 12-month follow-up visit. At the 12-month follow-up exam, 99.5% of eyes with the toric ICL had 2.0 D or less of

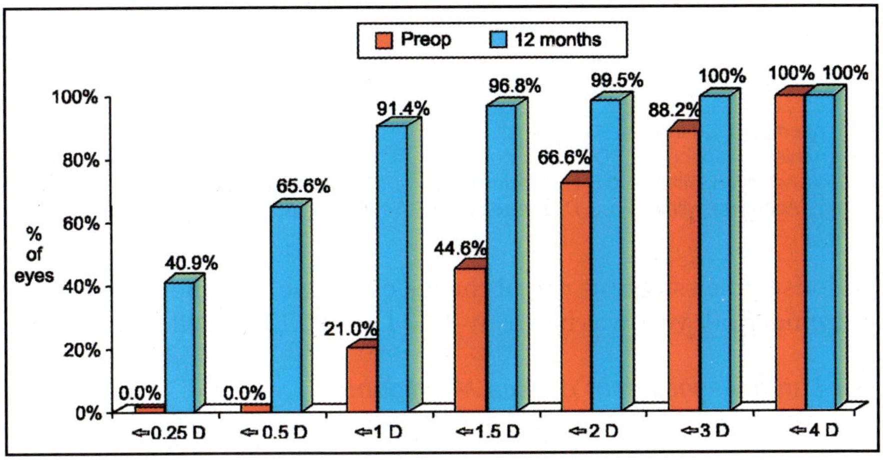

Fig. 42.2: Refractive cylinder

cylinder compared to 65.6% preoperatively. The mean manifest refractive cylinder dropped from 1.93 D (± 0.84) at baseline to 0.51 D (± 0.48) twelve months after toric ICL implantation, a 73.6% decrease in astigmatism. At 12 months, 83.9% of eyes achieved a reduction in their refractive cylinder compared to baseline values of at least 0.75 D and an additional 15.6% of cases were within ±0.5 D of their preoperative cylinder. Only one eye experienced an increase in refractive cylinder of $\geq$ 0.75 D at 12 months postoperatively, in this case there was a 0.75 D refractive cylinder increase which could be explained by a postoperative increase in corneal cylinder (keratometric cylinder increased by 1.4 D).

Predictability of Manifest Cylinder (Attempted vs Achieved)

In Table 42.2 we show how accurately the desired postoperative cylinder was achieved. The results were fairly consistent throughout the entire study period. The mean attempted cylinder was 1.55 D to 1.56 D at 6 to 12 months postoperatively while the actual achieved cylinder was 1.50 D to 1.53 D. The percent of cases with cylinder within 0.5D of the target was between 48.4% and 53.4%, and within 1.0 D in between 85.5% and 86.2% at 6 to 12 months postoperatively.

Stability of Absolute Cylinder

The cylinder appears to be stable from the earliest reported interval. Between 98.2% and 99.4% of cases changed by 1 D or less, and between 84.3% and 89.6% of cases changed by 0.5 D or less at all reported intervals. The mean difference was between –0.03 D and 0.04 D at each reporting interval. The 95% confidence intervals encompass 0 at all time

Table 42.2: Accuracy of cylinder to traget: The Visian TICL

Cylinder	*6 Months (n=174)*	*12 Months (n=186)*
Attempted Change ± SD	1.55 ± 0.66	1.56 ± 0.69
Achieved Change ± SD	1.50 ± 0.75	1.53 ± 0.82
% Achieved within ± 0.5 D of Attempted	93/174 (53.4%)	90/186 (48.4%)
% Achieved within ± 1.0 D of Attempted	150/174 (86.2%)	159/186 (85.5%)

periods (which suggests to real change over time) and the mean change in cylinder per year was between –0.13 D and 0.10 D at all time periods.

Slit Lamp Assessment of Axis Misalignment

The mean of the absolute value of misalignment based upon slit lamp examination was between 1.2 and 2.2 degrees for all time intervals tested. It was 2.2 (±5.5) degrees between the 6 and 12 month follow-up visits. There was 5 degrees or less of misalignment between 6 and 12 months after toric ICL implantation in 86.9% of patients; 92.3% had 10 degrees or less. Additionally, 95.4% of cases were 15 degrees or less for the same time period. No eyes (0%) had a reported misalignment of more than 30 degrees between the 1 to 3, 3 to 6 and 6 to 12 months time ranges.

The mean of the signed value of misalignment was between –0.5 and 0.5 degrees for all time intervals tested. The 90% confidence interval for all time periods tested had a maximum range of less than 2 degrees and encompassed 0, which suggests no systematic clockwise or counterclockwise rotation.

A review of the 13 cases with ICL axis shift (misalignment) greater than 15 degrees at any time period demonstrates that in no case was there a change in refractive cylinder magnitude and axis corresponding to these slit lamp observations of axis shift. If these ICLs had truly shifted 15° or more, then one would have expected at least a 50% decrease in cylinder correction and possibly an axis shift.[28] This lack of correlation suggests an error in misalignment measurement and not a true axis shift.

Manifest Refraction Spherical Equivalent (MRSE)

The mean MRSE improved from –9.36 D (± 2.66) preoperatively to 0.05D (± 0.46) at 12 months postoperative. Preoperatively, no eyes (0.0%) had a MRSE within 2.0 D of emmetropia however 98.3% of eyes were within 1.0 D at 12 months postoperative. Only 1 eye (0.6%) had > 2.0 D of residual myopia (–2.25 D) at any postoperative follow-up period during the study. It should be noted that this eye had a pre-operative spherical equivalent of –19 D.

Table 42.3: Predictability of manifest refraction spherical equivalent attempted vs achieved

	1 Week *n/N (%)*	*1 Month* *n/N (%)*	*3 Months* *n/N (%)*	*6 Months* *n/N (%)*	*12 Months* *n/N (%)*
<= 0.50D	150/196 (76.5%)	150/193 (77.7%)	139/187 (74.3%)	124/174 (71.3%)	143/186 (76.9%)
<= 1.00D	190/196 (96.9%)	185/193 (95.9%)	181/187 (96.8%)	169/174 (97.1%)	181/186 (97.3%)
<= 2.00D	196/196 (100%)	193/193 (100%)	187/187 (100%)	173/174 (99.4%)	186/186 (100%)
Overcorrected > 1D	1/196 (0.5%)	1/193 (0.5%)	1/187 (0.5%)	0/174 (0%)	2/186 (1.1%)
Overcorrected > 2D	0/196 (0%)	0/193 (0%)	0/187 (0%)	0/174 (0%)	0/186 (0%)
Undercorrected > 1D	5/196 (2.6%)	7/193 (3.6%)	5/187 (2.7%)	5/174 (2.9%)	3/186 (1.6%)
Undercorrected > 2D	0/196 (0%)	0/193 (0%)	0/187 (0%)	1/174 (0.6%)	0/186 (0%)
Not Reported	4	2	1	1	0
TOTAL	200	195	188	175	186

Predictability of Manifest Refraction (Attempted vs Achieved)

Predictability (Table 42.3) was achieved very early with the toric ICL (96.9% within 1.0 D at the 1 week visit) and was maintained over the duration of the study follow-up. Predictability within 1.0 D at the 6 month and 12-month follow-up visits after implantation of the toric ICL was 97.1% and 97.3% of eyes respectively. Similarly, predictability within 0.50 D was 76.5% at 1 week after implantation of the ICL with 71.3% of eyes accurately predicted within 0.50 D at 6 months postoperative; 76.9% at the 12-month follow-up visit.

Patient Satisfaction

At 12 months postoperatively, 97.7% reported that they were very/ extremely satisfied with the results of their surgery, 2.3% were moderately to fairly satisfied, and none reported that they were unsatisfied.

Best Spectacle Corrected Visual Acuity (BSCVA)

BSCVA Over Time

BSCVA in the study cohort improved after ICL implantation compared to preoperative levels. At 12 months, 38% of eyes had a BSCVA of 20/ 12.5 or better; an improvement over the baseline level of 5% of eyes. Further, BSCVA 20/20 or better occurred in 97% at 12 months postoperative compared to 83% preoperatively (Fig. 42.3).

Change in BSCVA

Best spectacle corrected visual acuity was well preserved after ICL implantation with only 3 cases (1.6%) with loss of 2 or more lines of BSCVA at 12 months postoperative (Fig. 42.4). The first patient had preoperative BSCVA of 20/25 and at 12 months postoperatively had BSCVA of 20/50 due to a 2+ anterior subcapsular cataract. This patient had the only clinically significant lens opacity reported in the study cohort. In the second patient, the preoperative BSCVA was 20/12.5 and at all reported visits except the 12-month visit, the BSCVA was 20/ 16 or better. At 12-month the BSCVA was recorded as 20/20 (a 2 line loss). The patient's refractive error changed from -10.50 +1.00 x 118 preoperatively to –0.50 + 0.75 × 90 at 12-month associated with a change in UCVA from finger counting to 20/25. There were no lens opacities noted at any visit and the patient consistently rated her satisfaction with the procedure as very/extremely satisfied. The third patient was the amblyopia case that had 20/40 BSCVA preoperatively but was reported to have 20/60 at the 6-month and 12-month visits with no

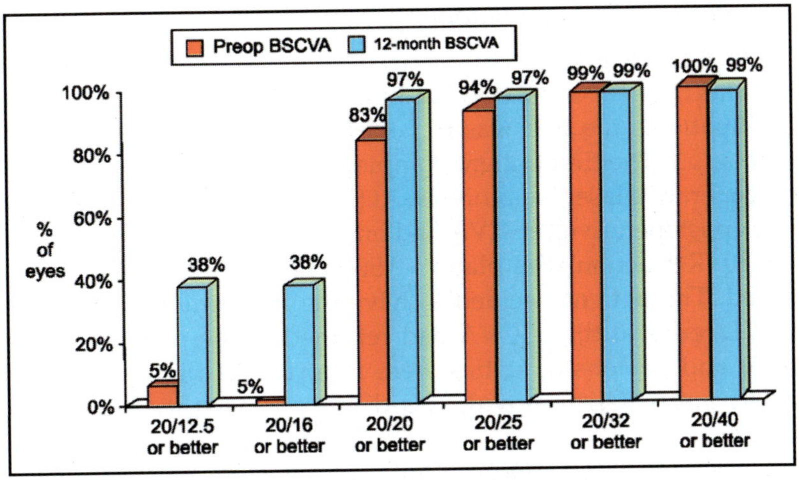

Fig. 42.3: Cumulative visual acuity

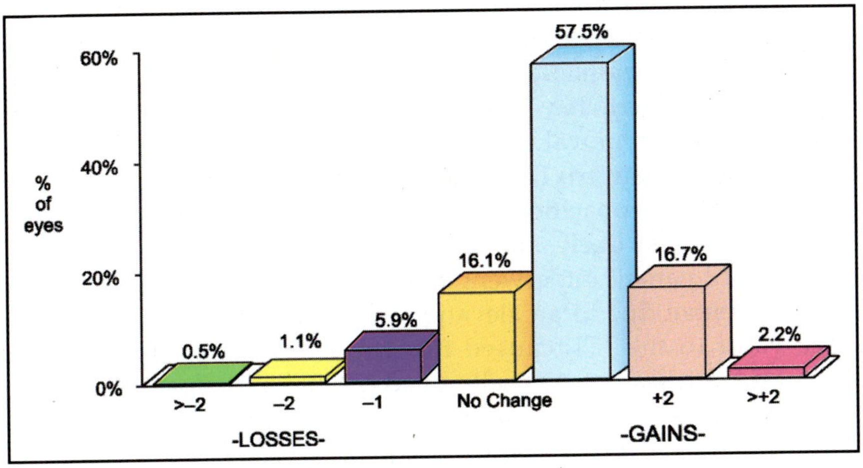

Fig. 42.4: BSCVA line changes

reason given, however, this patient was subsequently seen 5 months after the 12-month visit and was within 1 line of preoperative BSCVA. Only 1 other case had a visual loss of 2 or more lines of BSCVA at any time 3 months or later postoperatively and the loss of 2 lines was only transient (20/12.5 to 20/20 to 20/16).

BSCVA improved 2 lines in 16.7% of eyes at 12 months postoperative; a >2 line improvement was observed in 2.2%. The mean change in BSCVA at the 12-month follow-up visit after ICL implantation was 0.88 lines of improvement. At the 12-month follow-up, 76.3% of eyes had an increase in BSCVA in contrast to only 5.9% with a 1 line loss and 1.6% (3 eyes) with $\geq$ 2 lines of BSCVA loss (no change in 16.1%).

Secondary ICL-related Surgeries

Secondary surgical interventions were reported in 5 eyes (2.4% of the total cohort) in the toric ICL study cohort.

In 3 patients the ICL was removed with no subsequent IOL/ICL implantation. The first patient complained of a line in his vision from the preoperative laser iridotomies. At the last visit prior to ICL removal (1 week postoperative), BSCVA had improved from 20/16 preoperative to 20/10. Refraction was plano +0.50 x 139. No complications were reported. The patient decided to have the ICL removed. At 1 month post-ICL removal the BSCVA had returned to the preoperative level (20/16) and no lens opacities were reported. Although the patient insisted upon ICL removal, it did not correct for the line in his vision.

The second patient had an anterior subcapsular Lens Opacities Classification System III (LOCS III) score of 0.5 at 1 week postoperative, with BSCVA of 20/16. No complications were reported at this visit. The patient, an optometrist working in the investigator's practice, was concerned about possible future progression of this asymptomatic opacity and elected to have the ICL removed at 1 week postoperatively. At 2 weeks post removal the BSCVA remained at 20/16 and the lens opacity was unchanged. The patient's preoperative evaluation gave no indication of lens opacification, thus the cause of this asymptomatic opacity was most likely due to surgical trauma.

The third patient underwent an additional YAG iridotomy on day 1 postoperative due to an elevation of intraocular pressure (IOP). A large vault to the ICL caused the pupil to enlarge producing an anisocoria that was cosmetically unacceptable to the patient. The ICL was removed at 1 month postoperatively, and at one month after the removal, the IOP was 14 mm Hg and the BSCVA was within 1 line of baseline (20/25) with no subsequent complications.

The fourth patient underwent an ICL replacement because the lens was too long, causing iridocorneal touch secondary to excessive vault. Four months after ICL replacement with a shorter lens, the patient had an uncorrected visual acuity of 20/25 and 12 months from the original surgery, a BSCVA of 20/20 (a 1 line improvement) with no postoperative complications or lens opacities.

There was 1 patient that had an ICL repositioning that occurred on the day after surgery because of misalignment to the intended ICL axis. At 12 months postoperatively, this patient with a -14 -4 × 97 preoperative refraction, had no postoperative cylinder and demonstrated an improvement of 1 line of BSCVA to 20/16, and an UCVA of 20/20 with no postoperative complications or lens opacities.

Postoperative complications after implantation of the toric ICL have been minimal. Transient iritis in 2 patients was observed only at 1 week in 1 case and at 1-week persisting to 1-month postoperatively in the other. One (0.5% of total cohort) retinal detachment was reported six months after surgery. Three months after the retinal repair surgery, the patient was reported to have uncorrected visual acuity of 20/20 and best corrected visual acuity of 20/16 with no further complications. At the 12 month visit, this eye had an UCVA of 20/16, a BSCVA of 20/12.5, MRSE was within 0.50 D and the patient reported being very/ extremely satisfied with their ICL outcome.

Lens Opacities Classification System III (LOCS III)

There were no cases (0%) of nuclear color, nuclear opalescence or cortical changes preoperatively or at any postoperative visit. Furthermore, all eyes (100%) had no posterior subcapsular changes at the preoperative and all postoperative follow-up visits.

Six eyes (2.9% of the total cohort) reported anterior subcapsular opacities of trace or more postoperatively. Five cases were asymptomatic with 20/20 or better BSCVA and 20/25 or better UCVA at their last reported visits. The remaining case had a 2+ anterior subcapsular cataract (discussed previously in the 'Change in BSCVA' section); this was the only clinically significant lens opacity reported in the study cohort.

DISCUSSION

In December 2005, the ICL for spherical myopia -3D to -20D was approved for commercial use in the United States. The spherical myopia ICL study and the toric ICL study were similar with regard to preoperative myopia (10.1D vs 9.36D) and residual postoperative cylinder (0.61D vs 0.51D) however, as shown in Table 42.4, efficacy appeared better with the toric ICL. Postoperative UCVA was 20/20 or better in 50.4% of the spherical ICL series compared to 83.1% of the toric series. The spherical ICL study allowed patients with worse BSCVA, as poor as 20/100, compared to 20/40 in the toric study and a significant number of patients with preoperative myopia of more than 15D were not targeted for emmetropia in the spherical ICL study. Even correcting for these differences by only comparing patients with preoperative BSCVA of 20/20 or better and those eyes targeted for emmetropia, 60.7% of spherical ICL cases had UCVA of 20/20 or better postoperatively compared to 90.1% in the toric ICL group. Furthermore 57.5% of cases in the spherical ICL group had postoperative UCVA better than or equal to preoperative BSCVA compared to 76.5% in the toric ICL group. In

Table 42.4: Summary of key efficacy variables: the Toric ICL

	Visian TICL 12 Months Postoperative	*Spherical ICL 12 Months Postoperative*	*US FDA Targets*
UCVA			
20/20 or better	83.1%	50.4%#	
20/40 or better	95.6%	91%#	
UCVA (if preop BSCVA 20/20 or better)			
20/20 or better	90.1%	60.7%#	
20/40 or better	100%	93.7%#	85% (75% for laser refractive surgery >7D of Myopia)
Predictability (MRSE): Attempted vs Achieved			
+/– 0.50D	76.9%	67.5%	50% (30% for laser refractive surgery >7D of Myopia))
+/– 1.00D	97.3%	88.2%	75% (60% for laser refractive surgery >7D of Myopia)
+/– 2.00D	100%	98.1%	
Patient satisfaction			
Unsatisfied	0%	0.6%	
Very/extremely satisfied	97.7%	92.1%	

#Excludes patients with greater than 15D of myopia which were undercorrected
ICL: Implantable Collamer Lens; TICL: Toric ICL; UCVA: Uncorrected visual acuity; BSCVA: Best spectacle corrected visual acuity

the spherical ICL group 67.5% were within ±0.5 D and 88.2% were within ±1.0 D of attempted spherical equivalent vs. 76.9% and 97.3% respectively in the toric ICL group. Interestingly, both spherical and toric ICL series exceeded all FDA suggested target values for efficacy recommended for both phakic IOLs and laser refractive procedures.

The spherical ICL study was not intended to treat astigmatism. The mean preoperative astigmatism was 0.73 D while the 1 year postoperative cylinder was 0.61 D. Preoperative cylinder was < 1D in 66.8% of cases. Only 13.7% had a decrease in cylinder of 0.75 D or more postoperatively and 7.3% had an increase in cylinder of 0.75 D or more. The remainder (79%) had postoperative cylinder within ± 0.5 D of the preoperative value. In contrast, in the toric ICL study, the mean preoperative astigmatism was 1.93D while the 1 year postoperative cylinder was 0.51 D. No cases had a preoperative cylinder of less than 1 D. A total of 83.9% of cases had a decrease in cylinder of 0.75 D or more and only 1 case (0.5%) had an increase in cylinder of 0.75 D. The remainder (15.7%) had postoperative cylinder within ± 0.5 D of the preoperative value.

We believe that no further follow-up is required for the toric ICL series since its haptic design is identical to that of the spherical myopic

ICL and follow-up on a large series has already established its safety over a 3 year period.[14] Furthermore, as a condition of approval, the FDA is requiring an additional 2 year follow-up of the spherical myopic ICL series. The data reported here clearly establishes both the stability and efficacy of the toric ICL in treating myopia and astigmatism.

In one previous report[13] we compared the results of the US FDA spherical ICL series to US FDA clinical trials of photorefractive keratectomy (PRK) and laser assisted *in situ* keratomileusis (LASIK) with preoperative myopia of > 6D and > 7D since the ICL series had a mean preoperative myopia of > 10D. In a later report[14] we compared the US FDA spherical ICL series to corneal refractive surgery (LASIK) in the ≤ 7D preoperative myopia subset, a range generally accepted to be optimum for excimer refractive procedures. In both of these comparisons the ICL proved to be comparable or in some cases superior to the corneal refractive procedures. Given that the toric ICL performed even better than its spherical counterpart, when the toric ICL is approved for commercial use in the US, it should be seriously considered as an alternative to corneal refractive procedures throughout its full range of approved spherical and astigmatic correction.

Currently, the most common forms of refractive surgery, including photorefractive keratectomy (PRK), LASIK, and intra-corneal implants of either lenses or rings, assume that alteration of the natural shape (curvature) of the cornea is the best way to address myopic astigmatic refractive errors. While many patients who undergo these procedures ultimately achieve a good visual outcome, the final success of any of these techniques has been shown to be variable and dependent on surgeon experience and wound healing responses.[29] Furthermore, postoperative regression requiring re-treatment has occurred with varying rates dependent on the surgical procedure; exposing the patient to a second surgical procedure with its accompanying risks.

Phakic intraocular lenses are considered an attractive approach based in large part on the phenomenal acceptance of intraocular lenses for not only the aphakic or cataract patient but recently also for the refractive patient. The use of phakic IOLs offers the predictability and efficacy of IOL technology, yet is less invasive since the crystalline lens is left intact. In addition, the procedure is reversible/exchangeable, and should the crystalline lens be damaged during phakic IOL implantation, lensectomy with IOL implantation remains a good second option.

Future investigations may involve the use of the toric ICL to treat cases with higher refractive cylinder (> 4D). Patients that suffer from high astigmatism and high myopia are usually not suitable candidates for corneal-reshaping procedures because there is an increased risk of corneal ectasia, associated with poor visual quality and unpredictability.[30] These cases with high astigmatism may benefit from toric phakic IOL implantation.

REFERENCES

1. Gimbel HV, Ziemba SL. Management of myopic astigmatism with phakic intraocular lens implantation. J Cataract Refract Surg 2002 May;28(5):883-6.
2. Bartels MC, Saxena R, van den Berg TJ, et al. The influence of incision-induced astigmatism and axial lens position on the correction of myopic astigmatism with the Artisan toric phakic intraocular lens. Ophthalmology 2006; 113(7): 1110-7.
3. Tehrani M, Dick HB. Iris-fixated toric phakic intraocular lens: three-year follow-up. J Cataract Refract Surg 2006 Aug;32(8):1301-6.
4. Tahzib NG, Cheng YY, Nuijts RM. Three-year follow-up analysis of Artisan toric lens implantation for correction of postkeratoplasty ametropia in phakic and pseudophakic eyes. Ophthalmology 2006 Jun;113(6):976-84.
5. Bartels MC, Santana NT, Budo C, et al. Toric phakic intraocular lens for the correction of hyperopia and astigmatism. J Cataract Refract Surg. 2006 Feb;32(2):243-9.
6. Bartels MC, van Rij G, Luyten GP. Implantation of a toric phakic intraocular lens to correct high corneal astigmatism in a patient with bilateral marginal corneal degeneration. J Cataract Refract Surg. 2004 Feb;30(2):499-502.
7. Nuijts RM, Missier KA, Nabar VA. Phakic toric intraocular lens implantation after flap decentration in laser in situ keratomileusis. J Cataract Refract Surg 2004 Jan;30(1):266-8.
8. Alio JL, Galal A, Mulet ME. Surgical correction of high degrees of astigmatism with a phakic toric-iris claw intraocular lens. Int Ophthalmol Clin 2003 Summer;43(3):171-81.
9. Dick HB, Alio J, Bianchetti M, et al. Toric phakic intraocular lens: European multicenter study. Ophthalmol. 2003; 110 (1): 150-62.
10. Tehrani M, Dick HB, Schwenn O, et al. Postoperative astigmatism and rotational stability after artisan toric phakic intraocular lens implantation. J Cataract Refract Surg. 2003; 29(9): 1761-6.
11. Guell JL, Vazquez M, Malecaze F, et al. Artisan toric phakic intraocular lens for the correction of high astigmatism. Am J Ophthamol 2003; 136(3): 442-7.
12. Sanders DR, Brown DC, Martin RG, et al. Implantable contact lens for moderate to high myopia: Phase I FDA clinical study with 6 month follow-up. J Cataract Refract Surg 1998;24:607-11.
13. Sanders DR, Vukich JA, Doney K, Gaston M. Implantable Contact Lens in Treatment of Myopia Study Group. US Food and Drug Administration clinical trial of the Implantable Contact Lens for moderate to high myopia. Ophthalmology 2003 Feb; 110:255-66.
14. Sanders DR, Vukich JA, Doney K, Gaston M. Implantable Collamer Lens in Treatment of Myopia Study Group. US Food and Drug Administration clinical trial of the Implantable Contact Lens for moderate to high myopia; Three Year Follow-up. Ophthalmology 2004;111:1683-92.
15. Arne JL, Lesueur LC. Phakic posterior chamber lenses for high myopia: functional and anatomical outcomes. Cataract Refract Surg 2000;26:369-74.

16. Gonvers M, Othenin-Girard P, Barnet C, et al. Implantable contact lens for moderate to high myopia: short-term follow-up of 2 models. J Cataract Refract Surg 2001;27:380-8.
17. Menezo JL, Peris-Martinez C, Cisneros A, et al.. Posterior chamber phakic intraocular lenses to correct high myopia: a comparative study between STAAR and Adatomed models. J Refract Surg 2001;17:32-42.
18. Pesando PM, Ghiringhello MP, Tagliavacche P. Posterior chamber collamer phakic intraocular lens for myopia and hyperopia. J Refract Surg 1999;15:415-23.
19. Assetto V, Benedetti S, Pesando P. Collamer intraocular contact lens to correct high myopia. J Cataract Refract Surg 1996;22:551-6.
20. Zaldivar R, Davidorf JM, Oscherow S. Posterior chamber phakic intraocular lens for myopia of –8 to –19 diopters. J Refract Surg 1998;14:294-305.
21. BenEzra D, Cohen E, Karshai I. Phakic posterior chamber intraocular lens for the correction of anisometropia and treatment of amblyopia. Am J Ophthalmol 2000;130:292-6.
22. Fink AM, Gore C, Rosen E. Cataract development after implantation of the Staar Collamer posterior chamber phakic lens. J Cataract Refract Surg 1999;25:278-82.
23. Jimenez-Alfaro I, Benitez del Castillo JM, Garcia-Feijoo J, et al. Safety of posterior chamber phakic intraocular lenses for the correction of high myopia: anterior segment changes after posterior chamber phakic intraocular lens implantation. Ophthalmol 2001;108:90-9.
24. Kaya V, Kevser MA, Yilmaz OF. Phakic posterior chamber plate intraocular lenses for high myopia. J Refract Surg 1999;15:580-5.
25. Rosen E, Gore C. Staar Collamer posterior chamber phakic intraocular lens to correct myopia and hyperopia. J Cataract Refract Surg 1998;24:596-606.
26. Sarver EJ, Sanders DR. Astigmatic power calculations for intraocular lenses in the phakic and aphakic eye. J Refract Surg 2004;20: 472-7.
27. Martin RG, Gills JP. Evaluating Outcomes of Cataract Surgery. In Sanders DR, Koch DD, (Eds):. An Atlas of Corneal Topography. New Jersey: SLACK Incorporated, 1993; chap. 4.
28. Sanders DR, Grabow HB, Shepherd J, Raanan MR. STAAR AA 4203T Toric Silicone IOL. In: Martin RG, Gills JP, Sanders DR, eds. Foldable Intraocular Lenses. New Jersey: SLACK Incorporated, 1993; chap 14.
29. Durrie D, Lesher M, Cavanaugh T. Classification of Variable Clinical Response After Photorefractive Keratectomy. J Ref & Corn Surg, Sept/Oct 1995; 11(5):341-7.
30. Marcos S. Aberrations and visual performance following standard laser vision correction. J Refract Surg 2001; 17: 596 – 601.

CHAPTER

43

Swati Phuljhele, Lalit Alok,
Anand Aggarwal, Tanuj Dada (India)

Clinical Profile of Blue Light Filtering Intraocular Lenses

INTRODUCTION

Ultraviolet (UV) radiation comprises invisible high energy rays (200-400 nm) from the sun that lie just beyond the blue end of the visible spectrum. Violet (400-440 nm) and blue (440-500 nm) light comprise the shorter wavelength part of the visible spectrum. The UV radiation present in sunlight is not useful for vision. There are good scientific reasons to consider that UV absorption by the eye may contribute to age-related changes in the eye and a number of other serious eye diseases.

UV-RELATED EYE DISEASES

Ultraviolet radiation has a contributory role to play in the development of various ocular disorders such as cataract, pterygium, cancer of the skin around the eye, photokeratitis and corneal degenerative changes, solar retinopathy, and may contribute to age-related macular degeneration. The bright illumination of ophthalmic instruments, such as the indirect ophthalmic instruments may also cause retinal damage.[1]

There are several evidences to suggest that wavelengths between 350 nm in the UV spectrum and 441 nm in the visible spectrum are potentially the most dangerous in causing retinal phototoxicity, which can lead to or accelerate age related macular degeneration.[2-4] There is now considerable evidence that it is the loss of retinal pigment epithelial cells that leads to secondary photoreceptor cell degeneration in AMD. The most pronounced aging change in the retinal pigment epithelium (RPE) is the accumulation of a fluorescent material that constitutes the lipofuscin of the cell. This increased accumulation of the photosensitiser lipofuscin may impair free radical control mechanisms leading to apoptosis. A major fluorophore of RPE lipofuscin, the compound A2E, is maximally excited by blue light of the spectrum and has been shown to be capable of mediating blue light damage.[5-7]

PROTECTIVE MECHANISMS IN THE HUMAN EYE

The human eye has its own naturally protecting mechanisms like pupil constriction, lid squinting, and eye movements. An essential component of an eye's light filtering system are the cornea and crystalline lens.[8] The cornea protects from UV radiation shorter than 300 nm while the crystalline lens blocks most UV radiation between 300 nm and 400 nm.[8-10] The age related nuclear sclerosis causes yellowing of lens thereby attenuating blue light.[10-12] Removal of the cataractous lens in elderly patients followed by implantation of an IOL that does not attenuate blue light may leave RPE cells vulnerable at an age when their content of blue light sensitive lipofuscin is the highest. This has led to the development of an IOL that can block UV as well as short wavelength blue-violet light.

The first PMMA intraocular lenses transmitted UV light in addition to visible light. The incorporation of UV blocking chromophores began in 1986.[13] The introduction of IOLs blocking visible light (blue-violet spectrum) is the latest development in the field of cataract surgery.

MECHANISM OF ACTION OF FILTERING IOLs

These IOLs consist of polymers (chromophores) that are photochromic and are capable of filtering at least a portion of blue light incident thereon. The photochromic and light-filtering property of the polymers is activated by light having wavelengths in the blue range, i.e. from about 400 nm to about 500 nm. Upon being activated, the polymer also absorbs, thus filters out, a portion of incident light having different wavelengths in the blue range. In one aspect, the polymer is also capable of filtering at least a portion of UV radiation (i.e., radiation having wavelengths in the range from about 180 nm to about 400 nm) incident thereon.

TYPES OF FILTERING IOLs

1. UV only blocking IOLs—block only the UV rays and transmit the blue light which is potentially harmful to retina, e.g. conventional IOLs.
2. UV + blue + violet blocking IOLs— these lenses block UV rays as well as shortwave lengths of visible spectrum. These lenses provide complete photoprotection but at the cost of scotopic vision; e.g. AcrySof® Natural IOL, AcrySof ® IQ IOL, Hoya® AF-1 UY.
3. UV + violet blocking IOLs— these lenses block the UV rays and violet rays. They provide less photoprotection than the above group but the scotopic vision is better, e.g AMO® Optiblue.

AcrySof Natural® IOL SN60AT® (Fig. 43.1), Alcon laboratories, was the first one to be introduced in this category. The lens is made up of hydrophobic acrylic with UV light and blue light chromophores. Rodriguez-Galietero A et al[14] compared the AcrySof Natural IOL (SN60AT) with AcrySof SA60AT in diabetic patients and concluded that the AcrySof Natural IOL provides better contrast sensitivity than the AcrySof SA60AT. The blue-light filter of the AcrySof Natural IOL did not cause chromatic discrimination defects based on total error scores and improved color vision in the blue-yellow chromatic axis in diabetic patients. Cionni[15] compared color vision in patients with bilateral AcrySof Natural IOL implants with bilateral AcrySof single-piece UV-blocking lenses using the Farnsworth 100-hue magnetic color

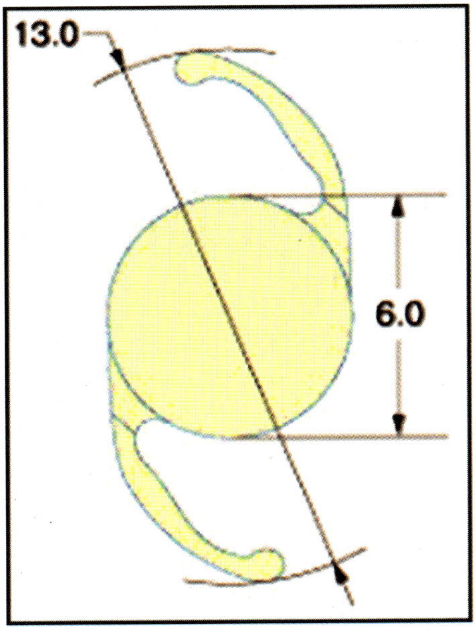

Fig. 43.1: AcrySof SN60AT

perception test and found no difference in color perception between these groups. There was also no impact on color perception if the patients underwent implantation with the AcrySof Natural IOL in 1 eye and the AcrySof single-piece lens in the other.

This lens is now modified to accommodate a special feature in the form of a posterior aspheric surface and is now available **as AcrySof® IQ IOL SNWF®** The multifocal version of the lens is available in form **of AcrySof® ReSTOR®** natural IOL.

Hoya® AF-1 UY (Fig. 43.2) is a high quality UV-absorbent single-piece acrylic foldable intraocular lens. This lens uses a safe and uniform soft acrylic resin for the optics; the PMMA haptics are specifically designed to be stable within the capsule. The yellow-filter is incorporated into the acrylic material. Hoya AF-1 UY admits natural color tones similar to the human crystalline lens. It protects the retina by absorbing UV-light and a part of visible short wavelength light.

AMO® Optiblue is a violet blocking IOL that provides less photoprotection than the blue light blocking lens but a better photoreception.

CLINICAL USE

Age-related macular degeneration and diseases affecting macula like diabetes are the major indications for the implantation of blue light filtering IOLs.

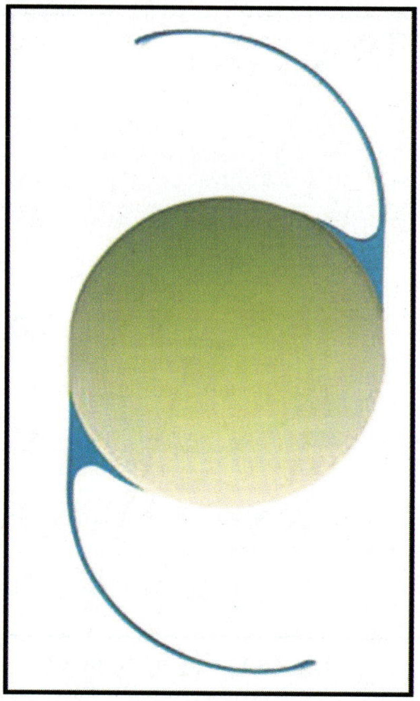

Fig. 43.2: Hoya® AF-1 UY

A few recently published clinical trials have evaluated the efficacy with regard to the blue filtering IOLs vis a vis the standard hydrophobic acrylic lenses. Mayer S et al[16] did an intraindividual comparison in 14 patients of the contrast sensitivity under mesopic conditions with one eye being implanted the AcrySof natural IOL and the other eye the conventional AcrySof IOL. They reported no significant differences in contrast sensitivity under different lighting conditions using the FACT test (Functional Acuity Contrast Test). A projected cost benefit analysis in preventing the potential treatment of ARMD developing after cataract surgery was recently published by Reddy P et al.[17] Estimated savings with blue light filtering IOLs per 100 eyes were $4275, $29 997, and $111 734 in the 55 to 64-year-old, 65 to 74-year-old, and > or= 75-year-old cohorts, respectively. They did acknowledge the current limitations with regard to the lack of proven evidence against AMD protection. Moreover the data used for the model were derived from the animal and lab studies that may not be directly extrapolated onto human beings. But these cost benefits analyses will no doubt be increasingly coming to clinical practice in the future especially in resource poor countries like India especially while formulating public health policies on the management and prevention of AMD as the life expectancy of the people here also increase with improved health resources.

LIMITATIONS

The most important draw back of blue light filtering IOLs is the reduced scotopic vision. The data regarding scotopic contrast sensitivity as of present are controversial with different authorities having different opinion on the issue. IOLs blocking UV and blue light reduce the phototoxicity but they also reduce the light reaching the photoreceptors, especially the S cones, and rods which are best stimulated by short wavelength light. As a result the scotopic vision in these eyes is affected.[18] Moreover these are the eyes that already have compromised rod function due to age-related photoreceptor degeneration. This may add to the disability of night vision in such patients. Mainster MA[19] compared the various types of IOL in his study and he concluded that UV, violet and blue light are responsible for 67%, 18% and 14% of UV-blue phototoxicity, respectively, in the spectral region from 350-700 nm where optical radiation can potentially reach the retina of a pseudophakic eye. The violet light blocking IOL provides better aphakic scotopic photosensitivity. However in a recent clinical study on scotopic contrast sensitivity with the use of blue filtering IOLs, Schwiegerling J et al[20] reported a 52% improvement in light entering the eyes in pseudophakic patients in scotopic conditions. The apparent discrepancies between the recent and the previous clinical studies comes from the data interpretation of the rod spectral sensitivity curves in phakes and aphakes/pseudophakes, there being no internationally accepted standards that are available for aphakes/pseudophakes.

CONCLUSION

All the above lenses are still under trial, and while a few early reports regarding their performance are available, their long term follow up effects are yet to evaluated and reported. Their will be ongoing clinical evaluation with regard to the efficacy both in terms of reducing the incidence of AMD after cataract surgery with the use of new blue blocking IOLs vis a vis the apparent reduction in mesopic contrast sensitivity. The present studies are limited with regard to the limited follow-up, small series of patients in which these IOLs have been implanted, the confounding effect of pupil size on retinal illuminance, and optimal methods of data acquisition regarding light transmittance by these IOLs. The future studies will also have to address the issues of posterior capsular opacification in degrading the optical qualities of these IOLs especially under low illuminance conditions. Further prospective studies are required before these IOLs become accepted as the standard method for optical rehabilitation after phacoemulsification.

REFERENCES

1. Fruednab E, Kuwabara T. The retinal pigment epithelium-IV. The damaging effects of radiant energy. Arch Opthalmol 1968;80:265-79.
2. Van der Hoeve J. Eye lesions produced by light rich in ultraviolet rays: senile cataract, senile degeneration of the macula. Am J Ophthalmol 1920;3:178-94.
3. Tso MO. Pathogenetic factors of aging macular degeneration. Ophthalmology 1985;92:628-35.
4. Burkle A. Mechanisms of ageing. Eye 2001;15:371-5.
5. Sparrow JR, Nakanishi K, Parish CA. The lipofuscin fluorophore A2E mediates blue light-induced damage to retinal pigmented epithelial cells. Invest Ophthalmol Vis Sci 2000;41:1981-9.
6. Sparrow JR, Cai B. Blue light-induced apoptosis of A2E-containing RPE: involvement of caspase-3 and protection by Bcl-2. Invest Ophthalmol Vis Sci 2001;42:1356-62.
7. Sparrow JR, Zhou J, Ben-Shabat S, Vollmer H, Itagaki Y, Nakanishi K. Involvement of oxidative mechanisms in blue light induced damage to A2E-laden RPE. Invest Ophthalmol Vis Sci 2002;43:1222-7.
8. Boettner EA, Walter JR. Transmission of the ocular media. Invest Ophthalmol 1962; 1:776-83.
9. van Norren D, Vas JJ. Spectral transmission of the human ocular media. Vis Res 1974;14:1237-44.
10. Mellerio J. Yellowing of the human lens: nuclear and cortical contributions. Vis Res 1987;27:1581-7.
11. Gaillard ER, Zheng L, Merriam JC, Dillon J. Age-related changes in the absorption characteristics of the primate lens. Invest Ophthalmol Vis Sci 2000;41:1454-9.
12. Weale RA. Aging and vision. Vision Res 1986;26:1507-12.
13. Mainster MA. The spectra, classification, and rationale of ultraviolet protective intraocular lenses. Am J Ophthalmol 1986;102:727-32.
14. Rodriguez-Galietero A, Montes-Mico R, Munoz G, Albarran-Diego C.Blue-light filtering intraocular lens in patients with diabetes: vontrast sensitivity and chromatic discrimination. J Cataract Refract Surg 2005 Nov;31(11):2088-92.
15. Cionni RJ, Tsai JH. Color perception with AcrySof natural and AcrySof single-piece intraocular lenses under photopic and mesopic conditions. J Cataract Refract Surg. 2006;32(2):236-42.
16. Mayer S, Wirbelauer C, Pham DT. Functional results after intraocular lens implantation with or without blue light filter: An intraindividual comparison. Klin Monatsbl Augenheilkd. 2006;223(2):142-6.
17. Reddy P, Gao X, Barnes R, Fairchild C, Boci K, Waycaster C, Pashos C. The economic impact of blue-light filtering intraocular lenses on age-related macular degeneration associated with cataract surgery: a third-party payer's perspective. Curr Med Res Opin. 2006;22(7):1311-8.
18. Werner JS. Night vision in the elderly: consequences for seeing through a "blue filtering" intraocular lens. Br J Ophthalmol 2005;89(11):1518-21.
19. Mainster MA. Violet and blue light blocking intraocular lenses: photoprotection versus photoreception. Br J Ophthalmol 2006;90:784-92.
20. Schwiegerling J. Blue-light-absorbing lenses and their effect on scotopic vision. J Cataract Refract Surg 2006;32:141-4.

CHAPTER

44

K Takhchidi, Boris Malyugin, T Morozova
O Kravchuk, V Cherednik (Russia)

IOL with Gradient Refractive Index Optics

BASIC TENDENCIES IN MULTIFOCAL INTRAOCULAR APHAKIA CORRECTION

Multifocal intraocular lenses proved to be highly effective in restoring near visual function. Nowadays they are widely used for refractive lens exchange and presbyopia correction (Lindstorm RL, 1993, 2003; Eisenmann D et al, 1996; Bleckmann H et al, 1996; Featherstone KA et al, 1999; Javitt JC, Steinert RF, 2000; Kamath GG et al, 2000; Brydon KW et al, 2000; Knorz MC, 2000; Lesueur L et al, 2000; Cagini Ñ. et al, 2002).

In multifocal IOL light coming into the eye is divided on a couple of components forming focal zone of certain depth. Multifocal lenses from the optical point of view is definitely a compromise between opportunity to get high quality visual functions and capability to see at various distances. Basic issue of multifocal correction is obviously a correlation between focus depth and modulation transfer functions of the optical system. Which multifocal IOL (MIOL) design provides better quality of vision and independence of additional correction is a matter of ongoing research.

In our studies we took in mind fundamental optical studies of crystalline lens, accommodation and mechanisms of presbyopia development (Jain IS, 1982; Fisher RF, 1986; Hiejde GL, 1986; Ursell PG et al, 1998; Strenk SA et al, 1999; Schachar RA, 1992, 1994; Schachar RA et al, 1995; Glasser A, 1999, 2000). Now a days lenticular theory of presbyopia is dominating. According to it the main cause of presbyopia development is natural crystalline lens optical parameters changing with age.

The concept incorporates well established data including crystalline lens annual growth rate (0.02 mm/year), changes in mean equivalent refractive index (1.427 ÷ 1.418) and surface refractive index (1.386 ÷ 1.394) (Garner LF, Ooi CS, Smith G, 1996; Glasser A,Campbell MC, 1997, 1998, 1999; BK Piercionek, 1997).

The abovementioned results in optical total aberrations change from negative values in younger age to positive ones in the elder person. It is known that aberrations nature determines optical parameters including depth of focal zone. Depth of focus increase leads to "passive" ability to see at various distances without active change of lens optical power during accommodation (Hamasaki et al, 1956; Koretz J F et al, 1989).

We tried to embody this physiological process which can be modelled by gradient optics while developing our multifocal IOL. Our goal was to create the lens with sufficient pseudo-accommodation volume of 4.0–5.0 D which corresponds to normal accommodation values of 40–44 years old subject (Milder B, Ruben ML, 1978).

Unlike currently available multifocal IOLs with variable refractive power due to complex shape of their anterior and/or posterior surfaces, gradient optics is characterized by various refractive power resulted from change of refractive index in lens inner structure. This circumstance defines a number of its optical and structural advantages. We assume possibility to improve functional results as well as to diminish optical side effects in patients with implanted MIOL. The idea of gradient multifocal IOLs design has prospects from several points of view.

Apart from good imitation of normal physiology we formulate the following benefits of gradient multifocal IOLs over other types of MIOLs:

- Smooth optical surface decreases the possibility of mechanical optics trauma during IOL implantation
- In cases of YAG–laser capsulotomy in postoperative period possibility of functional efficacy loss due to optic damage is substantially decreased. This gives surgeon an opportunity to avoid intraoperative opening of fibrotic posterior capsule thus minimizing risk and volume of the surgery
- Postoperative functional vision is achieved in a wide range including near and intermediate distances which is utmost important for computer work and driving
- High visual functions in various luminance (photopic, mesopic, and scotopic)
- Opportunity to perform wide ophthalmoscopy in postoperative period and to conduct pan retinal laser coagulation and vitreoretinal surgery if indicated.

Considering all abovementioned the purpose of our study was theoretical research, development and clinical approbation of multifocal intraocular lens with gradient optics.

CLASSIFICATION OF MULTIFOCAL IOLs

20 years depth patent search revealed great variety in shape, optical part design and materials of multifocal intraocular lenses. A large number of pre-existing and theoretically possible models stimulated us to elaborate classification scheme describing characteristics of optical part structure and design.

The classification enables to systematize information, to set position of the gradient optics and to evaluate prospects of future research (Fig. 44.1).

Depending on number of optical components forming optical part structure we classify multifocal IOLs on monocomponent, i.e. consisting

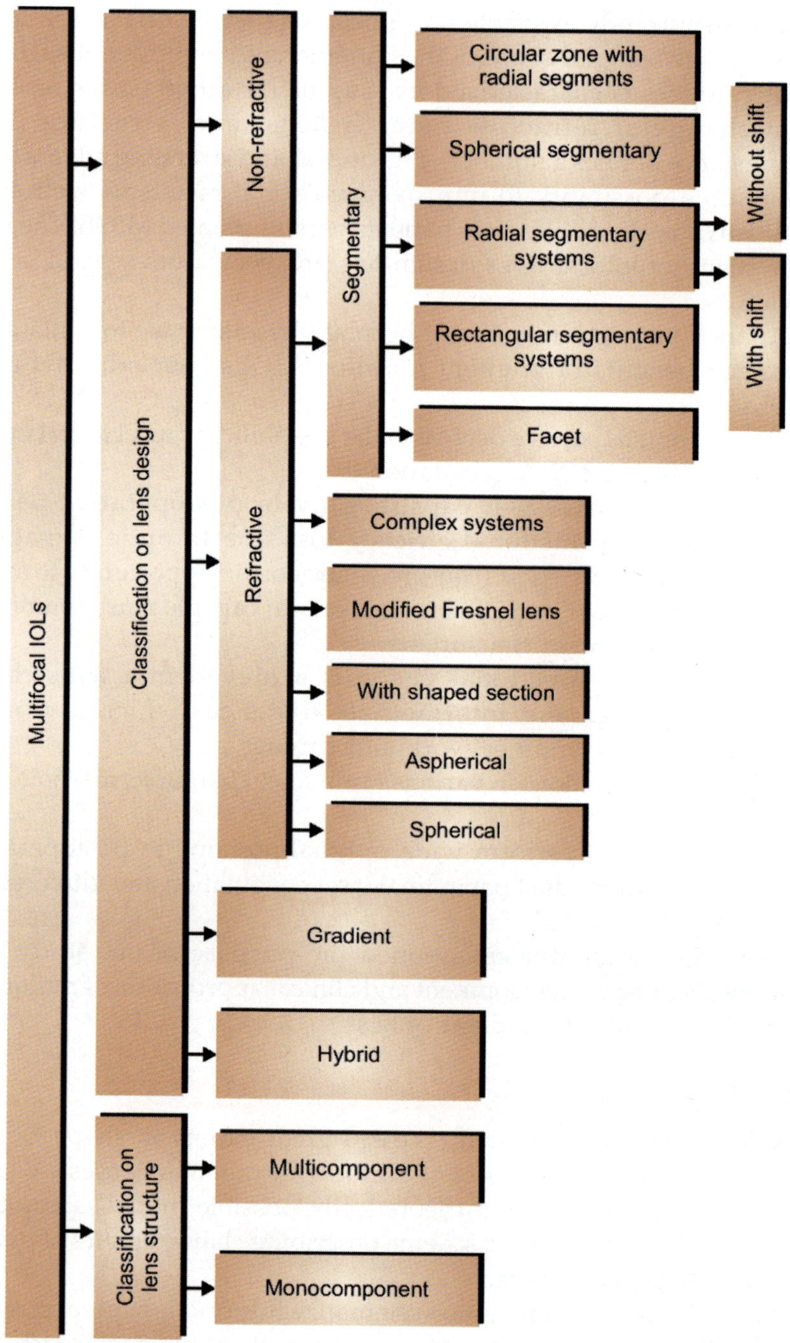

Fig. 44.1: Multifocal IOLs classification on structure and design

of one optical element and multicomponent, i.e. consisting of two and more optical components (Fig. 44.2).

Multifocal IOLs are graded in four major groups depending on the design: refractive, gradient, non-refractive and hybrid.

Most of presently existing models can be attributed to the first group (Fig. 44.3).

Group of refractive IOLs is utmost diverse. It includes spheric and aspheric designs, optical systems with shaped section, modified Fresnel lens, segmentary and complex systems (Fig. 44.4).

Segmentary optical systems subgroup incorporates facet designs, rectangular segmentary systems, radial segmentary systems (with and without shift in frontal plane), circular zone with radial segments, spherical segmentary systems (2,3,4 components) and complex optical systems (Fig. 44.5). Non-refractive IOLs group is less representative. It includes diffractive lenses with theoretical possibility to develop new models using wave image and holographic technologies.

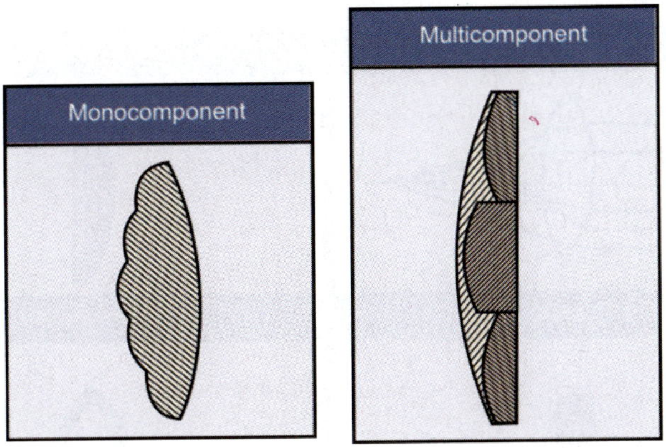

Fig. 44.2: Multifocal IOLs classification on lens structure

HUMAN EYE OPTICAL SYSTEM COMPUTER MODELING WITH MULTIFOCAL GRADIENT INTRAOCULAR LENSES IMPLANTED

Aiming to get the highest quality image and to select gradient intraocular lens optimal parameters the original mathematical modeling software was developed based on fundamental optic laws. The software is set for calculations of the human eye optical system. It enables to make and analyze test objects images by ray tracing in axial and transverse planes, to model and visualize test objects color images projected on the retina. Also it provides opportunity to conduct comparative quantitative analysis of lens optical characteristics

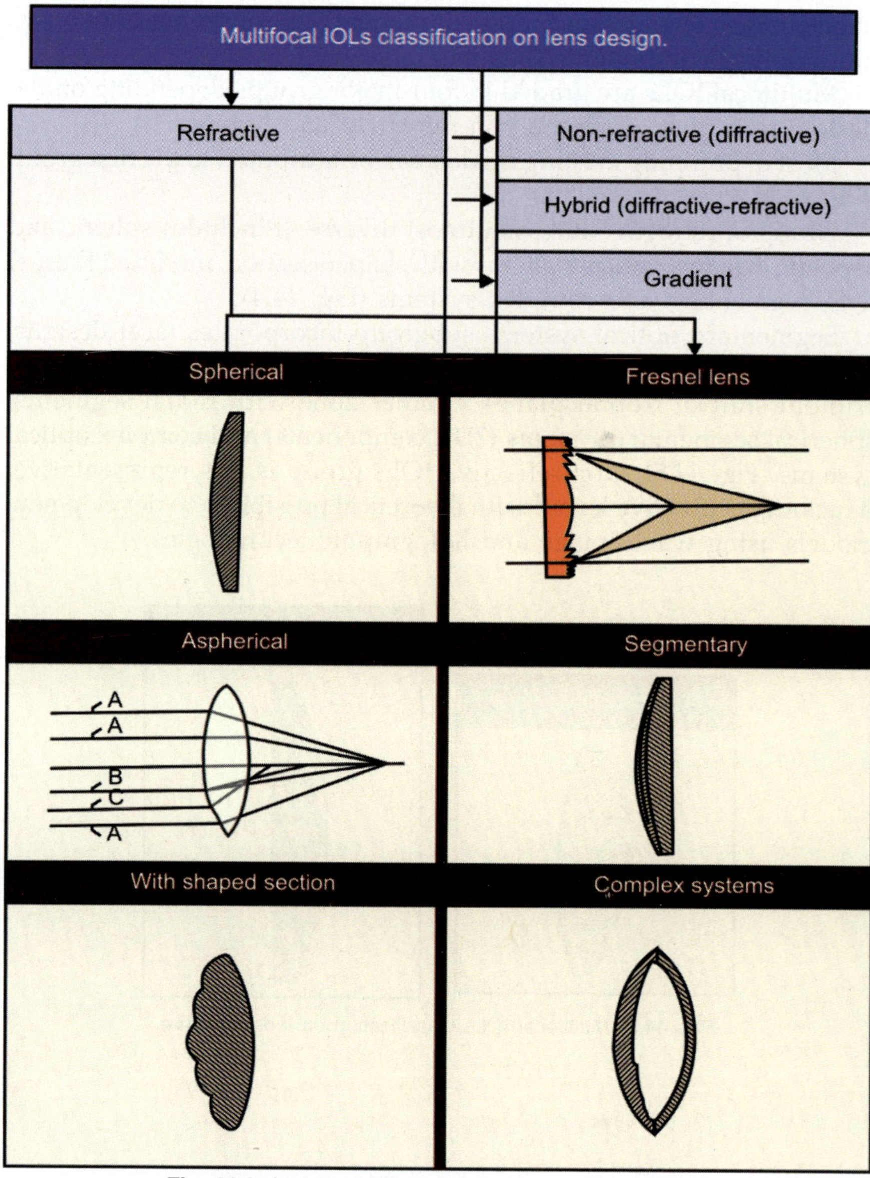

Fig. 44.3: Multifocal IOLs classification on lens design

(Modulation transfer and scattering functions) considering its parameters variability (diameter, surface curvature radius, refractive index).

Theoretical Basis and Software Working Algorithm

The software is based on calculation of light rays beam transmission each of those is incident on the lens surface at arbitrary point under

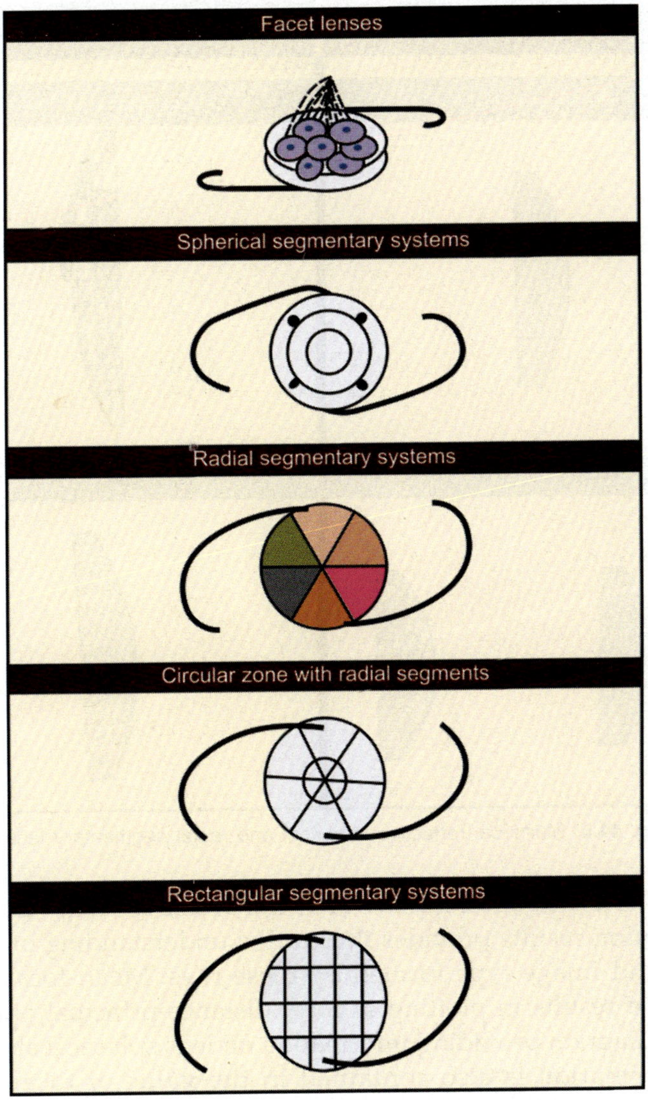

Fig. 44.4: Multifocal refractive segmentary lenses

variable angles. The only one simplifying assumption fully fulfilled in all real designs is lens axial symmetry.

Surfaces of the intraocular lenses can be spheric, ellipsoid, hyperboloic or paraboloic. The software calculates convex, concave, convex-concave and concave-convex lenses. Calculation of each ray is performed according to laws of geometrical optics in three-dimensional space.

In order to get point light source image it is necessary to calculate data of the rays' beam emitting from the given source and passing

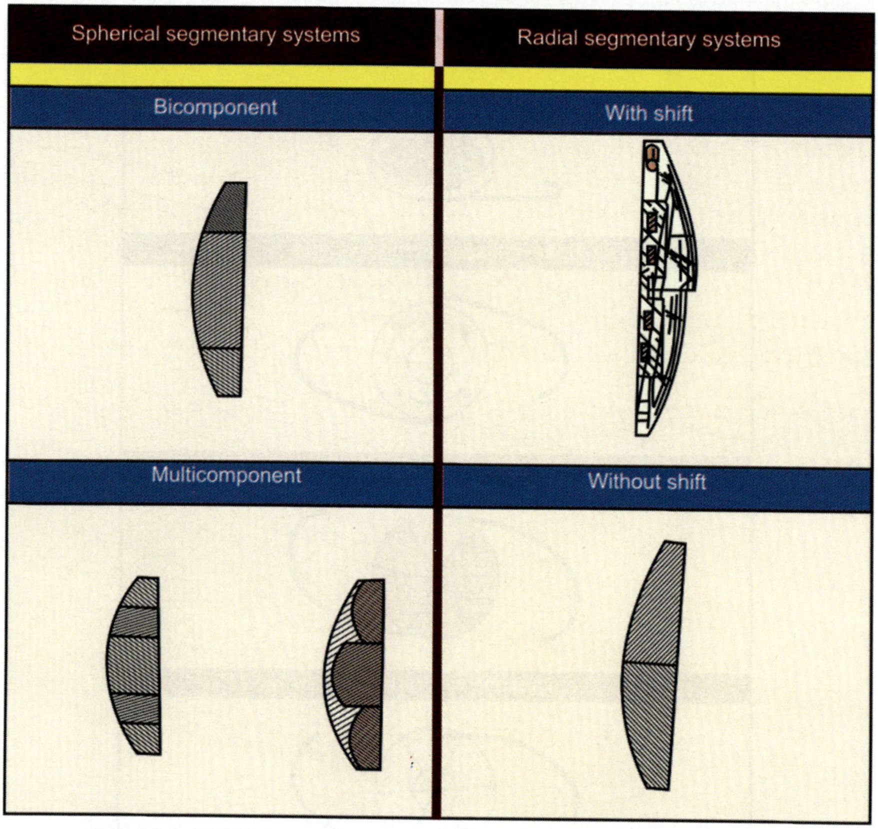

Fig. 44.5: Multifocal refractive spherical and radial segmentary lenses

through the lens at different sites of its transverse section. Visualization of calculation results provides illustrative understanding of emission pattern and image type formed by these rays. Mean focal distance calculation results in plotting of focal distance-principal optical axis distance diagram providing information on lens spherical aberrations. This information is also contained in the value of focal distance standard deviation. Spherical and higher order aberrations are calculated according to the software algorithm. The algorithm is easily extrapolated at system of lenses and can be modified for calculation of lenses with complex surface structure including gradient optic lenses.

Software Operating Window: Determination of Gradient Multifocal IOL Optimal Optical Parameters

The calculations were performed by software consisting of visual programming environment Borland C++ Builder (version 6) under Windows XP operation system.

Program operating window is presented at Figure 44.6 which demonstrates software version for particular gradient lens calculation which consists of outer and inner components. The latter has less diameter differing from the outer one by external surfaces radii and refraction index. On the whole the software takes into account considerable number of optical system parameters including cornea, aqueous humor, artificial lens, vitreous body and retina. Intraocular lens parameters are set either such as optical components diameter, curvature radius, refraction index, intraocular lens thickness, lens sphericity in relation to optical axis, and diaphragm diameter (pupil).

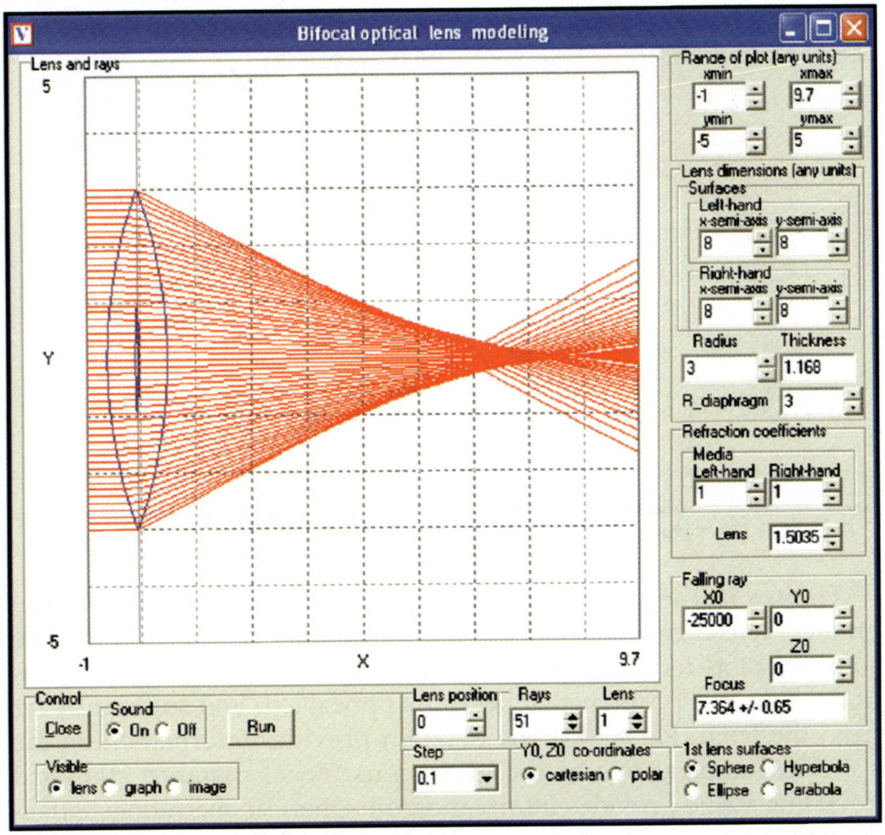

Fig. 44.6: Software operating window. Modeling rays passes through gradient lens thus determining focal zone parameters

Human eye optical parameters include curvature radius of outer corneal surface (7.7 mm), inner corneal surface (6.8 mm), outer corneal surface-retina distance (24.0 mm), retinal curvature radius (12.0 mm), cornea refraction index (1.376), aqueous humor (1.336), and vitreous body (1.337).

Computer modeling software enables to analyze distribution and rays pattern in the principal focus neighborhood and aberrations type (Figs 44.7 and 44.8).

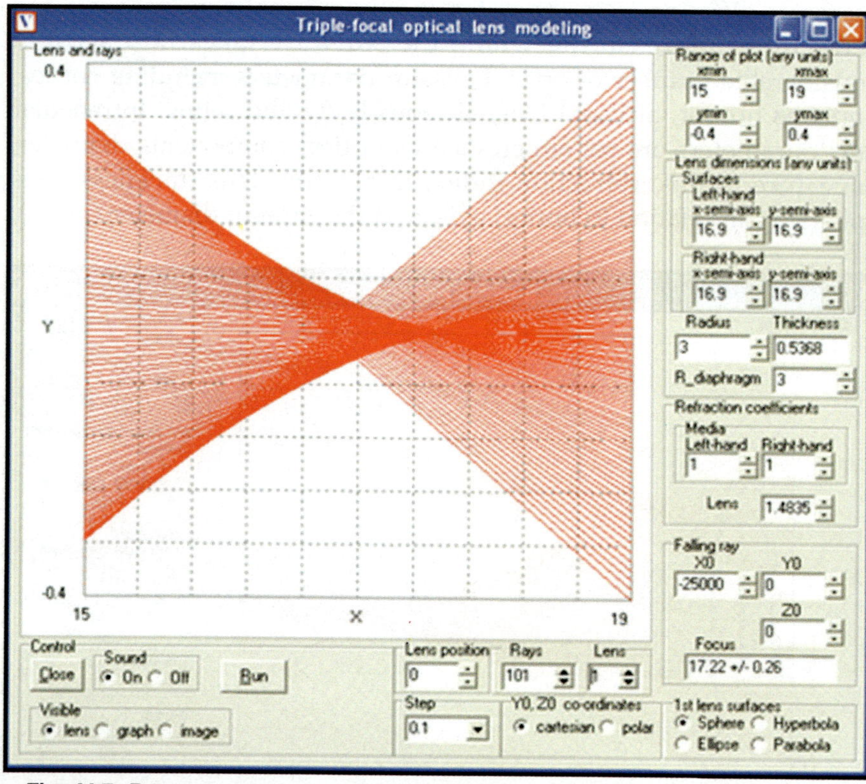

Fig. 44.7: Rays transmission nearby monofocal lens focus (refraction index-1.4835)

Figures 44.9 and 44.10 demonstrate ray transmission near multifocal gradient lens focus reflecting optimal lens parameters correlation. The software plots focal distance-ray position to lens optical axis diagram (if the source is positioned at principal optical axis and sufficiently far from the lens) (Fig. 44.11).The diagram provides information on the spherical aberrations of the given lens. Focal distance standard deviation value provides information on spherical aberrations either. All other lens aberrations are calculated according to the software algorithm.

The software enables to get and analyze point light sources located at various distances from lens principal optical axis. Figure 44.12 demonstrates light scattering sources around the light beam maximum concentration zone attributed to one of the multifocal lens focus.

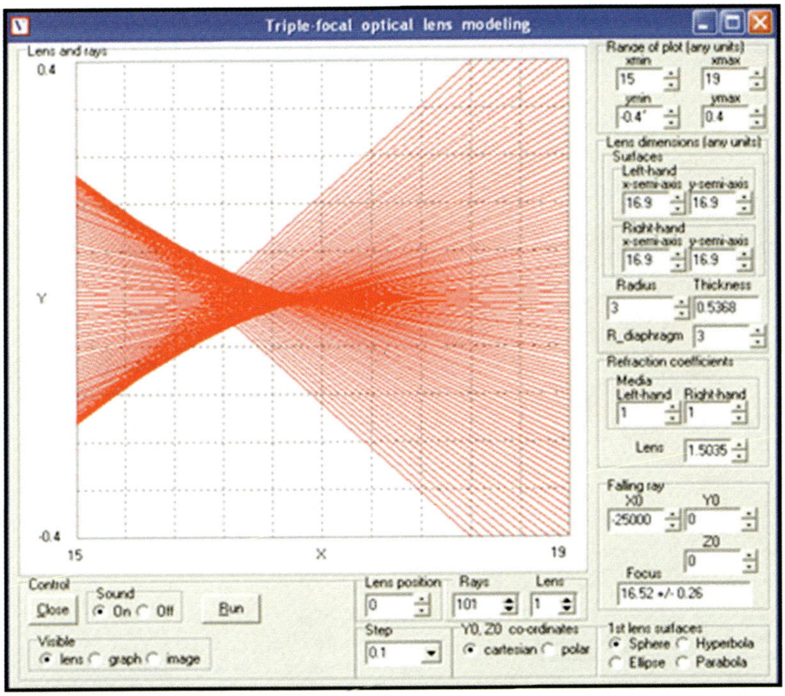

Fig. 44.8: Rays transmission nearby monofocal lens focus (refraction index-1.5035)

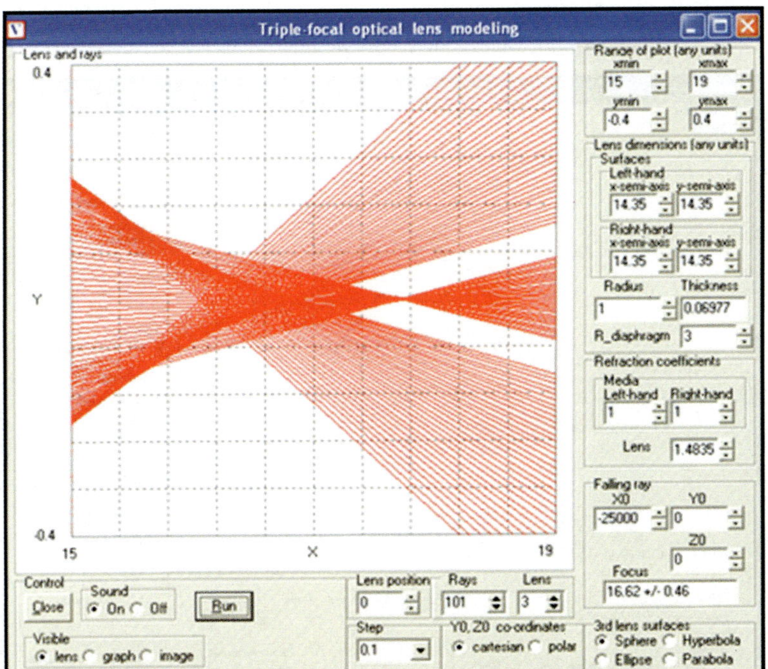

Fig. 44.9: Rays transmission nearby multifocal gradient lens focus. Outer lens component refraction index 1.5035, inner component-1.4835

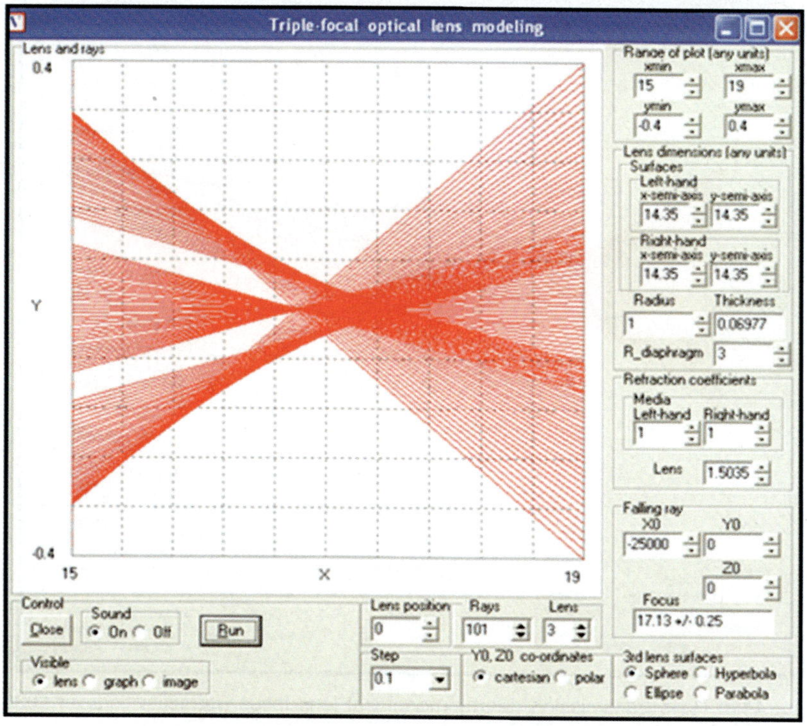

Fig. 44.10: Rays transmission nearby multifocal gradient lens focus. Outer lens component refraction index 1.4835, inner component-1.5035

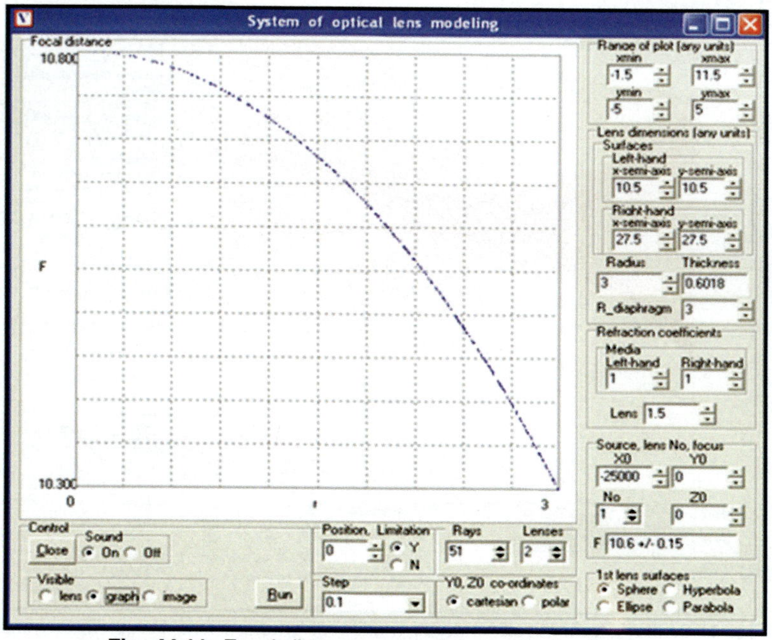

Fig. 44.11: Focal distance-ray radial coordinate diagram

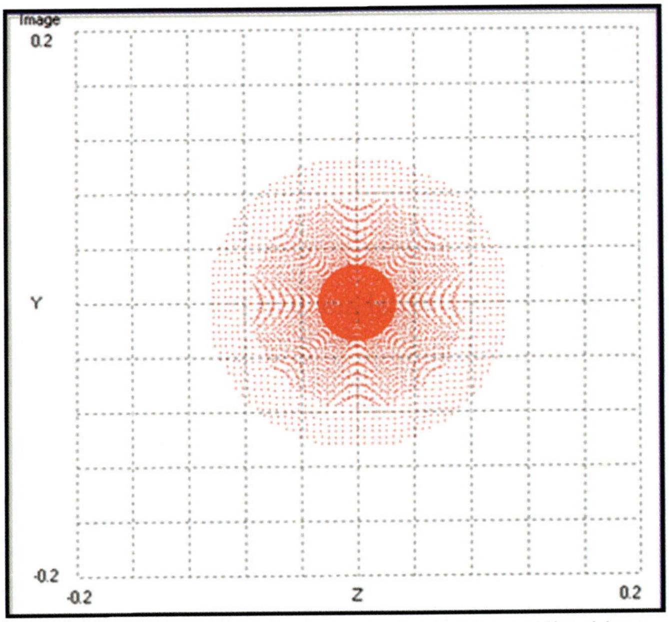

Fig. 44.12: Point light source image formed by multifocal lens

Simultaneous analysis and visualization of spherical and chromatic aberrations by the software allows building color images of test objects formed on the retina of pseudophakic eye. To obtain image quantitative estimation computer modeling software calculates modulation transfer function (MTF) and scattering function as well.

In order to calculate and select multifocal gradient IOL optimal parameters we performed comprehensive computer modeling data evaluation. Additional optical power (difference in refractive power between zones for far and near) was specified by optimal distance for near vision (30/33 cm) and was determined by refraction index (1.520 and 1.4795 for outer and inner components correspondingly) and by components curvature radius (15.11 mm outer lens component, 13.66 mm inner). Optimal calculated value of refractive power difference for far and near (outer and inner components of the lens) was 3.0 D.

Taking in mind retinal image computer modeling data, priority of vision for far in pseudophakic patients, safe driving (especially in acute miosis under bright light) and possibility of senile miosis, IOL central optical zone was designed for far vision. Diameter of inner component was calculated with consideration of light beams optimal redistribution under various luminance conditions (variable pupil diameters).

Optimal calculated value of inner component diameter made up 2.0 mm (pupil diameter 3.0 mm). Under photopic conditions light beam distribution between zones for far and near was 45% and 55%

correspondingly (inner component diameter 2.0 mm). Under bright light and 2.5 mm miosis light beam redistribution occurs at 65% and 35% correspondingly. Under mesopic conditions and 3.5-4.0 mm pupil diameter light beam for far and near zones was distributed at 30% and 70% correspondingly. Overall diameter of the intraocular lens is 6.0 mm. Inner component is placed in the center of outer one on radius and thickness. Overall intraocular lens thickness is 1.0 mm, its central component– 0.4 mm.

Monobloc foldable multifocal gradient IOL was manufactured with step-by-step polymerization technology in transfer molds of photohardening material (UV light) with various refraction indexes (oligourethanmethacrylate). This technology enables to produce multifocal artificial lenses with gradient optics. Relative simplicity is advantage of manufacturing process hence it is possible to combine stages of material polymerization with lens manufacturing at the same time. Besides, polymerization in the forms method determines better lens optical characteristics in comparison with milling method by achieving higher surface quality and minimizing optics aberrations.

"Gradiol" intraocular lens is a joint work out of the S Fyodorov Eye Microsurgery Complex (K P Takhchidi, B E Malyugin, T A Morozova) and REPER-NN lens manufacturing company (V M Treushnikov, E A Viktorova).

Figures 44.13 and 44.14 demonstrate overall view of pseudoaccommodating multifocal intraocular lens with gradient optics "Gradiol".

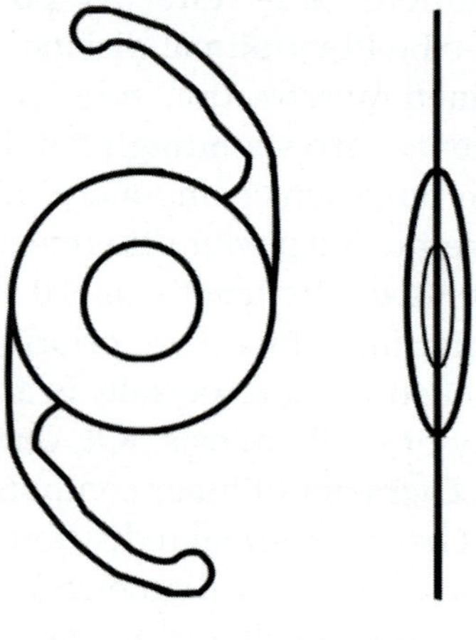

Fig. 44.13: Overall view and side view of multifocal gradient intraocular lens (blueprint)

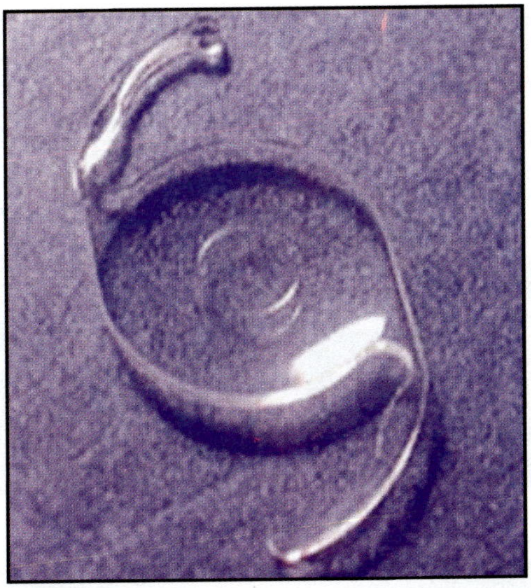

Fig. 44.14: Overall view of multifocal intraocular lens with gradient optic (photo)

CLINICAL RESULTS

Methods

25 patients (28 eyes) were prospectively enrolled with age ranging 60-82 years. Surgery included phacoemulsification with 2.75 mm clear corneal incision using Millenium® CCS (B&L). We implanted IOL in the capsular bag using forceps or injector. At the end of the surgery incisions were hydrated (Figs 44.15 and 44.16).

No complications were observed in early and long-term follow-up.

Visual Acuity for Far

Visual acuity improved in all cases after phacoemulsification with implantation of gradient multifocal IOL. Analysis of data on uncorrected and with correction visual acuity for far at various follow-up periods (1,3,6 months) proves stability and high level of the functions received (Table 44.1).

Table 44.1: Mean visual acuity (VA) for far in postoperative

Mean VA	*1 month*	*3 months*	*6 months*
Uncorrected	0.73 ± 0,16	0.72 ± 0.20	0.73 ± 0.18
With correction	0.77 ± 0,19	0.88 ± 0.13	0.89 ± 0.15

Better functional results were obtained in patients with slight hyperopia equal to ±0.5 D sphere, ±0.5 D of against-the-rule corneal

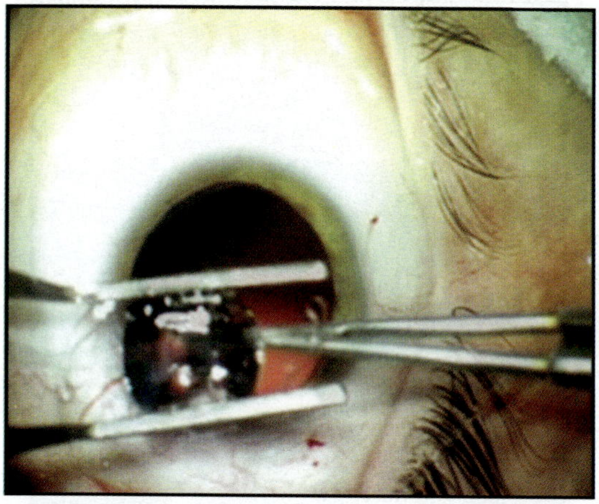

Fig. 44.15: IOL folding before implantation

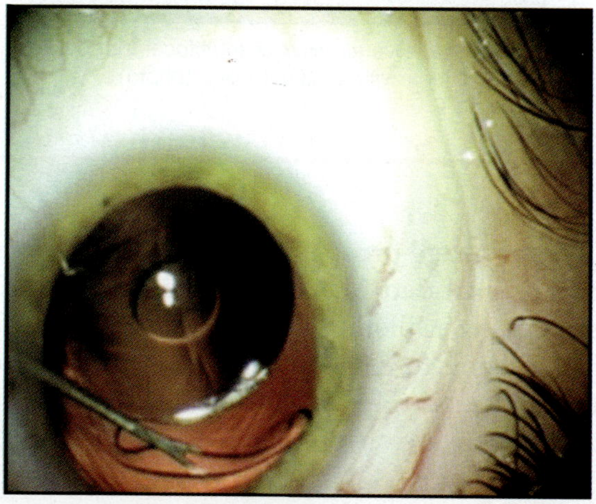

Fig. 44.16: Implantation of trailing haptic element in the capsular bag

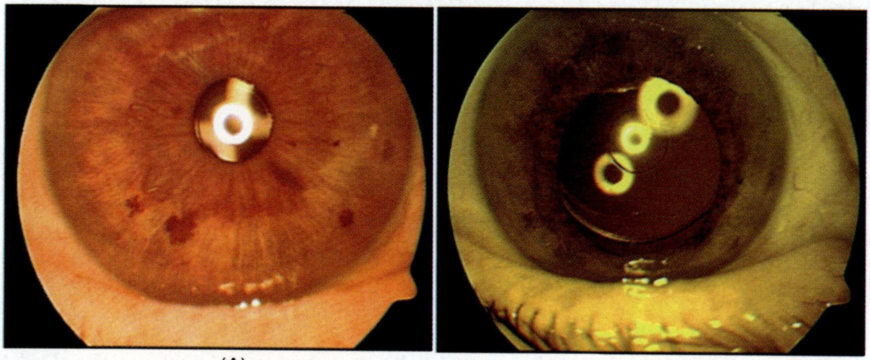

(A) (B)

Fig. 44.17: First day postoperation: (A) narrow pupil, (B) after instillation of mydriatic drops astigmatism and 1.0 D with-the-rule corneal astigmatism. Mean spheric equivalent in the group was equal to ±0.09 D.

Visual Acuity for Near

Analysis of data on uncorrected and with correction visual acuity for near at various follow-up periods (1, 3, 6 months) also proved stability and high level of visual functions achieved (Table 44.2). These data determine full visual rehabilitation and high scoring after subjective evaluation postoperative Outcomes of VA for near also provide possibility of intensive reading without additional spectacle correction.

Table 44.2: Mean visual acuity (VA) for near postoperation

Mean VA	*1 month*	*3 months*	*6 months*
Uncorrected	0.62 ± 0.16	0.60 ± 0.21	0.57 ± 0.19
With correction	0.70 ± 0.20	0.76 ± 0.18	0.84 ± 0.07

Study of VA for near with correction for far (Table 44.3) gives visual functions features specific for multifocal gradient IOLs. Additional correction for far in cases of residual myopic refraction decreases visual acuity for near compared to uncorrected VA for near. Additional correction for far in cases of residual hyperopic refraction either increases or has no effect on VA for near compared to VA for near without correction. The latter determines residual hyperopic refraction in postoperative which is more preferable.

Table 44.3: Visual acuity for near with correction for far (16 cases) and patients refractive postoperative

VA for near without correction	*VA for near with correction for far*	*Refraction*
0.5	0.4	M
0.8	1	H
0.7	0.7-0.8	H
0.8	0.4	M
0.8	0.4	M
0.5	0.8	H
0.6	0.8	H
0.7	0.3	M
0.4	0.5	H
0.5	0.3	M
0.9	0.6	M
0.3	0.5	H
0.4	0.2	M
0.3	0.8	H
0.3	0.1	M
0.5	0.3	M

Pseudoaccommodation Volume

With consideration of optical zones power difference calculated pseudoaccommodation volume should be equal at least 3.0 D. Methods used for pseudoaccommodation testing included:

- Spheres addition-assisted defocusing with 1.0 D step at corrected VA for far 0.8 using accommodometer;
- Spheres addition-assisted defocusing with 0.5 D step at corrected VA 0.5 using conventional optotypes.

We found pseudoaccommodation volume after gradient IOL implantation to be 4.75±0.5 D (Fig. 44.18).

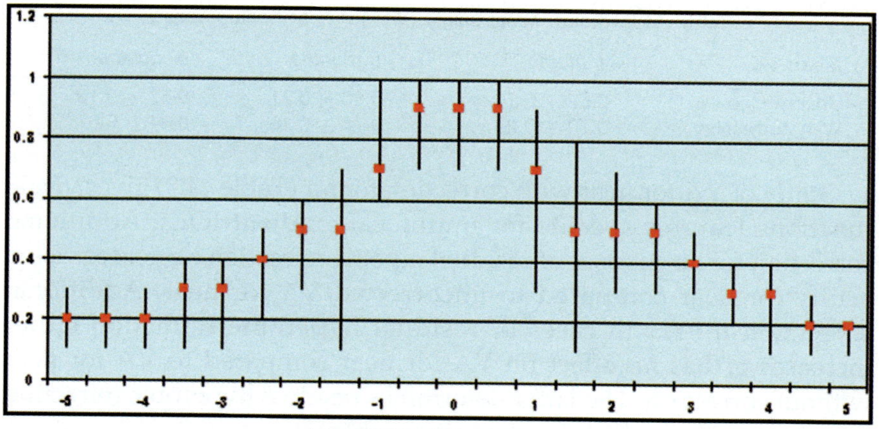

Fig. 44.18: Defocus curve

There was even distribution of light energy among all optical zones (for far, near and intermediate distances). Hence, the resultant defocus curve was smooth with peak at the point of maximum corrected visual acuity for far.

Contrast Sensitivity Testing

Contrast sensitivity testing is one of the basic components in comprehensive clinical evaluation of patient's visual outcomes in post-operation. Earlier clinical studies confirm that contrast sensitivity under conditions of diminished contrast and high spatial frequencies and mesopic visual acuity (with/without glare) are both less after multifocal implantation compared to normal values.

Our studies found specific characteristic of multifocal gradient IOLs which is even statistically insignificant decrease of contrast sensitivity at all spatial frequencies 1.5,3.0,6.0,12.0,18.0 cycl/deg compared to normal values (Fig. 44.19).

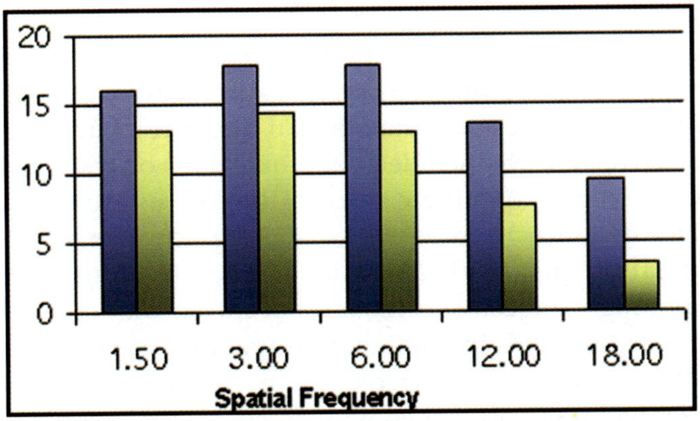

Fig. 44.19: Data on spatial contrast sensitivity testing after "Gradiol" implantation. 3 months postoperation

Optical Phenomenons

Optical phenomenons included light streaks, halos, flare, flashes, glare (Haring G et al, 2001). Halos and glare were the most frequent complaints. The grades varied from subtle to pronounce. There was no tendency for those optical phenomena to decrease on long-term follow-up.

We assume that after gradient IOL implantation the rationale of those phenomena is light beam separation at focus zone as well as presence of distinct border between inner and outer optics components. Majority of patients (57.1%) mentioned optical phenomena under thorough history taking, and only in 10.7% cases these symptoms were functionally significant. Mostly patients complained on halos in darkness and "blinding" effect at night driving when exposed to the headlights of vehicles. We did not observe optical phenomena to the extent which would substantiate IOL explantation (Table 44.4).

Table 44.4: Optical phenomenons

Type	*Total (abs.)*	*Total (%)*
Pronounced (halos only)	3	10.7
Moderate	-	-
Subtle (halos, glare)	13	46.4
Total	16	57.1
Halos	13	46.4
Glare	3	10.7

If we take patients with optical phenomenons as 100% patients with residual myopic refraction will constitute the prevailing share (81.3%). Residual myopia augments light scattering leading to more pronounced optical phenomenons thus decreasing patient's quality of life.

Subjective Visual Functions Testing

To perform quantitative analysis of visual dysfunctions we employed P Steinberg Visual Function–14 questionnaires (VF-14). With consideration of functional needs and specific characteristics of multifocal correction we included extra questions on the ability to use computer without spectacle correction (to evaluate vision at intermediate distances) and details of optical phenomena (type, level).

In our study mean VF-14 value was equivalent to 100 thus determining high subjective estimation of intraocular correction after multifocal gradient IOL implantation. Capability of effective work at near without extra spectacle correction in postoperation was present in 80% cases including prolonged work at near, small print text reading as well as working with computer under various luminance conditions (bright and dim light).

DISCUSSION

We can theoretically calculate light beams distribution in optical models of the human eye, modulation transfer and scattering functions as well as to perform retinal image modeling. But the final conclusion on efficacy of particular pseudoaccommodating IOL design can be made after clinical trials only. It is almost impossible to predict whether human brain is capable to analyze visual information altered by multifocal lens of certain design. Functional outcomes for far and near at long-term follow-up and pseudoaccommodation volume obtained prove efficacy of multifocal gradient IOL.

We received data on visual acuity for far at "Gradiol" group comparable to groups with diffractive and refractive MIOLs. For instance, in ReSTOR® lens (diffractive/refractive; Alcon) uncorrected visual acuity for far reaches 0.8 in 54% cases, for near- 0.5 in 100% and 0.8 in 52% cases (L Balashevich, Y Takhtayev, 2005; Packard R, 2006). AMO Array® (refractive IOL) multicenter clinical trial reports uncorrected visual acuity for far 0.7 and better in 73%, visual acuity for near 0.5 and better in 85%. According to H B Dick (2005), mean binocular uncorrected visual acuity for far after ReZoom® refractive multifocal IOL implantation is equal to 1.0, for near- 0.5.

Unlike patients with refractive and gradient IOLs people with diffractive IOLs complain on substantial visual impairment at intermediate distances (from 40 cm to 1 m) the latter essential for driving (dashboard control) and computer work.

Contrast sensitivity testing in our study showed data comparability with previous results of diffractive MIOLs 3M (825 LE model) and refractive AMO Array® (SSM 26 NB model) (Pieh S et al, 1998). In those studies contrast sensitivity in both groups at low and high spatial frequencies was identical ranging in recommended age normal values. Compared to refractive MIOLs contrast sensitivity in patients with diffractive MIOLs was lower at moderate frequencies. At glare testing contrast sensitivity in the first group was significantly less than recommended normal value.

We consider subtle decrease of contrast sensitivity at all spatial frequencies as an important specific feature of multifocal gradient IOLs. We believe this characteristic enables visual work under variable luminance and adequate functional rehabilitation of patients in post-operative period. Having compared contrast sensitivity testing outcomes in our and other trials we assume that gradient and refractive MIOLs have advantage over diffractive intraocular lenses as the latter are accompanied by impaired contrast sensitivity and increased glare.

Optical phenomenons postoperative study is an important part of functional outcomes research. We registered clinically significant symptoms in 10.7% only. There is no regression of symptoms in long-term follow-up. However, brain is capable to ignore this information therefore most of the patients note optical phenomenons only after meticulous discussion (57%). Theoretically mechanisms of this phenomenons can be explained by light reflection from transitional zone and IOL surface and light diffraction at the border of optical components.

During comparative analysis obtained data were similar in different types of MIOLs, e.g. G.Haring (2001) reports of side optical effects in 9% cases after monofocal IOL implantation and in 41% cases after refractive multifocals. Halos and flare are more frequent in patients after multifocal implantation compared to monofocal. In Acrysof ReSTOR® (Alcon) L Balashevich and Y Takhtayev (2005) observed visual impairment in twilight conditions in 8% cases, optical side effects near point light source in 11%, impairment on glare testing in 14%. Symptoms were of moderate grade. Obvious prospective solution of optical side effects is probably in further IOL design refinements including elimination and smoothening of transitional zones.

Conventional visual acuity testing is the most widely used in evaluation of functional outcomes. Nevertheless this testing neither reflects pertinently patient's satisfaction nor provides information on his quality of life and work. Subjective testing in all MIOLs groups demonstrates high level of patient's satisfaction postoperation. According to various publications dealing with functional results evaluation after multifocal implantation 32-81% patients did not require extra spectacle correction (Roy F H, Tindall R, 1993; Wiemer C et al, 1994; Pearce J L, 1996; Javitt J C et al, 1997; Jacobi F K et al, 1999; Javitt

J C, Steinert R F, 2000; Sasaki A, 2000; Slagsvold J E, 2000). In our study 86% patients did not use extra spectacle correction for work at far and near including prolonged activity and driving.

Consequently, our clinical trial proves safety, efficacy and stability of results determining adequate visual rehabilitation and high level of satisfaction. Having excellent prospects, idea of multifocal correction drives scientists and manufacturers to keep on searching for design refinements of existing IOLs, creation of new models stipulating interest to this field in future.

Our initial results are essential in development of optics with gradient change in refraction index. The most significant disadvantage of "Gradiol" multifocal intraocular lens lies in postoperative optical phenomena which is common for the whole group of multifocals. Prospective solutions can be found in elimination and smoothening of transitional zone between two optical components. Currently we conduct clinical trial of new generation of multifocal gradient intraocular lenses with no transitional border between two optical zones.

REFERENCES

1. Bleckmann H, Schmidt O, Sunde T, Kaluzny J. Visual results of progressive multifocal posterior chamber intraocular lens implantation. J Cataract Refract Surg 1996, Vol. 22 (8), pp 1102-7.
2. Brydon K W, Tokarewicz A C, Nichols BD. AMO Array multifocal lens versus monofocal correction in cataract surgery. J Cataract Refract. Surg, 2000 (26), pp 96-100.
3. Eisenmann D, Jacobi F K, Dick B, Jacobi KW Related. The "Array" silicone multi-focal lens: experiences after 150 implantations. Klin Monatsbl Augenheilkd, 1996, Vol 208 (5), pp 270-2.
4. Featherstone K A, Bloomfield J R, Lang A J, Miller-Meeks M J, Woodworth G., Steinert R F. Driving simulation study: bilateral array multifocal versus bilateral AMO monofocal intraocular lenses. J Cataract Refract Surg, 1999, Vol 25 (9), pp 1254-62.
5. Fisher R F. The ciliary body in accommodation. Trans Ophthalmol Soc UK, 1986, Vol 105, pp 208-19.
6. Garner L, Ooi C, Smith G, Refractive index of the crystalline lens in young and aged eyes. Clin Exp Optometry, 1998, Vol 81 (4), pp 145-50.
7. Giardini P, Mazzilli S, Hauranieh N, Frialdi F. PRELEX to correct hyperopia and presbyopia: our experience nongress of the ESCRS, 20th: Abstracts–France, 2002, pp 139.
8. Glasser A. Can accommodation be surgically restored in human presbyopia?. Optometry and Vision Science, 1999, Vol 3 (9).
9. Glasser A. Thoughts on surgical correction of presbyopia. Refractive surgery: Theses of Subspecialty Day of AAO Annual Meeting. Dallas, 2000, pp 177-80.
10. Glasser A, Campbell C W. Presbyopia and the optical changes in the human crystalline lens with age. Vision Res, 1998, Vol 38, (2), pp 209-29.

11. Hamasaki D, Ong J, Marg E. The amplitude of accommodation in presbyopia. Am. J Optom, 1956, Vol 33, pp 3-14.
12. Haring G, Dick H B, Krummenauer F, Weissmantel U, Kroncke W. Subjective photic phenomena with refractive multifocal and monofocal intraocular lenses results of a multicenter questionnaire. J Cataract Refract Surg, 2001, Vol 27 (2), pp 245-9.
13. Hiejde G L. Age-related changes in the accommodation mechanism. Optom. Vis Sci 1996, Vol 73, pp 235-42.
14. Jain I S, Ram J, Bupta A. Early onset of presbyopia Am. J Optom Physiol Opt 1982, Vol 59, pp 1002-4.
15. Javitt J C, Steinert R F. Cataract extraction with multifocal intraocular lens implantation: a multinational clinical trial evaluating clinical, functional, and quality-of-life outcomes. Ophthalmology, 2000, Vol 107 (11), pp 2040-8.
16. Javitt J C, Wang F, Trentacost D J, Rowe M, Tarantino N. Outcomes of cataract extraction with multifocal intraocular lens implantation: functional status and quality of life. Ophthalmology, 1997, Vol 104 (4), pp 589-99.
17. Kamath G G, Prasad S, Danson A, Phillips R P. Visual outcome with the array multifocal intraocular lens in patients with concurrent eye disease. J Cataract Refract Surg, 2000, Vol 26 (4), pp 576-81.
18. Knorz M C. Presbyopic lens exchange (PRELEX) using the Arrày multifocal IOL. Congress of the ESCRS, 20th: Abstracts– France, 2002, pp 159.
19. Lesueur L, Gajan B, Nardin M, Chapotot E, Arne J L. Ñomparison of visual results and quality of vision between two multifocal intraocular lenses. Multifocal silicone and bifocal PMMA. J Fr Ophtalmol, 2000, Vol 23 (4), pp 355-9.
20. Milder B, Ruben M L. Accommodation. In: The fine art of prescribing glasses without making a spectical of Gainesville: Triad Scientific Publishes, 1978, pp 18-41.
21. Packard R. Lifestyle considerations for patients bilaterally implanted with a diffractive refractive intraocular lens: long-term follow-up// Ñongress of the ESCRS, 24-th: Abstracts. London, 2006, pp 113.
22. Pearce J. Multifocal intraoculare lenses. Curr Opin Ophthalmol, 1996, Vol 7 (1), pp 2-10.
23. Pieh S, Weghaupt H, Skorpik C. Contrast sensitivity and glare disability with diffractive and refractive multifocal intraocular lenses. J Cataract Refract Surg, 1998, Vol 24 (5), pp 659-62.
24. Piercionek BK. Presbyopia - effect of refractive index. Clin Exp Optom, 1999, Vol 73, pp 23-30.
25. Pierscionek B. Refractive index in the human lens. Exp Eye Res, 1997, Vol 64, pp 887-93.
26. Roy F H, Tindall R. Multifocal intraocular lens technology and clinical applications. J Ophthalmic Nurs Technol, 1993, Vol 12 (4), pp 172-4.
27. Sasaki A. Initial experience with a refractive multifocal intraocular lens in a Japanese population. J Cataract Refract Surg, 2000, Vol 26 (7), pp 1001-7.
28. Schachar R A. Cause and treatment of presbyopia with a method for increasing the amplitude of accommodation. Ann Ophthalmol, 1992, Vol 271 pp 445-52.
29. Schachar R A. Is Helmholtz's theory of accommodation correct? Ann Ophthalmol, 1999, Vol 31, pp 10-17.

30. Schachar R A. Pathophysiology of accommodation and presbyopia: understanding the clinical implications. J Florida Med Assoc, 1994, Vol 81. pp 268-71.
31. Schachar R A, Black T D, Kash R L, Cudmore D P, Schanzlin D J. The mechanism of accommodation and presbyopia in the primate Ann Îphthalmol, 1995, Vol 27, pp 58-67.
32. Slagsvold J E. 3M diffractive multifocal intraocular lens: eight year follow-up. J Cataract Refract Surg, 2000. Vol 26 (3), pp 402-407.
33. Strenk S A, Semmlow J L, Strenk L M, Munoz P, Gronlund-Jacob J, DeMarco K J. Age-related changes in human ciliary muscle and lens: a magnetic resonance imaging study. Invest Ophthalmol Vis Sci, 1999, Vol 40, pp 1162-9.

CHAPTER

45

I Howard Fine, Mark Packer, Richard S Hoffman (USA)

Refractive Lens Exchange: Current Perspectives

INTRODUCTION

The treatment of presbyopia has many suboptimal modalities including progressive-lens spectacles, bifocal contact lenses, monovision IOLs, and conductive keratoplasty. There are also investigational modalities including scleral implants, multifocal excimer ablation and corneal inserts.

In 2001, my partners and I published a paper documenting that we could, with power modulations, reduce the energy input into the eye to a tenth of one percent of previously used levels, remove all grades of nuclear density cataracts, and still have dramatic improvements in visual outcomes, as noted by very high levels of totally clear corneas and uncorrected visual acuities of 20/40 or better in the immediate, two to 24 hour, postoperative period.[1] This study also documented that uncorrected visual acuities were inversely proportional to the amount of energy introduced in the course of cataract surgery: the lowest levels of energy resulted in the best levels of uncorrected visual acuities, independent of patient age or cataract density. We subsequently surveyed all of the new phacoemulsification technologies and showed that once again, with utilization of these technologies, we had dramatic further improvements in outcomes.[2] We have also refined our technique for refractive lens exchange in clear lenses and soft cataracts.[3]

The procedure is performed under topical anesthesia after appropriate informed consent, preoperative measurements for IOL determination, and preoperative dilation and antibiotics. A Mastel Paratrap diamond keratome (Mastel Precision Surgical Instruments, Rapid City, SD) is utilized to create two 1.2 mm clear corneal incisions 30-45° from the temporal limbus (60-90° from each other) (Fig. 45.1). One-half cc of non-preserved lidocaine 1% is instilled into the anterior chamber followed by complete expansion of the anterior chamber with Viscoat®. A straight 25 gauge needle is then inserted through the right-handed microincision to perforate the central anterior lens capsule while simultaneously lifting a flap edge to begin a capsulorhexis (Fig. 45.2). Needles routinely bent at the tip for conventional capsulorhexis initiation have been found to lacerate the roof of the microincision during withdrawal of the needle. The straight unaltered 25 gauge needle is less likely to result in this complication. After removal of the needle, a capsulorhexis forceps, specially designed to fit and function through a 1 mm incision is then inserted through the same incision and used to complete a 5-6 mm rhexis (Fig. 45.3).

Cortical cleaving hydrodissection[4] with decompression is then performed in two separate distal quadrants followed by a third round

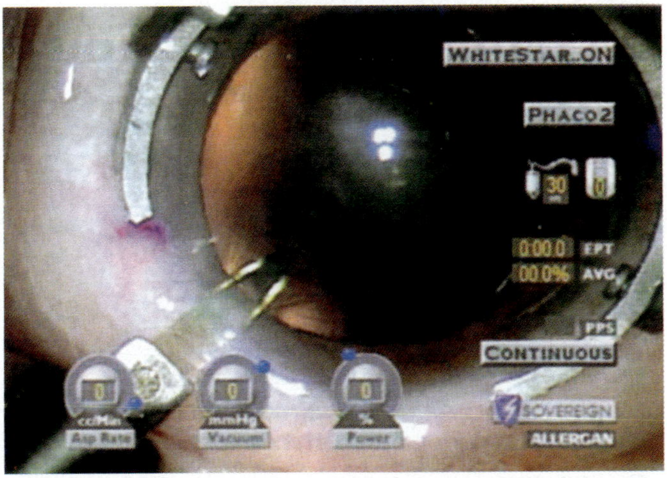

Fig. 45.1: Left-handed 1.2 mm clear corneal microincision placed 45° from the temporal limbus utilizing a Mastel Paratrap diamond knife

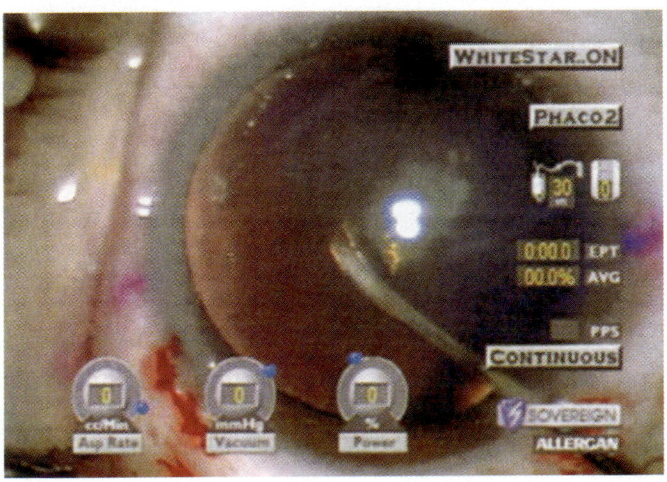

Fig. 45.2: A straight 25 gauge needle begins the capsulorhexis by perforating the central anterior lens capsule while simultaneously lifting a flap edge

of hydrodissection to prolapse the entire lens or at least one-half of the lens out of the capsular bag. The microincision irrigating handpiece (Fig. 45.4) is placed in the left-hand incision and the unsleeved phaco needle is inserted through the right-hand incision. Lens extraction is then performed in most cases without phaco power, utilizing high levels of vacuum while carouselling the relatively soft lens in the plane of the iris until it is consumed (Fig. 45.5). Small amounts of ultrasound energy can be utilized when needed. Care should be taken to avoid directing the infusion flow towards the phaco needle tip so as to prevent dislodging nuclear material from the tip. While maintaining

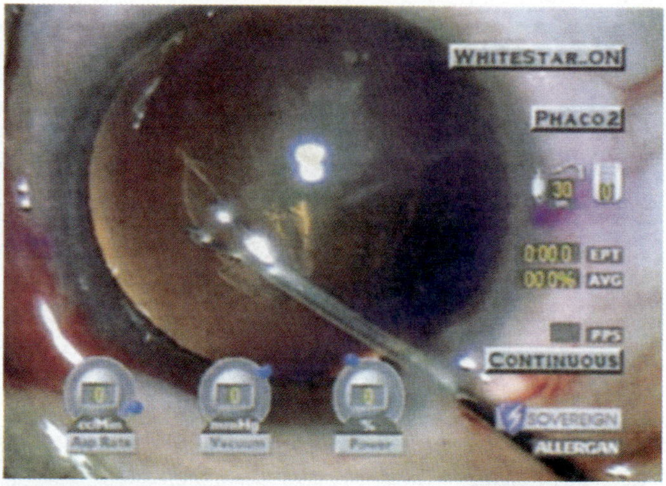

Fig. 45.3: Capsulorhexis formation utilizing an ASICO microincision capsulorhexis forceps

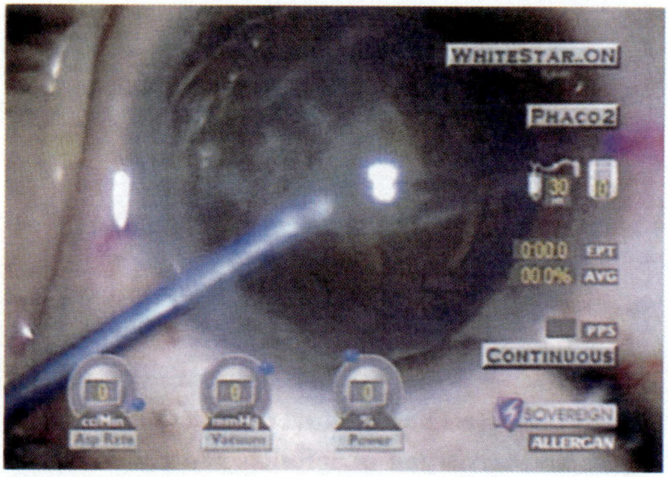

Fig. 45.4: The Duet System (MST Microsurgical Technology) beveled irrigating handpiece within the left-handed microincision

infusion with the irrigating handpiece, the phaco needle is removed and the aspiration handpiece is inserted to remove residual cortex and polish the posterior capsule. If subincisional cortex is difficult to extract, the I/A handpieces can be alternated between the two incisions in order to gain easier access to the subincisional capsular fornix (Fig. 45.6).

Once all cortex has been removed, the aspiration handpiece is removed and viscoelastic is injected into the capsular bag and anterior chamber while withdrawing the irrigating handpiece (Fig. 45.7). Following this, the viscoelastic cannula is removed from the eye and a new 2.5 mm clear corneal incision is placed between the two

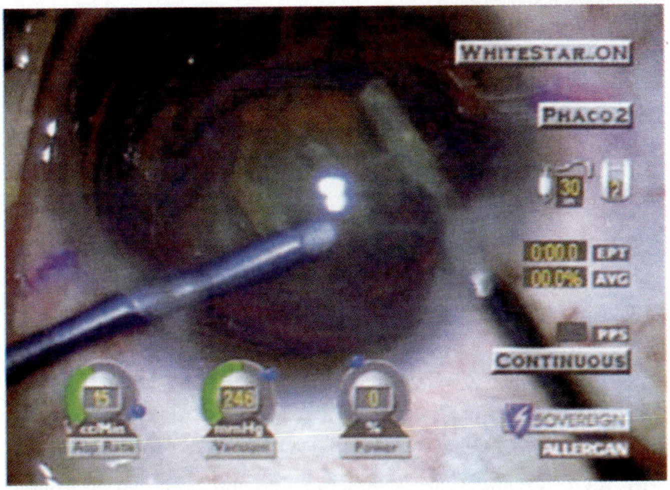

Fig. 45.5: The soft lens is carouselled in the iris plane and consumed utilizing high vacuum levels. Forward movement of the lens is prevented with the irrigating handpiece

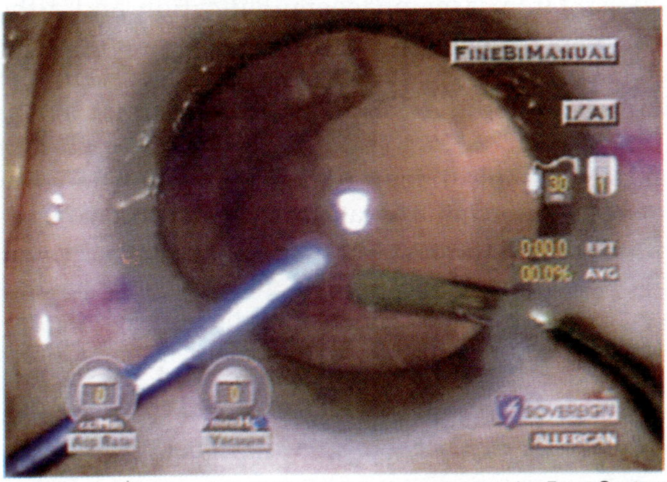

Fig. 45.6: Subincisional cortex is easily removed using the Duet System (MST) bimanual irrigation and aspiration handpieces. (Note the Effective Phaco Time EPT = 0 and Average Percent Phaco Power AVG = 0 following lens removal)

microincisions for IOL insertion. After IOL insertion, stromal hydration of the 2.5 mm incision is performed to assist in its self-sealing. Bimanual I/A is performed to remove all viscoelastic. The aspiration handpiece is then removed and irrigation of the anterior chamber maintained. Stromal hydration of the empty incision is performed to assist in closure of the microincision. The irrigation handpiece is then removed followed by stromal hydration of that incision. In this manner, the eye is fully formed and pressurized throughout the procedure avoiding hypotony and shallowing of the anterior chamber.

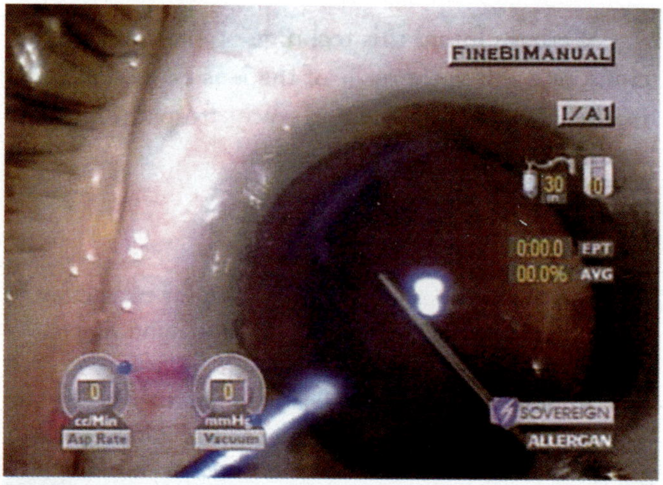

Fig. 45.7: Viscoelastic is injected into the capsular bag while maintaining infusion with the irrigating handpiece

We investigated laser phacoemulsification and although we achieved excellent results, we realized that we were limited to very soft nuclei. We used equivalent or greater levels of energy than ultrasound with modulations. We put three times as much fluid through the eye and the surgeries took two to three times as long as ultrasound phacoemulsification with power modulations. As a result, at this time, laser phacoemulsification is no competition for ultrasound.

Based on these studies, we concluded that cataract/lens extraction is incredibly safe and efficacious. In 2002, we published a paper in which we described our participation in the FDA-monitored study of the IOL Master documenting that partial coherence interferometry was as accurate as immersion ultrasound axial length measurements, using the Quantel Axis-II system.[5] The coefficient of correlation of these two modalities was .996. During that study, we documented fully that 48% of our patients outcomes achieved precisely the spherical equivalent for which were aiming, 92% were within a quarter of a diopter of the desired spherical equivalent, and the mean absolute error was .21 diopters. This leads us to conclude that preoperative measurements and calculations today allow for excellent results and continue to improve.

Improved cataract surgery outcomes as a result of lower energy, smaller incisions, and adjunctive astigmatic techniques with increased accuracy and safety, has lead to an evolution of lens surgery into refractive surgery. We also have to recognize that corneal refractive surgery has certain limitations. These include high hyperopes, higher myopes, patients with thin corneas and with cataracts, and also

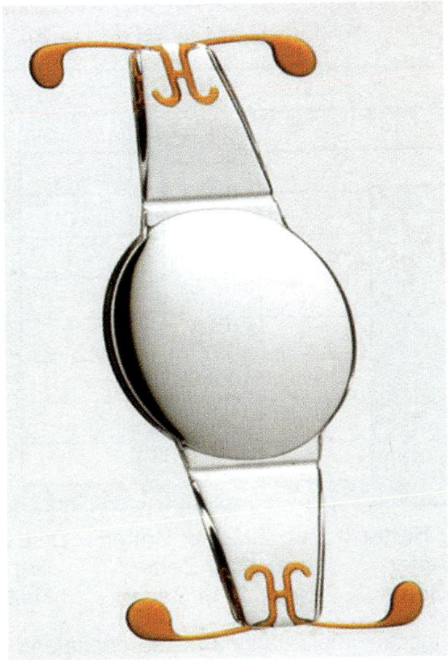

Fig. 45.8: The eyeonics crystalens™ SE

presbyopes. We also have to recognize that spherical aberration remains stable in the cornea but increases in the crystalline lens with increasing age. Anything that is done to the cornea as a refractive surgery modality will degrade over time as the spherical aberration in the human crystalline lens changes.

When we look at the available IOLs for refractive lens exchange, we realize that options are becoming increasingly larger in number and better in what they offer. New lenses include the eyeonics crystalens™ (Aliso Viejo, CA) which is the first accommodative IOL that has become available in the United States (Fig. 45.8). With its improved 360° square posterior edge and ability to be injected through a 2.5 mm incision, this is an extremely attractive option. One hundred percent of our patients in the FDA-monitored study who were binocularly implanted with the crystalens™ were at least 20/30 or better at all distance and 71% were 20/20 or better at all distances (Fig. 45.9). Figure 45.10 demonstrates the stability of these results over three years.

We have noted, however, that 15.7% of our patients, all of whom were hyperopes, were more than one diopter from the desired spherical equivalent. We believe this is related to an inability to predict the final position of the optic within the eye. A small capsular bag will compress the haptics and result in a more posteriorly located optic, resulting in hyperopia, and a large bag will compress it less resulting in an anteriorly located optic, which will result in myopia (Fig. 45.11). We

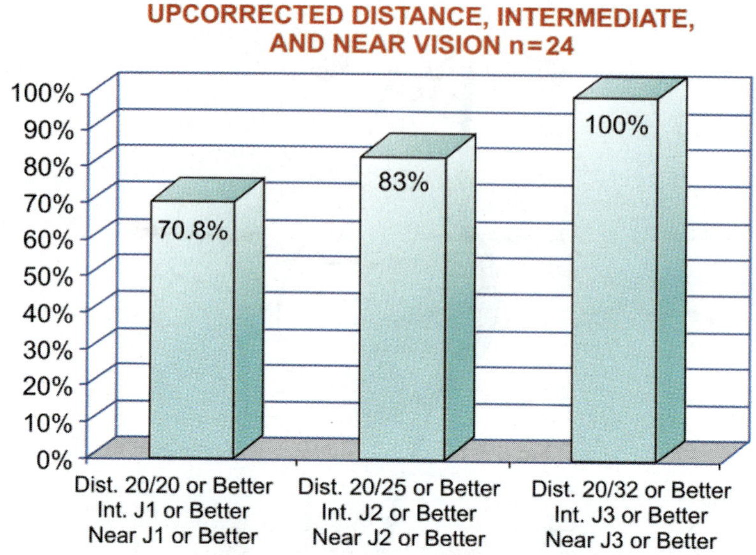

Fig. 45.9: Results for binocular implantations of the crystalens at Drs Fine, Hoffman and Packer as part of the FDA-monitored study

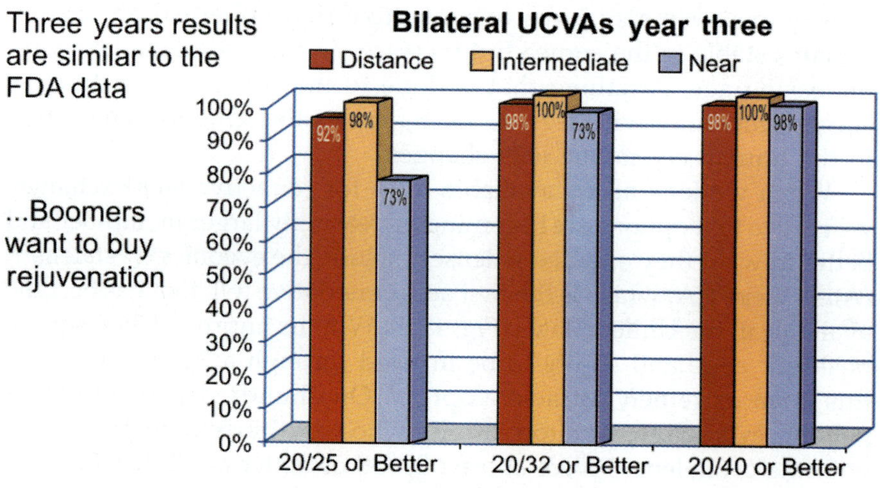

Fig. 45.10: Three results of binocular implantations of the crystalens

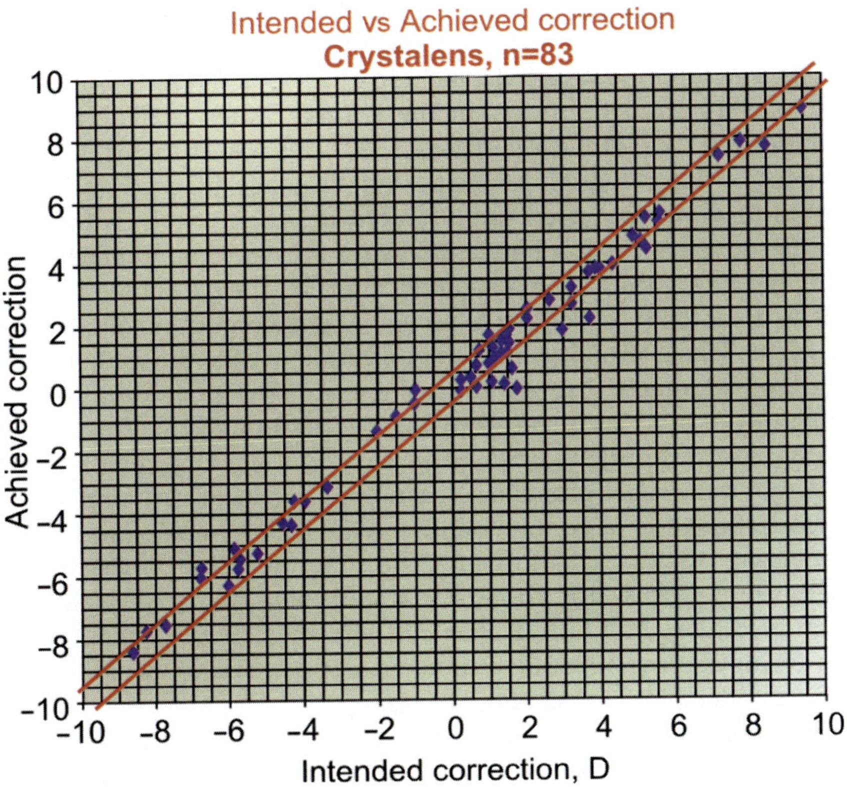

Fig. 45.11: Scatterplot of intended versus achieved spherical equivalent for implantations of the crystalens™

enhanced all of these patients with excellent results by implanting a piggyback IOL in the ciliary sulcus which is quite far in front of the crystalens™ and does not appear to impede the mechanism of accommodation of the lens.

We have completed quality of life surveys on our crystalens™ patients and have found that spectacle independence is achieved in 73% of our patients and that is exactly the percentage of our patients that were at least 20/25 or better at all distances. This mirrors the experience we have had earlier with the Array Multifocal IOL[6,7] (Advanced Medical Optics, Santa Ana, CA). In that group of patients, 44% were at least 20/25 or better at all distances and that is exactly the same percentage of patients who were spectacle independent. This may be what Richard Lindstrom, MD, has previously indicated as 20/"happy," that visual acuity that will allow for complete spectacle independence.

Other lenses that move in the eye include the Kellen TretraFlex (Lenstec, St Petersburg, FL) and the Human Optics 1CU (Human Optics

AG, Erlangen Germany), both of which have been tested in Europe, but we have had no experience within the United States.

Other accommodative IOLs include dual-optic IOLs. The first that has come to clinical studies in the United States is the Visiogen Synchrony™ Dual-Optic IOL (Irvine, CA). This is a lens with a minus-powered optic located against the posterior capsule attached by flexible haptics to a plus-powered optic located more anteriorly within the capsular bag. The flexible haptics allow for greater separation between the two optics during accommodative effort on the part of the patient. This is essentially a Galilean telescope and theoretical evaluation of dual-optic lenses promises greater amplitude of accommodation than single-optic lenses that move in the eye.[8] The early data for the Synchrony™ IOL has been good (Figs. 45.12 and 45.13). This lens is also injectable through a 3.5 mm incision by a new injection system.

Perhaps the most promising technology for increased amplitudes of accommodation in accommodative IOLs is deformable optic IOLs. The Power Vision IOL (Power Vision, Santa Barbara, CA) has a reservoir that allows for fluid to be stored there during relaxation of accommodation. The fluid is pumped into the central portion of the lens during accommodation, resulting in a greater curvature of the optic and a greater plus power (Fig. 45.14).

One of the most exciting technologies is the NuLens Accommodating IOL from Herzliya, Israel. The manufacturers of this

Feb 2005 - synchrony (24 eyes)	6 months
BCVA 20/40 or better	100% (24/24)
DCNVA 20/40 or better	96% (23/24)
Defocus curves	3.22 D

Fig. 45.12: Summary of six-month data for the Visiogen Synchrony™ Dual-optic IOL

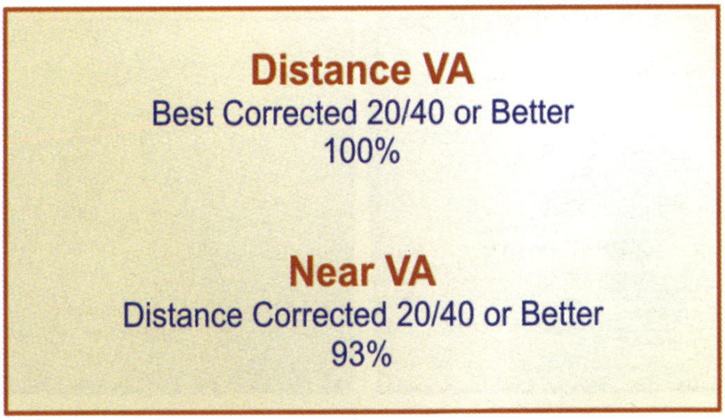

Fig. 45.13: Best corrected near and distance visual acuities for the most recent implantations of the Visiogen Synchrony™ Dual-optic IOL

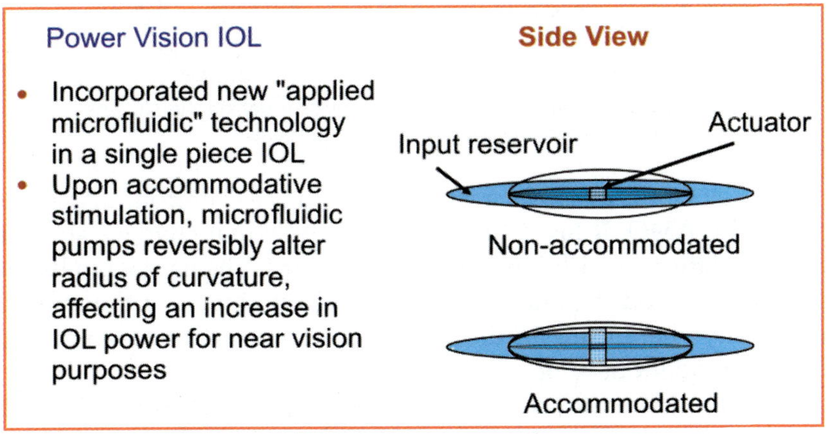

Fig. 45.14: Schematic of the Power Vision IOL

lens believe that at least eight diopters of accommodation are required for comfortable, continuous activity: one diopter for adjustment of the far plane, three diopters for near and an accommodative amplitude of twice that, resulting in a need for eight diopters of accommodation in order to avoid accommodative fatigue. The lens is based on a naturally occurring system of deformable optics which is present in the Merganser. This is a bird that flies but also fishes for food and is able to see under water by forcing the anterior surface of the lens through a stiff pupil, resulting in a marked increased curvature of the lens (Fig. 45.15). The NuLens is essentially built by putting a compressible polymer between two firm plates. Accommodation results in a pressing of that polymer through the aperture in the anterior plate and an increased curvature, which theoretically can give up to 30 diopters of accommodation.

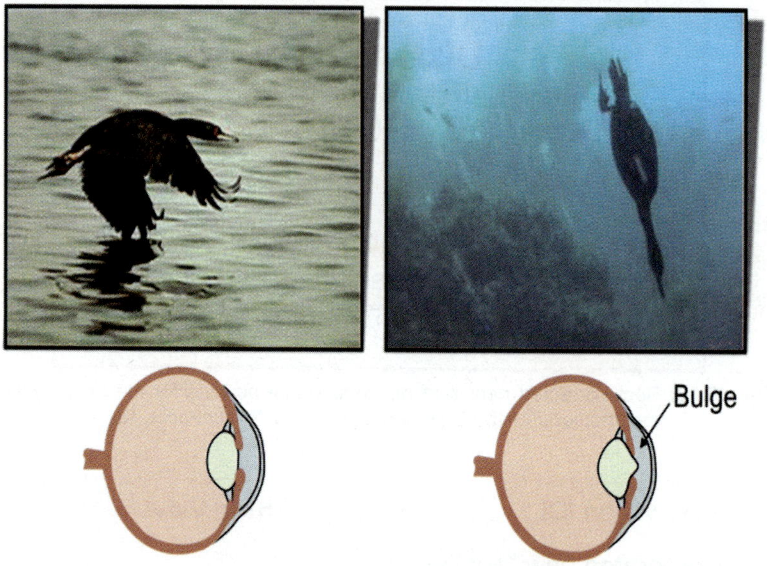

Fig. 45.15: Illustration of the physical principle behind the NuLens Accommodating IOL: The Merganser

The Flex Optic, by Quest Vision Technologies (Tiburon, CA), is now licensed by AMO. It has a plus-powered optic that changes shape on accommodation in addition to moving forward. The haptic is a balloon configuration and depending on the refractive index of the material, there is anywhere from 3.3 diopters of accommodation to 4.5 diopters of accommodations (Fig. 45.16).

In addition, there are several injectible polymer IOLs on the horizon. The most promising is the Smart IOL (Medennium, Inc, Irvine, CA), which is a hydrophobic acrylic that is designed to completely fill the capsular bag so there will be no decentration or edge effects. It is convertible, at room temperature, to a stiff rod and when it is implanted through a small incision into the eye, the thermodynamically active material reconstitutes to its original, size, shape, and dioptric power. At body temperature, it is a very flexible polymer and with a high refractive index, has a large amplitude of accommodation. This lens also has the advantage of being a stable gel so that if a YAG laser capsulotomy became necessary, it could be performed because the lens would not extrude into the vitreous cavity (Fig. 45.17).

A new and unusual solution is the LiquiLens (Vision Solution Technologies, Rockville, MD), which is a lens that has a fluid filled central aperture containing two immiscible liquids, one with a lower refractive index that fills the pupillary space with the patient in an upright position, and a higher refractive index fluid above that. When the patient tilts his head down, as for reading, there is a redistribution

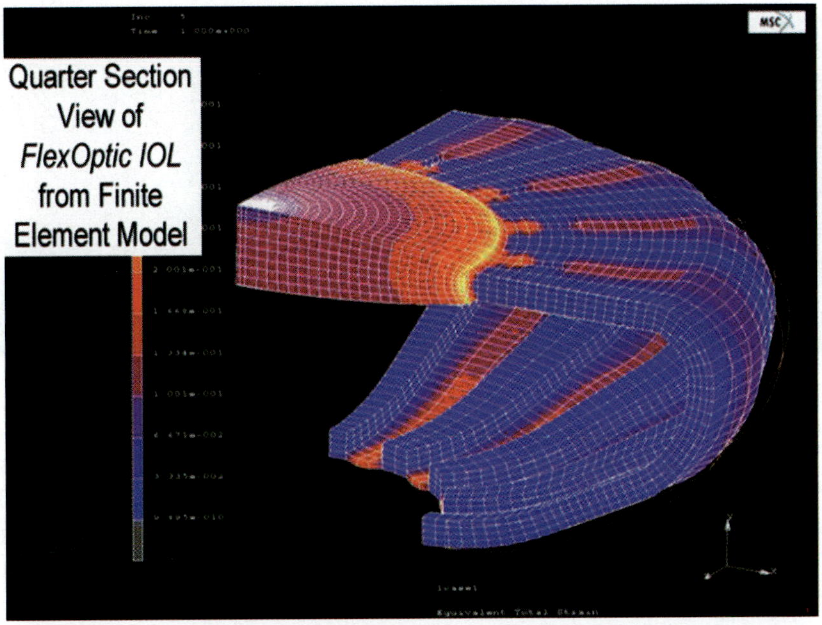

Fig. 45.16: Schematic of the Flex Optic IOL

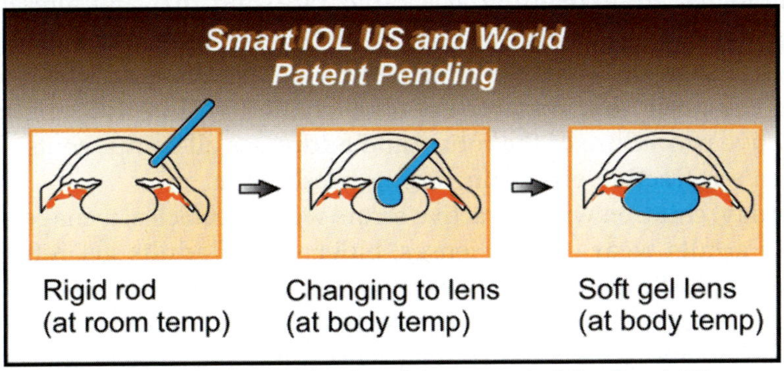

Fig. 45.17: Schematic drawing of the concept of the Smart IOL

of the polymers so that some of the high-refractive index falls within the pupillary space and allows for a more plus-powered lens (Fig. 45.18).

Light adjustability, as in the Calhoun lens (Calhoun Vision, Pasadena, CA), is a technology that may be applicable to all other IOLs, either in the form of thin lens that can be piggybacked on top of other IOLs, or with an incorporation of the photosensitive macromers into other lenses.

An interesting new technology from Medennium (Irvine, CA) is the Photochromatic Matrix IOL, which would be a blue-blocking IOL under high levels of UV light, but would revert back to a clear lens under

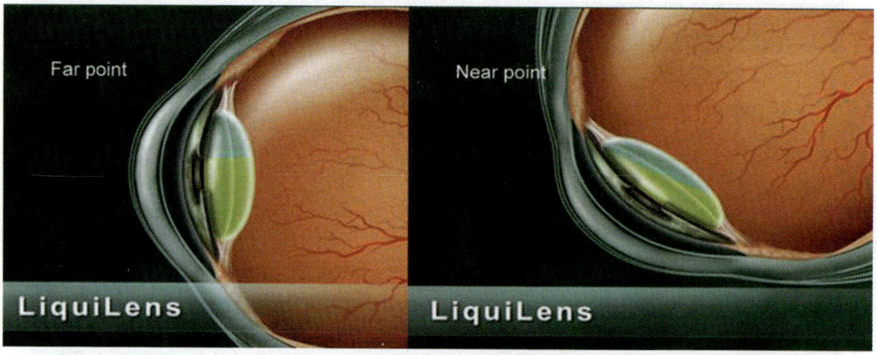

Fig. 45.18: Demonstration of the physical principles underlying the LiquiLens

scotopic and mesopic conditions of illumination.

Finally, the Vision Membrane (Vision Membrane Technologies, Carlsbad, CA) has multiorder diffractive optics (Fig. 45.19) and, like other anterior chamber multifocal IOLs, is capable of being implanted into the anterior chamber of people who are already monofocally implanted pseudophakes, seeking relief from presbyopia.

It is essential to emphasize that new phacoemulsification and IOL technologies are expanding at a rapid rate, and that any alterations to the cornea for refractive purposes will be compromised by changing spherical aberration of the crystalline lens as the patient ages. This leads us to conclude that refractive lens exchange will be the dominant refractive procedure of the future and addresses all components of the patient's refractive errors, including presbyopia.

Today, children with refractive errors wear spectacles, teenagers and young adults wear contact lenses, older young adults get refractive surgery, middle aged adults wear bifocals, and senior citizens undergo cataract surgery. We believe that tomorrow, children will wear spectacles, and teenagers, contact lenses, but the groups that today

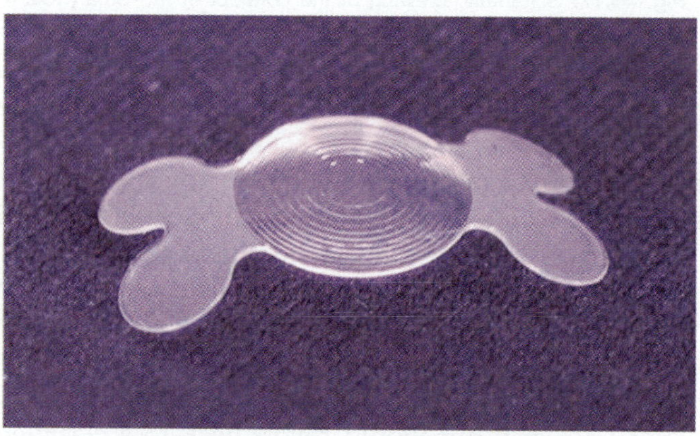

Fig. 45.19: The Vision Membrane Phakic IOL

undergo corneal refractive surgery, wear bifocals and undergo cataract surgery will all opt for refractive lens exchange.

This represents a quadruple-win. Patients can enjoy a predictable refractive procedure with a rapid recovery that addresses all types of refractive errors including presbyopia and never develop cataracts. That is a significant advantage because of the changing spherical aberration in so-called clinically insignificant cataracts. The second win is that surgeons can offer these procedures without the intrusion of private or government insurance and establish a less disruptive relationship with their patients. The third win is that ophthalmic industry can anticipate profits from their research and regulatory expenses which can further expand the emerging IOL technology. Finally, the government can enjoy the decreased financial burden from their number one health-care expense, cataract surgery, for the ever increasing ranks of baby boomers as more and more of these patients opt for lens exchange to address their refractive goals, ultimately reaching Medicare coverage as pseudophakes.

REFERENCES

1. Fine IH, Packer M, Hoffman RS. Use of power modulations in phacoemulsification: Choo-choo chop and flip phacoemulsification. J Cataract Refract Surg 2001; 27(2):188-97.
2. Fine IH, Packer M, Hoffman RS. Power modulations in new technology: Improved outcomes. J Cataract Refract Surg 2004; 30:1014-9.
3. Fine IH, Hoffman RS, Packer M. Optimizing refractive lens exchange with bimanual microincision phacoemulsification. J Cataract Refract Surg 2004; 30:550-4.
4. Fine IH. Cortical cleaving hydrodissection. J Cataract Refract Surg 1992; 18:508-12.
5. Packer M, Fine IH, Hoffman RS, Coffman PG, Brown LK. Immersion A-scan compared to partial coherence interferometry: outcome analysis. J Cataract Refract Surg 2002; 28 (2):239-42.
6. Hoffman RS, Fine IH, Packer M. Refractive lens exchange with a multifocal intraocular lens. Current Opinion in Ophthalmology 2003; 14:24-30.
7. Packer M, Fine IH, Hoffman RS. Refractive lens exchange with the array multifocal intraocular lens. J Cataract Refract Surg 2002; 28:421-4.
8. McLeod SD, Portney V, Ting A. A dual optic accommodating foldable intraocular lens. Br J Ophthalmol 2003; 87:1083-5.

CHAPTER

46

Antonio Calossi, Carlo F Lovisolo, (Italy)

Orthokeratology

INTRODUCTION

Orthokeratology (also known as OK, ortho-k, corneal reshaping, and corneal refractive therapy) is not a new procedure,[1, 2] but it has undergone a resurgence of clinical and research interest in the last decade. In 1971 the International Orthokeratology Section of the National Eye Research Foundation defined orthokeratology as the "reduction, modification, or elimination of refractive anomalies by the programmed application of contact lenses." This early definition is still valid, although successful orthokeratology outcomes are now often achieved with a single lens rather than a series of progressively flatter lenses applied during a period of weeks or months.[3]

HOW IT WORKS?

Orthokeratology contact lenses induce a temporary reduction of myopia by changing the shape of the cornea, taking advantage from corneal plasticity, particularly that of epithelial layer.[4, 5] If the amount of corneal molding is properly controlled, it is possible to bring the eye into correct focus to compensate the refractive error.

Conventional contact lenses are designed to cause little or no effect on the corneal shape, while orthokeratology lenses are designed to intentionally flatten the cornea in a controlled way. When the lens is on the eye, the patient can see clearly, like with a conventional lens. After the contact lens is removed, the cornea retains its modified shape for a certain amount of time, and the patient continues to see well, even without the lens. During the first days, the effect lasts for a short time, but in the following days, the effect stabilizes for the whole day. This treatment is reversible and, if the patient stops wearing the lenses completely, the refractive state of the eye will regress to the pre-treatment level.[6] The corneal topographies of Figures 46.1A to C show the reversibility of ortho-k procedure.

It is now recognized that orthokeratology is an effective treatment for low to moderate myopia. With overnight wear of modern contact lenses for orthokeratology, usually changes are very rapid: already after few nights of wearing we observe a significant improvement of unaided vision and, in most cases, the final result can be achieved with only one pair of lenses, in a period of time between one and two weeks.[7]

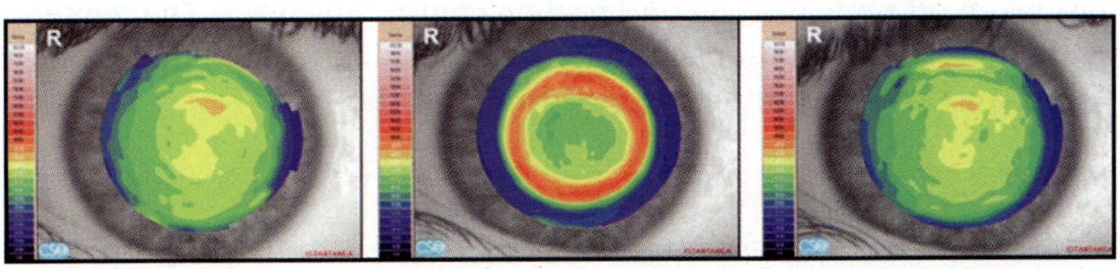

Figs 46.1A to C: (A) Prefit, (B) Postortho-K, (C) Two weeks after suspending

Treatment of astigmatism is controversial. Work is in progress to design toric reverse-geometry lenses for the specific treatment of astigmatism, and results are awaited with interest. Treatment of hyperopia and possibly presbyopia through corneal steepening is also under current investigation; preliminary studies suggest that corneal steepening with apical clearance lens designs may be possible, although the time scale and limits to this procedure require further study.

OVERNIGHT ORTHOKERATOLOGY

In the last years, orthokeratology procedures involve the overnight use of contact lenses: the cornea is reshaped during the sleeping time and lenses are taken off when the patient wakes up. In most cases, the effect lasts until the evening. This procedure has the advantage of eliminating some environmental factors (dust, wind, conditioned air, sports) that can give trouble during the day; in addition, the pressure of closed lids improves the rapidity of corneal molding.

For overnight wear, high oxygen permeable materials are necessary to provide sufficient oxygenation to the cornea, even if lids are closed.[8,9] When rigid gas permeable (RGP) lenses are worn during waking hours, oxygen can reach the cornea via two mechanisms: by circulation of oxygen-rich tears behind the lens, driven by a lid-activated tear pump, and by diffusion through the lens material. An estimated 10-20% tear exchange occurs with each blink under a rigid lens.[10, 11] Polse[12] estimates a tear exchange per blink of only 1% under soft lenses, due to their greater diameter and flexibility. On the contrary, both lens types provide oxygen to the cornea during closed-eye wear by diffusion through the lens material. Thus, soft and RGP lenses of comparable Dk/t will induce similar levels of overnight edema. On awaking, the lid-activated tear pump is much more efficient with RGP compared to soft lenses, so oxygen is supplied in more quantity, facilitating rapid corneal recovery from overnight hypoxic stress. Andrasko[13] and Holden et al.[14] have demonstrated that the cornea deswells more rapidly after overnight wear of RGP lenses than with soft lenses, because of the greater tear pumping efficiency of rigid lenses. This recovery is even more rapid if we talk about overnight wear, with the lens taken off on wakening, rather than continuous wear. The removal of the lens allows both cleansing of the lens and the elimination of debris and waste products trapped behind the lens.

REVERSE GEOMETRY CONTACT LENS DESIGN

Modern contact lenses for orthokeratology have a curvature profile that is "reversed" from traditional rigid lens design, so they are usually

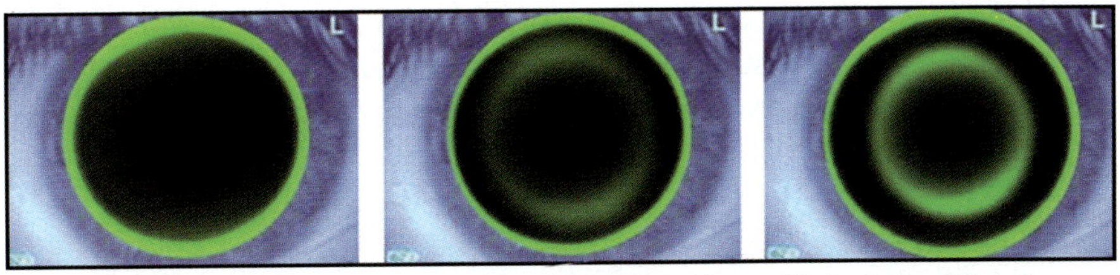

Figs 46.2A to C: (A) 1st generation flat conventional lens, (B) 2nd generation three-zone reverse-geometry, (C) 3rd generation four-zone reverse-geometry

defined "reverse-geometry contact lenses."[15, 16] Traditional lens designs have secondary and peripheral curves flatter than the central curve of the lens. On the contrary, reverse-geometry lenses have one or more peripheral curves steeper than the curve of the optical zone.

In modern reverse-geometry lenses for orthokeratology, we can identify four main functional zones: optical zone, reverse zone, alignment zone and peripheral zone. Usually reverse-geometry lenses for orthokeratology have a diameter larger than traditional RGP lenses (Figs 46.2 A to C).

The back optical zone determines the shape that the cornea will assume after the corneal molding, and so it determines the amount of refractive error corrected by the orthokeratological treatment.

Usually, it is a spherical curve. The radius of curvature of this zone is calculated in order to get the desired orthokeratological effect. The lift of peripheral curves over the cornea around the optical zone creates a tear reservoir.

The reverse zone allows the joining of the optical zone with the alignment zone. In the reverse zone, there are one or more curves steeper than the back optical zone.

The alignment zone is the bearing zone of the lens; it gives stability to the lens and keeps it centered on the cornea. In some particular lens design,[17,18] it also enhances the corneal molding, putting a pressure in the periphery of the cornea that aids the redistribution of corneal tissue towards the optical zone. The curvature of the alignment zone is flatter than the reverse zone, but steeper than the optical zone.

The peripheral zone allows the lens edge to lift from the cornea, to achieve an adequate tear turnover under the lens. This tear exchange is necessary for two reasons: to get in new tear liquid to oxygenate the cornea, and to get out the debris and metabolic residuals formed under the lens. If the lens has a proper alignment and a right lift in the peripheral disengagement zone, during the blinking we have an effective pumping action of tear fluid. Besides this primary function, the tear meniscus under the peripheral curves allows a capillary attraction helping the lens to keep centered. The edge lift has other functions too: it controls the pressure of the edge of the lens minimizing the risks of corneal insult and helps the removal of the lens by mean of lid tension. The curvature of the peripheral zone is flatter than the alignment zone.

THE IDEAL FITTING

Reverse-geometry contact lenses are designed in order to produce a hydrodynamic force on the cornea, that aims at causing epithelial cells to migrate, so as to obtain a change in the first cellular layers.[4,19,20] In order for this force to work efficaciously, the fitting should have definite characteristics as regards the position of the lens, its movement and the clearance between the cornea and the lens. Let us analyse them in detail.

- *Positioning:* The centration of the lens is critical for the efficacy of orthokeratological effect. Decentred lenses cannot produce the desired myopia reduction; it may cause an increase in astigmatism and corneal distortion. A poorly centred lens can induce poor visual acuity after lens removal.
- *Movement:* The lens should have a 0.2-1.0 mm blink induced movement. Orthokeratology contact lenses should show less movement than conventional lenses.
- *Fluorescein pattern:* The typical fluorescein pattern of reverse-geometry lens fitting should show an image characterised by concentric rings: dark centre (minimal apical clearance, without touch), green ring (tear reservoir, with variable thickness, depending on the corrective effect, usually between 30 and 50 microns), dark ring (mid-periphery touch, alignment zone), thin green ring (edge lift, 80-100 micron) (Fig. 46.3). The transition between the different zones should be blended. After first adaptation, there should not be air bubbles. This would indicate an excessive lift in the tear reservoir zone.

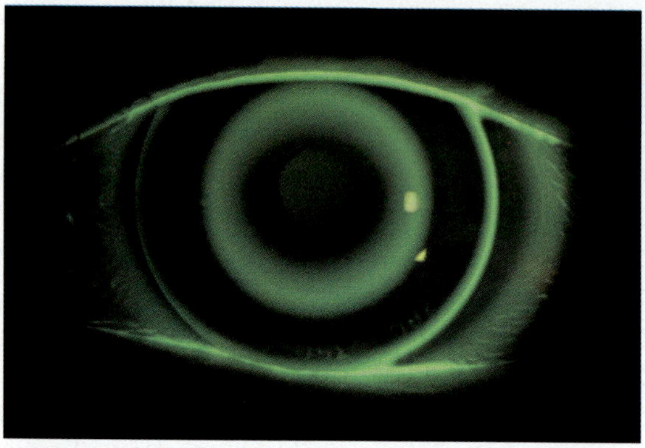

Fig. 46.3: Typical fluorescein pattern (ESA-ortho6)

SELECTION OF PATIENTS

Usually orthokeratology can be used in low and moderate myopia, up to 6.00 D, even if associated with low astigmatism. In higher myopias, orthokeratology can reduce the refractive error, without correcting it totally. This kind of correction can be useful as well, in people who wish either less dependence on optical aids, or who wish to wear more functional and well-designed spectacles. In most cases, this technique is contraindicated in high astigmatism.

Primarily, orthokeratology is indicated when myopic patients are contraindicated to refractive surgery or they are unwilling to undergo any surgery. Not all myopic patients are willing to undergo an operation, however safe it is, and however low the risks of failure or complications may be.

Besides not all myopic are suitable for surgery, for example due to their age or because they have a myopic progression: refractive surgery is not advisable until myopia is not stable definitely. Refractive surgery should not be performed on young people or teenagers. Also in cases of young adults we have to be sure that there are not functional conditions promoting a future myopic progression.

As well, some patients have a low refractive error and wish more independence from standard corrective aids, spectacles or contact lenses. Pilots, athletes, police officers, fire fighters, etc. might need more independence from corrective aids, without undergoing surgery.

LIMITS

Orthokeratology is not suitable to every patient, because it has some contraindications and limits. Orthokeratology is contraindicated in all those ocular conditions that do not allow the use of conventional contact lenses. These are: acute and subacute inflammations or infection of the anterior segment of the eye; any eye disease, injury, or abnormality that affects the cornea, conjunctiva or eyelids, which may be exacerbated by wearing contact lenses; any systemic disease, which may affect contact lens wear, as immune system diseases, or metabolic dysfunctions; allergic reactions of ocular surfaces or adnexa which may be induced or exaggerated by wearing contact lenses or by the use of contact lens solutions; alterations of tears (dry eyes).

Limits of orthokeratology treatment have to be explained in detail to each candidate. At the beginning, it is necessary to adapt to rigid contact lenses, which in a few cases can be troublesome in the initial period, even if this trouble is reduced to the minimum in overnight wear.

Then, results depend on pretreatment ocular conditions: corneal shape, lid position and action, corneal tissue response, presence or absence of astigmatism, etc. and usually 20/20 can be achieved only for low or middle myopia.

For some patients, the main limitation of orthokeratology is that results are temporary. Actually, changes achieved with orthokeratology do not last forever. To maintain the reduction of myopia, lens wear have to be continued on a prescribed wearing schedule. At the beginning of treatment, the clear vision period may last few hours, and then visual acuity begins to decrease progressively. With time, we have an increase of the clear vision period after lens removal. When vision is no longer acceptable, the patient needs to wear retainer lenses. For people who wish to get rid of any correction for good, the temporary results are definitely a limitation. However, in some cases, reversibility of treatment can be an advantage.

RISK ANALYSIS

Even if the recent literature reports a series of cases of microbial keratitis,[21] we do not expect that contact lenses for orthokeratology may provide a risk that is greater than other contact lenses.[22] The incidence and prevalence of microbial keratitis related to corneal reshaping contact lens wear is not known. Any overnight wear of contact lenses increases the risk of infection, but it is not known whether the risks of microbial keratitis are greater for corneal reshaping overnight contact lens wearers than other form of overnight contact lens wear.[23]

However, besides the side effects that are common to all rigid contact lenses, there are some specific complications due to corneal distortion.

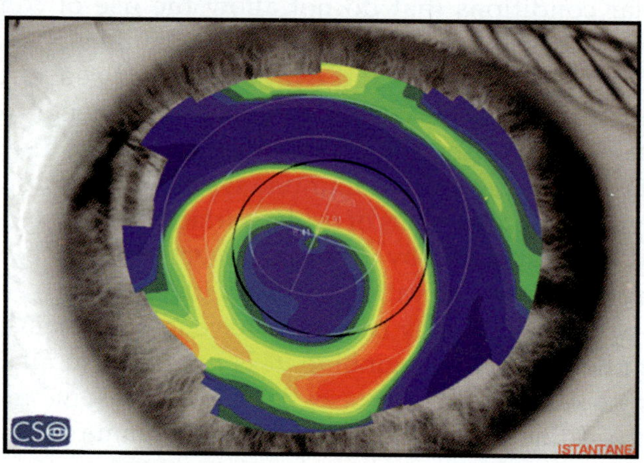

Fig. 46.4: Decentration of the molded area due to dislocation of the lens

Sometimes we observe some corneal irregularities that can be due to lens displacement. Usually, they are slight and do not affect quality of vision. Sometimes we have a greater decentration of the molded area (Fig. 46.4). This decentration may be due to dislocation or binding of the lens. In this case, strong irregularity of corneal profile may cause an inadequate refractive condition and high order aberration, troubling effects in twilight and night vision. Since orthokeratology does not produce permanent and irreversible corneal changes, when such a problem occurs, we can modify lens parameters until we obtain a satisfactory result in terms of both positioning and correction. In most problematic cases, we have to stop lens wear.

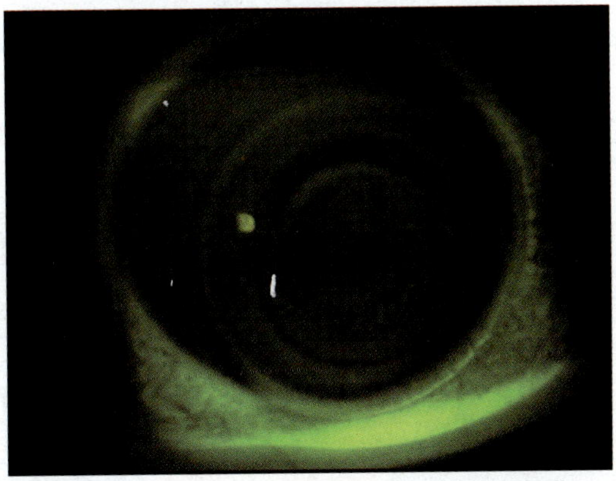

Fig. 46.5: Corneal warpage due to lens binding

As regards corneal staining, we can have this problem because of both a loose lens, which causes mechanical abrasion on corneal epithelium, and a tight lens, which adheres to the cornea (Fig. 46.5). Moreover staining may be due to debris trapped behind the lens or to deposits on the lens. Finally, it is recommended that ongoing education be provided to practitioners and staff regarding safety, informed consent, and prevention of potential problems, with special emphasis on the critical need to properly and thoroughly disinfect lenses that will be worn overnight.

SOME CASES

Figures 46.6 to 46.8 show some successful cases.

Efficacy and Safety of Overnight Orthokeratology by means of a Customized Hexa-curve Reverse Geometry Lens

A growing number of clinical studies have reported on the efficacy of modern orthokeratology using a range of different reverse-geometry lens designs. [7, 24-29]

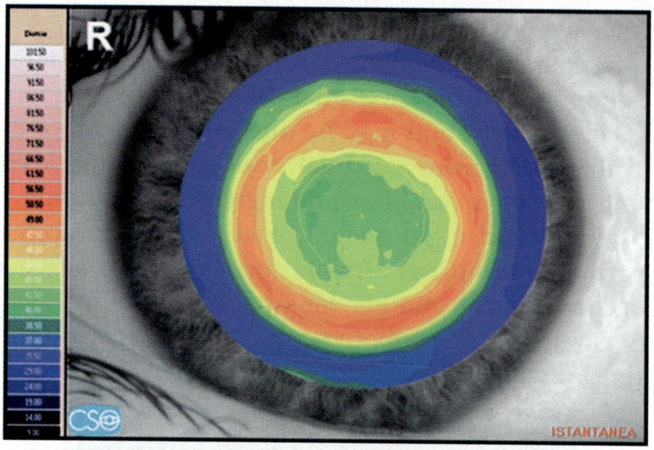

Fig. 46.6: Pre: RX Sf. – 2.25; Post: UCVA 12/10

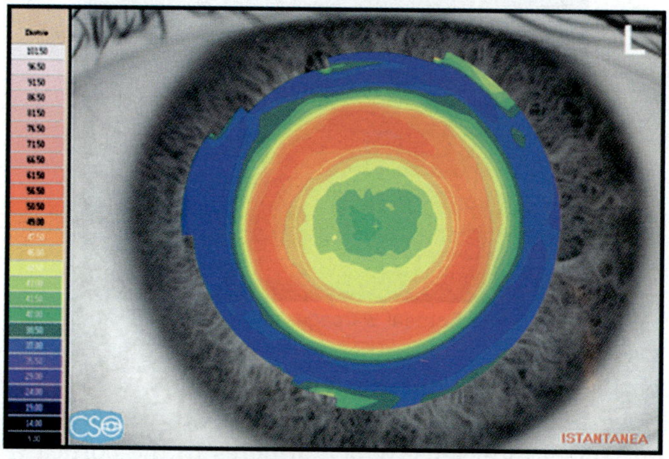

Fig. 46.7: Pre: RX Sph. – 6.00; Post: Sph. – 0.75

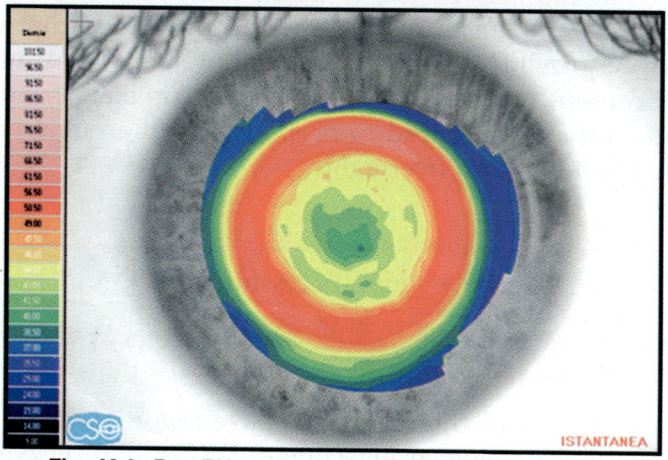

Fig. 46.8: Pre: RX – 7.50 –0.50 x 180 ; Post: UCVA 9/10

One of us (AC) patented a new design and calculation method to customize a multicurve reverse geometry lens.[17,18] A prospective, randomized study to evaluate the safety, efficacy, predictability, stability, quality of vision and adverse reactions of overnight orthokeratology by means of this customized hexacurve reverse geometry lenses (ESA ortho-6) in hyper-Dk gas-permeable material (Boston XO, hexafocon-A).[30, 31]

Fifty eyes of 25 myopic patients aged from 11 to 44 years, without any tear, corneal, ocular and/or systemic disease at the baseline time and without any previous ocular surgery were treated. The baseline refractive error was from –1.00 to –6.00 D spherical equivalent, WTR astigmatism up to 1.50 D and ATR astigmatism up to 1.00 D. The results showed that the cornea responds rapidly with significant ($p<0.05$) central corneal flattening and improvement in visual acuity after just 60 min of lens wear. The corneal shape changes from prolate to oblate asphericity after 1 night of wear; in the majority of cases improvement in unaided visual acuity up to 0.1 LogMAR can be obtained for at least 12 h after lens removal in the first week of treatment. These changes were sustained at 1 and 3 months.

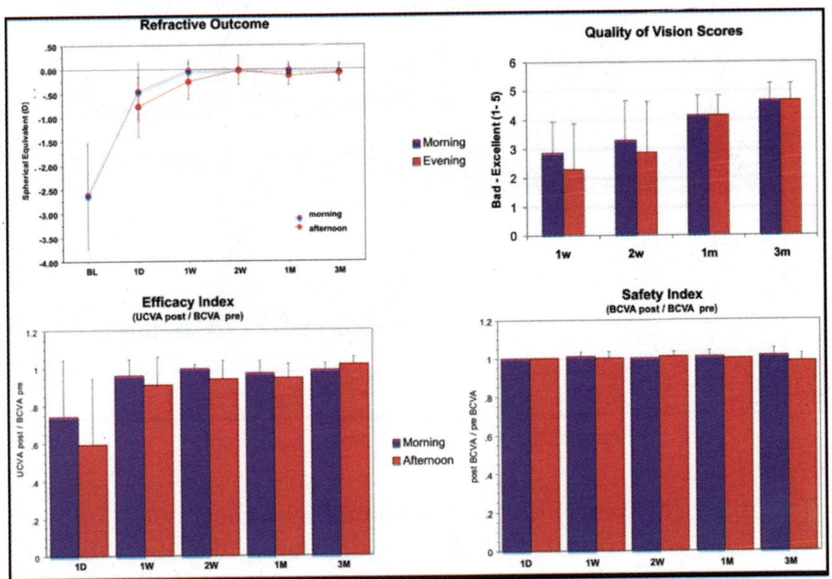

Fig. 46.9: Refractive outcome, quality of vision score, efficacy index, and safety index[30, 31]

In the first week, there was a significant improvement in subjective ratings of quality of day and night vision ($p < 0.05$) but a significant increase of corneal spherical aberration ($p < 0.05$) due to post-treatment oblate shape of the cornea (Figs 46.9 and 46.10A and B).

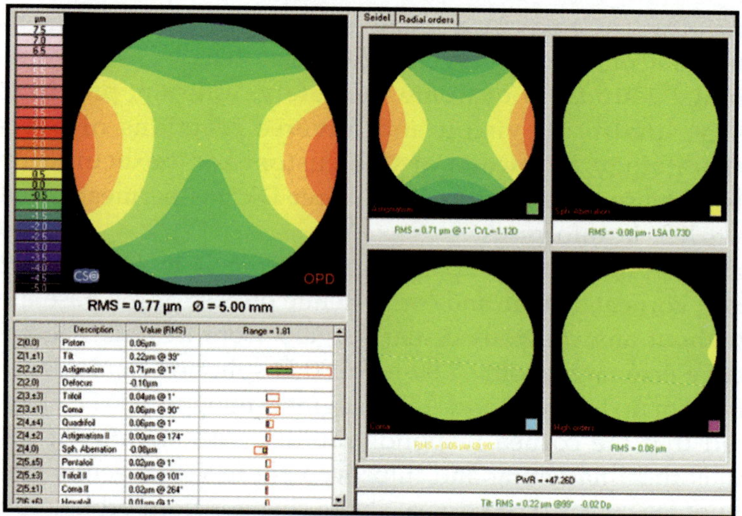

Fig. 46.10A: Pretreatment corneal wave-front

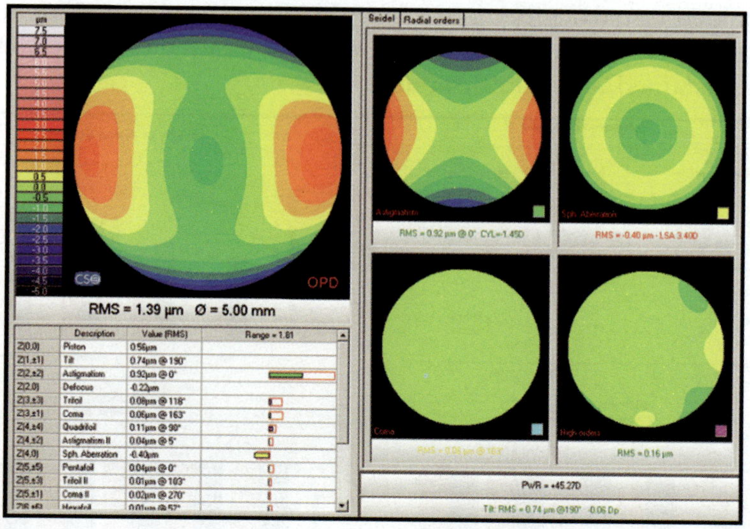

Fig. 46.10B: Postortho-k corneal wave-front

The spherical aberration was correlated with the amount of treated myopia and with pupil diameter, while coma-like aberration was correlated with the displacement of the pupil as regards the geometric center of the cornea. Subjective ratings continued to improve after objective measures stabilized at 1-week. Biomicroscopy showed no corneal infiltrates or ulcers; there were some observations of grade 1 fluorescein staining of the cornea, and imprinting in the morning that disappeared in the evening; no other significant ocular adverse events were observed during the trial. No significant change was observed in the central thickness of the cornea ($p > 0.28$). No significant change was found in the intraocular pressure ($p > 0.08$). Specular microscope showed no measurable changes in the endothelium. Confocal microscopy: in several subjects, basal layer of the epithelium showed larger and less regular cells after the treatment (Fig. 46.11). We can explain this phenomenon with a mild cellular edema due to the hypoxia or the mechanical effect of the treatment. A few subjects showed a slight increasing in reflectivity of Bowman's layer and of anterior stroma. The appearance and the activation rate of keratocytes were not modified. Therefore, the slight increase in reflectivity could be explained by a mild increasing of corneal glycosaminoglycans production, that is a reversible phenomenon due to an aspecific reaction of anterior stroma to different traumas. No other significant alterations were observed in the anterior epithelium, sub basal nerve plexus, mid and deep stroma and endothelium.The results of this study suggest that the corneal epithelium can be molded or redistributed very rapidly in response to the tear film forces generated behind this reverse-geometry lens design. Safety and efficacy of the procedure appear to be favorable without significant adverse reactions.

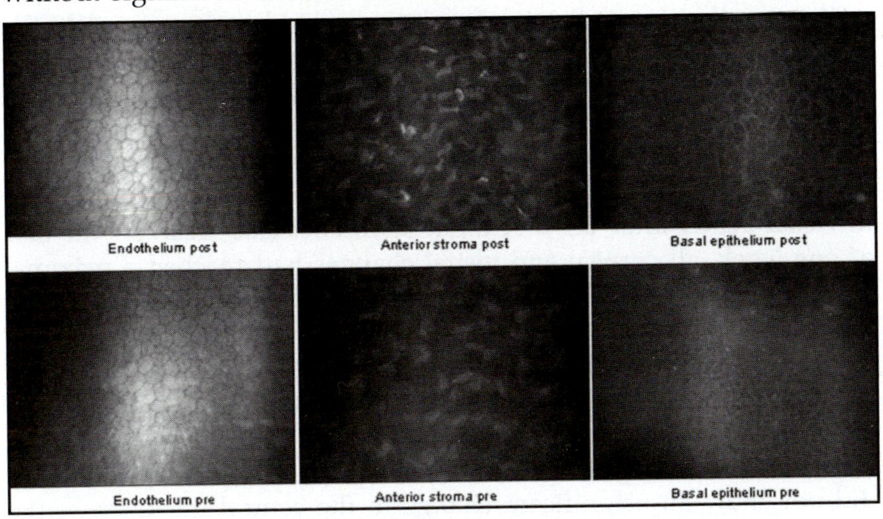

Fig. 46.11: Confocal microscopy[30, 31]

Corneal Thickness

One of the concerns of myopia correction by corneal molding is the thinning of central epithelium of the cornea induced by a direct compression of the optical zone. As it happened in the radial keratotomy or intrastromal corneal rings procedures, we think that it is possible to bring on a central flattening, working in the periphery of the cornea and we designed a lens geometry that would aid the displacement of peripheral epithelium towards the optical zone. Our biomechanical hypothesis is that the central flattening might be secondary to a mid-peripheral steepening, induced by a displacement of the epithelium that results from a proper compression in the alignment zone of this lens. The hexacurve reverse geometry lens design (ESA ortho-6) we mention above attempts to mold the periphery of the cornea with a minimum compression in the centre of the lens.[17,18]

A prospective, consecutive study was performed to evaluate the corneal response and central corneal thickness (CCT) changes after overnight orthokeratology by means of this customized hexacurve reverse geometry lens in hyper-Dk gas-permeable material (Boston-XO).[32]

Twenty-eight eyes of 14 myopic patients (ranging from –1.00 to – 4.25 D sph, and astigmatism up to 1.00 D) were enrolled in the study. Assessment criteria included uncorrected visual acuity, best-corrected visual acuity, manifest refraction, ultrasound pachymetry, corneal topography, and biomicroscopic data. These data were collected at baseline, and then after one night, one week, two weeks, one month, and three months of lens wear. All the examinations were performed in the morning immediately after lens removal and repeated in the evening of the same day. An ultrasound pachymeter (Allergan Humphrey model 850, Carl Zeiss Meditec, Dublin, CA), using a velocity of 1640 m/s, was used to measure central corneal thickness.

The results of this study showed that the cornea responded rapidly with significant ($p < 0.05$) central corneal flattening and improvement in visual acuity after the first night of contact lens wear. By the end of one week, all corneal and visual changes had reached a maximal level and remained stable during the day. These changes were sustained at the following visits. After the first molding, the fluorescein pattern showed a clearance under the center of the lens that demonstrated a minimal central touch. Biomicroscopy showed no significant ocular adverse events. The average pretreatment CCT was 533 ± 31 µm. During the period of the study, ultrasound pachymetry did not show any significant change in the central thickness of the cornea (Fig. 46.12) (repeated measures ANOVA: $p = 0.978$), both in the morning and in the evening (Bonferroni/Dunn post-hoc test: $p > 0.414$). Fig. 46.1 show the details of the difference in CCT.

The lack of change found in the central pachymetry data suggests that the overnight contact lens can successfully flatten the cornea without direct compression of the center of the cornea. The absence of change in CCT during the day may exclude a masking effect due to edema.[33] Contrary to these finding, the majority of previous studies reported that orthokeratology and corneal refractive therapy causes

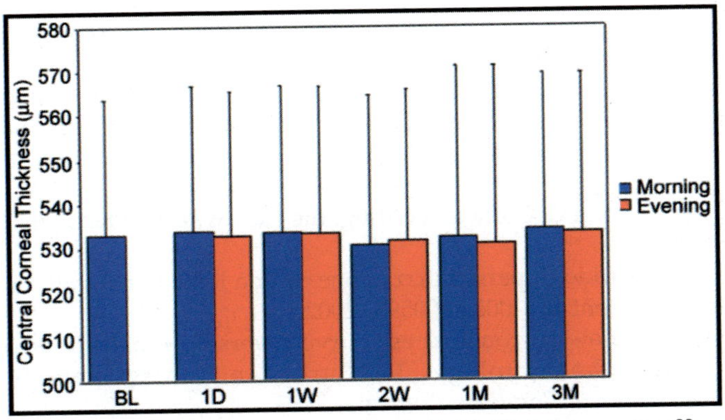

Fig. 46.12: Changes in central corneal thickness over time[32]

central epithelial and total corneal thinning.[34-38] This difference could be caused by the different geometry and behavior of the lenses.

These results seem to confirm the biomechanical hypothesis that the central flattening of the cornea might be achieved as secondary to a midperipheral steepening, induced by a displacement of the epithelium that results from a proper compression in the alignment zone of this lens.

REFERENCES

1. Jessen GN. Orthofocus techniques. Contacto 1962;6:200-204.
2. Grant SC, May CH. Orthokeratology: a therapeutic approach to contact lens proceduress. Contacto 1970;14:3-16.
3. Swarbrick HA. Orthokeratology (corneal refractive therapy): what is it and how does it work? Eye Contact Lens 2004;30:181-5; discussion 205-6.
4. Matsubara M, Kamei Y, Takeda S, Mukai K, Ishii Y, Ito S. Histologic and histochemical changes in rabbit cornea produced by an orthokeratology lens. Eye Contact Lens 2004;30:198-204; 205-6.
5. Choo J, Caroline P, Harlin D. How does the cornea change under corneal reshaping contact lenses? Eye Contact Lens 2004;30:211-3; 218.
6. Soni PS, Nguyen TT, Bonanno JA. Overnight orthokeratology: refractive and corneal recovery after discontinuation of reverse-geometry lenses. Eye Contact Lens 2004;30:254-62; discussion 263-4.
7. Swarbrick HA. Orthokeratology review and update. Clin Exp Optom 2006;89:124-43.
8. Holden B, Mertz G. Critical oxygen level to avoid corneal edema for daily and extended wear contact lenses. Invest Ophtalmol 1984;63.
9. Swabrick H, Holden B. Extended wear lenses. In Phillips A, Speedwell L, (Eds): Contact Lenses: Butterworth-Heinemann, 1997:494-6.
10. Cuklanz H, Hill R. Oxygen requirements of corneal contact lens system. Am J Optom 1969;46:228-30.
11. Fatt I, Hill R. Oxygen tension under a contact lens during blinking: a comparision of theory and experimental observation. Am J Optom 1970;47:50-55.
12. Polse K. Tear flow under hydrogel conctact lenses. Invest Ophtalmol Vis Sci 1979;18:409-13.

13. Andrasko G. Corneal deswelling response to hard and hydrogel extended wear lenses. Invest Ophtalmol Vis Sci 1986;27:20-23.
14. Holden B, Sweeny D, La Hood D, Kenyon E. Corneal deswelling following overnight wear of rigid and hydrogel contact lenses. Current Eye Res 1988;7:49-53.
15. Fontana AA. Orthoeratology using the one piece bifocal. Contacto 1972;16:45-7.
16. Wlodyga R, Bryla C. Corneal molding: the easy way. Contact Lens Spectrum 1989;4:58-62.
17. Calossi A. Metodo di personalizzazione di una lente per il trattamento della miopia. IT Patent BO2002A000595, 2002.
18. Calossi A. A new customized esa-curve reverse geometry lens design for overnight orthokeratology. 33° European Contact Lens Society of Ophthalmologists Congress, Venezia, 2003.
19. Choo JD, Caroline PJ, Harlin DD, Meyers W. Morphologic Changes in Cat Epithelium Following Overnight Lens Wear with the Paragon CRT Lens for Corneal Reshaping. Invest Ophthalmol Vis Sci 2004;45:1552.
20. Matsubara M, Takeda S, Hirowatari T, Mukai K, Ishii Y. Histological Findings of Rabbit Cornea Produced by an Orthokeratology Lens. Invest Ophthalmol Vis Sci 2005;46:2058.
21. Watt K, Swarbrick HA. Microbial keratitis in overnight orthokeratology: review of the first 50 cases. Eye Contact Lens 2005;31:201-8.
22. Morgan PB, Efron N, Hill EA, Raynor MK, Whiting MA, Tullo AB. Incidence of keratitis of varying severity among contact lens wearers. Br J Ophthalmol 2005;89:430-6.
23. Walline JJ, Holden BA, Bullimore MA, et al. The current state of corneal reshaping. Eye Contact Lens 2005;31:209-14.
24. Nichols JJ, Marsich MM, Nguyen M, Barr JT, Bullimore MA. Overnight orthokeratology. Optom Vis Sci 2000;77:252-9.
25. Rah MJ, Jackson JM, Jones LA, Marsden HJ, Bailey MD, Barr JT. Overnight orthokeratology: preliminary results of the Lenses and Overnight Orthokeratology (LOOK) study. Optom Vis Sci 2002;79:598-605.
26. Barr JT, Rah MJ, Jackson JM, Jones LA. Orthokeratology and corneal refractive therapy: a review and recent findings. Eye Contact Lens 2003;29:S49-53; discussion S57-9, S192-4.
27. Soni PS, Nguyen TT, Bonanno JA. Overnight orthokeratology: visual and corneal changes. Eye Contact Lens 2003;29:137-45.
28. Tahhan N, Du Toit R, Papas E, Chung H, La Hood D, Holden AB. Comparison of reverse-geometry lens designs for overnight orthokeratology. Optom Vis Sci 2003;80:796-804.
29. Cheung SW, Cho P. Subjective and objective assessments of the effect of orthokeratology: a cross-sectional study. Curr Eye Res 2004;28:121-7.
30. Calossi A. Refractive outcome and corneal response to a customized esa-curve reverse-geometry lens designs for overnight orthokeratology. Abstracts of the 28th BCLA Annual Clinical Conference, Birmingham, 2004. Cont Lens Anterior Eye 2004;27:87-107.
31. Calossi A. Efficacy and safety of overnight orthokeratology by means of a customized ESA Curve reverse geometry lens. 2nd annual Global Orthokeratology Symposium, Toronto, 2004.
32. Calossi A, Romano M, Romano F, Ferraioli G. Overnight Orthokeratology Flattening the Cornea Without Direct Compression of the Center. Invest Ophthalmol Vis Sci 2006;47:100.

33. Nguyen T, Soni S, Carter D, Biehl T. Corneal Changes Associated With Overnight Orthokeratology. Invest. Ophthalmol. Vis. Sci. 2002;43:3092.
34. Alharbi A, Swarbrick HA. The effects of overnight orthokeratology lens wear on corneal thickness. Invest Ophthalmol Vis Sci 2003;44:2518-23.
35. Choo J, Caroline P, Harlin D, Meyers B. Morphologic changes in cat epithelium following overnight lens wear with Paragon CRT lens for corneal reshaping. 2nd annual Global Orthokeratology Symposium, Toronto, 2004.
36. Haque S, Fonn D, Simpson T, Jones L. Corneal and epithelial thickness changes after 4 weeks of overnight corneal refractive therapy lens wear, measured with optical coherence tomography. Eye Contact Lens 2004;30:189-93; discussion 205-6.
37. Swarbrick HA, Wong G, O'Leary DJ. Corneal response to orthokeratology. Optom Vis Sci 1998;75:791-9.
38. Wang J, Fonn D, Simpson TL, Sorbara L, Kort R, Jones L. Topographical thickness of the epithelium and total cornea after overnight wear of reverse-geometry rigid contact lenses for myopia reduction. Invest Ophthalmol Vis Sci 2003;44:4742-6.

CHAPTER

47

Tanuj Dada, Harinder S Sethi,
Swati Phuljhele, Manoj Gupta (India)

Update on IOL Technologies

INTRODUCTION

The evolution of the cataract surgery with the introduction of intraocular lens implantation has been one of the major achievements of modern medicine. The intraocular lens technology has come a long way since the use of standard PMMA lenses for extracapsular surgery. The intraocular lenses provide a precise pseudophakic optical rehabilitation with minimal magnification and excellent optical properties. The advent of small incision surgery made possible by phacoemulsification and foldable IOLs represents another major milestone in cataract surgery.

The art and science of cataract surgery is undergoing a rapid evolution. In the last decade emphasis has shifted to lens based refractive surgery with the use of Phakic IOLs and recently the new technique of Micoincision cataract surgery (MICS) or Phakonit has been introduced with use of ultrathin lenses which can be inserted via sub 1.5 mm incisions. In addition to these advancements new IOL materials such as collagen polymers, specific blue light blocking IOLs, IOLs to decrease aberrations and restore accommodation have come into vogue. It is important for the ophthalmologists to have an in depth knowledge of the basic design and optical features of the various IOLs currently in use. Efforts are being continuously put to create custom made IOLs for each individual, based on wave front technology. The present text highlights the basic design and optical features of new IOL technologies.

CLASSIFICATION OF IOLs

The various characteristics of intraocular lenses are given in Table 47.1.

1. **Site of implantation**
   - i. Posterior chamber IOLs.
   - ii. Iris plane IOLs.
   - iii. Anterior chamber IOLs.
   - iv. Scleral fixated IOLs.
2. **Flexibility of lenses**
   - i. Rigid IOLs — PMMA.
   - ii. Foldable IOLs — Silicone, hydrogel, acrylic, collamer.
3. **Material of optic**
   - i. Polymethyl methacrylate (PMMA) optic.
   - ii. Silicone optic.
   - iii. Hydrogel or hydrophilic acrylic.
   - iv. Hydrophobic acrylic.
   - v. Thermoset (memory lens).
   - vi. Collamer.

Table 47.1: Characteristics of intraocular lenses

Characteristics	*Variations*
Number of pieces	• One piece (disc or plate haptic) • Three piece (disc)
IOL material	• PMMA • Silicone • Hydrogel/hydrophilic acrylic • Hydrophobic acrylic • Thermoset • Collamer
Loop material	• Polypropylene (flexible, possible higher incidence of endophthalmitis) • PMMA (rigid) • Polyacrylic • PVDF
Loop shape	• Angulation (forward angulation increases pressure on posterior capsule and may decrease PCO, and increases distance of optic from iris. Less angulation may facilitate insertion) • J or C loops • Plate haptics
Optic design	• Convex plano, plano convex, biconvex (Biconvex associated with the least image degradation with decentration and tilt and less PCO), aspheric (gives better contrast sensitivity) • Length of the IOL (14 mm for sulcus fixation, 12-12.5 mm for in-the-bag fixation) • Size of optic (4.5-7 mm. Larger optics may be better for patients with large pupils but need bigger incisions. Smaller optics for bag fixation) • Holes (to facilitate dialling into capsular bag) • Ridges (designed to facilitate laser capsulotomy, but associated with more PCO) • Sharp or round optic edge (less PCO when optic has a square edge than round, due to barrier to lens epithelial cell migration, e.g. Alcon AcrySof IOL;
Surfacemodification	• Binding of hydrogels or heparin to the IOL surface (tomake IOL more hydrophilic, found to reduce inflammatory cell precipitate) • Surface passivation (to make IOL more hydrophobic and oleophilic, aiming to repel lipids such as cell membranes and ocular tissues)

4. **Combination of optic and haptic material**
   i. Single-piece IOL — haptic and optic made of same material, e.g. All PMMA single-piece IOL, all acrylic single piece IOL.
   ii. Three piece IOL — where optic and haptic are made up of different materials, e.g. three piece PMMA IOL (optic made of PMMA and haptics of polypropylene), acrysol multipiece IOL (optic made of hydrophobic acrylic and haptics of PMMA.

Table 47.2: Characteristics of optic materials

IOL Type	*Advantages*	*Disadvantages*
PMMA	Long term experience Good biocompatibility Cheap	Rigid so need large incision Pits with YAG laser High incidence of PCO
Silicone - Low refractive index	Foldable - small incision High refractive index - thinner IOLs (second generation silicone) Fairly low incidence of PCO	Thicker IOLs (first generation silicone) Pits with YAG laser Dislocation after YAG Rapid unfolding in the eye More decentration More anterior capsule contraction Slippery when wet Cannot use with silicone oil
AcrySoft	Foldable—small incision High refractive index - thin IOLs Very low incidence of PCO LEC regression Biocompatible Fewer pits with YAG laser Slow uncontrolled folding	Short experience Tacky surface - sticks to forceps More difficult to fold ?Glistenings ?Glare
Hydroview	Foldable—small incision Good biocompatibility low inflammatory cell reaction Fewer pits with YAG laser Controlled unfolding Less endothelial cell damage with cornea touch	LECs on anterior IOL surface High incidence of PCO
Thermoset (MMA+HEMA)	Rollable-microincison easy insertion	Requires cold chain maintenance
Collamer	Most biocompatible	

OPTIC MATERIALS FOR IOLs (TABLE 47.2)

An ideal IOL material should have following properties:

- High optical quality
- High index of refraction
- Light weight
- Durable, resistant to mechanical stress
- Easy fabrication
- Non-antigenic/non-allergic
- Non-carcinogenic
- Easy sterilization
- Lack of inflammatory reaction, foreign body reaction, or tissue chaffing
- Blocking UV radiation
- Implantable through a small incision.

Polymethylmethacrylate (PMMA)

PMMA is an inert polymer of methylmethacrylate monomer. It is manufactured through addition polymerization of methacrylic acid methylester, which is derived from acrylic acid. It was the first material to be used for intraocular implants by Harold Ridley. The idea of this material being used for IOLs came from the fact that it had been noticed that during World War II, intraocular fragments of PMMA in the eyes of the pilots (which came from the shattered canopies of fighter aircrafts), demonstrated inert properties. This material is light, hard and transparent and transmits a broader spectrum of light than the human lens, thereby allowing the transmission of UV rays. Hence, UV absorbing materials have been incorporated as covalently bonded or entrapped chromophores to prevent retinal damage. The agents commonly used as UV absorbers are benzotriazoles and benzophenones. The material is hydrophobic and may damage corneal endothelium on contact. The main disadvantage of PMMA lenses is that they are non-flexible and have to be inserted through a larger incision. The specific gravity of PMMA is 1.19 and the refractive index of 1.497. PMMA has the longest track record as an intraocular lens material and has given an excellent optical performance till date. Surface modification by heparin and other chemicals can be done to reduce the deposits over the IOL and capsule opacification.

Silicone

It is composed of repeating chains of cross-linked dimethyl siloxane. The major advantages of this material are the autoclavibility and decreased trauma to the intraocular structures. Silicone has affinity for proteins, which may account for the build up of the surface proteins on to the IOL optic. The material has a low tensile strength and must be handled carefully to avoid tearing. It is compressible and has an excellent memory (the ability to return to original shape after deformation). The refractive index is 1.41–1.46 and specific gravity is 1.01–1.06. Due to low refractive index, their relative thickness is more for the same dioptric power and hence high power silicone lenses are thick and cumbersome to handle with an uncontrolled opening inside the eye. Discoloration to a tan brown color had been reported in the first generation lenses and these lenses cannot be used in the presence of silicone oil within the eye as it chemically adheres to these lenses.

Recently, second generation silicone material has been introduced which has a higher refractive index and is increasingly becoming popular. The AMO CeeOn Edge 911 IOL and Tecnis, represent the second generation silicone IOLs. The edge of the optic is square or truncated and it uses polyvinylidine fluoride haptic material with a well-designed Capular C haptic configuration design providing an excellent memory. It has an optic diameter of 6 mm with an overall diameter of 12 mm (Table 47.3).

Table 47.3: Three-piece silicone intraocular lenses

Properties	*Elastimide IOL*	*SI 30 NB*	*SI 40 NB*	*SI 55 NB*	*Array SA 40 N*
Design	3-piece silicone-IOL	3-piece silicone-IOL	3-piece silicone-IOL	3-piece silicone-IOL	3-piece silicone-IOL
Model	AQ-1016/ AQ –2010/ AQ - 2003	SI 30 NB	SI 40 NB	SI 55 NB	SA 40 N
Manufacturer	Staar surgical, Inc.	Allergan Inc.	Allergan Inc.	Allergan Inc.	Allergan Inc.
Overal diameter (mm)	13.5/13.5/12.5	13.0	13.0	13.0	13.0
Optic diameter (mm)	Biconvex 6.3	Biconvex 6.0	Biconvex 6.0	Biconvex 5.5	Biconvex 6.0
Optic diamter	Silicone polymer	Silicone polymer	Silicone polymer	Silicone polymer	Silicone polymer
Water content	< 1%	< 1%	< 1%	< 1%	< 1%
Refractive index	NA	1.46	1.46	1.46	1.46
Haptic material	Polyimide	Polypropylene	PMMA	PMMA	PMMA
Haptic angulation	10 deg	10 deg	10 deg	10 deg	10 deg
A–constant	119	117.4	118	118	118
ACD (mm)	5.55	4.4	4.7	4.7	4.7
Diopter (range)	+14.5 to +28.5	+6.0 to +30	+6.0 to +30	+6.0 to +30	+16.0 to +24
Incision (mm)	NA	NA	NA	2.6	3.0

Properties	*Cee On 912*	*Cee On Edge 911*
Design	3-piece silicone - IOL	3 piece silicone - IOL
Model	CeeOn 912	CeeOn 912
Manufacturer	Pharmacia - Upjohn, Inc.	Pharmacia - Upjohn, Inc.
Overal diameter (mm)	12.0	12.0
Optic diameter (mm)	Biconvex 6.0	Biconvex 6.0
Optic diamter	Silicone polymer	Silicone polymer
Water content	< 1%	< 1%
Refractive index	1.43	1.46
Haptic material	PMMA	PVDF (polyvinylidine fluoride)
Haptic angulation	6 deg	6 deg
A–constant	117.8	118.3
ACD (mm)	4.6	4.9
Diopter (range)	+10 to +30.0	+12.0 to +28.0
Incision (mm)	NA	NA

Hydrogel

The optic of hydrogel lenses is made up polyhydoxyethylmethacrylate (HEMA) with a 38 % water content and bonded with an UV absorber. They are lathe cut in the dry state and require polishing. They are rigid in the dehydrated state and become soft and rubbery on hydration. Since they are hydrophilic, they are less damaging to the corneal endothelium on contact. These lenses have a low tensile strength and can get torn on insertion. This IOL material they may accumulate protein deposits and can be deformed by tissue pressures, leading to optical changes and changes in effective power. Their refractive index is 1.43 and specific gravity is 1.19. This group of polymers resembles the living tissue in their physical properties more than any other class of materials and is the easiest to insert. Recently, high grades of posterior capsular opacification have been reported with these lenses.

Thermoset Intraocular Lens

Thermoset IOLs created by the Optical Radiation Company (ORC) is a hydrophilic polymer consisting of methylmethacrylate and HEMA (Table 47.4). Popularly known as the "Memory Lens," it can be rolled into a diameter of 2.35 mm and easily inserted with any forceps into the capsular bag. At temperatures lower than 25 degree C, the polymer is rigid and thus available in a pre-rolled form. At temperatures higher than 25 degree C, the polymer begins to soften and the lens unrolls. Thus the hard pre-rolled lens is inserted through a standard phacoemulsification incision and as it warms up inside the capsular bag, it unrolls and assumes its original lenticular shape. It is the easiest foldable IOL to insert as it does not require any special instruments for holding or folding of the optic. The refractive index is 1.47 and the

Table 47.4: Memory thermoset IOL

Properties	*Memory Lens*
Design	3-piece –hydrogel-IOL
Model	Memory lens U940A
Manufacturer	Ciba vision, Inc.
Overal diameter (mm)	130
Optic diameter (mm)	6.0
Optic diamter	Hydrogel polymer
Water content	20 %
Refractive index	1.47
Haptic material	polypropylene
Haptic angulation	10 deg
A–constant	119
ACD (mm)	5.6
Diopter (range)	N/A

lens can be sterilized by autoclaving. The major draw back of these lenses is that they require a cold chain to be maintained which is sometimes difficult in our setup.

Acrylic

Flexible acrylic is a co-polymer of phenylethylacrylate and phenylethylmethacrylate. The cross linking imparts it a good three dimensional stability and temperture dependent viscoelasticity. Lenses made of this material are softer and more easily foldable at body temperature than room temperature. Unfolding is much slower and more controlled than silicone lenses. It has high refractive index of 1.55 making it the thinnest lens possible. It has a unique surface characteristic, i.e tackiness (tendency to adhere to surgical instruments and posterior capsule. These are available as single piece (all acrylic) and 3-piece lenses (PMMA haptics) and are currently the most popular foldable lens materials with the minimum incidence of posterior capsular opacification (Table 47.5). The decreased rate of posterior capsular opacification (PCO) has been attributed to the square edge design of the lens optic which has a barrier effect on proliferating lens epithelial cells.

The Alcon AcrySof is the most popular IOL in this group. It has an optic made up of flexible acrylic available in 2 diameters of 5.5 mm (MA30BA) and 6 mm (MA60BM) and open loop haptics made of PMMA. The overall diameter of the IOL is 12.5 mm (smaller optic) and 13 mm (larger optic).

Single piece AcrySof lenses have both the optic and haptic made up of acrylic and offer the best option for the capsular bag. These lenses (SA 30 AL, SA 30 AT, and SA 60 AT) from Alcon have a "modified L" haptic configuration with 0 degree angulation. The refractive index is 1.55, A constant is 118.4, they have an anterior asymmetric biconvex optic available in two sizes (5.5 mm and 6 mm), overall diameters of 12.5 to 13 mm and can be implanted with the Monarch II delivery system.

Various studies have documented that PCO rates are least with the AcrySof lenses which has been related to the good biocompatibility of this IOL. This is due to the "sticky" characteristic of the IOL and its close adherence with both the anterior and posterior capsules and the square truncated optic edge.

AMO has introduced an acrylic IOL with a new edge design. This is called the Sensar IOL with an "OptiEdge." The IOL has a rounded anterior edge, a sloping side edge and a square posterior edge. The rounded anterior edge helps to minimize glare as it allows light to be

Table 47.5A: Acrylic foldable IOLs

Design	*3-piece acrylic- IOL*	*3-piece acrylic- IOL*
Model	AcrySof MA30BA(5.5 mm optic), MA60BM (6.0 mm optic).	AR-40
Manufacturer	Alcon laboratories, Inc.	Allergan, Inc.
Overal diameter (mm)	12.5 and 13.0	13.0
Optic diameter (mm)	Biconvex 5.5 and 6.0	Biconvex 6.0
Optic diamter	Hydrophobic acrylic polymer	Hydrophobic acrylic polymer
Water content	< 0.5%	NA
Refractive index	1.55	1.47
Haptic material	PMMA	PMMA
Haptic angulation	5 and 10 deg	5 deg
A–constant	118.9	118.4
ACD (mm)	5.49	5.2
Diopter (range)	+10.0 to +30 MA30BA +6 to +30 MA60BM	+10.0 to +30
Incision (mm)	3.0 to 3.5 and 3.5 to 4.0	3.2

Table 47.5B: Single piece acrylic lenses

Model	*SA 30 AL*	*SA 60 AT*
Material (Haptic + Optic)	UV absorbing acrylate/ methacrylate polymer	UV absorbing acrylate/ methacrylate polymer
Manufacturer	Alcon laboratories, Inc.	Alcon laboratories, Inc.
Overal diameter (mm)	12.5 mm	13.0 mm
Optic diameter (mm)	5.5 mm	6.0 mm
Optic edge thickness	0.3 mm	0.21 mm, 0.3 mm
Diopter range	+10 to +30	+6 to +34
Refractive index	1.55	1.55
Haptic material	Acrylic	Acrylic
Haptic angulation	0 deg	0 deg
A–constant	118.4	118.4
Forceps implantation	Burratto forceps 3.2 mm	Burratto forceps 3.2-3.5 mm
Injector implantation	Monarch II B cartridge 3.2 mm	Monarch II B cartridge 3.2 mm
Incision (mm)	3.2 mm	3.2 to 3.5 mm

Table 47.5C: Various AcrySof foldable IOLs and the cartridges used for the insertion

ACRYSOF® Acrylic Foldable IOL					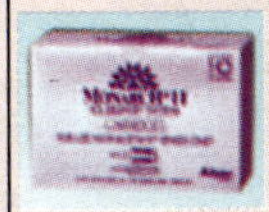	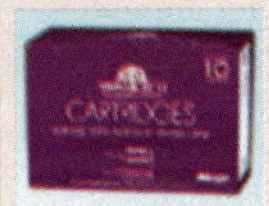	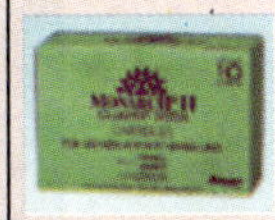
Model Number	*Optic size (mm)*	*Overall length (mm)*	*A-Constant range*	*Power cartridge (D)*	*"A" cartridge 8065977757*	*"B" cartridge 8065977758*	*"C" 8065977759*
SA60AT	6.0	13.0	118.4	+6-30 +31-40; 1.0		✓	
SA30AT	5.5	13.0	118.4	+10-30			✓
SA30AL	5.5	12.5	118.4	+10-30		✓	
MA60AC	6.0	13.0	118.4	+6-30	✓		
MA30AC	5.5	12.5	118.4	+10-30		✓	
MA50BM	6.5	13.0	118.9	+6-30	✓		
MA60MA	6.0	13.0	118.9	minus 5 - plus 5; 1.0	✓		

diffused from the front edge. The sloping side edge reduces the surface area that reflects the rays of light and generates an edge glare. The square posterior edge creates a barrier for epithelial cell migration. The optic of the lens does not have to be warmed in the operative room prior to insertion. The IOL can be inserted with the "Unfolder" implantation system through a 3.2 mm incision.

Collamer

The collamer IOL from Staar surgical Inc (USA) is a pure polymer of collagen and thus may be the most biocompatible IOL (Fig. 47.1). The collagen attracts a monolayer of fibronectin on the surface of the lens, which in turn inhibits the deposition of other proteins on the surface of the lens. Once the monolayer is formed the lens is not recognized as a foreign body inside the eye and thus it is the most biocompatible IOL. The material has a refractive index of 1.44 and is available both as a single piece and multipiece IOL.

HAPTIC MATERIALS FOR IOLs

Polymethylmethacrylate (PMMA)

The advantage of PMMA haptics is the total lack of degradation in vivo. Since they are stiffer than polypropylene, they can be easily dialled in the bag. Moreover they have better memory than polypropylene, with better fixation and centration. Three piece silicone IOL with polypropylene haptics have a higher incidence of

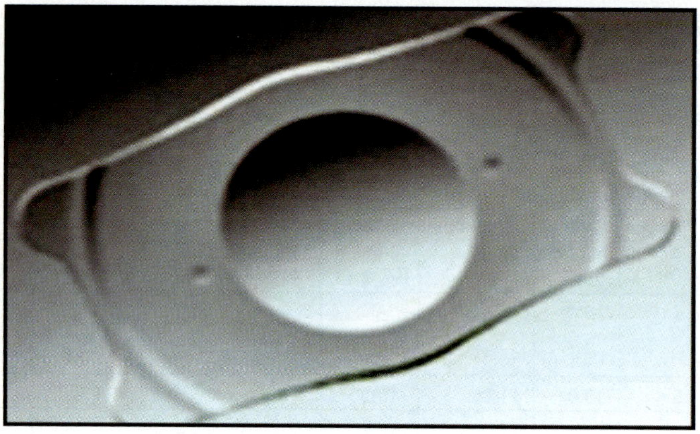

Fig. 47.1: The Staar Collamer IOL

decentration, pigment adherence and capsule opacification compared with PMMA haptics. Single piece all-PMMA exhibits the best loop memory. It is currently the most popular haptic material. An angulation of the haptics, 10 degrees anterior to the optic is done to minimize pupillary capture and iris chaffing and also allows a closer contact with the posterior capsule preventing epithelial proliferation under the optic.

Polypropylene (Prolene)

It is polymer derived from propane. Its main advantage is its hydrophobic nature making it very resistant to hydrolysis. However, a full spectrum UV light irradiation leads to loss of tensile strength. It is commonly used in the three-piece lenses because of its biological compatibility, resistance to biodegradation, flexibility and tensile strength. It is usually dyed blue or purple for better visibility. A tendency to lose memory with time when deformed by tissue is noted, with higher incidence of decentration. Prolene loops are more flexible making insertion easier. The main disadvantage of these haptics is that they activate the complement pathway leading to neutrophil chemotaxis with more postoperative inflammation. Bacteria also adhere better to polypropylene and this leads to a greater risk of endophthalmitis. Hence, this material is no longer used for making IOL haptics.

Polyvinylidine Fluoride (PVDF)

This is the latest IOL haptic material that has recently been introduced with some of the new generation silicone lenses. It provides a good memory and very stable fixation.

Table 47.6: Plate haptic lenses

Properties	*Bausch and lomb surgical, Inc.*	*Staar surgical, Inc.*	*Bausch and lomb surgical, Inc.*	*Staar surgical, Inc.*
Design	1 - piece silicone IOL	1 - piece silicone IOL	1 - piece silicone IOL	1 - piece silicone IOL
Model	C10 UB (small holes 0.3 mm)	AA-4203V (small holes 0.3 mm)	C11 UB (large holes 1.15 mm)	AA-4203 VF (Large holes 1.15 mm)
Manufacturer	Bauch and lomb surgical,Inc (Formerly chiron vision)c	Staar surgical, Inc.	Bauch and lomb surgical,Inc. (Formerly chiron vision)c	Staar Surgical, Inc. (Formerly chiron vision)c
Overal diameter (mm)	10.5	10.5	10.5	10.5
Optic diameter (mm)	Biconvex 6.0 mm	Biconvex 6.0 mm	Biconvex 6.0 mm	Biconvex 6.0 mm
Optic diamter	Silicone polymer	Silicone polymer	Silicone polymer	Silicone polymer
Water content	< 1%	< 1%	< 1%	< 1%
Refractive index	1.413	1.413	1.413	1.413
Haptic material	Silicone	Silicone	Silicone	Silicone
Haptic angulation	O deg	O deg	O deg	O deg
A - constant	119	118.5	119	118.5
ACD (mm)	5.59	5.26	5.59	5.26
Diopter (range)	+4 to +31	+14.5 to +28.5	+4 to +31	+14.5 to +28.5
Incision (mm)	3.2	3.5	3.2	3.2

Acrylic

In the new generation single piece acrylic lenses, the haptics are also made up of the same acrylic material as the optics and also have a square edge. These haptics are quite thick and can lead to iris chaffing if placed on the capsulorhexis in the ciliary sulcus.

Haptic Design

There are basically three types of haptic designs currently in use:

1. Open loop (such as modified C loop design).
2. Plate haptic (Chiron C10UB and C11UB) (Table 47.6)
3. Mini loop plate haptic design

PROFILE OF RIGID IOLs USED FOR PHACOEMULSIFICATION

Conventially an optic size of 6.5 mm and an overall diameter of 13 mm have been used for cataract surgery with IOL implantation in the ciliary sulcus. With the advent of small incision cataract surgery and capsulorhexis it has become possible to place the lenses within the capsular bag and hence smaller lenses are now being used. These lenses are essentially one-piece PMMA implants with either of two kinds of optic designs, round or oval. The round optic lenses have a diameter ranging from 5.0 mm to 5.5 mm, while the oval optic lenses have a horizontal diameter of 5.0 mm and a vertical diameter of 6.0 mm. The overall diameter of these lenses ranges from 11.5 to 12.5 mm, approximately the diameter of the empty capsular sac. The oval lens optic is no longer used as it is more prone to decentration and an increased incidence of postoperative glare and diplopia has been reported with these lenses.

The main disadvantage of using these lenses is that since they are rigid, implantation of these lenses requires an enlargement of the incision size equal to optic diameter. Once the incision is enlarged to 5-5.5 mm it no longer remains astigmatically neutral and there is an increased chance of postoperative leakage from the wound if left unsutured. Even if there is no leakage of fluid after applying pressure on the cornea/sclera at the operating table one should always apply a suture. This is important because there can be a long term slippage of the wound lip and progressive against the rule astigmatism in such cases. Therefore, one must apply at least one 10-0 monofilament nylon suture when rigid IOLs are used for small incision cataract surgery. Another problem with these lenses is that due to the smaller optic size, there can be problems of glare/diplopia in patients with large pupils and during night vision. There is also a higher incidence of posterior capsular opacification and decentration. These lenses should not be used if the capsulorhexis has been torn or if there is a large posterior capsular rupture so that the lens has to be placed over the margin of the capsulorhexis. Currently, these are the most popular lenses used for small incision cataract surgery due to the low cost.

FOLDABLE IOLs

These lenses made a major landmark in the history of IOLs and as the name suggests these lenses can be folded and enabling insertion through small incisions in cataract surgery.

Advantages

1. Require a small incision (2.5-3.5 mm) for insertion.
2. This decreases postoperative astigmatism, increases wound stability and allows rapid visual rehabilitation.
3. These lenses have a decreased incidence of posterior capsular opacification and cellular precipitates on the lens surface as compared to PMMA lenses.
4. These lenses are relatively easy to explant due to decreased perilenticular fibrosis. In addition due to a soft lens material the optic can be cut into two and removed easily.
5. Currently used foldable lenses also have a better Nd-YAG laser compatibility and put decreased strain on the zonules because of their reduced weight.

Disadvantages

1. Foldable lenses have a shorter track record and their long term biocompatibility within the ocular tissues has not been fully evaluated.
2. These lenses have a low tensile strength and are thus more prone to damage during implantation. Permanent fold marks and creases from holding, folding and inserting these lenses may produce disturbances in vision. In a cold temperature ccrylic lenses may even crack when folded.
3. Some of the foldable IOLs such as the memory IOL, require a cold chain to be maintained in a foldable form.
4. Lens discoloration has been reported with silicone IOLs.
5. It is difficult to use foldable IOL in the presence of a posterior capsular rent.
6. If vitreoretinal surgery is required in an eye with a silicone implant, silicone oil cannot be used as a vitreous substitute.
7. Currently foldable lenses are also much more expensive than rigid PMMA lenses.

SURGICAL CONSIDERATIONS IN THE INSERTION OF FOLDABLE IOLs

There are two basic techniques for foldable IOL insertion. These IOLs can be inserted into the capsular bag by using a passport/insertor/ injector system or a holder-folder system. The former system requires the smallest incision size for IOL implantation. The holder-folder method is the most popular method for IOL insertion.

The IOL can be folded by using either of the following two principles:

1. Horizontal or longitudinal principle which allows for a two-step implantation technique ensuring control and safety. This is folding along the 6 to 12 o'clock meridian such that the haptics form a "moustache." The anterior haptic goes in first under the capsulorhexis margin while the posterior haptic stays outside the wound. After the IOL is released inside the capsular bag, the posterior optic is dialed into the capsular bag (Figs 47.2 and 47.3).
2. Vertical or transverse principle which allows the lens to be placed in the bag in one maneuver. This is folding along the 3 to 9 o'clock meridian such that both haptics are placed together in the capsular bag and do not need to be dialed after the lens opens up in the capsular bag (Figs 47.4 and 47.5).

It is important to remember that silicone IOLs should be dried before handling with the holder/folder, while acrylic lenses should be wetted during folding.

In the event of a zonular dialysis the IOL should be inserted after putting an endocapsular ring (ECR) made of PMMA to stabilize the capsular bag or else put in the ciliary sulcus, orienting the haptics away from the area of dialysis.

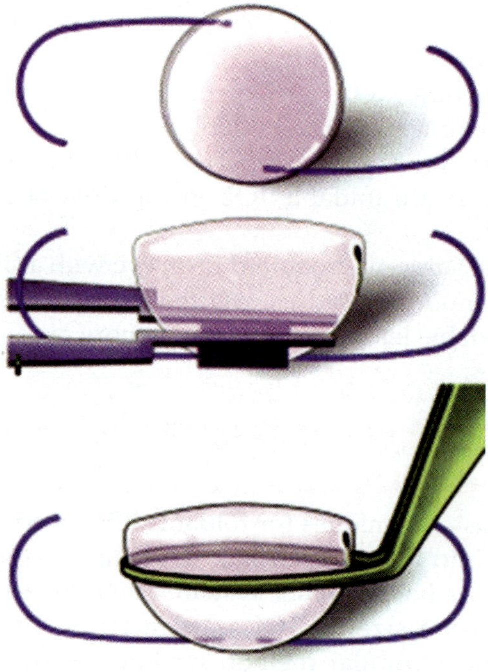

Fig. 47.2: Horizontal or longitudinal principle of foldable IOL insertion with forceps

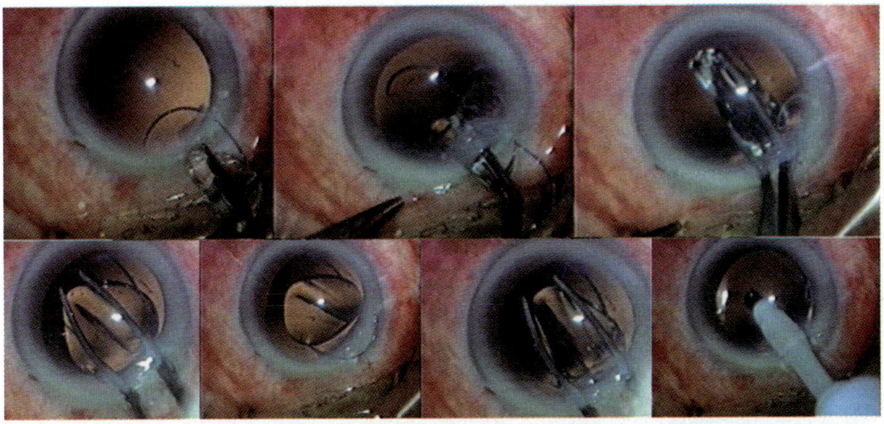

Fig. 47.3: AcrySof three-piece IOL insertion by horizontal or longitudinal principle of foldable IOL insertion with holding and folding forceps

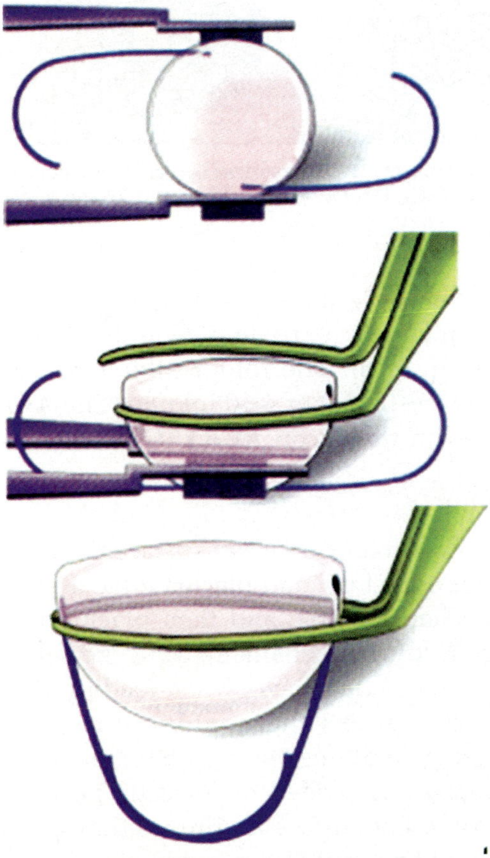

Fig. 47.4: Vertical or transverse principle of foldable IOL insertion with forceps

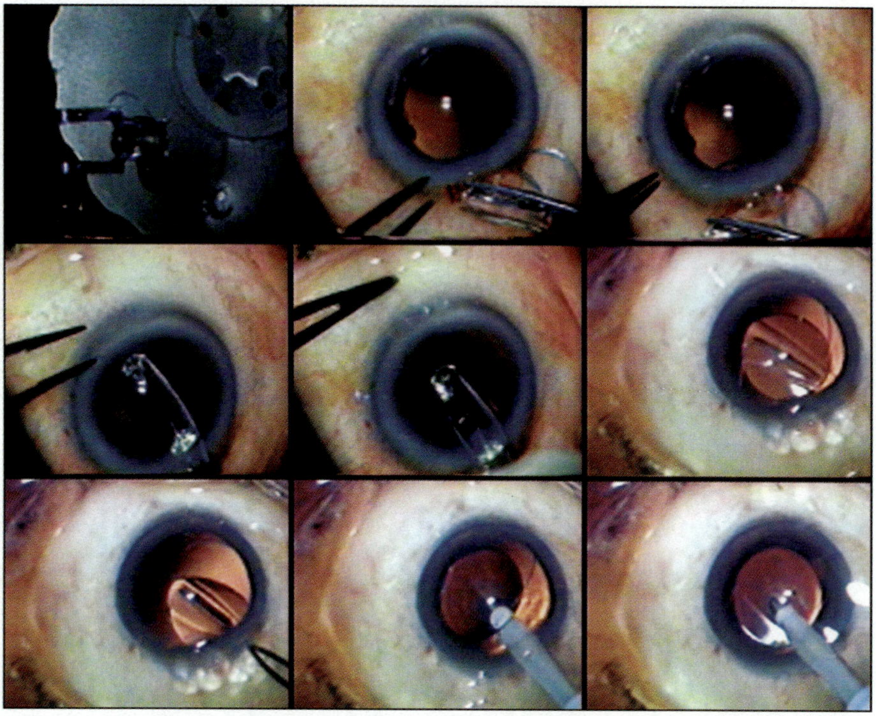

Fig. 47.5: AcrySof three piece IOL insertion by vertical or transverse principle of foldable IOL insertion with holding and folding forceps

ACRYPAK® FOLDER

The **ACRYPAK®** folder is a sterile, single use folder molded from polypropylene (Fig. 47.6). The folder allows the user to load the **ACRYSOF®** lens for 6-12, 3-9 or 4-10 folding. The **ACRYPAK®** folder is meant for use with the Alcon **ACRYSOF®** acrylic foldable IOL.

Folding Instructions

Place the ACRYPAK® folder on a flat surface. Load lens by grasping the haptic, anterior aspect up, and placing edge of the optic under the lower folding mechanism first, and then placing the opposite edge under the upper folding mechanism. Squeeze folder slightly with thumb and forefinger to open jaws when loading the 6.0 mm lens as shown at left. Wet the lens thoroughly by irrigating with sterile intraocular irrigating solutions (such as BSS® or BSS PLUS®). Nudge haptics or optic edges as needed to correctly position lens in folder. Place the folder on a flat surface and reposition grip to place thumb and forefinger on folder arms. Using gentle pressure, slowly compress folder arms until lens is folded. *Do not* release pressure on arms until

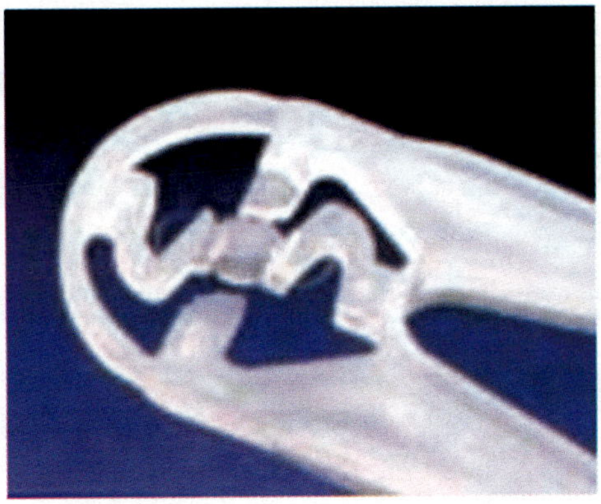

Fig. 47.6: The ACRYPAK® folder

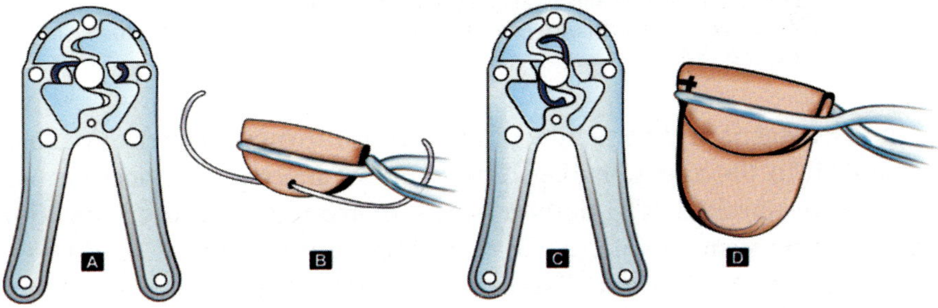

Fig. 47.7: The ACRYPAK® folder. A,B: Loaded position for 6-12 fold and C,D: Loaded position for 3-9 fold

lens is removed. Center open implantation forceps over lens. Position the forceps flat on the folder surface. Close forceps on folded lens, release folder arms and remove lens from folder (Fig. 47.7).

IMPLANTATION DEVICES FOR FOLDABLE IOLs

Implantation devices were developed to provide uniform folding of the IOL and to allow the IOL to be inserted through smaller incisions than are possible with forceps. Unlike the holding and folding technique, the inserters isolate the IOL from the external environment, reducing the risk of introducing surface pathogens into the eye at the time of implantation. The injector systems use a disposable cartridge wherein the IOL is placed. There is usually a drawing of the IOL outlined on the cartridge which tells the surgeon as to which direction the IOL should be placed. The IOL is placed in the cartridge coated with a viscoelastic, the catridge is then is closed and inserted into the injector. The screw of the injector is slowly turned and one can visualize the haptic of the IOL coming into the nozzle of the cartridge. The nozzle is then placed inside the capsular bag which has already been filled

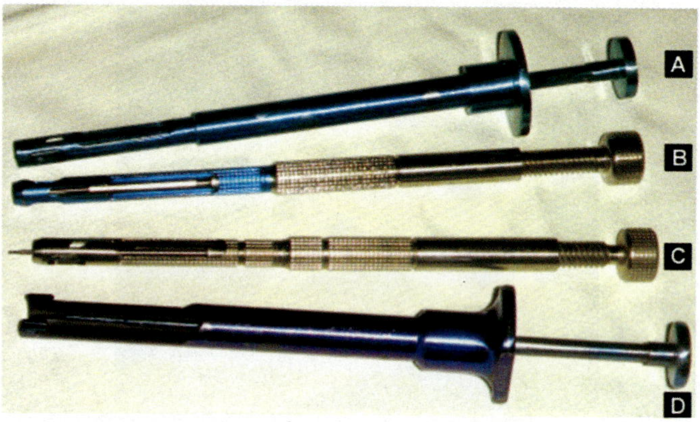

Fig. 47.8: Foldable IOL Injectors. A to D: A: Injector for Tecnis IOL. B. The sapphire unfolder implantation system for Sensar IOL . C. The silver series unfolder implantation system for SI 40 . D: The Monarch II injector for AcrySof IOL

with viscoelastic and the screw of the injector turned further to release the IOL into the capsular bag. The primary insertion devices in use are the Monarch II IOL delivery system from Alcon, the Unfolder implantation systems (Silver, Gold, and Sapphire) from the AMO (Fig. 47.8), and the M-Port and Passport II injector delivery systems from Bausch and Lomb.

MONARCH II DELIVERY SYSTEM

The Monarch II delivery system is designed to insert the three piece (MA30BA) and one-piece (SA30A) AcrySof acrylic IOLs into the capsular bag (Table 47.5C). The Monarch II has a reusable, titanium handpiece and single-use insertion cartridge. The Monarch 1 delivery system is used for implantation of the 5.5 mm AcrySof MA30BA IOL into the capsular bag. The Monarch system requires less manipulation and provides better control of IOL than folding and insertion with forceps. The Monarch II is designed to implant AcrySof IOLs through a 3 to 3.2 mm incision.

Lens Loading and Folding for Multipiece and Single-piece ACRYSOF® Lens with Standard Forceps (Fig. 47.9)

Inspect the cartridge pouch for any damage. If damage is observed, use another cartridge. Open the pouch using standard sterile procedures and transfer the cartridge to the sterile field. If, after inspection, the cartridge nozzle tip has damage, particulates, or deformation,use another cartridge. Use room temperature viscoelastic Ophthalmic Viscosurgical Device or BSS to fill the cartridge. Use

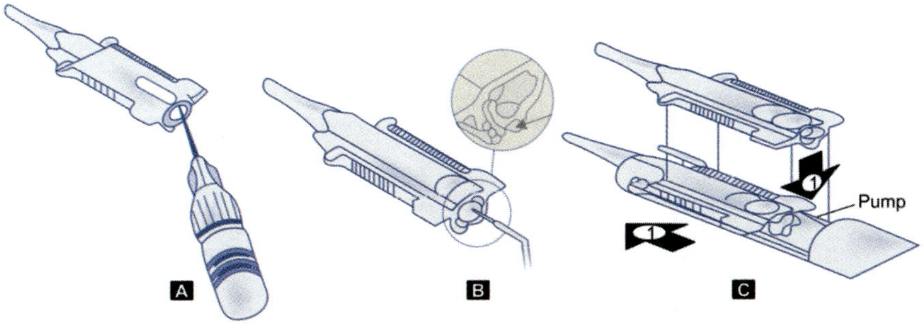

Fig. 47.9: Insertion of AcrySof IOL into cartridge

holding forceps to grasp the lens by the optic edge and place the lens anterior side up into the back of the cartridge as shown in the Figure 47.9. The lens should be inserted until it is centered with or slightly past the outline etched into the top of the cartridge. Lenses with a 6.5 mm optic diameter may need to be pre-folded for easy entry into the back of the cartridge. Lens may be pre-folded by applying pressure to the edge of the lens while holding the central optic with forceps. The trailing haptic will extend from the proximal end of the cartridge. Position the trailing haptic to the left of the haptic post. This will allow the plunger to go past the haptic during the initial advancement of the plunger into the cartridge. Verify that the lens is positioned on the bottom surface of the cartridge. The haptic should be maintained to the left of the post when the lens is loaded correctly. Accurate positioning of the lens will decrease the potential for optic and haptic damage.

Alternate Loading and Folding Technique for ACRYSOF® Single-piece Lens

Inspect the cartridge and fill it with room temperature viscosurgical device or BSS. Follow initial steps as described above and then grasp the lens by the optic edge and place the lens anterior side up into the back of the cartridge as shown in Figure 47.10. The lens should be inserted until the optic is a little more than half-way inside the cartridge. Use the holding forceps to gently push down on the lens, verifying that the lens is on the bottom surface of the cartridge. Using holding forceps, take the trailing haptic, and gently fold the haptic onto the anterior side of the optic. As shown in the Figure 47.10, grip or push the optic edge to position the lens as far into the cartridge as the forceps will permit, while ensuring the lens remains on the bottom surface of the cartridge and the trailing haptic remains on the optic.

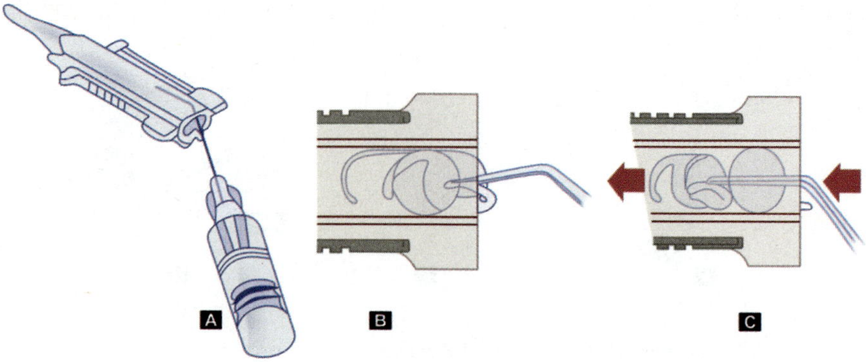

Fig. 47.10: Insertion of AcrySof IOL into cartridge (Alternative technique)

IOL Delivery

As shown in the Figures 47.9 and 47.10, insert the cartridge into the handpiece and fully slide the cartridge forward into the handpiece slot. Advance the plunger in one slow motion. If the haptic has not been placed on the optic, ensure that the plunger goes past the trailing haptic. The plunger should make initial contact with the cartridge at the ramp. In the event the plunger does not contact the cartridge at the ramp, do not use the handpiece. Slowly advance the plunger forward. Verify that the lens moves forward at the same rate as the plunger. To complete the delivery, slowly push the plunger forward to advance and fold the optic. When the threads on the knob make contact with the barrel, turn the knob clockwise to engage the threads. Once the threads are engaged, continue and complete the remaining steps of the delivery. As the lens moves through the cartridge, verify that the plunger tip is behind the optic and the leading haptic is looped in front of the optic. For the single-piece lenses, the leading haptic may become looped back between the folded halves of the optic. Insert the tip of the cartridge through the incision. Position the tip at the anterior capsule opening. If the leading haptic is looped in front of the optic, rotate the cartridge to be slightly bevel left to facilitate placement of the leading haptic into its normal orientation in the bag. Advance the lens only until the optic exits the nozzle, rotating the cartridge towards bevel right as needed to place the lens anterior side up. Unscrew and retract the plunger if needed until it has cleared the trailing haptic. Withdraw the cartridge nozzle while verifying that the trailing haptic exits from the nozzle. Place and center the lens using a suitable positioning instrument (Fig. 47.11).

Difficulties during Insertion of the AcrySof Single-piece IOL

We routinely use the single-piece AcrySof intraocular lens (IOL) (SA60AT, Alcon Laboratories, Inc.) with a 6.0 mm optic and an overall

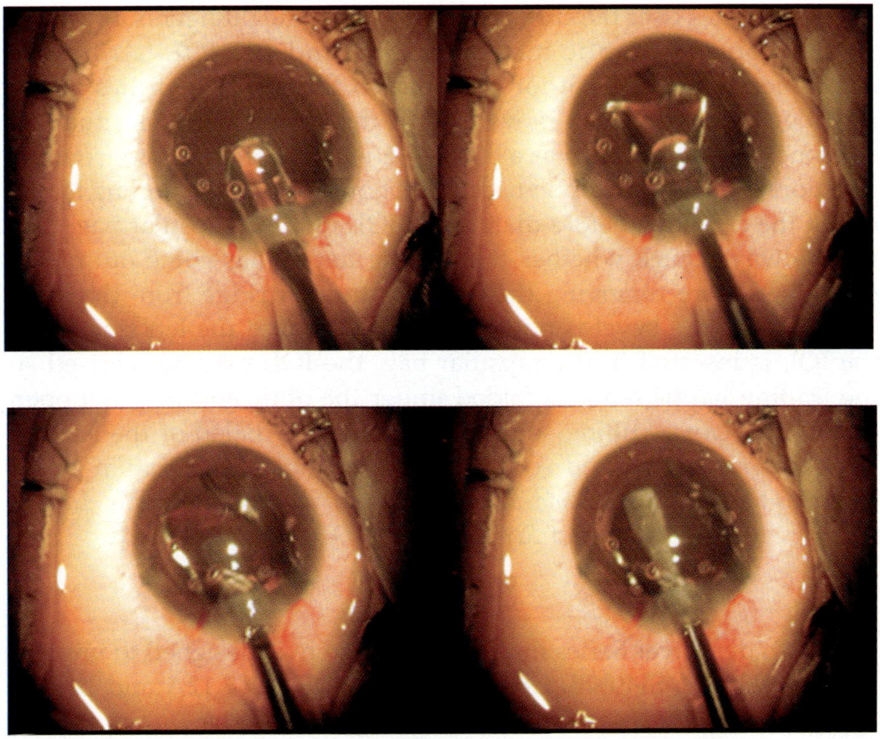

Figs 47.11A and B: Injection of AcrySof single piece IOL

diameter of 13.0 mm during phacoemulsification. The IOL is inserted in the capsular bag with the help of the Monarch II (B) IOL delivery system. According to product information from Alcon, the cartridge should be filled with an ophthalmic viscosurgical device (OVD) before the IOL is inserted. We have noticed that if an OVD is used, the IOL often sticks to the top of the cartridge, allowing the plunger to go beneath the IOL optic without engaging it. Balanced salt solution (BSS) can be used instead of an OVD for this purpose. We have found that using BSS to fill the cartridge makes IOL insertion, movement inside the cartridge, and engagement by the plunger much easier. However, the cartridge must be held in the horizontal plane, as BSS easily flows out.

The second problem we have encountered is imperfect engagement of the plunger with the IOL inside the cartridge. The IOL should be inserted into the cartridge so it lies on the bottom surface, and the trailing haptic must be placed on the anterior side of the optic. The IOL is then pushed farther down the cartridge and left in place until the plunger is forwarded to engage it.

In some cases, the plunger may engage the IOL between the optic and folded haptic and not at the optic edge as desired. In such a case, the plunger lies over the surface of the optic. If the plunger is advanced at this point, the optic may tag along and the IOL is released incompletely in the anterior chamber so the lower loop lies in the cartridge despite the full movement of the plunger. In this situation, a second instrument such as a Sinskey hook must be inserted from the side port to engage the optic-haptic junction and pull the trailing haptic out of the cartridge before dialing the IOL into the capsular bag. One must always check whether the trailing haptic has come out of the cartridge before removing the plunger and cartridge from the eye.

Finally, if the bevel is not kept slightly toward the left side when the IOL is inserted in the capsular bag, the IOL may be released so the leading haptic remains folded under the optic and may not open easily. This causes tilting, and the IOL must be dialed or the leading haptic manually opened so it takes its normal configuration at the capsular bag equator. *(Dada T. Difficulties during insertion of the AcrySof single-piece IOL. J Cataract Refract Surg 2004 Dec;30(12):2645).*

THE UNFOLDER IMPLANTATION SYSTEM

The Unfolder Silver Series implantation system is designed to implant AMO's SI30NB, SI40NB, ClariFlex, Tecnis (Figs 47.12A and B) and Array multifocal lenses through a 3 mm incision. The Unfolder Gold is designed to implant the SI 55NB silicone IOL through a 2.8 mm incision, and the Unfolder Sapphire is designed to implant the Sensar (AR40) and Sensar with OptiEdge (AR40e) acrylic IOLs through a 3.2-mm incision. All three systems have a reusable handpiece with disposable cartridges. The Silver and Gold Series have an additional sheath and tip, both of which are disposable. The UNFOLDER® Silver-T is a refinement of The UNFOLDER® Silver Series, which is even easier to use. The UNFOLDER® Silver-T requires fewer twists and delivers the lens 2-1/2 times faster than The UNFOLDER® Silver Series. The IOL optic body is implanted with a single twist provides the surgeon with total control during the delivery of the IOL. As the handpiece rod is advanced, the silicone SofTip™ Sheath "grips" the IOL. The SofTip™ Sheath continues to hold the IOL firmly throughout the unfolding—the surgeon decides the speed at which the IOL unfolds. Delivery can be stopped at any time, allowing the surgeon to adjust the placement. Even after the IOL is unfolded, the surgeon maintains control of the haptic and placement. The UNFOLDER® Silver-T also prevents IOL contact with the wound and the exterior of the eye, reducing the potential for postoperative inflammation. In addition to above, AMO has also introduced, the new Emerald Ease unfolder for the sensar acrylic IOL with OptiEdge This makes insertion further easier by

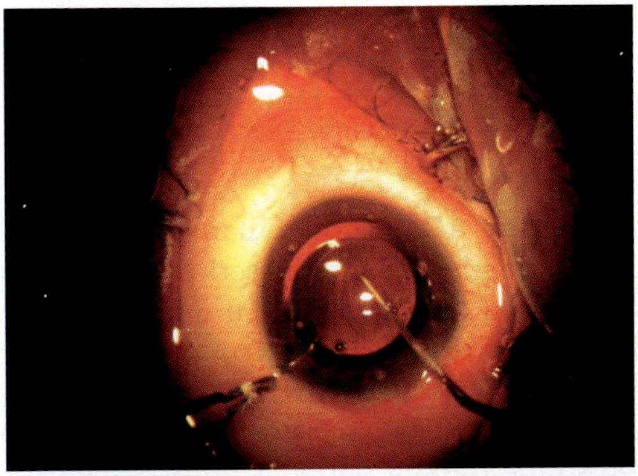

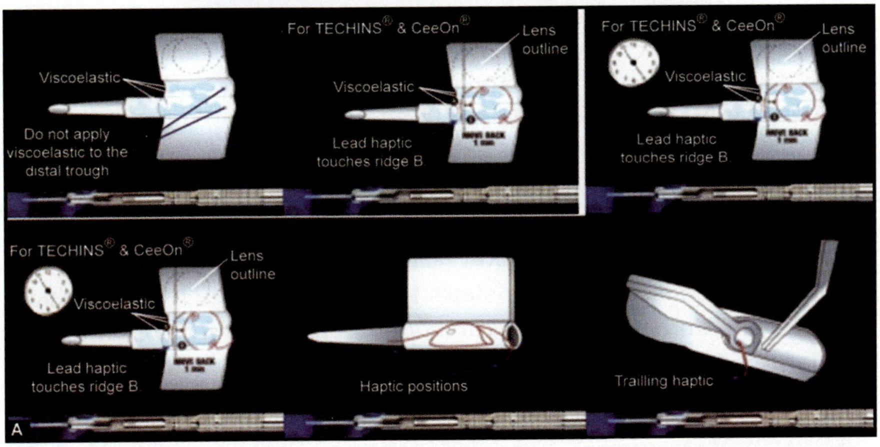

Fig. 47.12A: Diagrammatic representation of insertion of Technis silicone foldable IOL by the unfolder implantation system

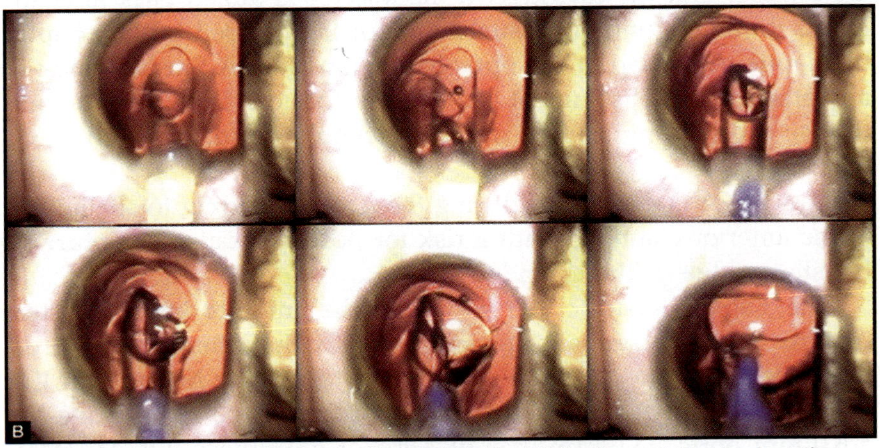

Fig. 47.12B: Insertion of Tecnis silicone foldable IOL by the unfolder implantation system

reducing rotations to only one axis with a single-handed syringe style. Surgeons can insert a three-piece, 6 mm-optic IOL through an unenlarged phaco incision of 2.6 mm.

Insertion of the Sensar IOL via the Monarch II Delivery System

The multipiece Sensar AR40 intraocular lens (IOL) (AMO Inc.) is inserted routinely through the Sapphire series unfolder delivery system. This IOL has a 6.0 mm optic and is 13.0 mm overall. With a trainee surgeon, errors can occur during 3 crucial steps when using this delivery system. The disposable cartridge is filled with methylcellulose 2% (or any other ophthalmic viscosurgical device) and the IOL placed in the cartridge so the trailing haptic is outside the cartridge and the leading haptic is inside the nozzle of the cartridge. The flaps of the cartridge are then closed, and one must ensure that the leading haptic is not caught between the flanges. If it gets caught and the surgeon pushes the plunger, the haptic can break. The surgeon may realize this only after the IOL has been injected into the eye, thus requiring subsequent explantation.

The second error can occur when the IOL is unfolded. During insertion of the IOL, the surgeon has to insert the cartridge inside the eye; when the leading haptic starts to come out, the Unfolder has to be rotated in an anticlockwise direction to ensure proper opening and orientation of the optic. If this anticlockwise rotation is not performed, the IOL will open upside down and may have to be flipped inside the capsular bag for optimal visual results.

The third error can occur if the trailing haptic gets stuck between the plunger and the cartridge. If the injector is pulled back after the IOL is unfolded, without visualization of the trapped trailing haptic, the haptic may snap at the optic-haptic junction. A Sinskey hook or any other second instrument has to be introduced from the side port to free the trailing haptic, and only then should the plunger be withdrawn.

Loss of OVD may occur during these steps, leading to shallowing of the anterior chamber, with a risk for posterior capsule rupture by the sharp edge of the cartridge tip.

The 3 steps illustrate that the use of the unfolder injector system requires several essential steps and dexterity that often lead to errors by trainee surgeons. A simpler option is to use the Monarch II IOL delivery system (Alcon Laboratories) with the Type A cartridge (for a 6.0 mm optic, 13.0 mm overall AcrySof multipiece IOL MA60AC [Alcon]). In this system, the cartridge is filled with an OVD and the IOL is placed according to the orientation drawn on the cartridge and pushed deep inside the cartridge with a forceps. The cartridge is then loaded onto the Monarch system and inserted into the eye. The IOL is pushed into the capsular bag with a simple forward motion of the plunger, no rotation being required. This system is much easier to use, and there is less chance of error by the trainee surgeon. The only point to remember is that with the unfolder, one can go through a 3.2 mm incision, while the Type A cartridge of the Monarch delivery system requires a 3.4 to 3.5 mm incision for a smooth insertion into the eye and placement of the IOL directly in the capsular bag. *(Dada T, Muralidhar R. Insertion of the Sensar IOL via the Monarch II delivery system. J Cataract Refract Surg 2005 Sep;31(9):1684.)*

M-PORT AND PASSPORT INJECTOR SYSTEMS

Bausch and Lomb's M-Port is a disposable injector system designed to implant the SoFlex LI61U, C3IUB, and Silens 6, multipiece silicone IOls. It provides uniform folding of the IOL into an M-fold and allows the IOL to be inserted through a 3 to 3.3 mm incision. The Passport II injector is a syringe-type system designed to propel the ChiroFlex Cll UB single-piece silicone IOL into the capsular bag.

Problems Encountered during Foldable IOL Insertion

i. The optic may slip if it is wet, especially if it is a silicone IOL.
ii. Flipping out of the IOL may result from inappropriate instruments and technique.
iii. Breakage of the haptic can occur from incorrect tucking of the haptic during insertion.
iv. Tearing of the optic can occur if the handling is not gentle, especially during the use of hydrogel IOLs.
v. The optic may crack when folded. This is usually seen with acrylic IOLs if they are used in a cold environment.
vi. The IOL may unfold with a sudden jerk within the capsular bag. This can lead to a loss of capsular integrity and a posterior capsular tear.
vii. Delayed unfolding may be been during the insertion of AcrySof or memory lens.
viii. The IOL optic may be indented/damaged by pressure from the holding/folding instrument.
ix. Incomplete opening of the holder may occur and the IOL may not be released into the capsular bag. In such cases the IOL needs to be disengaged from the holder with the help of a Sinskey hook introduced from the side port incision.
x. Detachment of the Descemet's membrane may occur during IOL insertion.

MULTIFOCAL AND ACCOMMODATING INTRAOCULAR LENSES

Traditional IOLs are monofocal, meaning they offer vision at one distance only (far, intermediate, or near). Multifocal IOLs are based on the simultaneous vision principle — if the power difference between two optical systems is 3.00DS or more, then the images are dissimilar enough for the brain to interpret them as separate. They are definitely an improvement over the cataractous lens that is replaced during surgery, which provides only cloudy, blurred vision at any distance. But traditional IOLs mean that you must wear eyeglasses or contact lenses in order to read, use a computer, or view objects in the middle distance, especially if you are already experiencing presbyopia before cataract surgery. The new multifocal and accommodating IOLs offer the possibility of seeing well at more than one distance, without glasses or contact lenses.

Presbyopic Lens Exchange

PRELEX^{SM} is a term used to describe presbyopic lens exchange with a multifocal intraocular lens. The onset of presbyopia has traditionally meant that use of glasses for clear vision. Even those individuals who have received laser vision correction will eventually become presbyopic and need glasses or contacts to restore their full range of sight. Unlike procedures that focus on changing the shape of the cornea, PRELEX^{SM} works on the lens inside the eye. Consequently, vision after the procedure will be stable and unlikely to change over time. In addition, cataract surgery will not be necessary later in life. The multifocal lenses that are used to replace eye's natural lens will provide with clearer vision at all distances, giving little or no dependence on traditional or progressive bifocal glasses.

The multifocal intraocular lenses can be classified into following types.

Refractive MIOLs

Two-zone/Target or Center Surround MIOL

The IOLAB NuVue^{TM} is an example of an MIOL with the central near add in the middle of the optic surrounded by a distance optical power. A new model made of silicone with PMMA haptics has shown surprisingly good clinical results despite the potential for visual blur with pupillary miosis. The NuVue^{TM} is considered to be a "near dominant" MIOL and some surgeons use it in a monovision capacity for the near eye. It has a 2 mm near zone in the center of a 5.5 mm optic which provides 4.0D of added power.

Three-zone MIOL

A variety of three-zone MIOLs providing distance and near vision by using a near annulus at various distance from the central distance component have been popular. The Storz True Vista™ and the Domilens Progress Three™ are examples of this style. Normal pupil patients do enjoy both near and distance vision but smaller pupils can obstruct the near component with some three zone MIOLs. One advantage of this lens design is that even though there is pupil dependency, distance vision is always preserved despite the loss of near acuity with miosis. The Storz True Vista IOL has a 1.5 mm central zone, 2.6 mm midperipheral zone and an overall diameter of 6 mm. Thus these lenses have 3 concentric refractive zones. Central and peripheral zones provide distance power while the midperipheral zone provides near add power.

Five-zone Spherical Curve MIOL

i. AMO Array® SA40N is a lens designed with *five zones* of near and distance powers on the anterior surface of the optic (Figs 47.13A and B). These power rings help to reduce pupillary dependency. The Array is considered a "distance dominant" lens and provides near acuities without correction in the J-3 range or better, offering good midrange and near acuity for most tasks. The lens has a 4.7 mm central zone with 5 annular refractive zones. Some patients will prefer the addition of a bifocal add for finer print and especially under low-light conditions. The AMO Array is available in a foldable silicone material with PMMA haptics. A new injectable delivery system allows for greater ease of insertion. The AMO Array lens is currently the most popular multifocal IOL in current use.

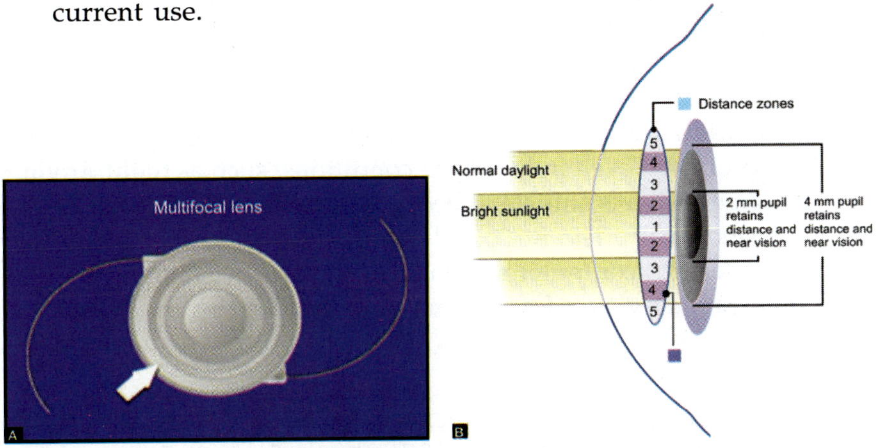

Figs 47.13A and B: Array multifocal IOL

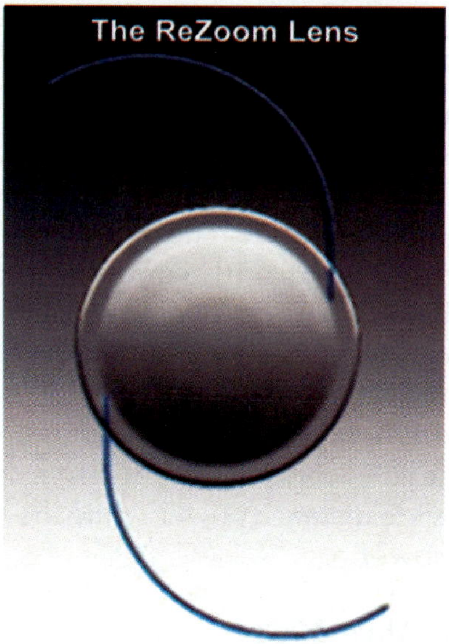

Fig. 47.14: Rezoom® IOL

ii. Rezoom® was developed as a successor to the Array IOL. It features five optical zones devoted to distance and near vision: (1) a central distance zone, (2) a paracentral near-dominant zone, (3) another distance zone, (4) another near-dominant zone, and (5) a peripheral distance zone (Fig. 47.14). The zones provide good distance vision under all light levels (pupil sizes). It gives near (1-2 feet), arm's length (2-3 feet), and distance vision simultaneously. The Rezoom® IOL is a distance-vision–dominant multifocal IOL; the distant focus has a higher image contrast than the near focus, because more incoming light is directed to distance versus near focus. With a small pupil, about 80% of light is directed to the distance focus, and approximately 20% to the near focus. With a 5 mm pupil, approximately 60% of light is directed to the distance, 30% to the near, and 10% to the intermediate focus. This light-distribution advantage is that distance vision is not compromised even in low-light conditions, such as night driving. Reading vision is sufficient, because individual light levels can be adjusted easily. The ReZoom™ lens gives generally satisfactory arm's length (computer screen, arm's length) vision but may not yield perfect vision for reading very small print up-close.

Diffractive MIOLs

Diffractive optics multifocal technology is slowly gaining wide acceptance. The major advantage of this lens is less pupil dependency and the ability to provide an even distribution of near and distance vision. However, manufacturing techniques are more difficult and critical with these lenses due to difficulties with making of the diffractive plate.

Alcon ReSTOR® diffractive multifocal IOL (Figs 47.15A to C) is one such IOL. The lens has anterior conventional refractive surface which provides the distant power and a posterior concentric diffractive plate which provides additional power ranging from 2.5 to 4.5 D. Rather than having three separate focusing zones like ReZoom™, however, the ReSTOR® lens focuses vision using an "apodized" surface. Apodization is a gradual reduction or blending of the diffractive step heights. This unique technology optimally manages light energy delivered to the retina because it distributes the appropriate amount of light to near and distant focal points, regardless of the lighting situation. The apodized diffractive optic is designed to improve image quality while minimizing visual disturbances. The result is an increased range of quality vision that delivers a high level of spectacle freedom. With the ReSTOR® lens, 97% of people can see both distance objects (road signs) and near objects (reading material within 1-2 feet) without difficulty, especially in good light. Arm's length vision (the computer screen, for example) at 2-3 feet is less clear, and most people will need glasses for these kinds of tasks.

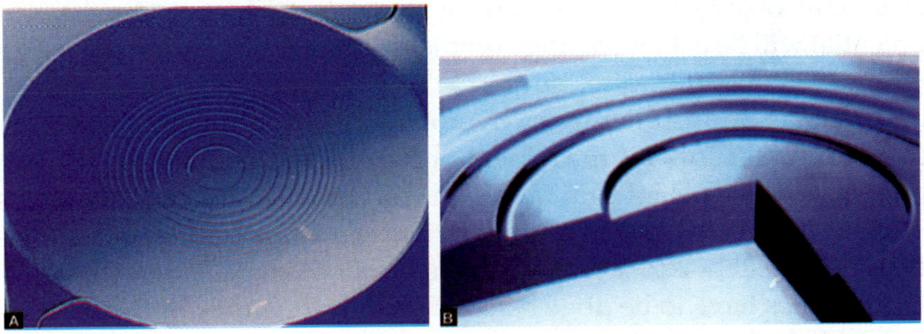

Figs 47.15A and B: A: ReSTOR® Multifocal IOL and B: Optics of ReSTOR® IOL

Pharmacia has also developed a diffractive MIOL, the Ceeon™ 811E. Addition of a diffractive component to the popular AcrySof™ acrylic IOL is also under consideration.

The disadvantages of multifocal lenses are glare and haloes from oncoming headlights at night and found night driving more difficult than the patients with monofocal IOLs. This "halo-effect" can also occur with other bright/dark contrast situations. An additional disadvantage of multifocal lenses is that they reduce contrast sensitivity resulting in loss of sharpness of vision particularly under poor visibility conditions such as low light or fog. Therefore, patients who spend their lives in a twilight environment and night-time work conditions may be disturbed by this loss of contrast sensitivity. Patient selection is a crucial step when considering whether a multifocal or monofocal lens should be implanted.

ACCOMMODATING INTRAOCULAR LENS

The ability to implant a new lens within the original capsular bag of the crystalline lens and restore the physiologic accommodation is a concept being investigated by many research workers all over the globe. The concept of an "accommodating" intraocular lens, a lens that would take advantage of the continued functionality of the ciliary muscle after cataract removal, with resulting forward movement of the optic to provide good, consistent near vision, was developed by cumming. The stimulus of accommodation leads to contraction of the ciliary muscle and relaxation of the zonules. The resultant mechanical energy stored in the capsular bag is transmitted to the implant during accommodation. This leads to a specific posterior deformation of the implant that increases its optical power, allowing near objects to focus on the retina. When accommodation ends, the ciliary muscle relaxes and zonular tension increases. The capsular bag is stretched and the accommodative IOL returns to its unaccommodative state. This results in distant objects being focused on the retina. The accommodative potential will be achieved after complete capsular bag shrinkage which takes about 4 weeks after surgery.

Kamman and Cumming have modifed the traditional plate haptic silicon IOL to allow for movement of the IOL within the capsular bag after insertion. This intriguing design has demonstrated initial success in restoring presbyopic accommodation. Accommodative amplitudes of approximately 2 to 3 diopters have been observed. However, long-term studies have to be done before the clinical efficacy of these lenses is established.

i. C and C Vision Crsytalens model AT-45® (Fig. 47.15C) is a modified plate-haptic lens manufactured from a high refractive index (RI = 1.430), third-generation nonreflective silicone material (Biosil), which contains an ultraviolet (UV) filter. The lens is hinged adjacent to the optic and has small looped polyimide haptics, which have been shown to fixate firmly in the capsular bag. The grooves across the plates adjacent to the optic make the junction of the optic with the plate haptic the most flexible part of the haptic/optic design. The overall length of the lens is 11.5 mm (loop tip to loop tip measurement), while the overall length as measured

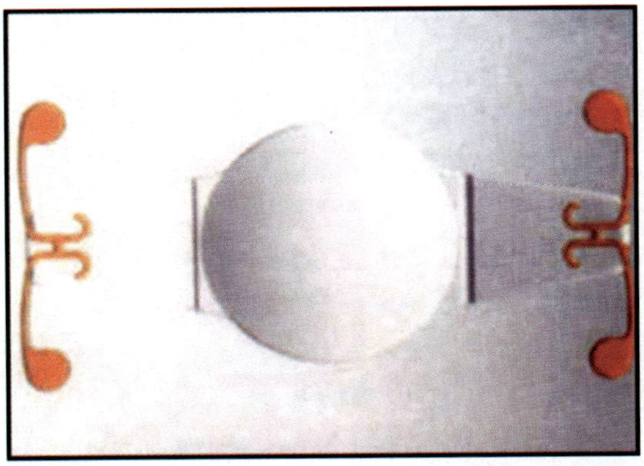

Fig. 47.15C: C and C Vision Crsytalens model AT - 45 accommodating IOL

from the ends of the plate haptics is 10.5 mm. The optic is biconvex and is 4.5 mm in diameter. The A-constant is 119.0, and the lens is designed for placement into the capsular bag has been shown in initial studies to provide 2.5 to 2.75 D of accomodation. The lens flexes back and forth and moves upto 1.5 mm with contraction of the ciliary muscle.

ii. Accommodative 1CU® Humanoptics (Fig. 47.16), a new pseudophakic accommodating foldable IOL has been developed by a German company. It is a hydrophilic acrylic lens with a refractive index of 1.46. It has an integrated ultraviolet inhibitor. The lens has four square edge dynamic transition elements with an overall diameter of 9.8 mm and a biconvex optic of 5.5 mm. It comes in a diopter range of +16 to +26 D in 0.5 D increments. The lens functions by dynamic transition elements that enable the optical power of the lens to change during accommodation.

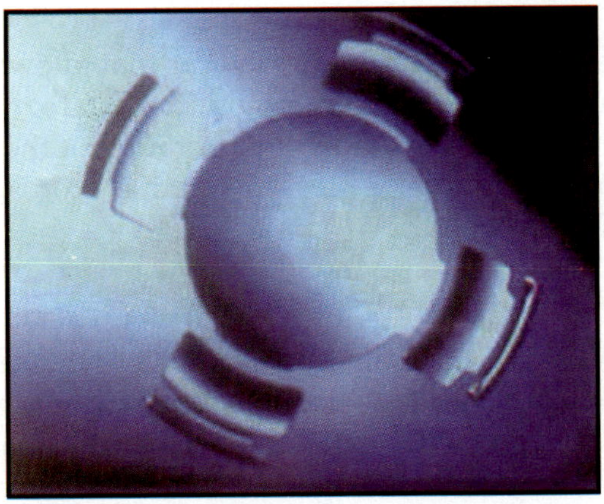

Fig. 47.16: Humanoptics accommodative 1CU IOL (Human optics, Germany)

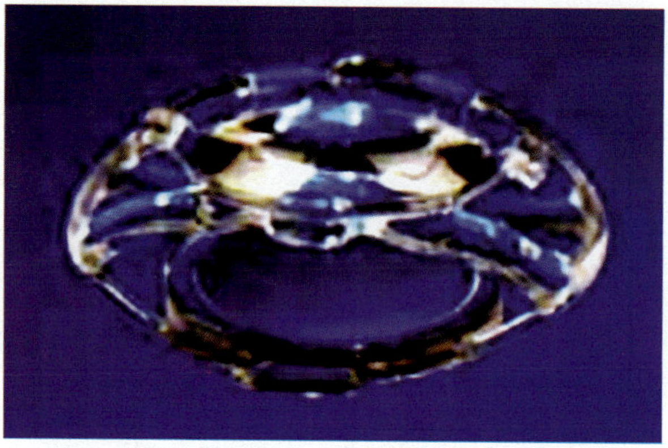

Fig.47.17: Synchrony® (Visiogen, Inc, California)

iii. Synchrony® (Visiogen, Inc, California) (Fig. 47.17) accommodating intraocular lens has dual optics, meaning that the ciliary muscles do not have to move it as much as other IOLs. The result, the company claims, is more accommodative power that translates into better vision at all distances. This is a one-piece, silicone lens, consisting of a high plus-powered (front) optic attached by flexible bridges to a low minus-powered (back) optic, fits within the capsular bag. In a nonaccommodated state, the distance between the two optics is shorter than in an accommodative state, when the bag slackens and the compressible haptics push the plus-powered optic forward.

A similar IOL, the Sarfarazi lens, has been licensed by Bausch and Lomb. It is also comprised of a minus-powered optic positioned posteriorly to a positive-powered optic, joined by compressible bridges.

Deformable IOLs

The Power Vision IOL has a fluid reservoir that allows for peripheral location of fluid in the nonaccommodative state, and the central movement of that fluid, increasing the curvature of the central portion of the optic, making it a more plus-powered lens on accommodation, e.g NuLens, FlexOptic IOL.

Light Adjustable IOL

Calhoun Vision (Sanfrancisco, USA) is developing a new IOL whose power can be adjusted postoperatively with laser energy. It is a foldable silicone IOL embedded with photosensitive silicone macromers. These macromers polymerize after being hit by a low energy laser. The power adjustments can be made by causing a polymerization of these macromers in different regions of the lens. If the laser is fired in the center of the lens then polymerization at the center leads to an increase in the IOL power. Polymerization in the periphery decreases the power of the lens while polymerization in one meridian can be used to treat residual astigmatism after cataract surgery. After the surgeon has achieved a satisfactory refractive result, the remaining photosensitive polymers are destroyed, thereby "locking" the lens at the desired refraction.

The Smart IOL, a **thermodynamic** accommodating IOL, which is a thin rod at room temperature and gains its original size, shape, and power at body temperature.

The main drawback of these lenses is that over long term, there is a significant fibrosis of the capsular bag which will not allow any movement and thus the IOL loses its ability to flex and accommodate. Performance of a YAG capsulotomy also opens up the capsular bag and disturbs the mechanics of these lenses.

TORIC INTRAOCULAR LENSES

The plate haptic IOL (Fig. 47.18) design has been modified to produce a toric IOL with the correction cylinder added along the long axis of the IOL. This is marked on the surface of the lens optic. For the toric design to be effective, the lens should not rotate within the eye after implantation. Rotation is relatively unusual but can occur during the first 4 to 6 weeks after implantation, prior to fibrosis around the lens and through the large positioning holes. After this 4 to 6 week period the lens fixates in the capsular bag via the fibrosis through the positioning holes and fusion of the anterior and posterior capsules. This helps to prevent long-term rotation as well as decentration and

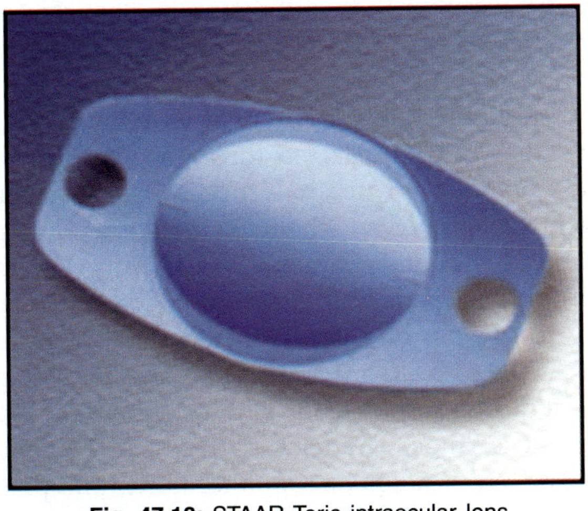

Fig. 47.18: STAAR Toric intraocular lens

dislocation of the IOL. One needs a proper capsulorhexis for this lens to have its effect and implantation should not be done if there is a breach in the capsulorhexis.

PIGGYBACK INTRAOCULAR LENSES

This concept involves the use of two intraocular lenses placed one on top of the other (piggyback). This may be done as a primary procedure to obtain an optimal refractive result in highly ametropic eyes, e.g. High Hypermetropia when sufficiently high power in a single IOL may not be available. The second IOL can also be implanted at a later date as a secondary procedure to correct for a poor refractive result of the previous cataract surgery. Either the lenses can be placed in the capsular bag or one can be placed in the bag and the second IOL in the ciliary sulcus. The main complication with use of piggyback lenses is *Interlenticular opacification* or interpseudophakic opacification of polypseudophakia (opacification between the two IOLs) which may require both IOLs to be explanted. This methodology is now rarely used as high hyperopic powers are available.

NEW IOLs FOR MICROINCISION CATARACT SURGERY

For microincision cataract surgery (MICS), new IOLs are being developed for insertion through an incision of 1.2 to 1.4 mm. Two such IOLs are the dehydrated acrylic IOL manufactured by AcriTec (Germany), and the hydrophilic acrylic IOL manufactured by ThinOptX®, Inc (USA). However, it remains to be seen whether these new ultrasmall incision IOLs will provide satisfactory visual performance, and whether they will maintain a satisfactory long-term stability within the eye. Various IOLs for microincision cataract surgery are:-

i. ThinOptx® Rollable IOLis an innovative IOL material (Figs 47.19 and 47.20) that can be inserted through a 0.9 mm incision. It is the latest advancement in small incision surgery that allows for complete phaco surgery via the two side ports. The optic diameter is 5.5 mm and the total diameter is 11.2 mm. The material is an 18% hydrophilic acrylic with a 50 μm to 400 μm optic and 50 um plate haptics. It can be manufactured in powers ranging from +30D to – 30D. The front surface of the lens is a curve that resembles a radius and the back surface has a series of 50 μm steps with concentric rings. The back surface can be concave, convex or plano. The lens is taken out of its container and placed in a bowl of BSS to make it pliable. It is then taken into the surgeons hand

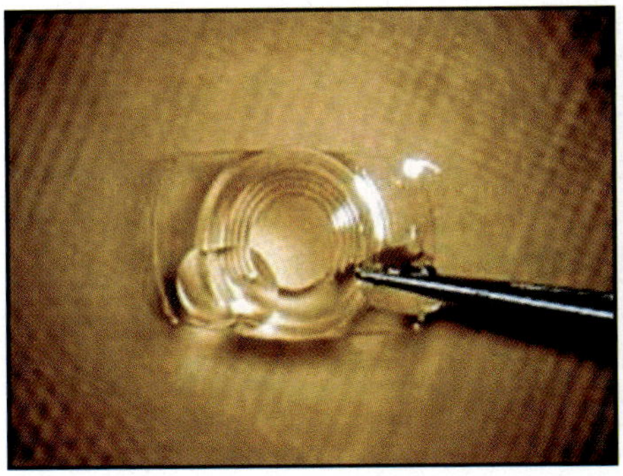
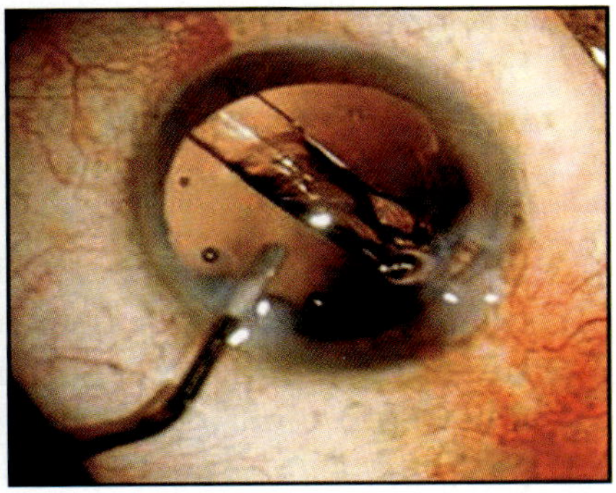

Figs 47.19 and 47.20: ThinOptx® Rollable IOL

between the index finger and the thumb. The lens is then rolled in a rubbing motion and held with a forceps for insertion through the side port incision. Once inside the bag the lens open up gradually as it warms up to the body temperature. Alternatively this lens can be implanted with the help of an injector.

ii. Acri Smart (Acri.Tec) IOL: This lens is a sterile foldable intraocular lens made of hydrophilic acrylic material with a hydrophobic coating (Fig. 47.21). Both the optics and haptics have a square edge design to prevent posterior capsule opacification. The method of insertion of this IOL is relatively simple. The injector tip is fitted with a sponge tip which comes with the cartridge and this prevents the injector tip from damaging the lens while inserting it inside the eye. Viscoelastic is injected in the cartridge and once the flanges of the IOL are in the groove of the cartridge, the cartridge is closed

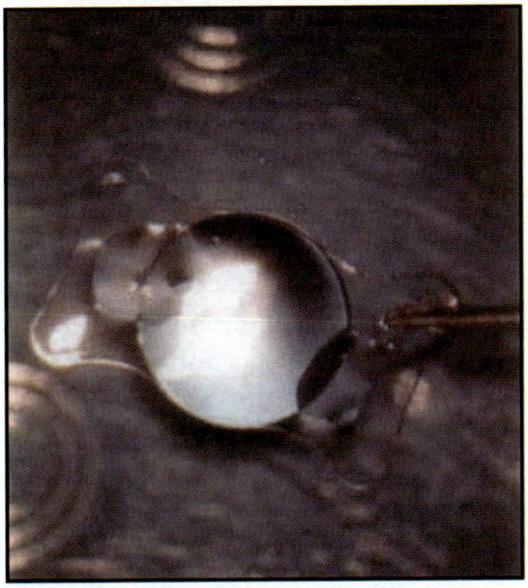

Fig. 47.21: The AcriTec® (Acri Smart) foldable IOL

and then inserted in the injector. The injection of the lens is done by the spongy tip. After the Phakonit procedure is completed, the incision is increased to 1.5 mm. Then the tip of the cartridge is kept at the site of the incision without being inserted into the anterior chamber. The IOL is gradually inserted through the incision and it unfolds inside the capsular bag. One has to be careful as implantation maneuvers can create marks on the delicate surface of the IOL. The lens is available with two optic sizes – 5 mm and 6 mm, the latter being more appropriate for younger patients. The 5 mm optic lens has now been redesigned to eliminate spherical aberration.

iii. Acri Flex IOL: The Acrimed Acriflex 46 CSE is a 25% hydrophilic acrylic IOL with a hydrophobic coating, a 5.5 mm optic and a total diameter of 11 mm. It is designed to be implanted with a special self blocking capsular tension ring. The ring is inserted in the capsular bag and once it is positioned only then the IOL is injected through the same incision. Approximately a 2 mm incision is required, and the ring stabilizes the lens capsule during IOL implantation, decreases capsular folds and improves IOL centration. This IOL can be implanted in eyes with weak zonules.

iv. Hydriol Slim: The Physiol Hydriol Slim IOL is made of a 26% water content hydrophilic acrylic material. It has a 6 mm optic and a total diameter of 10.5 mm. The lens can be injected through an incision of 2.2 mm. The IOL has a four point arched haptic design that ensures better centration and long term stability. The new version of the lens is preloaded in the cartridge and thus avoids any IOL manipulation before implantation.

WAVEFRONT BASED INTRAOCULAR LENSES

The development of wavefront aberrometry has not only influenced refractive surgery but has affected cataract surgery also, thus blurring the demarcation line between the two. It has been noted and reported that the pseudophakic patients still complain of dissatisfaction due to decreased contrast sensitivity and presence of glare and halos especially in dim light, in spite of having excellent visual acuity. There are two important factors, namely aberrations and scatter that affect the quality of the retinal image and therefore the quality of vision. The cornea has positive spherical aberration (peripheral rays focusing before the central rays). In young age the crystalline lens corrects this defect by producing the negative spherical aberration (central rays focusing before the peripheral rays). As the age advances the corneal aberration remains unchanged but the crystalline lens undergoes changes that cause a shift

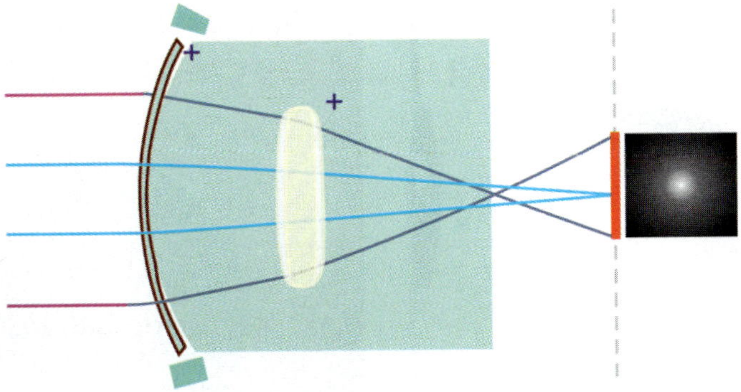

Fig. 47.22: Positive spherical aberration of conventional spherical IOL

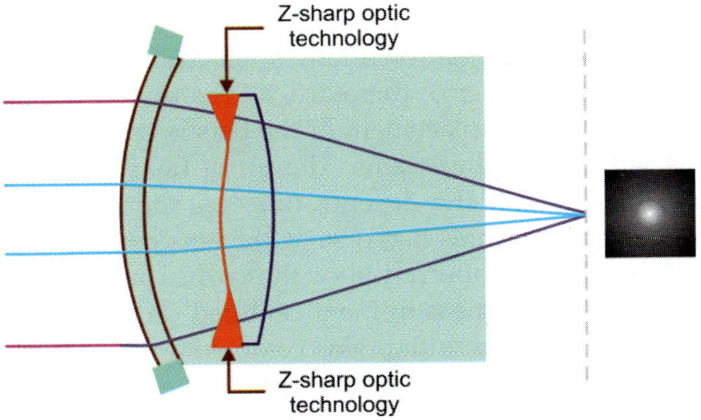

Fig. 47.23: Negative spherical aberration of aspheric IOL (Tecnis®), prolate anterior surface

of spherical aberration toward positive. This change adds to the positive spherical aberration of the cornea, with possible increased sensitivity to glare and reduced appreciation of contrast. The IOLs, which replace the natural lens, available today have spherical biconvex shape, they tend to attribute to the increased positive spherical aberrations of the human optical system (Fig. 47.22), thus reducing the quality of image in terms of contrast sensitivity. The aspheric IOL has modified surface that compensates for the positive spherical aberration of cornea (Fig. 47.23).

i. Tecnis Z9000® (Pfizer) is the first lens of this genre (Fig. 47.24A). Jack Holladay, Patricia A et al in 2002 designed and evaluated in laboratory this new intraocular lens. Tecnis is a foldable three-piece silicone lens similar to Ceeon Edge in every aspect expect for its anterior aspheric surface or more specifically, a "modified anterior prolate" surface. The lens has less refractive power at the periphery

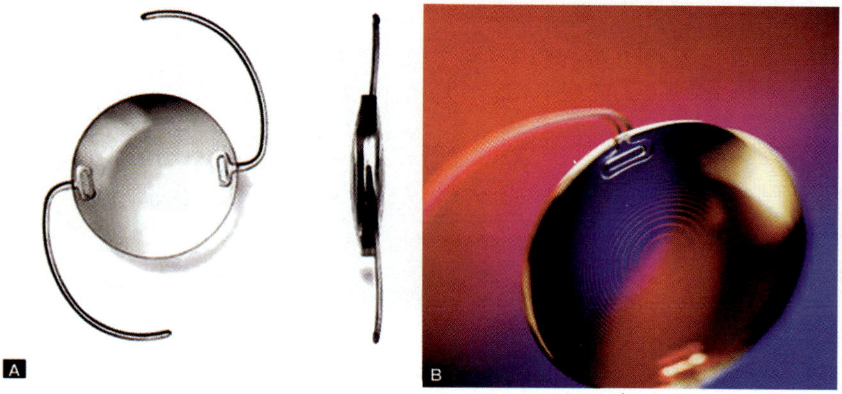

Figs 47.24A and B: A: Tecnis monofocal IOL B: Tecnis multifocal IOL

(contrary to the conventional lenses which have more refractive power at the periphery); therefore, all the rays come to focus at the same point. The placement of the lens is critical for optimum results with the aspheric lens. The tilt of the IOL has to be less than 7 degrees and the decentration less than 0.5 mm. This is because contrast values decrease as the lens gets increasingly off axis. The spherical aberration of the cornea used to design the Tecnis is based on measurement centered on the visual axis, so it has to be corrected with a lens centered on the same axis. The effort to lower spherical aberrations with the prolate design does not affect other aberrations. Since the Tecnis is a silicone lens, it should not be used in someone who has or may require silicone oil. In someone with proliferative retinopathy, for example, an acrylic lens is still the best choice. Clinical trials have shown a uniform improvement of contrast sensitivity over a variety of spherical IOLs in intra- and inter-individual studies. The multifocal variant of Tecnis is also available (Fig. 47.24B).

ii. AcrySof aspheric optic SN50WF HOA® IOL (Alcon) is a variant of popular lens AcrySof SA60AT with blue-light filtering material and a posterior aspheric surface to reduce spherical aberration as compared to standard spherical IOLs (Fig. 47.25).

iii. SofPort AO IOL (Bausch and Lomb) (Fig. 47.26). This aberration-free aspheric is a foldable silicone IOL with PMMA haptics and square edges and offers aspheric anterior and posterior surfaces, as well as uniform power from the center to the edge of the optic. This lens unlike Tecnis does not lead to increased aberrations even when decentered or tilted.

iv. Thin Optx Rollable IOL (see Fig. 47.19). The lens has three to five concentric optical zones with steps of 50 micrometers. Each Fresnel-like ring or segment of the lens has a small change in the

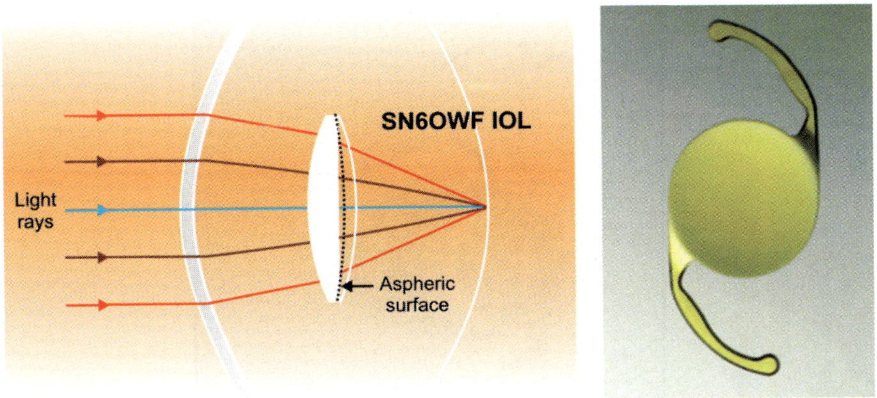

Fig. 47.25: AcrySof HOA®, aspheric posterior surface

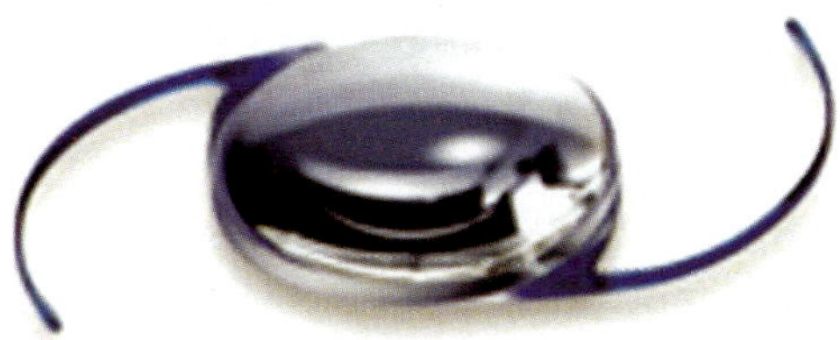

Fig. 47.26: The SofPort AOIOL®, both anterior and posterior surface are aspheric

radius to correct for spherical aberration. The difference in radius ensures that each ring of the lens focuses light at nearly the same point as the prime meridian. The edge of the lens is also 50 microns thick, which is thought to reduce the potential for halos and glare.

IMPLANTABLE MINIATURIZED TELESCOPE (IMT)

Vision Care ophthalmic technologies has developed the IMT device (Fig.47.27) which is basically a miniature implantable Galilean telescope which can restore central vision in patients with age related macular degeneration (ARMD). IMT is the first intraocular magnifying system proposed for optical correction in patients with age-related macular degeneration (ARMD). The optical component is embedded in a carrying device designed as an intraocular lens that is implanted after cataract surgery It contains a number of microlenses which magnify objects in the central visual field and allow the patient to see without external low vision aids. It is implanted in the posterior chamber after routine cataract surgery and held in position by haptic loops similar to ordinary IOLs. The IMT provides a nominal magnification of 3.0x and a field-of-view of 6.6 degrees (9.2 degrees for the 2.2x magnification version).

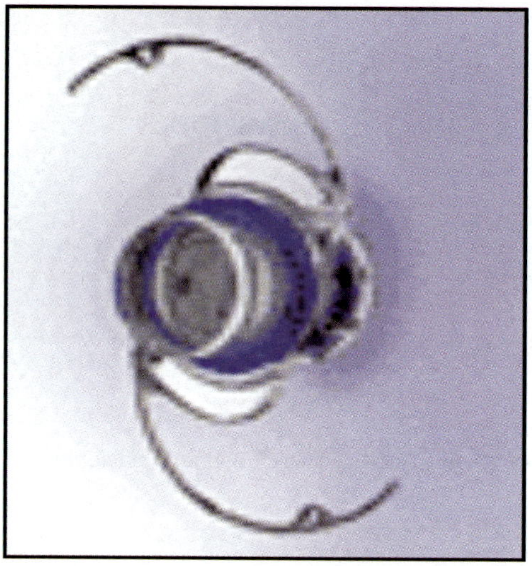

Fig. 47.27: Implantable miniaturized telescope (IMT)

THE PRISMATIC IOL

This prototype prismatic IOL developed in conjunction with IOL TECH LA Rochelle, France is fabricated from PMMA and is designed to shift the location of retinal images away from the nonfunctional fovea to enhance visual performance. Colin et al from University of Bordeaux, France reported results from a small pilot study in which patients with age-related macular degeneration underwent piggyback implantation with a new prismatic implant. The pilot study included 4 eyes of four patients implanted piggyback fashion, first with a Standard posterior chamber IOL and then with the new prismatic lens. They reported improvement in reading speed and near vision after the surgery. During the piggyback implantation, the PMMA posterior chamber IOL with a 5 mm optic is implanted in the bag through a slightly enlarged 5 mm incision. After this the prismatic IOL with a power of 22 degrees (5 D) is implanted through the same incision either in the same surgery session or later on. The next step is to constrict the pupil which is problematic due to very thick edge of this prototype lens.

The preoperative retinal function is evaluated with the scanning laser ophthalmoscope (SLO). This is very important because it allows us to determine the residual retinal function outside the fovea and to calculate the axis and power of the prismatic IOL which is required to deviate the light towards the still functioning area. Another advantage of this approach is that it is reversible and the prismatic IOL can be removed if the patient finds it intolerable. The prismatic IOL used in the French study is still a prototype and new designs are under development which will increase the angulation of the loops to create more space between the IOL and the iris. The newly designed lens will also be thinner to reduce the problems associated with constricting the pupil.

BLUE LIGHT-FILTERING IOL

This is the new AcrySof single-piece blue-blocking IOL (SN60AT or AcrySof Natural IOL). This IOL has transmission characteristics similar to those of the natural crystalline lens of a 53-year-old human. A yellow chromophore (Figs 47.28 A and B) has been added in the IOL which absorbs the blue light. Therefore, in addition to blocking ultraviolet light, wavelengths between 400 and 450 nm are only partially transmitted. The high-frequency blue wavelength light may be more likely to damage the retina through release of free radicals. The AcrySof Natural IOL blocks the unnatural transmission of this blue light and thereby may protect the retina better than standard UV-blocking IOLs. The yellow colored lens is also more easily visible inside the cartridge and thus easier to load and implant.

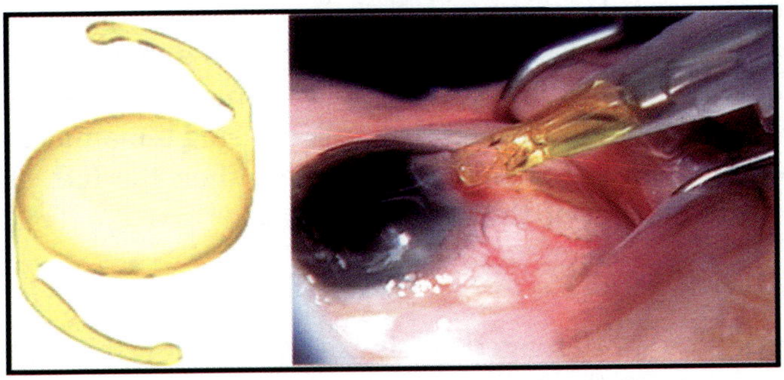

Figs 47.28A and B: AcrySof Natural IOL SN60AT

ANIRIDIA IOL

Morcher has developed special IOLs for use in patients with aniridia or a severe post-traumatic defeciency of the iris. These IOLs are available in various designs with an overall length ranging from 12.5 mm to 14 mm and an optic diameter of 3.5 mm to 5 mm. There is a central optic made up of clear PMMA surrounded by an aperture of black PMMA material with a size ranging from 3.5 to 10 mm.These IOLs have an A constant of 118.1 and are available in a dioptric range of 10-30 dioptres.

COMPLICATIONS OF FOLDABLE INTRAOCULAR LENSES

Descemet's Membrane Detachment Caused by IOL during Insertion

When inserting an IOL the lower edge of the optic can cause a Descement's membrane detachment. This Descemet's membrane detachment is likely to occur if IOL is inserted just parallel to the scleral tunnel incision and where a detached scroll of membrane is already present. In such cases the membrane can be repositioned through the injection of air or expanding gas into the anterior chamber.

Posterior Capsular Rupture during IOL Insertion

The posterior capsule can be ruptured during IOL insertion and a if there is a pre-existing tear in the posterior capsule, it can extend. Such a complication can occur if adequate quantity of viscoelastic has not been inserted in the bag or there is considerable leakage of viscoelastic substance during IOL insertion. The use of a passport system with plate haptic lenses is more likely to cause this problem. If there is a tear in the posterior capsule prior to IOL insertion, the injector/passport system should not be used at all. If a tear occurs during IOL insertion, the IOL may be left in the bag if the tear is small and the viscoelastic removed manually with a simcoe cannula or using bimanual irrigation-aspiration. However, if there is a large tear then the IOL should be placed on the margin of the capsulorhexis.

IOL Damage during Insertion

The haptics may be damaged during IOL insertion through a small wound and one of the haptics may be broken. In such cases it is essential to remove and replace the IOL. During insertion care should be taken to adequately extend the incision so as not to force the IOL through a small and tight wound. Special caution is warranted when a high power IOL is injected. Use of a wrong forceps for holding the IOL may cause compression marks on the IOL optic and may even crack the IOL requiring explantation of the IOL. *(Bala R, Rani A, Dada T. Forceps-induced cracking of a single-piece acrylic foldable intraocular lens. Ophthalmic Surg Lasers Imaging. 2003 Jul-Aug;34(4):306-7.)*

Bag Sulcus Fixation

During insertion of the IOL, the lower haptic may be placed in the bag and the upper haptic may lie in the ciliary sulcus. This can lead to IOL decentration and the haptic may also cause a chronic uveitis/pigment dispersion by rubbing on the iris tissue. Asymmetric loop placement can also cause the *windshield wiper syndrome* with the superior loop and optic shifting position with eye movements and causing damage to the corneal endothelium. To avoid this complication the upper loop of the IOL should be carefully dialed in the bag and the surgeon should check that both haptics are in the bag before concluding the surgery.

Capsular Bag Distension Syndrome

This problem arises when a small capsulorhexis completely covers the optic and thereby seals the capsular bag. There is sequesteration of fluid secreted from the remnant epithelial cells within the capsular bag and a progressive inflation of the capsular bag. Retained viscoelastic material behind the IOL can also lead to this condition by creating an osmotic gradient and drawing more fluid from across the capsule. This creates an anterior shift of the IOL and progressive myopia. The condition can be prevented by performing a large capsulorhexis. The treatment of this capsular distension syndrome is done by doing Nd-YAG laser capsulotomy of the anterior capsule. A nick is created at the edge of the capsulorhexis at 2/3 locations which allows fluid trapped within the capsular bag to escape into the anterior chamber.

IOL Decentration

Implanting a small diameter IOL in the ciliary sulcus (which is meant to go in the capsular bag) can lead to a severe decentration of the IOL. This is especially seen when a rent in the posterior capsule occurs and the small diameter IOL is placed over the margin of the capsulorhexis by the surgeon. It is important to remember that Plate haptic lenses which do not have open loops should never be placed over the capsulorhexis. The surgeon should always have a large diameter (6.5 mm optic, overall diameter 13 mm) IOL available for implanting in the ciliary sulcus in the event of a large posterior capsular rupture. In cases of zonular dehiscence, a PMMA endocapsular ring should be implanted within the capsular bag and then the IOL inserted, to prevent decentration of the IOL.

Lens Dislocation

Complete lens dislocation into the vitreous is a rare complication. It may occur due to the presence of an unrecognized zonular dialysis during surgery or the presence of pre-existing zonular deficiency such as in post-traumatic eyes or eyes that have undergone previous vitreo-retinal surgery. Such a complication has also been reported after YAG capsulotomy, especially with plate haptic lenses. Pars plana victrectomy is necessary for removal of lenses dislocated into the vitreous and the intraocular lens may than be repositioned with iris or scleral suturing or substituted with an anterior chamber IOL.

Silicone Oil Adherence to IOL

Irreversible silicone oil adhesion to the optic of a silicone foldable IOL may occur during vitreoretinal surgery. The silicone oil droplets condense on to the optic of the IOL and lead to a severe degradation of the optics of the IOL. This condition can be avoided by not implanting silicone IOLs in eyes with present or potential vitreoretinal disease.

Capsular Contracture Syndrome

The anterior capsulorhexis can undergo a progressive contracture leading to a capsular phimosis with obscuration of the visual axis and decentration of the IOL. This occurs due to a fibrous metaplasia of the residual lens epithelial cells and is aggravated if the original capsulorhexis is small. This complication is most frequently seen with the silicone plate haptic lenses. The contracture can be relieved by performing a YAG capsulotomy at the margin of the anterior capsule.

Uveitis

Polypropylene haptics can activate complement and induce white cell chemotaxis and thus incite an inflammatory reaction. IOLs with polypropylene haptics are also a risk factor for endophthalmitis with a risk 4 ½ times that of all PMMA posterior chamber lenses.

Endophthalmitis

Delayed onset endophthalmitis, which has a delayed onset and an indolent course, has been described in eyes with intraocular lenses. The most common organism responsible is *Staphylococcus epidermidis.* A more idolent form caused by *Propionibacterium acnes* may present as chronic granulomatous uveitis with white plaques on the posterior capsule. This infection appears to be enhanced by localized entrapment of organisms within the capsule and has been reported only in eyes with intraocular lenses. Adherence of organisms to lenses may play some role. If *Propionibacterium* is suspected, vancomycin is the treatment of choice, although some cases may not respond to medical management and require an IOL explantation with excision of the involved capsule.

IOL Discoloration

IOL discoloration has been reported with the first generation silicone IOLs. The discoloration of the optic varies from light tan to a brown color and appears from 15 months to 5 years after implantation. It can also be seen in the IOLs *in vitro* if the lenses have not been used for a long time. Although this coloration does not affect the visual acuity, it can cause a fall in the contrast sensitivity.

IOL Glistenings

This complication has been reported with the AcrySof IOL especially if AcryPak packaging has been used instead of the traditional wagon wheel packaging. These glistenings are basically microvacuole formation within the lens optic and are influenced by temperature changes. The can cause a significant decrease in the contrast sensitivity and induce glare.

Glare

Use of small optics (< 5.5 mm) can cause an edge glare, especially during conditions of decreased illumination, which cause a pupillary dilatation. This is a serious problem with square edge lenses such as the AcrySof with a 5.5 mm optic. It can cause a significant visual disability to the patients, especially during night driving. A trial of 0.5-1% pilocarpine may be done to decrease the symptoms in such patients, although the IOL may even have to be explanted due to this problem.

Posterior Capsule Opacification

Posterior capsular opacification (PCO) is currently the most important issue in modern day cataract surgery. Residual lens epithelial cells at the equator and the anterior capsule proliferate and cause an opacification of the posterior capsule after cataract surgery. This leads to a decrease in the visual acuity, contrast sensivity and causes glare. Silicone and PMMA lenses have higher rates of PCO as compared to acrylic lenses. A YAG laser capsulotomy has to be performed in such cases but it can cause damage to the optic of the IOL. Opening up of the posterior capsule increases the risk of a subsequent retinal detachment. PCO can be reduced by the following factors:

1. Adequate hydrodissection for facilitating a complete cortical clean up
2. An in-the-bag fixation of the IOL
3. Diameter of the capsulorhexis slightly smaller than the optic (seals the bag)
4. High biocompatibility of the IOL

5. Maximal IOL optic-posterior capsule contact
6. Square truncated edge of the IOL optic
7. Primary posterior capsulorhexis with optic capture in pediatric cases.

SUGGESTED READING

1. Agarwal S, Agarwal A, Agarwal A, Fine F, Sachdev MS, Mehta KR, Pandey SK. Phacoemulsification (3rd edn). Jaypee Brothers Medical Publishers (P) Ltd, New Delhi,2004.
2. Altmann GE, Nichamin LD, Lane SS, Pepose JS. Optical performance of 3 intraocular lens designs in the presence of decentration. J Cataract Refract Surg. 2005 Mar;31(3):574-85.
3. Apple DG, Solomon KD, Tetz MR, et al. Posteior capsule opacification. Surv Ophthalmol 1992;37(2):73-116.
4. Artal P, Guirao A. Contributions of the cornea and the lens to the aberrations of the human eye. Opt Lett 1998;23:1713-15.
5. Balasubramanya R, Rani A, Dada T. Forceps-induced cracking of a single-piece acrylic foldable intraocular lens. Ophthalmic Surg Lasers Imaging 2003;34(4):306-7.
6. Brown DC, Grabow HB, Martin RG, Rowen SL, Shepherd JR, Williamson CH, Ziemba SL. Staar Collamer intraocular lens: clinical results from the phase I FDA corestudy. J Cataract Refract Surg 1998; 24(8):1032-8.
7. Brown DC, Ziemba SL. Collamer IOL FDA Study Group. Collamer intraocular lens: clinical results from the US FDA core study. J Cataract Refract Surg 2001, 27(6):833-40.
8. Chehade M, Elder MJ. Intraocular lens materials and styles : A review . Aust N Z J Ophthalmol 1997;25(94):255-63.
9. Cumming JS, Ritter J. The measurement of vitreous cavity length and its comparison pre- and postoperatively. Eur J Implant Refract Surg 1994;6:261-272.
10. Dada T, Dada VK. Secrets of ECCE and IOL (3rd edn). Jaypee Brothers Medical Publishers, New Delhi, 2001.
11. Dada T, Muralidhar R. Insertion of the Sensar IOL via the Monarch II delivery system. J Cataract Refract Surg 2005;31(9):1684.
12. Dada T. Difficulties during insertion of the AcrySof single-piece IOL. J Cataract Refract Surg. 2004;30(12):2645.
13. Davison JA. Capsule contraction syndrome.J Cataract Refract Surg 1993;19(5):582-9.
14. Dogru M, Honda R, Omoto M, Toda I, Fujishima H, Arai H, Matsuyama M, Nishijima S, Hida Y, Yagi Y, Tsubota K. Early visual results with the 1CU accommodating intraocular lens. J Cataract Refract Surg 2005;31(5):895-902.
15. Elies Amat D, Coret Moreno A, Mauricio Casanovas J, Rombouts Matamala A,Gatell Tortajada J. Surgical management of the capsular contraction syndrome. Arch Soc Esp Oftalmol 2002;77(7):377-80.
16. Federico, Gianluca, et al. Low contrast visual acuity in pseudophakic patients implanted with an anterior surface modified prolate intraocular lens. Acta Ophthalmol Scand 2004;82:718-22.
17. Fine H, Hoffman RS, Packer M.The story of IOLs is still unfolding. EyeWorld 2004;9(8);36-7.

18. Fruscella S, Ducoli P, Manni GL. Decenteration of posterior chamber IOL: Effects of loop material and fixation technique. Eur J Ophthalmol 1994: 4(2): 111–4.
19. Gerten G, Michels A, Olmes A. Toric intraocular lenses. Clinical results and rotational stability. Ophthalmologe. 2001;98(8):715-20. German. Erratum in: Ophthalmologe 2001;98(10):954.
20. Gills JP, Fenzl RE. Minus-power intraocular lenses to correct refractive errors in myopic pseudophakia. J Cataract Refract Surg 1999; 25(9):1205-8.
21. Gills JP, Van der Karr MA. Correcting high astigmatism with piggyback toric intraocular lens implantation. J Cataract Refract Surg 2002;28(3): 547-9.
22. Gills JP, Van der Karr MA. Correcting high astigmatism with piggyback toric intraocular lens implantation. J Cataract Refract Surg 2002;28(3): 547-9.
23. Gills JP. Sutured piggyback toric intraocular lenses to correct high astigmatism. J Cataract Refract Surg 2003 Feb;29(2):402-4.
24. H. Burkhard Dick. Accommodative intraocular lenses:current status. Curr Opin Ophthalmol 2005;16(1):8-26.
25. Henahen JF.Piggyback implantaion of new prismatic IOL can improve visual functioning in ARMD patients. Eurotimes2001:6(1):18.
26. Hoffman RS, Fine IH, Packer M. Refractive lens exchange with a multifocal intraocular lens. Curr Opin Ophthalmol 2003;14(21):24-30. Review.
27. Jack Holladay, Patricia A, Gabor Koranyi, Marrie can der Mppren, NE Sverker Norrby. A new intraocular lens design to reduce spherical aberration of pseudophakic eyes. J Refract Surg 2002;18:683-91.
28. Kaskaloglu M, Uretmen O, Yagci A. Medium-term results of implantable miniaturized telescopes in eyes with age-related macular degeneration.J Cataract Refract Surg 2001;27(11):1751-5.
29. Kershner RM. Retinal image contrast and functional visual performance with aspheric, silicone, and acrylic intraocular lenses. Prospective evaluation. J Cataract Refract Surg 2003;29(9):1684-94.
30. Kershner RM. Silicone intraocular lens implant discoloration in humans Arch Ophthalmol 1991;109:913-914.
31. Kuroda T, Fujikado T, Ninomiya S, et al. Effect of aging on ocular light scatter and higher order aberrations. J Refract Surg 2002; 18:S598–S602.
32. Kurosaka D, Ando I, Kato K, Oshima T, Kurosaka H, Yoshino M, Nagamoto T,Ando N. Fibrous membrane formation at the capsular margin in capsule contraction syndrome. J Cataract Refract Surg 1999;25(7):930-5.
33. Leccisotti A. Secondary procedures after presbyopic lens exchange. J Cataract Refract Surg 2004;30(7):1461-5.
34. Leyland M, Zinicola E. Multifocal versus monofocal intraocular lenses in cataract surgery: a systematic review. Ophthalmology 2003 Sep;110(9):1789-98. Review.
35. Mamalis N, Spencer TS. Hayashi K, Harada M, Hayashi H, et al . Decenteration and tilt of polymethyl methacrylate, silicone and acrylic soft intraocular lenses. Ophjthalmology 1997;104(5):793-8.
36. Meacock WR, Spalton DJ, Boycee JF, Jose RM. Effect of optic size on posterior capsule opacification: 5.5 mm versus 6.0 mm AcrySof intraocular lenses. J of cataract Refract Surg 2001;27(8):1194-1198.

37. Mester U, Dillinger P, Anterist N. Impact of a modified optic design on visual function: clinical comparative study. J Cataract Refract Surg 2003;29(4):652-60.
38. Montes-Mico R, Alio JL. Distance and near contrast sensitivity function after multifocal intraocular lens implantation.J Cataract Refract Surg 2003 Apr;29(4):703-11.
39. Nichamin LD. Treating astigmatism at the time of cataract surgery.Curr Opin Ophthalmol 2003;14(1):35-8. Review.
40. Pieh S, Weghaupt H, Skorpik C. Contrast sensitivity and glare disability with diffractive and refractive multifocal intraocular lenses. J Cataract Refract Surg. 1998;24(5):659-62.
41. Schwartz DM, Jethmalani JM, Sandstedt CA, Kornfield JA, Grubbs RH. Post implantation adjustable intraocular lenses. Ophthalmol Clin North Am. 2001; 14(2):339-45, viii. Review.
42. Souza CE, Gerente VM, Chalita MR, Soriano ES, Freitas LL, Belfort R Jr. Visual acuity, contrast sensitivity, reading speed, and wavefront analysis: pseudophakic eye with multifocal IOL (ReSTOR) versus fellow phakic eye in non-presbyopic patients. J Cataract Refract Surg 2006;22(3):303-5.
43. Souza CE, Muccioli C, Soriano ES, Chalita MR, Oliveira F, Freitas LL, Meire LP, Tamaki C, Belfort R Jr. Visual Performance of AcrySof ReSTOR Apodized Diffractive IOL: A Prospective Comparative Trial. Am J Ophthalmol 2006 Mar17.
44. Theng JT, Jap A, Chee SP. Capsular block syndrome: A case series. J Cataract Refract Surg 2000;26(3):462-7.
45. Till JS, Yoder PR Jr, Wilcox TK, Spielman JL. Toric intraocular lens implantation: 100 consecutive cases. J Cataract Refract Surg. 2002; 28(2):295-301.
46. Till JS. Piggyback silicone intraocular lenses of opposite power. J Cataract Refract Surg 2001;27(1):165-8.
47. Tu KL, Gaskell A. Capsular bag distension syndrome.Br J Ophthalmol 1997;81(7):610.
48. Ulrich Mester, Patrick Dillinger, Nicola Anterist. Impact of a modified optic design on visual function: Clinical comparative study. J Cataract Refract Surg 2003;29:652-60.
49. Williamson W, Poirier L, Coulon P, Verin P. Compared optical performances of multifocal and monofocal intraocular lenses (contrast sensitivity and dynamic visual acuity). Br J Ophthalmol 1994;78(4):249-51.

CHAPTER

48

Rishi Mohan (India)

Recent Advances in IOL Materials

INTRODUCTION

The intraocular lens has certainly been the most significant ophthalmic invention in the last 50 years. The sheer impact on the visual recovery following cataract surgery, in a large percentage of the world's population, has been tremendous. However, the development of intraocular lens technology to its present levels has required a continuous effort by the physicists, biochemists, biomedical engineers and ophthalmologists so as to achieve the qualities currently available.

Perspex (PMMA or Poly-methyl-methacrylate), an acrylic material used in the manufacture of aircraft windscreens during World War II, was discovered by chance to be a relatively inert compound intraocularly. Pilots who sustained injury by shattered windscreens during the War tolerated its presence inside the eye, without significant inflammation.

Sir Harold Ridley, the pioneer and father of intraocular lens development and implantation, utilised this accidental discovery to produce the first intraocular lens from PMMA. He was inspired by the passing comment of a medical student observing a cataract extraction, regarding replacement of the lens after its removal. He designed and performed his first IOL implant in 1950. The surgery was done as a two-step procedure, in an attempt to allow the eye to become quiet and stable. The cataract extraction was performed in November 1949 (ECCE) followed by the IOL implantation secondarily in February 1950. The disc-shaped, biconvex, posterior chamber prototype IOL was manufactured by Rayner Ltd., U.K.

Since then the quest for better materials and designs for IOL manufacture has been unending. Various factors have guided and directed this evolution. Ophthalmologists have been plagued primarily by the problems of posterior capsular opacification, lens movement and intraocular inflammation and these factors, amongst others, have dictated the changes brought about in IOL materials and design.

The initial observations by Sir Harold Ridley, with regards to the contact of plastic material and edges of the IOL with sensitive ocular tissues and the tissue reactions elicited thereby, are important till this date. Improvements in lens quality with smoother contours and polished surfaces and designs which sequester the IOL away from the "sensitive" parts of the eye has led to improved outcomes in terms of acceptability by the patients and ophthalmologists.

IMPORTANT FACTORS

The important factors which governed the direction of the evolution of IOL design and materials have been:

1. Intraocular inflammation—membrane formation, secondary glaucoma.
2. Posterior capsular opacification (PCO).
3. IOL decentration—loops material biodegradation, tissue erosion, weight of the IOL.
4. Corneal endothelial decompensation.
5. Retinal light damage—UV, near-blue light toxicity.
6. Optical quality—aberrations, refractive index, clarity.
7. Late opacification of the IOL—unstable polymerization, biodegradation, chromophores.
8. Flexibility and "memory" of various materials—plasticity of foldable and injectable materials.
9. Lack of accommodation—development of accommodative IOLs.
10. Compatibility with other materials—for example silicon oil, hydrophobic/hydrophilicity.
11. Limitations of various materials in terms of sterilization techniques.

Inflammation

Inflammation amongst the earliest problems encountered with IOL implantation, was that of excessive inflammation, with fibrinous reactions, uveitis, pupillary membrane formation, pupillary block, secondary glaucoma and PCO. Many of these were possibly related to retained lenticular cortical material, adhesion of sterilising chemicals or polishing compounds on the IOL, poor finish and edges with resultant chafing of uveal tissue and unpolymerised acrylic (monomer) as an irritant.

Significant improvements in surgical techniques, equipment and microsurgical methods have led to a realm of excellent cortical clean-up. Similarly, intraocular lens material and finish have now ceased to be an important contributory factor in inflammation following IOL implantation.

The recognition of inadequate removal of residual sterilising agents such as cetrimide and sodium hydroxide, as also inadequate removal of the acrylic monomer (MMA) and possible retention of polymerizing chemicals such as benzoyl peroxide, and the realization that these might be responsible for inflammation was an important step. Measures were taken to minimize this and deal with the problem. Additionally, serial improvements in polymer technology have led to hugely improved biocompatibilities and lower inflammation levels and will be dealt with latter in the chapter.

Posterior Capsular Opacification

The late onset of capsular opacification has been an important factor in governing the lens design and creation of materials for IOL optics. Numerous studies have been conducted comparing PCO and Nd: YAG capsulotomy rates using different kinds of IOLs. Polyacrylic elastomer materials provided the least rates of PCO, followed by silicone and PMMA.[1,2] Polyacrylic lenses showed PCO regression as against progression with PMMA and silicone.[3] Ram et al [4] concluded that the implantation of a polyacrylic elastomer IOL reduced the incidence of PCO and need for Nd:YAG laser capsulotomies.

IOL Decentration/Dislocation

One of the earliest problem faced by Sir Ridley and the first generation IOLs was of dislocation, primarily due to the weight of the IOL, the disc design, and the poor techniques of ECCE with zonular and capsular bags that were not intact. With the advent of capsulorhexis as the standard, and in-the-bag implantation, this problem has been alleviated largely.

In a study examining the adhesion of IOL materials to labeled fibronectin, laminin and collagen type IV, Linnola et al [5] found polyacrylic elastomers to attract the greatest adhesion followed by PMMA, silicon, hydrogel and Heparin surface modified PMMA. They concluded that the stronger binding of fibronectin and laminin to the acrylate IOLs could explain the better adhesion of this material to the anterior and posterior capsules.

The change in the capsulorhexis opening with time has been used as an indicator of IOL stability with respect to the capsular bag. Various studies conducted have concluded that the polyacrylic elastomer IOLs show the least "movement" within the capsular bag, followed by the hydroxyl and PMMA IOLs. The silicon IOLs exhibit the most capsular fibrosis and decentration.[6-10]

Corneal Endothelial Decompensation

The complication of corneal endothelial decompensation has, most likely, been a problem related to surgical technique, irrigating fluids and viscoelastics as well as the lens position, placement and design, rather than the lens material per se. The better understanding of endothelial physiology and improvements in surgical techniques, the universal acceptance of the posterior chamber as the ideal site for routine IOL implantation and improved designs of anterior chamber IOLs, have vastly minimized the incidence of this complication.

Retinal Light Damage

Blue and near blue light have much higher energy levels than other wavelengths in the visible spectrum and are a component of solar and artificial light and radiation from computer display terminals. The human natural crystalline lens has the capacity to filter out these harmful rays, with the efficacy in filtering shorter wavelengths increasing as the lens ages.[11]

In the 1970's, the phenomenon of erythropsia was noted by patients receiving IOL implants. This was thought to be the earliest symptom of phototoxicity to the macular receptors and led to the addition of UV-blocking chromophores to IOL materials. UV blocking IOLs thus became the standard within a decade. However, blue light-related retinal toxicity was not adequately addressed.

With aging processes, there is an accumulation of lipofuscin in the retinal pigment epithelium (RPE) and the absorption of blue light energy by the lipofuscin fluorophore A2E may lead to free radical formation. This may, in turn, initiate cell death or apoptosis of the RPE.[12] The spectral dependence of reactive oxygen species generation by lipofuscin may explain the so-called 'blue-light' hazard to the retina.[13]

The clinical association between advancing AMD and cataract extraction is strong, even with the use of UV-blocking filters in IOLs.[14,15] In an attempt to minimize blue light induced retinal damage, IOL manufacturers have now incorporated blue-light filtering chromophores (0.04%) into the lens material, bonded covalently to polyacrylic elastomers and other materials, with light transmission spectrums closely matching those of the human crystalline lens.

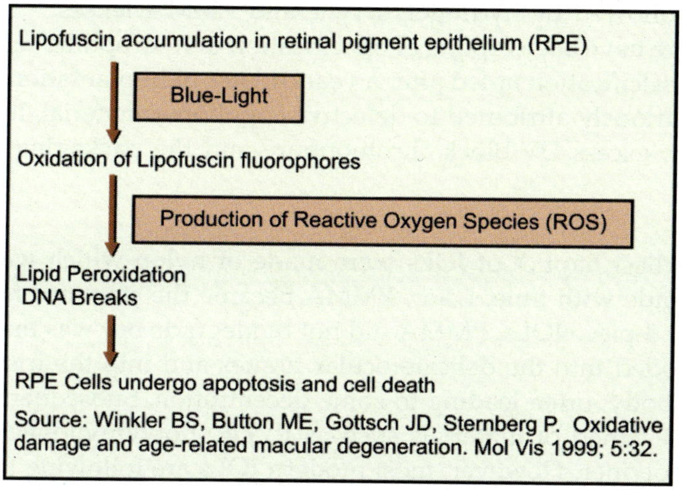

Fig. 48.1: Blue-light may be toxic to the aging retina. The production of reactive oxygen species in RPE cells can lead to apoptosis and cell death

Optical Quality

The 1st generation silicone materials had refractive indices ranging from 1.41-1.43 whereas acrylics have a refractive index of 1.55. Owing to the convexity of IOL surfaces, this tended to make the silicon IOL much thicker than the polyacrylic IOLs for any given dioptric power. This made the silicone IOL more difficult to fold and also necessitated a larger incision. With very high dioptric powers, there was a reduction in the effective optic size to ensure the IOL remained of manageable thickness. The 2nd generation silicone IOLs, with a higher refractive index of 1.47 have reduced these problems to some extent and helped with foldability and reduction in incision size. However, despite these improvements, there has been a decrease in popularity for the use of silicone IOLs amongst most ophthalmic surgeons.

All optical components of the various IOLs, whether of Perspex CQ (PMMA), silicone, hydrogels (hydrophilic acrylic) or hydrophobic polyacrylic elastomers, maintain excellent standards of light transmission. High levels of surface polishing, advancements in edge designs and treatments, and, more recently, the minimization or negation of spherical aberrations by incorporating changes in surface optics, are design features which are dealt with in other chapters.

Lens Opacification/Glistenings

Glistenings or water vacuoles may be found in many IOL materials some time after the surgery. In a retrospective study on the prevalence of glistenings in implanted IOLs presented at the ASCRS in 2001, Ahuja and Mintsoulis [16] found the maximum number of glistenings in silicon IOLs, followed by hydrogel, acrylic and PMMA lenses.

There have been reports of opacification of hydrophilic acrylic IOLs due to calcification noted after a year or later of implantation. This has been variously attributed to defective copolymer material, high water content, excess UV-block chromophore and the packaging system.

Haptics

The earliest haptics of IOLs were made of nylon which was known to degrade with time. Later, PMMA became the standard for haptics in most 3-piece IOLs. PMMA did not biodegrade but was much stiffer and eroded into the delicate ocular tissues and into the iris root and ciliary body, often leading to some decentration. Subsequently, loops were designed of materials such as PVDF (polyvinylidene fluoride) homopolymer. However, most modern IOLs are following the single-piece design with the haptics and optic material being identical.

BIOCOMPATIBILITY OF INTRAOCULAR LENSES

Biocompatibility can be defined as " not having toxic or injurious effects on biologic function"[17] and can be considered in 3 categories. ***Biostimulatory*** suggest stimulation of normal cell growth and proliferation. ***Biostatic*** or ***bioinert*** supports survival of cells but allows lens epithelial cells to die naturally. ***Biotoxicity*** suggests killing of cells or allowing changes into fibroblasts and thereby subsequent collagen formation. Biotoxicity also stimulates a blood-aqueous barrier breakdown and an inflammatory response.

Biocompatibility may be further divided into *uveal* and *capsular*.[18] Cellular reaction, small and giant cells on the IOL surface and aqueous flare are the measures of uveal compatibility. Lens epithelial cell (LEC) proliferation, Anterior capsular opacification (ACO), Posterior capsular opacification (PCO), Nd: YAG capsulotomy rates, capsular adhesion and capsular stability are indicators of the latter.

Numerous studies have been conducted evaluating the above parameters, albeit with slightly contradictory findings. However, in general, the majority views are listed below. The most often used indicators of biocompatibility clinically, have been the PCO & Nd: YAG rates. Polyacrylic elastomer IOLs resulted in the least incidence of PCO[1,2,19,24] and consequently, the least rates of Nd: YAG capsulotomies.[20] This conclusion was notwithstanding the fact that the lens design (square-edge) significantly affects PCO rates as well.[24]

With regards to proliferation of LECs on the IOL surface, the highest incidence was found with hydrogel lenses [21] (Biostimulatory effect). LECs tended to regress more on polyacrylic elastomers than on other surfaces. [3,22]

Polyacrylic elastomer material adheres more firmly to capsule like tissues.[23] This property probably contributes significantly to the low rates of PCO in these lenses.[1,2,4,19,20] PCO rates were significantly higher with hydrophilic acrylic as compared to hydrophobic, even though both material and design were found to be important.[24] Silicone materials provide the least stability of the capsule whereas the best stabilities were found to be achieved by polyacrylic elastomers and hydrogel IOLs.[8-10] Second generation silicones have improved in comparison to the first generation materials, but do not achieve performances in terms of ACO, capsular adhesion, PCO & Nd: YAG capsulotomy rates, equivalent to those of polyacrylic elastomers. [25]

The relative merits and demerits of various contemporary IOL materials are listed below:

Alcon Acrysof SA60AT, MA60BM (polyacrylic elastomer)

Copolymer 2 –Phenylethyl acrylate and 2 phenylethyl/methacrylates
Refractive index 1.55
Water content 0.3%

Structure

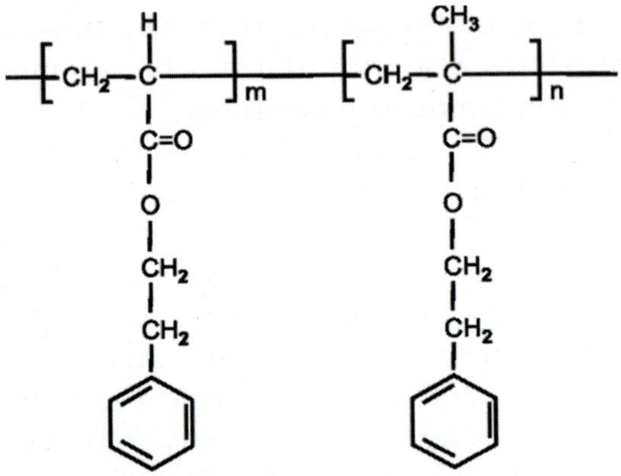

Material Features

- Low PCO, LEC growth, low Nd: YAG rates
- Material biocompatibility
- Capsular compatibility
- Cellular regression phenomenon
- Fully usable optic
- High refractive index
- Collagen adhesion (Capsular stability).

AMO Sensar AR40/AR 40e (hydrophobic acrylic)

Material	Terpolymer ethylacrylate, ethyl/ methacrylates and 2,2,2-trifluoroethylmethacrylate
Refractive index	1.47

Structure

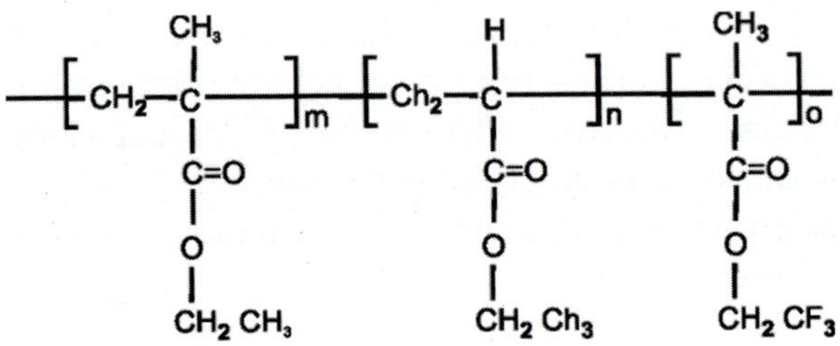

Material Features

- Biocompatibility
- PCO rates
- Surface tackiness
- Larger incision.

Hydrogel IOLs (hydrophilic acrylic)

Material	Hydroxyethylmethacrylate-methylmethacrylate copolymer and/or polyhydroxyethyl-methacrylate
Refractive index	1.46 -1.48
Water content	18% - 38 %

Structure

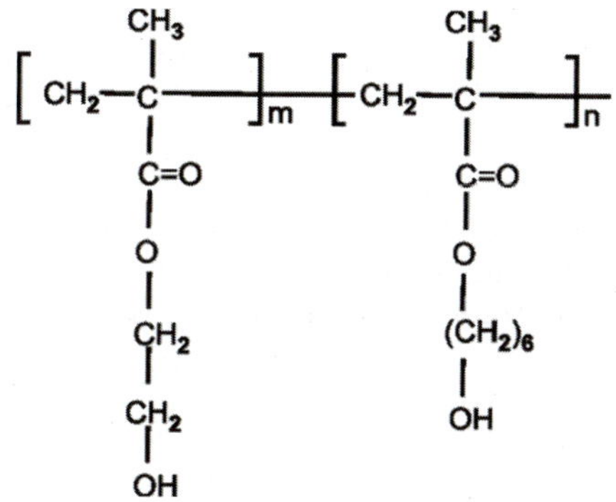

(HEMA – MMA Copolymer)

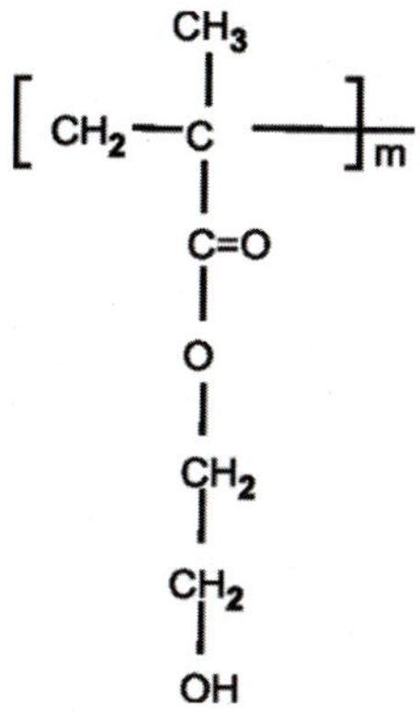

(PHEMA)

Material Features

- Higher PCO
- Anterior cell growth
- Higher lens thickness
- Cannot "dry" pack (needs storage under sterile solution).

Silicone IOLs

Material	1st generation	poly di-methyl siloxane
	2nd generation	poly di-phenyl siloxane
Refractive index	1st generation	1.41
	2nd generation	1.47

Structure

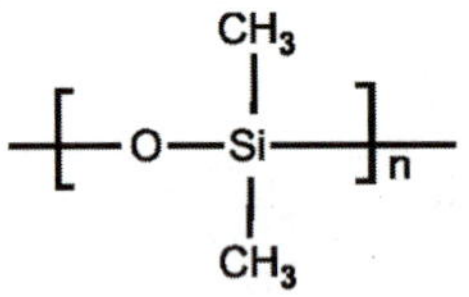

(1st generation)

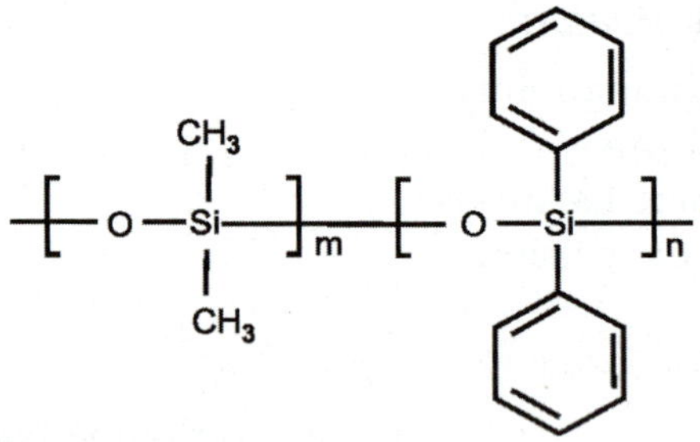

(2nd generation)

Material Features

- Higher PCO rates
- Anterior capsular fibrosis
- Increased thickness with larger incision
- Reduced usable optic
- Decentration
- Slipperiness when wetted
- Attachment to silicone oil.

REFERENCES

1. Ursell PG, Spalton DJ, Pande MV, et al. Relationship between intraocular lens biomaterials and posterior capsule opacification. J Cataract Refract Surg 1998; 24:352-60.
2. Hollick EJ, Spalton DJ, Ursell PG, et al. The effect of polymethyl- methacrylate, silicone, and polyacrylic intraocular lenses on posterior capsule opacification 3 years after cataract surgery. Ophthalmology 1999;106:49-55.
3. Hollick EJ, Spalton DJ, Ursell PG, et al. Lens epithelial cell regression on the posterior capsule with different intraocular lens materials. Br J Ophthalmol 1998;82:1182-8.
4. Ram J, Kaushik S, Brar GS, et al. Neodymium:Yag capsulotomy rates following phacoemulsification with implantation of PMMA, silicone, and acrylic intraocular lenses. Ophthalmic Surg Lasers 2001;32:375-82.
5. Linnola RJ, Sund M, Ylonen R, et al. Adhesion of soluble fibronectin, laminin and collagen type IV to intraocular lens materials. J Cataract Refract Surg 1999; 25:1486-91.
6. Hayashi K, Hayashi H, Nakao F, et al. Reduction in the area of the anterior capsule opening after polymethylmethacrylate, silicone, and soft acrylic intraocular lens implantation. Am J Ophthalmol 1997;123:441-7.
7. Schauersberger J, Amon M, Kruger A, et al. Comparison of the biocompatibility of 2 foldable intraocular lenses with sharp optic edges. J Cataract Refract Surg 2001;27:1579-85.
8. Ursell PG, Spalton DJ, Pande MV. Anterior capsular stability in eyes with intraocular lenses made of poly(methylmethacrylate), silicone, and AcrySof. J Cataract Refract Surg 1997;23:1532-8.
9. Georgopoulos M, Menapace R, Findl O, et al. Posterior continuous curvilinear capsulorhexis with hydrogel and silicone intraocular lens implantation. J Cataract Refract Surg 2001;27:825–32.

10. Sickenberg M, Gonvers M, van Melle G. Change in capsulorhexis size with four foldable loop-haptic lenses over 6 months. J Cataract Refract Surg 1998; 24:925-30.
11. Lerman S. Radiant Energy and the Eye. MacMillan Publisher, New York 1980.
12. Sparrow JR, Nakanishi K, Parish CA. The Lipofuscin Fluorophore A2E Mediates Blue Light – Induced Damage to Retinal Pigment Epithelial Cells. Invest Ophthalmol Vis Sci 2000;41:1981-9.
13. Winkler BS, Boulton ME, Gottsch JD, et al. Oxidative damage and age-related macular degeneration. Mol Vis 1999;5:32.
14. Pollack A, et al. Age-Related Macular Degeneration after Extracapsular Cataract Extraction (ECCE) with Intraocular Lens Implantation. Ophthalmology 1996;103:1546-54.
15. Klein RK, Klein BEK, Wong TY, et al. The Association of Cataract and Cataract Surgery with the Long-term incidence of Age-related Maculopathy. Arch Opthalmol 2002;120:1551-8.
16. Ahuja N, Mintsoulis G. Prevalence of Glistenings in Implanted IOLs. Paper Presentation, ASCRS 2001.
17. McCulley James P. Biocompatibility of Intraocular Lenses. Eye Contact Lens 2003;29(3):155-63.
18. Abela-Formanek C, Amon M, Schild G, et al. Uveal and capsular biocompatibility of hydrophilic acrylic, hydrophobic acrylic, and silicone intraocular lenses. J Cataract Refract Surg 2002;28:50-61.
19. Hayashi K, Hayashi H, Nakao F, et al. Changes in posterior capsule opacification after poly(methylmethacrylate), silicone, and acrylic intraocular lens implantation. J Cataract Refract Surg 2001;27:817-24.
20. Apple DJ, Peng Q, Visessook N, et al. Eradication of posterior capsule opacification; documentation of a marked decrease in Nd: YAG laser posterior capsulotomy rates noted in an analysis of 5416 pseudophakic human eyes obtained postmortem. Ophthalmology 2001; 108:505-18.
21. Schauersberger J, Amon M, Kruger A, et al. Lens epithelial cell outgrowth on 3 types of intraocular lenses. J Cataract Refract Surg 2001; 27:850-4.
22. Mullner-Eidenbock A, Amon M, Schauersberger J, et al. Cellular reaction on the anterior surface of 4 types of intraocular lenses. J Cataract Refract Surg 2001;27:734-40.
23. Oshika T, Nagata T, Ishii Y. Adhesion of lens capsule to intraocular lenses of polymethylmethacrylate, silicone, and acrylic foldable materials: an experimental study. Br J Ophthalmol 1998; 24:367-70.
24. Heatley CJ, Spalton DJ, Kumar A, et al. Comparison of posterior capsule opacification rates between hydrophilic andhydrophobic single-piece acrylic intraocular lenses. J Cataract Refract Surg 2005; 31:718-24.
25. Werner L, Pandey SK, Escobar-Gomez M, et al. Anterior capsule opacification, a histopathological study comparing different IOL styles. Ophthalmology 2000; 107:463-71.
26. Apple David L. Evolution of Intraocular Lenses. Centre for Intraocular Lens Research, Medical University of South Carolina, Storm Eye Institute, Charleston, S. Carolina.
27. Apple David L, Auffarth GU, Pevy Qun, et al. Foldable intraocular lenses - Evolution, Clinicopathologic Correlations and Complications. Pub Bond JH, SLACK Incorporated, USA 2000.
28. Laboratoire CORNEAL Acrylic Intraocular Lens Packaging Insert.
29. Pfizer Pharmacia TECNIS Foldable Lens Packaging Insert.
30. ALCON Acrysof IQ Acrylic Intraocular Lens Packaging Insert.
31. AMO Sensar AR4Oe Intraocular Lens Packaging Insert.

CHAPTER

49

Wolf Buehl, Oliver Findl (Austria)

Analysis of New Optic Designs to Reduce PCO

INTRODUCTION

Posterior capsule opacification (PCO, or after-cataract) remains a common problem after cataract surgery with implantation of an intraocular lens (IOL).[1,2] It resulted from the transition from intracapsular (ICCE) to extracapsular cataract extraction (ECCE), where the posterior lens capsule is left intact during surgery. Patients with PCO suffer from decreased visual acuity, impaired contrast sensitivity and from glare disability. Clinically, two different components of PCO can be differentiated, namely a regeneratory and a fibrotic component. *Regeneratory* PCO is much more common; it is caused by residual lens epithelium cells (LECs) from the lens equator region migrating and proliferating in the space between the posterior capsule and the IOL, forming layers of lens material and Elschnig pearls. *Fibrotic* PCO is caused by LECs from the anterior capsule that undergo transformation to myofibroblasts and gain access to the posterior capsule, causing whitening and wrinkling of the capsule.[2] This can lead to decentration of the IOL and hinder visualization of the peripheral retina. Both components of PCO lead to a decrease in visual function when they affect the central region around the visual axis.

PCO can easily be treated by Nd:YAG laser capsulotomy, however, this may lead to other complications, including an increase in intraocular pressure, ocular inflammation, cystoid macular edema, and retinal detachment.[3] Besides, Nd:YAG laser capsulotomy does not improve visualization of the peripheral retina, increases the costs for cataract treatment, and is not available in large parts of the developing world. Therefore, many efforts are made to prevent the formation of PCO. These efforts include mainly modifications in lens design and material as well as modifications in surgical technique, but also application of drugs, and others. While there is currently no commonly used surgical technique and/or drug which would lead to a significant reduction in PCO, the development of new IOL models in order to reduce PCO has made significant progress.

OPTIC EDGE DESIGN

During the past years it has become obvious that optic edge design plays an important role in the prevention of PCO. When the AcrySof MA60BM lens (Alcon Laboratories, Inc., Fort Worth, TX) was introduced in the early 1990s, several studies showed that PCO development was significantly less than with other IOLs.[4-9] First, this was attributed to the acrylic material and to the surface properties of the IOL.[10] Later it could be shown that the sharp edge design of the lens seemed to be the key factor for this effect.[11, 12] The sharp IOL edge

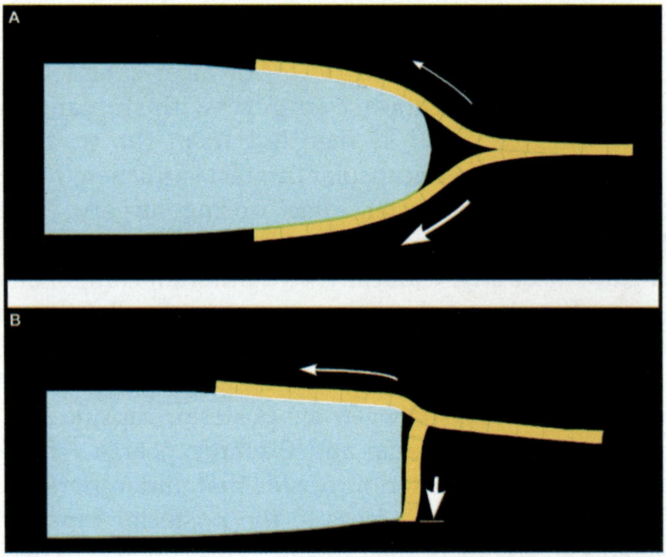

Figs 49.1A and B: Mechanism of the optic edge barrier effect. (A) An IOL with both anterior and posterior round optic edges allows lens epithelial cells to migrate and proliferate on the posterior capsule. (B) In an IOL with a sharp posterior optic edge, the capsular bend which is created at the sharp optic rim leads to contact inhibition and/or mechanical pressure between IOL and capsule

was a result of the manufacturing process, and its effect on lens epithelial cell migration, therefore, rather coincidental. Further studies confirmed that the rectangular shape of the IOL rim with its sharp edges, in combination with the acrylic material, was in fact the main reason for the reduced formation of PCO.[13] Studies by Nishi revealed that the discontinuous capsular bend seems to be a key factor for the preventative effect of a sharp edge optic.[14-16] There are two major theories to explain the barrier effect at a sharp posterior optic edge. The capsular bend at the posterior optic edge may cause mechanical pressure at the posterior capsule[17] and/or it leads to contact inhibition of LEC growth on the posterior capsule[39] (Figs 49.1A and B). The "fusion" process of the capsular bag at the IOL optic edge was also documented in studies by Sacu et al.[18,19] It is caused by contraction of the lens capsule in the first postoperative days and weeks, depending on the IOL type ("capsular sealing"). Anterior capsule fibrosis and a circumferential IOL/rhexis overlap have been shown to be important factors for this sealing process.

As a result of these findings, several new IOLs with a sharp optic edge design were introduced in the past years and compared in clinical trials. However, with some exceptions,[20-22] most of these trials were not randomized or compared IOLs differing not only in edge design but

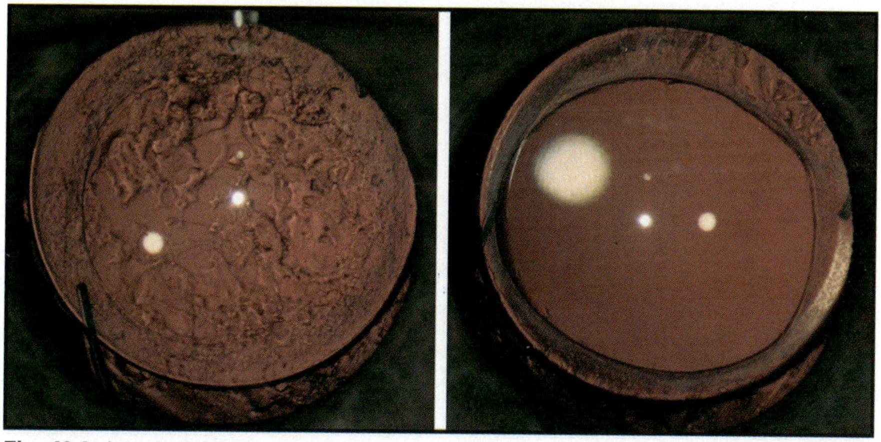

Fig. 49.2: Intra-individual comparison of round and sharp optic edges in an acrylic IOL. Retroillumination image of a round edge (left) and sharp edge (right) acrylic IOL 2 years after surgery. Right and left eye of the same patient; both IOLs differ only in optic edge design

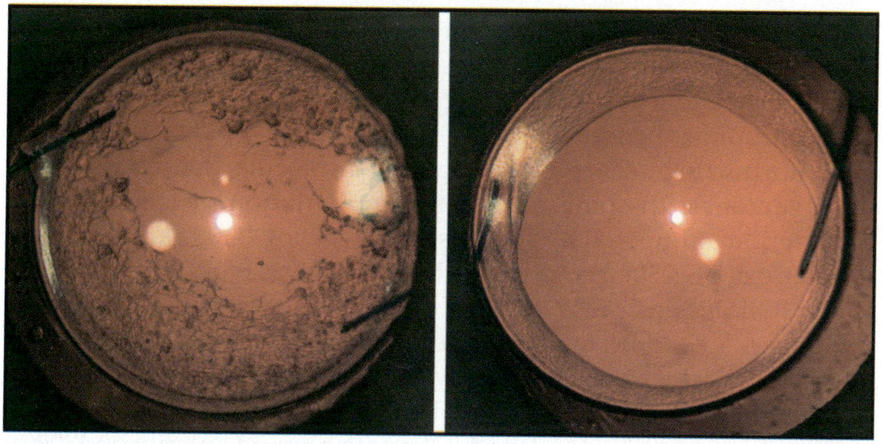

Fig. 49.3: Intra-individual comparison of round and sharp optic edges in a silicone IOL. Retroillumination image of a round edge (left) and sharp edge (right) acrylic IOL 2 years after surgery. Right and left eye of the same patient; both IOLs differ only in optic edge design

also in IOL material. As the effect of the optic material on PCO growth remains unclear, the exact reason for lower/higher PCO rates with certain IOL types could not be determined in many of these trials. Therefore, a number of studies varying only one parameter (either optic edge design or optic material) were performed also by our group. In one of these studies we compared 2 acrylic IOL types differing only in the design of the posterior optic edge.[23,24] (Fig. 49.2). An identical study was performed with 2 types of silicone IOLs[25] (Fig. 49.3) and a very similar study with 2 types of PMMA lenses[26] (Fig. 49.4). In all 3 studies there was significantly less PCO in eyes with sharp edge IOLs than in those with round edge IOLs. Nd:YAG laser capsulotomy rates

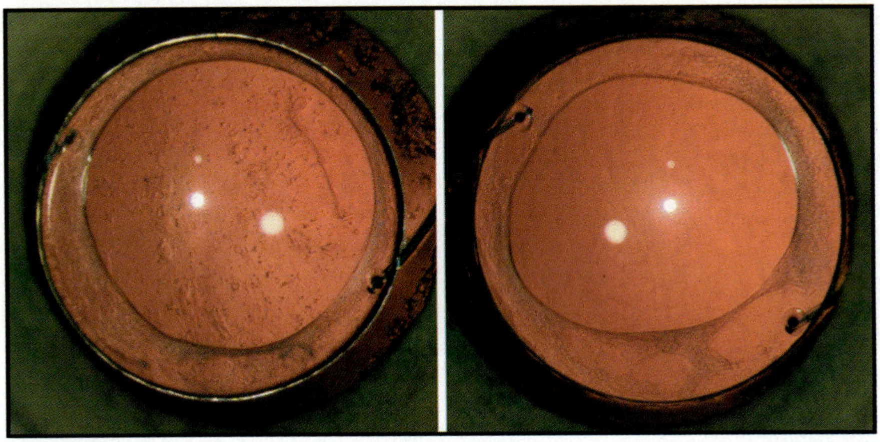

Fig. 49.4: Intra-individual comparison of round and sharp optic edges in a PMMA IOL. Retroillumination image of a round edge (left) and sharp edge (right) acrylic IOL 2 years after surgery. Right and left eye of the same patient; both IOLs differ only in optic edge design

were up to 10 times higher in the round edge groups.[23] This confirms that the sole modification of the posterior optic edge from a round edge to a sharp edge leads to a significant reduction of PCO by inducing a discontinuous bend at the posterior capsule.

Unfortunately, sharp optic edges of intraocular lenses also have disadvantages. In some cases after implantation of lenses with a rectangular edge shape (such as the AcrySof lens), an increased incidence of persistent edge glare phenomena was reported.[27,28] Sharp-edged IOL designs cause the light rays that are refracted through the peripheral IOL to be more intense on the peripheral retina. Round-edged IOL designs disperse the rays of light over a larger surface area of the retina, leading to less glare. However, the "half-rounded" edge profile of some newly developed IOLs with a round anterior and sharp posterior optic edge seems to avoid this disturbing side effect.[23]

IOL OPTIC MATERIAL

While the PCO inhibiting effect of a sharp posterior optic edge has been clearly demonstrated in several trials, the role of different IOL optic materials (i.e. PMMA, hydrophobic acrylic, hydrophilic acrylic = hydrogel, silicone) in reducing PCO remains uncertain. Although many studies comparing different IOL materials have been performed, significantly higher PCO rates have only been shown for hydrophilic acrylic (hydrogel)[29,30] and for PMMA IOLs[10,31-33] in comparison to other materials (i.e. acrylic and silicone IOLs). YAG capsulotomy rates of 24% were found for sharp-edge PMMA lenses compared to 71% for round-edge PMMA lenses between 3 and 5 years after surgery in a study by Findl et al.[26] However, in a similar study, YAG capsulotomy rates of less than 1% (sharp) and 39% (round) for acrylic IOLs and of less than 1% (sharp) and 15% (round) for silicone lenses were found 3 years after surgery.[24, 34] This shows that *sharp* edge PMMA IOLs lead to similar high or even higher capsulotomy rates than *round* edge acrylic or silicone IOLs.

A few studies comparing acrylic and silicone lenses did not find significant differences between these two materials.[21,35-37] The results of several other studies which found differences between acrylic and silicone IOLs or other IOL materials are questionable, because the compared IOLs differed not only in IOL material but also in IOL optic design (especially optic edge design), as already pointed out previously. First, the low PCO rates observed with the AcrySof IOL (Alcon, Fort Worth, USA) were attributed to the hydrophobic acrylic optic material used.[5] However, this study compared the sharp edge hydrophobic IOL to IOLs of silicone and PMMA material with round optic edges and edge design was, thus, not accounted for. Nishi and coauthors investigated the efficacy of the barrier created by a sharp edge optic in a rabbit model. They found a loss in barrier function in a round edge variant of the Acrysof IOL.[38] Also, in the animal model, the sharp edge 3-piece silicone CeeOn® 911 IOL (Pharmacia, Groningen, The Netherlands) and the 3-piece acrylic AcrySof MA60BM IOL (Alcon, Fort Worth, USA) were equally effective in preventing PCO.[39] Similar results were found in randomized clinical trials with intraindividual comparison of these IOLs by Prosdocimo et al and Findl et al.[35,36] Therefore, there is evidence that silicone and hydrophobic acrylate are at least equally effective in preventing PCO in the presence of a sharp optic edge up to 3 years after surgery.

There is even some evidence that silicone IOLs might produce less PCO than acrylic IOLs, however, there are too few randomized bilateral trials varying only the IOL optic material. Looking at 2 (randomized, bilateral) studies comparing sharp and round optic edges in acrylic and in silicone IOLs,[23,25] we also found lower PCO scores in the silicone IOL study, both in the sharp and in the round edge group. The IOL optic design was very similar in these 2 studies; however, the difference might also be a result of the different patient groups. Nevertheless, several authors independently found very low PCO rates in sharp edge silicone IOLs, also in the long-term follow-up.[40,41]

The reasons for the material effect on PCO rates are still unclear. Studies have shown that the speed of formation of a capsular bend at the optic edge is significantly faster with silicone and acrylic IOLs.[42] Linnola hypothesized that bioactive IOLs, such as acrylic IOLs, would prevent PCO better than PMMA or silicone IOLs, which have good biocompatibility but are bioinert. In a bioactive IOL, a single lens epithelial cell would act as a tie between IOL and posterior capsule, producing a "sandwich pattern" of IOL, cell monolayer, and posterior lens capsule, thus preventing further PCO growth (sandwich theory).[43] However, the theory is put into question by the low PCO rates in silicone IOLs.

IOL HAPTIC DESIGN

Haptic Angulation

The PCO preventative effect of sharp edge optics suggests that it might be useful to maximize the barrier effect at the posterior optic edge by pushing the IOL backwards against the posterior capsule. This can be achieved by angulated haptic designs. Consequently, such posterior vaulting characteristics can be found in many modern 3-piece IOLs. However, studies showed that these designs interestingly do not lead to a smaller lens/capsule distance[44] and do not seem to have a better PCO inhibiting effect than IOLs with little or no haptic angulation.[45] This might be explained by the fact that most angulated haptics lose their memory and the backward force against the posterior capsule thus might be too low for a significant effect, or the reduced contact to the anterior capsule, leading to less anterior fibrosis, might antagonize the PCO-inhibiting effect.

1-piece/3-piece IOLs

New manufacturing methods led to the introduction of single-piece IOLs some years ago. Unlike 3-piece IOLs, which usually consist of 2 different materials (optic and haptics), these IOLs are produced in a single step from one material. 1-piece IOLs tend to be more stable and the production process is cheaper. However, most 1-piece designs feature broad haptic shoulders at the transition to the IOL optic. This raised the question whether these lenses might weaken the PCO-preventative effect because of the incomplete sharp posterior optic rim and because of the compromised capsular bend formation due to reduced capsular fusion at the (thicker and broader) haptic-optic junction. Nevertheless, several clinical trials (some of them still ongoing) did not show significant differences in PCO rates between 1-piece and 3-piece optics.[37,46-48] (Fig. 49.5). However, the interrupted sharp optic rim might lead to problems in new ultra-thin 1-piece IOLs developed for (bimanual) micro-incision surgery. Additionally, some of these lens models also use plate haptics, which had almost disappeared before because of high PCO rates due to the missing barrier effect. Similar haptic designs have also been used for so-called "accommodating" IOLs over the past years. Most of these IOL models

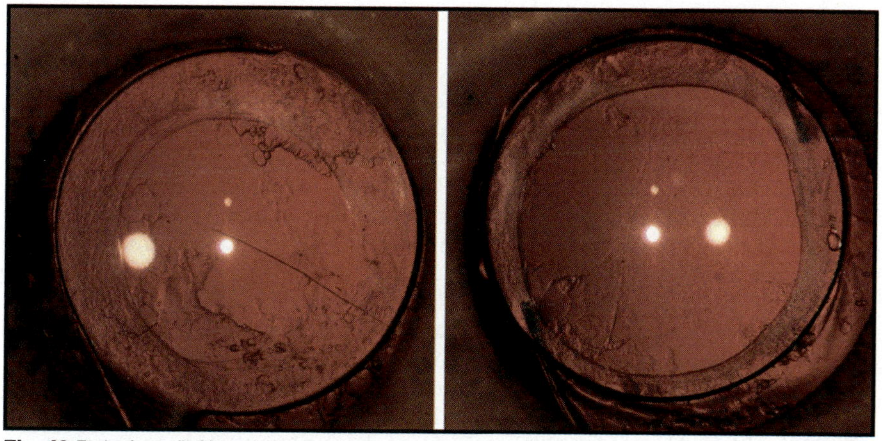

Fig. 49.5: 1-piece (left) and 3-piece (right) acrylic IOL 3 years after surgery. Pronounced PCO (lens epithelial cell ingrowth) can be observed near the haptic-optic junction. However, there is no significant difference in overall PCO intensity between the 2 IOL models (right and left eye of the same patient).

showed poor results concerning PCO rates, also primarily because of too many or too broad haptics and therefore reduced capsular bend formation.[49]

SUMMARY

Looking at modifications in IOL design, the concept of a sharp posterior optic edge has been proven to be the most effective method to reduce PCO up to now. As a result, round-edge IOLs practically have disappeared from the market. However, although drastically reduced, the problem of PCO has not entirely been eliminated. The role of IOL optic material remains unclear; while hydrogel and also PMMA lenses have been shown to have a high PCO incidence, there is still an ongoing debate whether acrylic or silicone IOLs should be preferred with respect to PCO development. Other concepts of modifying an IOL, such as extremely posteriorly vaulted IOLs, did not lead to a significant reduction of PCO. On the other hand, single-piece IOLs with an incomplete sharp optic rim also do not, as anticipated, show significantly higher PCO rates up to now. However, new ultra-thin IOLs which are currently being developed for micro-incision surgery might be a new challenge in the battle against PCO, due to their thin optic rim and therefore possibly weak barrier effect at the optic edge.

REFERENCES

1. Schaumberg DA, Dana MR, Christen WG, Glynn RJ. A systematic overview of the incidence of posterior capsule opacification. Ophthalmology 1998; 105:1213-21.

2. Kappelhof JP, Vrensen GF. The pathology of after-cataract. A minirevue. Acta Ophthalmol Suppl 1992;205:13-24.
3. Javitt MC, Tielsch JM, Canner KJ, Kolb MM, Sommer A, Steinberg EP et al. National outcomes of cataract extraction: increased risk of retinal complications associated with Nd:YAG laser capsulotomy. Ophthalmology 1992;99:1487-98.
4. Hollick EJ, Spalton DJ, Ursell PG, Pande MV, Barman SA, Boyce JF, Tilling K. The effect of polymethylmethacrylate, silicone, and polyacrylic intraocular lenses on posterior capsular opacification 3 years after cataract surgery. Ophthalmology 1999;106:49-55.
5. Ursell PG, Spalton DJ, Pande MV, Hollick EJ, Barman S, Boyce J, Tilling K. Relationship between intraocular lens biomaterials and posterior capsule opacification. J Cataract Refract Surg 1998;24:352-60.
6. Oshika T, Suzuki Y, Kizaki H, Yaguchi S. Two year clinical study of a soft acrylic intraocular lens. J Cataract Refract Surg 1996;22:104-9.
7. Hayashi H, Hayashi K, Nakao F, Hayashi F. Quantitative comparison of posterior capsule opacification after polymethylmethacrylate, silicone, and soft acrylic intraocular lens implantation. Arch Ophthalmol 1998; 116:1579-82.
8. Sundelin K, Friberg-Riad Y, Östberg A, Sjöstrand J. Posterior capsule opacification with AcrySof and poly(methyl methacrylate) intraocular lenses. Comparative study with a 3-year follow-up. J Cataract Refract Surg 2001; 27:1586-90.
9. Scaramuzza A, Fernando GT, Crayford BB. Posterior capsule opacification and lens epithelial cell layer formation: hydroview hydrogel versus AcrySof acrylic intraocular lenses. J Cataract Refract Surg 2001;27:1047-54.
10. Hollick EJ, Spalton DJ, Ursell PG, Pande MV. Lens epithelial cell regression on the posterior capsule with different intraocular lens materials. Br J Ophthalmology 1998;82:1182-88.
11. Nishi O. Posterior capsule opacification, Part 1: Experimental investigations. J Cataract Refract Surg 1999;25:106-17.
12. Ram J, Apple DJ, Peng Q, Visessook N, et al. Update on fixation of rigid and foldable posterior chamber intraocular lenses. Part II: Choosing the correct haptic fixation and intraocular lens design to help eradicate posterior capsule opacification. Ophthalmology 1999;106:891-900.
13. Nishi O, Nishi K, Sakanishi K. Inhibition of migrating lens epithelial cells at the capsular bend created by the rectangular optic edge of a posterior chamber intraocular lens. Ophthalmic Surg Lasers 1998; 29:587-94.
14. Nishi O, Nishi K, Menapace R, Akura J. Capsular bending ring to prevent posterior capsule opacification: 2 years follow-up. J Cataract Refract Surg 2001; 27:1359-65.
15. Nishi O, Nishi K. Preventing posterior capsule opacification by creating a discontinuous sharp bend in the capsule. J Cataract Refract Surg 1999;25:521-6.
16. Nishi O, Nishi K, Mano C, et al. The inhibition of lens epithelial cell migration by a discontinuous capsular bend created by a band-shaped circular loop or a capsular bending ring. Ophthalmic Surg Lasers 1998;29:119-25.
17. Boyce JF, Bhermi GS, Spalton DJ, El-Osta AR. Mathematical modeling of the forces between an intraocular lens and the capsule. J Cataract Refract Surg 2002;28:1853-59.

18. Sacu S, Findl O, Menapace R, Buehl W. Influence of optic edge design, optic material, and haptic design on capsular bend configuration. J Cataract Refract Surg 2005;31:1888-94.
19. Sacu S, Findl O, Linnola RJ. Optical coherence tomography assessment of capsule closure after cataract surgery. J Cataract Refract Surg 2005;31:330-6.
20. Hayashi K, Hayashi H. Posterior Capsule Opacification in the Presence of an Intraocular Lens with a Sharp versus Rounded Optic Edge. Ophthalmology 2005;112:1550-6.
21. Mester U, Fabian E, Gerl R, et al. Posterior capsule opacification after implantation of CeeOn Edge 911A, PhacoFlex SI40NB, and AcrySof MA60BM lenses: One-year results of an intra-individual comparison multicenter study. J Cataract Refract Surg 2004;30:978-85.
22. Sundelin K, Shams H, Stenevi U. Three-year follow-up of posterior capsule opacification with two different silicone intraocular lenses. Acta Ophthalmol Scand 2005;83:11-9.
23. Buehl W, Findl O, Menapace R, et al. Effect of an acrylic intraocular lens with a sharp posterior optic edge on posterior capsule opacification. J Cataract Refract Surg 2002;7:1105-11.
24. Buehl W, Findl O, Menapace R, et al. Long-term effect of optic edge design in an acrylic intraocular lens on posterior capsule opacification. J Cataract Refract Surg 2005;31:954-61.
25. Buehl W, Menapace R, Sacu S, et al. Effect of a silicone intraocular lens with a sharp posterior optic edge on posterior capsule opacification. J Cataract Refract Surg 2004;30:1661-7.
26. Findl O, Buehl W, Menapace R, et al. Long-term effect of sharp optic edges of a polymethyl methacrylate intraocular lens on posterior capsule opacification: a randomized trial. Ophthalmology 2005;112:2004-8.
27. Holladay JT, Lang A, Portney V. Analysis of edge glare phenomena in intraocular lens edge designs. J Cataract Refract Surg 1999;25:748-52.
28. Erie JC, Bandhauer MH, McLaren JW. Analysis of postoperative glare and intraocular lens design. J Cataract Refract Surg. 2001;27:614-21.
29. Heatley CJ, Spalton DJ, Kumar A, et al. Comparison of posterior capsule opacification rates between hydrophilic and hydrophobic single-piece acrylic intraocular lenses. J Cataract Refract Surg 2005;31:718-24.
30. Hayashi K, Hayashi H. Posterior capsule opacification after implantation of a hydrogel intraocular lens. Br J Ophthalmology 2004;88:182-5.
31. Hollick EJ, Spalton DJ, Ursell PG, Meacock WR, Barman SA, Boyce JF. Posterior capsular opacification with hydrogel, polymethylmethacrylate, and silicone intraocular lenses: two-year results of a randomized prospective trial. Am J Ophthalmol 2000;129:577-84.
32. Yoshida S, Senoo T, Fujikake F, Obara Y. Clinical evaluation of posterior capsule opacification in eyes with different small-incision intraocular lenses. Ophthalmic Surg Lasers 2002;33:450-5.
33. Hayashi K, Hayashi H, Nakao F, Hayashi F. Changes in posterior capsule opacification after poly(methylmethacrylate), silicone, and acrylic intraocular lens implantation. J Cataract Refract Surg 2001;27:817-24.
34. Buehl W, Menapace R, et al. Long-term effect of optic edge design in a silicone intraocular lens on posterior capsule opacification (awaiting publication).
35. Prosdocimo G, Tassinari G, Sala M, et al. Posterior capsule opacification after phacoemulsification: silicone CeeOn Edge versus acrylate AcrySof intraocular lens. J Cataract Refract Surg 2003;8:1551-5.

36. Findl O, Menapace R, Sacu S, Buehl W, Rainer G. Effect of Optic Material on Posterior Capsule Opacification in Intraocular Lenses with Sharp-edge Optics. Ophthalmology 2005;112:67-72.
37. Zemaitiene R, Jasinskas V, Barzdziukas V, Auffarth GU. Prevention of posterior capsule opacification using different intraocular lenses (results of one-year clinical study). Medicina (Kaunas, Lithuania) 2004;40:721-30.
38. Nishi O, Nishi K, Akura J, et al. Effect of round-edged acrylic intraocular lenses on preventing posterior capsule opacification. J Cataract Refract Surg 2001;4:608-13.
39. Nishi O, Nishi K and Wickstrom K. Preventing lens epithelial cell migration using intraocular lenses with sharp rectangular edges. J Cataract Refract Surg 2000; 10:1543-49.
40. Rabsilber TM, Reuland AJ, Entz BB, et al. Quantitative Nachstarevaluierung von Acrylat- und Silikonintraokularlinsen mit scharfem Kantendesign (Quantitative evaluation of acrylic and silicone intraocular lenses with a sharp optic edge design and the development of posterior capsule opacification). Ophthalmologe 2005.
41. Pohjalainen T, Vesti E, Uusitalo RJ, Laatikainen L. Posterior capsular opacification in pseudophakic eyes with a silicone or acrylic intraocular lens. Eur J Ophthalmol 2002;12:212-8.
42. Nishi O, Nishi K, Akura J. Speed of capsular bend formation at the optic edge of acrylic, silicone, and poly(methyl methacrylate) lenses. J Cataract Refract Surg 2002;28:431-7.
43. Linnola RJ. Sandwich theory: bioactivity-based explanation for posterior capsule opacification. J Cataract Refract Surg 1997;23:1539-42.
44. Findl O, Drexler W, Menapace R, et al. Accurate determination of effective lens position and lens-capsule distance with 4 intraocular lenses. J Cataract Refract Surg 1998;24:1094-8.
45. Menapace R. Posterior capsule opacification and capsulotomy rates with taco-style hydrogel intraocular lenses. J Cataract Refract Surg 1996; 22:1318-1330.
46. Leydolt C, Davidovic S, Sacu S, et al. Longterm effect of 1-piece and 3-piece hydrophobic acrylic intraocular lenses on posterior capsule opacification: A randomized trial (awaiting publication).
47. Bilge AH, Aykan U, Akin T, Unsal U. The effects of three-piece or single-piece acrylic intraocular lens implantation on posterior capsule opacification. Eur J Ophthalmol 2004;14:375-80.
48. Bender L, Nimsgern C, Jose R, Jayaram et al. Effect of 1-piece and 3-piece AcrySof intraocular lenses on the development of posterior capsule opacification after cataract surgery. J Cataract Refract Surg 2004;30:786-9.
49. Findl O. Accommodative IOLs. In Essentials in Ophthalmology – Cataract and Refractive Surgery; Springer 2005.

Index

L

M

N

O

P

U

V